INTERNATIONAL ENCYCLOPEDIA OF PHARMACOLOGY AND THERAPEUTICS

Sponsored by the International Union of Pharmacology (IUPHAR)
(Chairman: B. UvNäs, Stockholm)

Executive Editor: G. PETERS, Lausanne

Section 48

PHARMACOLOGY OF THE ENDOCRINE SYSTEM AND RELATED DRUGS:

PROGESTERONE, PROGESTATIONAL DRUGS AND ANTIFERTILITY AGENTS

Section Editor

M. TAUSK
Utrecht

VOLUME II

EDITORIAL BOARD

D. BOVET, *Rome*
A. S. V. BURGEN, *Cambridge*
J. CHEYMOL, *Paris*
G. B. KOELLE, *Philadelphia*
M. J. MICHELSON, *Leningrad*
G. PETERS, *Lausanne*
C. RADOUCO-THOMAS, *Quebec*
H. RAŠKOVÁ, *Prague*
V. V. ZAKUSOV, *Moscow*

INTERNATIONAL ENCYCLOPEDIA OF
PHARMACOLOGY AND THERAPEUTICS

Pharmacology of the Endocrine System and Related Drugs: Progesterone, Progestational Drugs and Antifertility Agents

VOLUME II

CONTRIBUTORS

C. C. CHANG
J. DE VISSER
J. FERIN
F. A. KINCL

H. W. RUDEL
K. SEMM
M. TAUSK
J. H. H. THIJSSEN

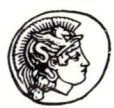

PERGAMON PRESS

OXFORD · NEW YORK · TORONTO
SYDNEY · BRAUNSCHWEIG

Pergamon Press Ltd., Headington Hill Hall, Oxford
Pergamon Press Inc., Maxwell House, Fairview Park, Elmsford,
New York 10523
Pergamon of Canada Ltd., 207 Queen's Quay West, Toronto 1
Pergamon Press (Aust.) Pty. Ltd., 19a Boundary Street,
Rushcutters Bay, N.S.W. 2011, Australia
Vieweg & Sohn GmbH, Burgplatz 1, Braunschweig

Copyright © 1972 Pergamon Press Ltd.

All Rights Reserved. No part of this publication may be reproduced, stored in a retrieval system, or transmitted, in any form or by any means, electronic, mechanical, photocopying, recording or otherwise, without the prior permission of Pergamon Press Ltd.

First edition 1972
Library of Congress Catalog Card No. 73-153797

Printed in Great Britain by A. Wheaton & Co., Exeter
08 016812 4

CONTENTS

CONTENTS OF VOLUME I	vii
LIST OF CONTRIBUTORS	ix
PREFACE	xi
KEY TO ABBREVIATIONS	xiii

SUBSECTION II
DERIVATIVES OF AND SUBSTITUTES FOR PROGESTERONE

PART 1
DRUGS FOR PARENTERAL ADMINISTRATION

CHAPTER 25. CHEMISTRY AND PHARMACOLOGY OF INJECTABLE COMPOUNDS   1
    C. C. Chang, New York, N.Y., U.S.A.

CHAPTER 26. EFFECTS IN MAN, DURATION OF ACTION AND METABOLISM   13
    J. Ferin, Louvain, Belgium

PART 2
ORALLY ACTIVE SUBSTITUTES FOR PROGESTERONE

CHAPTER 27. THE CHEMISTRY OF ORALLY ACTIVE SUBSTITUTES FOR PROGESTERONE AND CLASSIFICATION OF COMPOUNDS IN USE   25
    F. A. Kincl, New York, N.Y., U.S.A.

CHAPTER 28. PHARMACOLOGY OF ORALLY ACTIVE PROGESTATIONAL COMPOUNDS: ANIMAL STUDIES   35
    M. Tausk, Utrecht, The Netherlands and J. de Visser, Oss, The Netherlands

CHAPTER 29. THE METABOLISM OF ORALLY ACTIVE SYNTHETIC PROGESTATIONAL COMPOUNDS   217
    J. H. H. Thijssen, Utrecht, The Netherlands

CHAPTER 30. ORALLY ACTIVE PROGESTATIONAL COMPOUNDS. HUMAN STUDIES: EFFECTS ON THE UTERO-VAGINAL TRACT   275
    J. Ferin, Louvain, Belgium

CHAPTER 31. OTHER EFFECTS OF SYNTHETIC PROGESTATIONAL
COMPOUNDS IN THE HUMAN 275
M. Tausk, Utrecht, The Netherlands and
J. de Visser, Oss, The Netherlands

CHAPTER 32. THERAPEUTIC APPLICATION OF
PROGESTATIONAL DRUGS 303
K. Semm, Munich, Federal Republic of Germany

SUBSECTION III
THE ANTIFERTILITY EFFECTS OF ESTROGENS,
PROGESTATIONAL COMPOUNDS AND COMBINATIONS
OF THESE

CHAPTER 33. ESTROGENS AS ANTIFERTILITY AGENTS 347
F. A. Kincl, New York, N.Y., U.S.A.

CHAPTER 34. ORAL CONTRACEPTIVES. HUMAN FERTILITY
STUDIES AND SIDE EFFECTS 385
H. W. Rudel and F. A. Kincl, New York, N.Y., U.S.A

CHAPTER 35. GENERAL SUMMARY 471
M. Tausk, Utrecht, The Netherlands

AUTHOR INDEX 493

SUBJECT INDEX 515

CONTENTS OF VOLUME I

LIST OF CONTRIBUTORS   xi
PREFACE   xiii
HISTORICAL INTRODUCTION   1
   M. Tausk, Utrecht, The Netherlands

SUBSECTION I
THE CHEMISTRY AND PHARMACOLOGY OF PROGESTERONE
PART 1. ANIMAL STUDIES

CHAPTER 1. CHEMISTRY AND BIOCHEMISTRY OF PROGESTERONE   13
   F. A. Kincl, New York, N.Y., U.S.A.

CHAPTER 2. HISTOLOGICAL EFFECTS OF PROGESTERONE ON THE VAGINA AND THE UTERUS   65
   Z. S. Madjerek, Amsterdam, The Netherlands

CHAPTER 3. PROGESTERONE AND MAMMARY DEVELOPMENT   83
   J. M. M. Hilgers, Amsterdam, The Netherlands

CHAPTER 4. PHYSIOLOGICAL AND PHARMACOLOGICAL EFFECTS OF PROGESTERONE ON MYOMETRIAL CONTRACTILITY AND ACTIVITY IN ANIMALS   103
   L. P. Bengtsson, Lund, Sweden

CHAPTER 5. THE ELECTROPHYSIOLOGICAL MANIFESTATIONS OF THE PROGESTERONE EFFECT ON THE UTERUS   123
   A. Csapo, St. Louis, Missouri

CHAPTER 6. EFFECTS OF PROGESTERONE ON IMPLANTATION OF THE FERTILIZED OVUM AND THE FORMATION OF DECIDUOMATA   205
   Z. S. Madjerek, Amsterdam, The Netherlands

CHAPTER 7. EFFECTS OF PROGESTERONE ON THE STRUCTURE AND FUNCTION OF THE FALLOPIAN TUBES   251
   M. Tausk, Utrecht and J. de Visser, Oss, The Netherlands

CHAPTER 8. THE INFLUENCE OF PROGESTERONE ON TRANSPORT AND CAPACITATION OF SPERM IN THE FEMALE ORGANISM   265
   M. Tausk, Utrecht and J. de Visser, Oss, The Netherlands

CHAPTER 9. SYNERGISM WITH AND ANTAGONISM TO ESTROGENS   275
   F. A. Kincl, New York, N.Y., U.S.A.

CHAPTER 10. PROGESTERONE AND THE MAINTENANCE OF PREGNANCY   291
   Z. S. Madjerek, Amsterdam, The Netherlands

CHAPTER 11. PROTECTION AGAINST EARLY POSTNATAL
STEROID DAMAGE 319
    F. A. Kincl, New York, N.Y., U.S.A.
CHAPTER 12. PROGESTERONE AS TESTOSTERONE
ANTAGONIST 325
    F. A. Kincl, New York, N.Y., U.S.A.
CHAPTER 13. INDUCTION AND INHIBITION OF OVULATION
BY PROGESTERONE 331
    G. H. Zeilmaker, Amsterdam, The Netherlands
CHAPTER 14. THE EFFECTS OF PROGESTERONE ON BODY
TEMPERATURE 353
    M. Tausk, Utrecht and J. de Visser, Oss, The Netherlands
CHAPTER 15. EFFECTS OF PROGESTERONE ON BODY MASS
AND METABOLISM 361
    M. Tausk, Utrecht and J. de Visser, Oss, The Netherlands
CHAPTER 16. THE ROLE OF PROGESTERONE IN
MAMMALIAN REPRODUCTION 367
    M. Tausk, Utrecht and J. de Visser, Oss, The Netherlands
CHAPTER 17. VARIOUS OTHER EFFECTS OF PROGESTERONE 375
    M. Tausk, Utrecht and J. de Visser, Oss, The Netherlands
CHAPTER 18. BIOASSAYS 389
    Z. S. Madjerek, Amsterdam, The Netherlands
Section Editor's note replacing CHAPTER 19:
PROGESTERONE AND THE DEVELOPMENT OF
TUMORS 403
CHAPTER 20. THE TOXICITY OF PROGESTERONE 405
    H. W. Rudel and F. A. Kincl, New York, N.Y., U.S.A.

PART 2. PROGESTERONE: HUMAN STUDIES

CHAPTER 21. PROGESTERONE AND ITS METABOLITES IN
BLOOD AND URINE 413
    L. P. Bengtsson, Lund, Sweden
CHAPTER 22. THE EFFECTS OF PROGESTERONE ON THE
HUMAN UTEROVAGINAL TRACT 441
    J. Ferin, Louvain, Belgium
CHAPTER 23. HISTOCHEMISTRY OF THE EFFECTS OF GESTAGENS
ON THE HUMAN ENDOMETRIUM 457
    H. Schmidt-Matthiesen, Frankfurt on Main, Germany
CHAPTER 24. EFFECT OF PROGESTERONE ON THE ACTIVITY OF
THE HUMAN MYOMETRIUM 487
    L. P. Bengtsson, Lund, Sweden
Section Editor's note on THE THERAPEUTIC APPLICATION OF
PROGESTERONE 519
AUTHOR INDEX xv
SUBJECT INDEX xxxvii

LIST OF CONTRIBUTORS

CHANG, C. C. Biomedical Division, The Population Council, New York, N.Y., U.S.A.

DE VISSER, J. Group Leader, Endocrinological Research Laboratory, N.V. Organon, Oss, The Netherlands.

FERIN, J. Professor, Department of Obstetrics and Gynecology, University Hospital, Louvain, Belgium.

KINCL, F. A. Vice-President, Biological Concepts Inc., New York, N.Y., U.S.A.

RUDEL, H. W. Biological Concepts Inc., New York, N.Y., U.S.A.

SEMM, K. Department of Obstetrics and Gynecology, Universitäts-Frauenklinik, Kiel, Federal Republic of Germany.

TAUSK, M. Professor of Endocrinology, Faculty of Medicine, University of Utrecht, Utrecht, The Netherlands.

THIJSSEN, J. H. H. Head of Endocrinological Laboratory, Department of Medicine, University Hospital, Utrecht, The Netherlands.

PREFACE

IN AUGUST 1965 the present writer was invited to serve as editor for this section, which was to cover the whole pharmacology of progestational agents as well as their applications as antifertility drugs.

It seemed essential to separate progesterone, a natural hormone with physiological functions, from its synthetic substitutes and the latter from their combinations with estrogens as used in oral contraceptives.

Consequently Volume I was entirely devoted to progesterone and this provided a convenient basis for the classification and descriptions of synthetic compounds and their effects in animals and humans, as presented in Chapters 25 to 32 of the present volume.

Chapters 33 and 34 deal with antifertility drugs. Since most of these contain an estrogen, it was necessary to deal with the antifertility effects of estrogens, leaving aside other actions and uses of (natural or synthetic) estrogens which are thoroughly treated in Sections 44 and 45.

A general summary of Volumes I and II is presented in Chapter 35.

The present section editor is greatly indebted to the medical library of N.V. Organon, Oss, The Netherlands, for extensive services and to other departments of that company for help and assistance.

Bibliographical data and reprints were obtained from the following companies and persons, whose contributions are gratefully acknowledged, apart from those mentioned in the text:

BDH (Research) Limited, Godalming (Surrey) (Dr. D. K. Vallance).
Leo Pharmaceutical Products, Ballerup (Denmark).
The Lilly Research Laboratories, Indianapolis (Dr. D. M. Brennan).
Merck Institute, Rahway (NJ) (Dr. S. L. Steelman).
E. Merck, A.G., Darmstadt (Dr. M. G. Kraft, Prof. G. Hecht-Lucari).
Organon, Oss (Scientific Information Department).
Ormonoterapia Richter, Milan (Dr. Fugazza).
Philips Duphar, Weesp, The Netherlands (Dr. V. Claassen).
Roussel, Paris (Dr. Leguay).
Schering A.G., Berlin (Dr. F. Neumann).
Searle Co., Chicago (Dr. V. A. Drill).
Syntex Research, Palo Alto, Calif. (Dr. W. H. Rooks).
The Upjohn Company, Kalamazoo (Mich.) (Dr. G. W. Duncan).

The Subject Index of Volume II was prepared by Mr. P. L. M. Van de Voort, the Author Index by Mrs. Th. M. J. Van de Voort-te Riele.

I am particularly grateful to those authors who spent a great deal of work on updating their chapters, which became necessary when the completion of the whole volume appeared to be delayed beyond expectation.

M. TAUSK

KEY TO ABBREVIATIONS

Most of the abbreviations used in this book are defined in the text. For convenience the abbreviations are also listed here.

ACTH adenocorticotrophic hormone
AGD ano–genital distance
AI artificial insemination
AL allylestrenol
AN anagestone acetate
ATPase adenosine triphosphatase
BSP bromosulphophthalein
BW body weight
CA/CAP chlormadinone acetate
CBG cortisol binding globulin
CL corpora lutea
CNS central nervous system
DCR decidual cell response
DES diethylstilbestrol
DFFT dry fat-free tissue
DHA dehydro-*epi*-androsterone
DHAS dehydro-*epi*-androsterone sulphate
DM dimethisterone
DMBA 7,12-dimethylbenzanthracene
DMS dimethylstilbestrol
DMSO dimethylsulfoxide
DP-acetofuran 2-acetofuran derivative of 16α,17α-dihydroxyprogesterone
DP-acetonide acetonide derivative of 16α,17α-dihydroxyprogesterone
DP-acetophenone acetophenone derivative of 16α,17α-dihydroxyprogesterone
DNA deoxyribonucleic acid
DPS dimethyl polysiloxane
DY dydrogesterone
EB estradiol benzoate
EC enlarged clitoris
ECP estradiol cyclopentyl propionate
ED ethynodiol diacetate
EE/EED ethynyl estradiol (diacetate)
ET ethisterone
ETH ethynodiol diacetate
FC free cortisol

FI fertility index
Fib fibrinogen
FSH follicle-stimulating hormone
FSI fetal survival index
GH growth hormone
Glu β-glucuronidase
HAP haptoglobine
HCG human chorionic gonadotrophin
HHG human hypophyseal gonadotrophin
HMG human menopausal gonadotrophin
HP caproate 17α-hydroxyprogesterone caproate
ICSH interstitial cell stimulating hormone
IDV impaired development of vagina
i.p. intraperitoneal(ly)
I.U. international unit
i.v. intravenous(ly)
LH luteinizing hormone
LHRF luteinizing hormone-releasing factor
LHRH luteinizing hormone-releasing hormone
LTH luteotrophic hormone, prolactin
LYN lynestrenol
MAP medroxyprogesterone acetate
MED medrogestone
MEE median eminence extracts; ethynyl estradiol-methyl ether
MEG megestrol acetate
MET 17α-methyltestosterone
MGA melengestrol acetate
MLA levator ani muscle
NAC norethisterone acetate
NE/NET norethisterone
NG norgestrel
NGN norgesterone
NGT norgestrienone

NL norethynodrel
NM normethandrone
NSI net success index
NV norvinisterone
OAAD ovarian ascorbic acid depletion test
PB prostatic buds
PBI protein bound iodine
p.c. post coitum
PL plasminogen
PME posterior median eminence
PMS pregnant mares, serum gonadotrophin
p.o. per os
PPW part persistence of Wolffian ducts
PR pregnancy rate
Q quingestanol
s.c. subcutaneous(ly)
SGOT serum glutamate pyruvate transaminase
SGPT serum glutamate oxalacetate transaminase
SM sterile mating
TBG thyroxin binding globulin
TBPA thyroxin binding prealbumin
TEP testosterone propionate
TP total proteins
TPN triphosphopyridin nucleotide

SUBSECTION II

DERIVATIVES OF AND SUBSTITUTES FOR PROGESTERONE

PART 1
DRUGS FOR PARENTERAL ADMINISTRATION

CHAPTER 25

CHEMISTRY AND PHARMACOLOGY OF INJECTABLE COMPOUNDS

C. C. Chang

Biomedical Division, The Population Council, New York

I. INTRODUCTION

A large number of new progestational steroids have been synthesized in the past two decades and some of them are successfully used in clinical therapy. In this review the scope will be confined to the group of substitutes for progesterone, which are more potent than progesterone when administered parenterally and have been used clinically. Thus, the following synthetic progestins are included (Fig. 1): medroxyprogesterone acetate (6α-methyl-17α-acetoxypregn-4-ene-3,20-dione (I))*; 17α-hydroxyprogesterone caproate (17α-hydroxypregn-4-ene-3,20-dione caproate (II)); the acetophenone derivative of 16α,17α-dihydroxyprogesterone (Droxone (III)); the acetonide derivative of 16α,17α-dihydroxyprogesterone (IV); and the 2-acetofuran derivative of 16α,17α-dihydroxyprogesterone (V).

It is well recognized that esterification of progestational steroids produces a markedly prolonged duration of action and sometimes a great increase in activity. For example, medroxyprogesterone acetate and 17α-hydroxyprogesterone caproate are derived from and structurally related to 17α-hydroxyprogesterone, which is known to be inactive. Likewise, 16α,17α-dihydroxyprogesterone is inactive as a progestin but its derivatives are more potent than progesterone.

To understand the biological activities of these synthetic progestins, a spectrum of endocrine responses, particularly their actions on the reproductive processes, will be examined, although the mechanisms by which they influence the endocrine functions are still not well elucidated.

---

* Since medroxyprogesterone acetate is mainly used orally it is also included in Chapter 28.

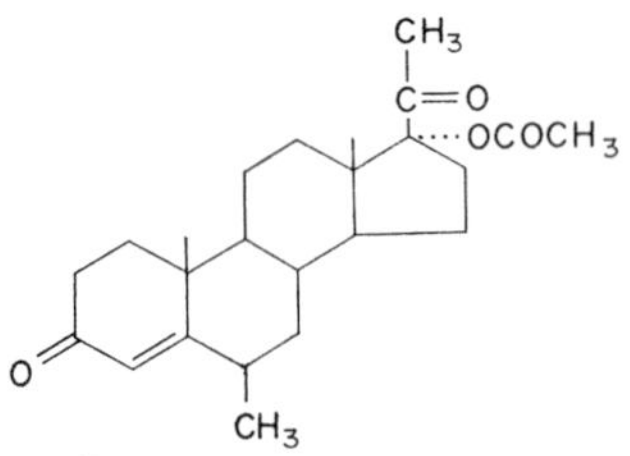

FIG. 1. Structural formulas of synthetic progestational agents active by injection.

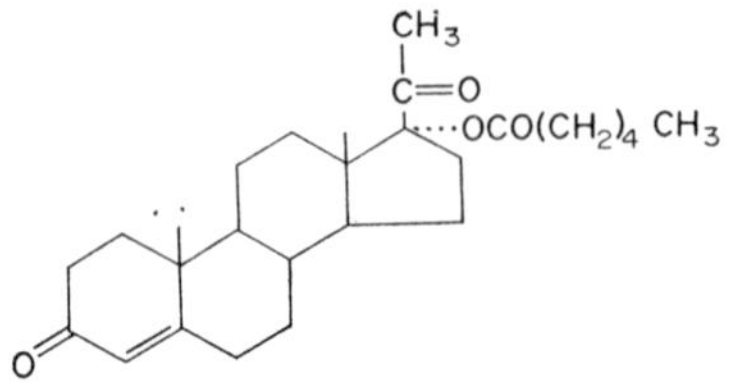

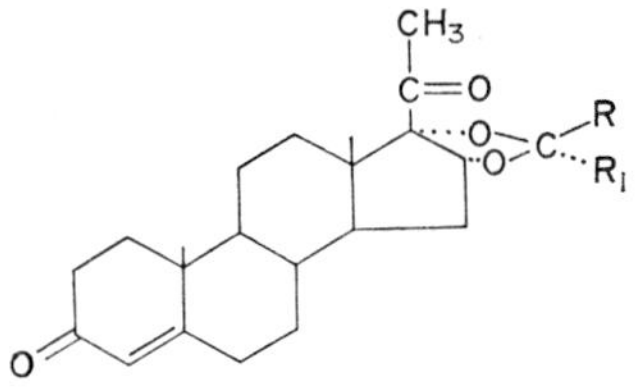

III	R = H; R₁ = phenyl
IV	R, R₁ = methyl
V	R = methyl; R₁ = furyl

For convenience' sake, the abbreviations commonly used for these synthetic progestins are employed in this survey: MAP stands for medroxyprogesterone acetate; HP caproate stands for 17α-hydroxyprogesterone caproate; DP-aceto-phenone stands for acetophenone derivative of 16α,17α-dihydroxyprogesterone; DP-acetonide stands for acetonide derivative of 16α,17α-dihydroxyprogesterone; and DP-acetofuran stands for 2-acetofuran derivative of 16α,17α-dihydroxyprogesterone.

II. CHEMISTRY

The preparation of esters of 17α-hydroxyprogesterone is simple; it involves essentially only esterification of the tertiary alcohol. This can be achieved readily at room temperature with the appropriate acid anhydride with *p*-toluene sulfonic acid as catalyst. In most processes the 17α-substituent is introduced prior to the establishment of the α,β-unsaturated

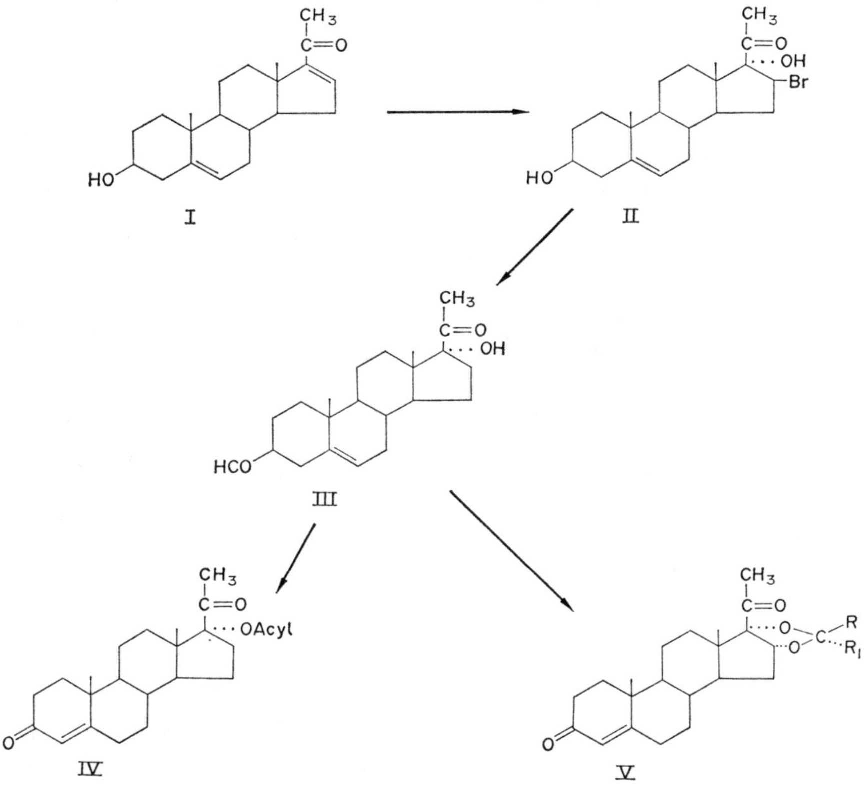

FIG. 2.

ketone moiety, and hence special manipulations are necessary to protect the double bond.

The most widely used route is probably that developed by Julian et al. (1950) from 3β-hydroxypregn-5,16-dien-20-one (see Chapter 1) in four steps (Fig. 2). Treatment of this key intermediate (I) with alkaline hydrogen peroxide leads to the formation of 16α,17α-epoxide which can be opened in methylene chloride solution with hydrogen bromide in acetic acid to the bromohydrin (II). Hydrogenation in methanol in the presence of ammonium acetate, followed by formylation of the 3-alcohol, affords the suitably protected intermediate (III). The 17α-hydroxyl group can now be esterified. An Oppenauer type of oxidation is used to introduce the Δ^4-3-ketone (IV).

The synthesis of acetals and ketals of 16α,17α-dihydroxyprogesterone (V) is achieved by stirring one part of (V) in ten parts of the appropriate ketone or aldehyde in the presence of 0.05 volume of 70% perchloric acid (Fried *et al.*, 1961). The 16α-hydroxyl group can be introduced either by osmium tetroxide hydroxylation of the 16-double bond of (I) (Allen and Bernstein, 1955) or directly by microbiological 16α-hydroxylation with *Streptomyces roseochromogenus* (Thoma *et al.*, 1957).

III. PROGESTATIONAL ACTIVITY

The progestational activity of derivatives of 16α,17α-dihydroxyprogesterone (DP), including those with acetophenone, acetone, and 2-acetofuran groups, was studied by Lerner and his associates (1961, 1963).

Both DP-acetophenone and DP-acetonide were 1–2 times as potent as progesterone while DP-acetofuran has 32–64 times its progestational activity when parenterally administered. If progesterone is defined as having a potency of 100%, a comparison of potencies of these steroids is shown in the order as follows:

DP-acetofuran > MAP > DP-acetophenone > Progesterone
              DP-acetonide
              HP-caproate

3200–6400   2000–3500   200   100

The progestational activity of MAP was approximately 20 times that of progesterone according to Revesz and Chappel (1966), but 35 times according to Edgren *et al.* (1967). Kessler and Borman (1958) reported that the progestational efficacy of 0.25 mg (total dose) of HP-caproate was equal to that of 0.5 mg of progesterone as evaluated by the method of McPhail.

All of these injectable steroids are highly potent and display long progestational activity. Administration of a single subcutaneous dose of HP-caproate (20 mg) to rabbits exhibited a depot action lasting for 20 days (Junkmann, 1957; Davis and Wied, 1955). This was confirmed by Kessler and Borman (1958). They also found that the delay in onset of action as compared with progesterone was overcome by using benzyl benzoate–sesame oil. Revesz and Chappel (1966) reported that when a single 10-mg subcutaneous injection of MAP was given to immature female rabbits, the endometrial response was demonstrable for 17 days. The activity found at that time was slightly more potent than that of HP-caproate. Similar studies on the duration of progestational activity of the derivatives of

16α,17α-dihydroxyprogesterone were performed by Lerner et al. (1961) and Lerner et al. (1963). They demonstrated that a single 10-mg intramuscular injection of DP-acetonide, DP-acetophenone and DP-acetofuran to ovariectomized rabbits produced a progestational response for 20, 25, and 35 days, respectively, whereas progesterone showed no residual effect 10 days following injection.

MAINTENANCE OF PREGNANCY

It has been firmly established that pregnancy is interrupted in rats and rabbits ovariectomized shortly after implantation of blastocyst and that administration of progesterone prevents the termination of pregnancy (Zarrow, 1961—see Chapter 10). Junkmann (1954) reported that treatment of ovariectomized rats with 10 mg of progesterone daily brought about normal development of the fetuses. Revesz and Chappel (1966) found a single subcutaneous injection of 200 mg progesterone to maintain pregnancy in ovariectomized rats with an activity index of 72 (which was calculated by the number of live fetuses per animal, divided by the number of implantation sites at the time of ovariectomy, multiplied by 100). They also found that a single subcutaneous dose of 10 mg of MAP produced better results with an index of 80.

Daily doses of 1.25 mg of MAP were effective in maintaining pregnancy (Lerner et al., 1962) (see Table 1).

TABLE 1. MAINTENANCE OF PREGNANCY IN OVARIECTOMIZED RATS BY SUBCUTANEOUS INJECTION OF PROGESTINS[a]

Treatment	Optimum daily dose (mg)	Average no. implantation sites per animal	% rats with live pups	Relative potency, %
Progesterone	20	10.7	100	100
DP-acetophenone	10	11.8	93	200
DP-acetonide	10	10.1	100	200
DP-acetofuran	5	11.1	83	400
MAP	1.25	10.6	100	1600
HP-caproate	20	6.1	0	< 100

[a] After Lerner et al. (1961, 1963).

It has been demonstrated by Velardo (1958) that intact rats given HP-caproate at doses ranging from 0.5 to 7.5 mg daily for 7 days had higher numbers of implantation sites than animals treated with equivalent doses of progesterone. A single subcutaneous dose of 9.0 mg or daily doses of 6.25 mg of HP-caproate produced a comparable number of implantation sites in PMS–HCG treated and mated prepuberal mice as was reported by Smithberg (1958). However, neither single 10–100 mg doses of HP-caproate (Junkmann, 1957) nor daily doses of 20 mg (Lerner et al., 1962) (see Table 1) could maintain pregnancy in spayed rats, although Suchowsky and Junkmann (1958) reported that HP-caproate (a single dose of 100 mg/100 g) maintained pregnancy in rabbits ovariectomized shortly after mating.

A comparison of the pregnancy-maintaining ability of the acetophenone, acetonide and 2-acetofuran derivatives of $16\alpha,17\alpha$-dihydroxyprogesterone and other progestational steroids in ovariectomized rats is shown in Table 1. As can be seen, the subcutaneous administration of DP-acetophenone, DP-acetonide and DP-acetofuran was effective in maintaining pregnancy. The optimum subcutaneous dose was 10 mg, 10 mg, and 5 mg or more for DP-acetophenone, DP-acetonide, and DP-acetofuran, respectively.

IV. ANTIFERTILITY ACTIVITY

Tests used for the evaluation of antifertility activity of synthetic progestins have included the suppression of production and/or release of gonadotropic hormone(s), interference with estrous cycle, mating, ovulation, or ovum implantation.

EFFECTS ON THE ESTROUS CYCLE, MATING, AND OVULATION

No delay of the estrous cycle was found by Velardo (1958) in rats treated with daily doses of 0.5 to 7.5 mg of HP-caproate for 7 days, whereas progesterone treatment (1 to 2 mg) prolonged the estrous cycles from the control mean of 4.5 days to 7.0 to 7.5 days.

Lerner et al. (1964) found that daily subcutaneous injections of 1, 5, or 25 mg of DP-acetophenone for 20 days arrested vaginal cycles in a diestrous state within 3–4 days. The animals treated with 1 mg of DP-acetophenone resumed normal cycling about 70 days after the termination of treatment. Furthermore, chronic treatment of 21-day-old rats with DP-acetophenone (1 or 5 mg daily for 88 days) produced ovarian atrophy and absence of mature follicles and corpora lutea after treatment.

The data of Velardo (1958) indicate that daily subcutaneous doses of 0.5 to 7.5 mg of HP-caproate for 7 days prior to cohabitation with males shortened the time for mating to occur (ranging 1–4 days) (while 0.5 to 7.5 mg progesterone have a delaying effect, ranging 6.7–9.2 days). This progestin does not interfere with ovulation or fertility, as evidenced by the numbers of corpora lutea and implantation sites present.

Barnes *et al.* (1959) demonstrated that MAP (0.05 mg) was about 20 times more potent than progesterone (1 mg) in inhibiting ovulation in rabbits.

Lerner *et al.* (1964) have found that daily subcutaneous administration of 0.8 mg of DP-acetophenone 5 days prior to and 10 days after cohabitation inhibits mating and fertility in rats. The treated animals which do not mate are capable of resuming fertile mating 80 days after withdrawal of treatment. Furthermore, Lerner *et al.* (1964), using successful pregnancy as the indicator, demonstrated DP-acetophenone and DP-acetofuran to be potent antifertility steroids in mice. The daily dose required to inhibit pregnancy in 100% of the animals was 200 mcg for the two synthetic steroids as compared to 1000 mcg for progesterone.

INHIBITION OF PITUITARY GONADOTROPIN SECRETION

1. *Anti-luteinizing effect*

Since progesterone has an inhibitory activity on the formation of corpora lutea in the ovaries and estrogens in suitable doses can provoke it, Junkmann (1957) devised an assay to determine the inhibition of luteinization elicited in immature rats (weighing 50–55 g) by a single dose of estradiol valerate (10 mcg). He reported that a single dose of 10 mg HP-caproate when given together with the estrogen was more effective in antiluteinizing activity than doses of 1 mg of progesterone per day for 8 days (see Table 2). It is interesting to note that 19-nor-17α-hydroxyprogesterone caproate possesses relatively weak pituitary inhibiting potency although it has a stronger progestational activity than progesterone (Neumann *et al.*, 1968). Shipley (1962) reinvestigated the Junkmann assay in examining antiluteinizing effects of progesterone and MAP and found that when 27–35-day-old female rats (Holtzman strain) received the progestional compounds daily for 7 days in addition to a single injection of 10 mcg estradiol valerate, the formation of corpora lutea was effectively inhibited with the various dose levels as shown in Table 2.

Labhsetwar (1966) evaluated the effects of MAP (subcutaneous injection of 12.5 mg twice a week for 5 weeks) on the ovaries of immature rats. While these organs were smaller than those of the controls and contained no corpora lutea, their response to injected PMS (10 I.U. for 3 injections in

TABLE 2. INHIBITION OF CORPORA LUTEA FORMATION WITH PROGESTERONE, MEDROXYPROGESTERONE ACETATE AND 17α-HYDROXY-PROGESTERONE CAPROATE

Treatment	Effective daily dose (mg)	Average no. of C.L. per animal	% rats with C.L.
0[a]	0	8.1	93
Progesterone[a]	0.5	1.4	12.5
	2	0	0
MAP[a]	0.05	1.9	14.3
	0.1	0	0
HP-caproate[b]	1	3	40
	10	0.2	10

[a] After Shipley (1962).
[b] A single dose; after Junkmann (1957).

3 days) as measured by weight increase was almost twice that of the controls. Furthermore, he measured the LH content of the pituitary by the ovarian ascorbic acid depletion test of Parlow (1958) and demonstrated that both the concentration and the total content of LH were significantly reduced. He suggested that MAP primarily blocked synthesis of LH in the pituitary.

2. Parabiotic test

Miyake (1961) studied the inhibition of pituitary gonadotropin secretion by using parabiotic mice. He found that MAP at a total dose level of 1 to 10 mcg had an antigonadotropin activity similar to that of progesterone in total doses of 10 mg as evaluated by the percentage of inhibition of ovarian growth of the intact partner.

DELAY OF NIDATION

It has been shown by Barnes and Meyer (1964) that daily injections of 2.4 mg of MAP to pregnant rats from day 1 through day 13 of pregnancy cause delay of nidation in 100% of the animals. Nidation can be initiated by the administration of estrone. They suggested that MAP suppresses LH production or release, resulting in preventing the secretion of sufficient endogenous estrogen to cause nidation. Similar results were obtained by Mayer and Duluc (1968). However, progesterone at a single daily dose of 16 mg or more did not cause delayed implantation in intact rats (Cochrane and Meyer, 1957; Nutting and Sollman, 1967).

V. ANTIHORMONAL ACTIVITY

ANTIESTROGENIC EFFECT

The mouse vaginal smear and the mouse uterine growth are commonly used as assays for comparative antiestrogenic evaluations for progestational steroids. Edgren et al. (1967) reported that MAP was active in the vaginal smear test compared at the ED_{50}, the dose estimated to reduce the expected response to a total of 2 mcg estrone over a 4-day period. Using the uterine growth test, they found that MAP exerted an antiestrone effect 3 times greater than that of progesterone when 0.3 mcg of estrone was given to induce uterine growth in immature mice.

Dorfman and Kincl (1963) found that MAP required a minimum of 150 mcg total dose compared to 25 mcg of 17α-acetoxyprogesterone to produce an antiuterotropic effect in mice when a total dose of 0.4 mcg of estrone was administered. The antiestrogenic activity of DP-acetophenone as well as DP-acetofuran in doses of 100 mcg and 1 mg was found by Lerner et al. (1961) and Lerner et al. (1963), respectively, to be equivalent to the activity of similar doses of progesterone when given simultaneously with 0.1 mcg of estradiol benzoate to immature female mice. The authors suggested that this antiestrogenic effect resulted in the arrest of the estrous cycles in the diestrous phase and the disturbance of mating.

HP-caproate showed no antiuterotropic activity in the immature mouse (Kessler and Borman, 1958) and in the ovariectomized rat (Velardo, 1958).

ANTIANDROGENIC EFFECT

Some progestational steroids are known to inhibit the growth responses of accessory sex organs to administered androgens in castrated rats (Dorfman, 1962). The studies by Revesz and Chappel (1966), using castrated immature male rats injected subcutaneously with MAP (2.0 mg/day) in combination with testosterone propionate (0.03 mg/day) for 7 days, show that this progestin has only a very slight antiandrogenic effect on the weight of the ventral prostate, while progesterone in the same dose has none at all and only a dose level of 25 mg significantly reduced the increase in weight of the ventral prostate, seminal vesicles and levator ani.

Lerner et al. (1961) and Lerner et al. (1963) found no antiandrogenic activity of DP-acetophenone and DP-acetofuran when 1 mg of DP-acetophenone or 5 mg of DP-acetofuran were injected daily with 25 mcg testoterone propionate.

TERATOLOGICAL EFFECTS

Of all the synthetic steroids discussed, only MAP has been found to produce masculinization of female fetuses in the rat. The ano–genital distance was used as the indicator and the compound was injected once daily during the latter part of pregnancy (Revesz et al., 1960; Schöler and de Wachter, 1961; Falconi et al., 1961; Lerner et al., 1962; Revesz and Chappel, 1966). Other progestational steroids such as HP-caproate (Suchowsky and Junkmann, 1960), the acetophenone and 2-acetofuran derivatives of 16α,17α-dihydroxyprogesterone (Lerner et al., 1962; Lerner et al., 1963) do not show any virilizing action on the external genitalia and the internal sex and accessory sex organs of the offspring on gross examination.

REFERENCES

ALLEN, W. S. and BERNSTEIN, S. (1955) Steroidal cyclic ketals. XII. The preparation of Δ^{16}-steroids. J. Amer. Chem. Soc. 77: 1028–1032.

BARNES, L. E., SCHMIDT, F. L. and DULIN, W. E. (1959) Progestational activity of 6α-methyl-17α-acetoxyprogesterone. Proc. Soc. Exp. Biol. and Med. 100: 820–822.

BARNES, L. E. and MEYER, R. K. (1964) Delayed implantation in intact rats treated with medroxyprogesterone acetate. J. Reprod. Fertil. 7: 139–143.

COCHRANE, R. L. and MEYER, R. K. (1957) Delayed nidation in the rat induced by progesterone. Proc. Soc. Exp. Biol. Med. 96: 155–159.

DAVIS, M. E. and WIED, G. L. (1955) 17α-hydroxyprogesterone-caproate: a new substance with prolonged progestational activity. A comparison with chemically pure progesterone. J. Clin. Endocr. 15: 923–930.

DORFMAN, R. I. (1962) Anti-androgenic substances. In: Methods in Hormone Research, Vol. II, pp. 315–323. Bioassay, Dorfman, R. I. (Ed.). Academic Press, New York.

DORFMAN, R. I. and KINCL, F. A. (1963) Steroid anti-estrogens. Steroids 1: 185–209.

EDGREN, R. A., JONES, R. C. and PETERSON, D. L. (1967) A biological classification of progestational agents. Fertil. Steril. 18: 238–256.

FALCONI, G., GARDI, R., BRUNI, G. and ERCOLI, A. (1961) Studies on steroidal enol ethers: An attempt to dissociate progestational from contraceptive activity in oral gestagens. Endocrinology 69: 638–647.

FRIED, J., SABO, E. F., GRABOWICH, P., LERNER, L. J., KESSLER, W. B., BRENNAN, D. M. and BORMAN, A. (1961) Progestationally active acetals and ketals of 16α,17α-dihydroxyprogesterone. Chemistry and Industry 465–466.

JULIAN, P. L., MEYER, E. W., KARPEL, W. J. and WALLER, I. R. (1950) 17α-hydroxy-11-desoxycorticosterone (Reichstein's substance S). J. Amer. Chem. Soc. 72: 5145–5147.

JUNKMANN, K. (1954) Über protrahiert wirksame Gestagene. Arch. Exp. Path. Pharmakol. 223: 244.

JUNKMANN, K. (1957) Long-acting steroids in reproduction. In: Recent Progress in Hormone Research, Vol. XIII, pp. 389–428. Pincus, G. (Ed.). Academic Press, New York.

KESSLER, W. B. and BORMAN, A. (1958) Some biological activities of certain progestogens: I. 17α-hydroxyprogesterone 17-n-caproate. Ann. N.Y. Acad. Sci. 71(5): 486–493.

LABHSETWAR, A. P. (1966) Mechanism of action at medroxyprogesterone (17α-acetoxy-6α-methyl progesterone) in the rat. J. Reprod. Fertil. 12: 445–451.

LERNER, L. J., BRENNAN, D. M. and BORMAN, A. (1961) Biological activities of 16α,17α-dihydroxyprogesterone derivatives. *Proc. Soc. Exp. Biol. Med.* **106**: 231–234.

LERNER, L. J., BRENNAN, D. M., YIACAS, E., DEPHILLIPO, M. and BORMAN, A. (1962) Pregnancy maintenance in ovariectomized rats with 16α,17α-dihydroxyprogesterone derivatives and other progestogens. *Endocrinology* **70**: 283–287.

LERNER, L. J., DEPHILLIPO, M., YIACAS, E., BRENNAN, D. and BORMAN, A. (1962) Comparison of the acetophenone derivative of 16α,17α-dihydroxyprogesterone with other progestational steroids for masculinization of the rat fetus. *Endocrinology* **71**: 448–451.

LERNER, L. J., YIACAS, E. and BORMAN, A. (1963) Biological activities of the 2-acetofuran derivative of 16α,17α-dihydroxyprogesterone. *Proc. Soc. Exp. Biol. Med.* **113**: 663–666.

LERNER, L. J., YIACAS, E., BIANCHI, A., TURKHEIMER, A. R., DEPHILLIPO, M. and BORMAN, A. (1964) Effect of the acetophenone derivative of 16α,17α-dihydroxyprogesterone on the estrous cycle, mating, and fertility in the rat. *Fertil. Steril.* **15(1)**: 63–73.

MAYER, M. G. and DULUC, ANNE-JOSETTE (1968) Action de l'acétate de médroxyprogestérone sur la nidation chez la ratte. *C.R. Acad. Sci. (Paris)* **266**: 1600–1603.

MIYAKE, T. (1961) Inhibitory effect of various steroids on gonadotropin hypersecretion in parabiotic mice. *Endocrinology* **69**: 534–546.

NEUMANN, F., KRAMER, M. and RASPÉ, G. 1968) Das endokrinologische Wirkungsspektrum von 19-nor-17α-hydroxyprogesteroncapronat (Gestonoroncapronat). *Arzneimittel-Forsch.* **18**: 1289–1297.

NUTTING, E. F. and SOLLMAN, P. B. (1967) Delay of implantation in intact rats treated with progestins. *Acta Endocr.* **54**: 8–18.

PARLOW, A. F. (1958) A rapid bioassay method for LH and factors stimulating LH secretion. *Fed. Proc.* **17**: 402.

REVESZ, C., CHAPPEL, C. I. and GANDRY, R. (1960) Masculinization of female fetuses in the rat by progestational compounds. *Endocrinology* **66**: 140–143.

REVESZ, C. and CHAPPEL, C. I. (1966) Biological activity of medrogestone: a new orally active progestin. *J. Reprod. Fertil.* **12**: 473–487.

SCHÖLER, H. F. L. and DE WACHTER, A. M. (1961) Evaluation of androgenic properties of progestational compounds in the rat by the female foetal masculinization test. *Acta Endocr.* **38**: 128–136.

SHIPLEY, E. G. (1962) Anti-gonadotropic steroids, inhibition of ovulation and mating. In: *Methods in Hormone Research*, Vol. II, pp. 179–274. Dorfman, R. I. (Ed.). Academic Press, New York.

SMITHBERG, M. (1958) Attempts to induce and maintain pregnancy in prepuberal mice following treatment with 17α-hydroxyprogesterone 17-n-caproate. *Ann. N.Y. Acad. Sci.* **17(5)**: 555–559.

SUCHOWSKY, G. and JUNKMANN, K. (1958) Untersuchungen der schwangerschaftserhaltenden Wirkung von 17α-hydroxyprogesteroncapronat an kastrierten trächtigen Kaninchen. *Acta Endocr.* **28**: 129–131.

SUCHOWSKY, G. and JUNKMANN, K. (1960) A study of the virilizing effect of progestogens on the female rat fetus. *Endocrinology* **68**: 341–349.

THOMA, R. W., FRIED, J., BONANNO, S. and GRABOWICH, P. (1957) Oxidation of steroids by microorganisms. IV. 16α-hydroxylation of 9α-fluorohydrocortisone and 9α-fluoroprednisolone by *Streptomyces roseochromogenus*. *J. Amer. Chem. Soc.* **79**: 4818.

VELARDO, J. T. (1958) Biological action of 17α-hydroxyprogesterone 17-n-caproate on the reproductive processes of the rat. *Ann. N.Y. Acad. Sci.* **71(5)**: 542–554.

ZARROW, M. X. (1961) Gestation. In: *Sex and Internal Secretions*, Vol. II, pp. 958–1031, 3rd ed. Young, W. C. (Ed.). Williams & Wilkins, Baltimore.

CHAPTER 26

EFFECTS, DURATION OF ACTION AND METABOLISM IN MAN

J. Ferin

Department of Obstetrics and Gynecology, University Hospital, Belgium

EFFECTS AND DURATION OF ACTION

Study of the effects of progesterone on the genital tract of women has shown that, as far as its epithelial lining is concerned, the secretory and decidual transformation of the endometrium is the only truly specific action of the hormone. In fact the term progestational compounds or progestogens applies to substances which in animals are able to produce endometrial changes ("la dentelle utérine") similar to those normally preceding nidation.

These effects are unquestionably the best measure of progestational activity. Any substance that can produce this transformation in the human endometrium will be considered as a progestogen for man.

Theoretically such progestational activity should always be demonstrated in ovariectomized women after adequate estrogen treatment. The experimental conditions so established are ideal. However, in practice it may be difficult to find such subjects and the investigator may have to resort to the study of women whose ovaries do not function—either permanently or even only temporarily, in which case one should guard against a spontaneous abrupt revival of ovarian function.

It has been shown that a number of substances can induce progestational transformation of the endometrium after injection—in oily solution or aqueous suspension—into ovariectomized estrogen-treated women. These are:

1. 17α-hydroxyprogesterone caproate (Boschann, 1954; Davis and Wied, 1957).
2. 17α-hydroxyprogesterone acetate (Davis and Wied, 1957).
3. 6α-methyl-17α-hydroxyprogesterone acetate (Davis and Wied, 1957).

4. 17α-hydroxy-19-nor-progesterone caproate (Nevinny-Stickel, 1962)
5. 19-nor-testosterone-17β-methyl ether (Nevinny-Stickel, 1963).
6. 17α-ethynyl-19-nor-testosterone-enanthate (Boschann and Kur, 1957; Davis and Wied, 1957).
7. 17α-ethynyl-estrenol phenyl-propionate (Ferin and Schlikker, unpublished).
8. 16α-ethyl progesterone (Linthorst, unpublished).

The following substances have, at least in the doses used, been found in ovariectomized women to produce only the first phase of secretory transformation of the endometrium, the *massive glandular deposition of glycogen*, which is not really a specific effect of progesterone (see Chapter 22, page 447):

1. 11-dehydro progesterone (Ferin, 1950).
2. 19-nor-progesterone (Ferin, 1957).
3. 20-α-hydroxy-pregn-4-ene-3-one cyclopentyl propionate (20α-progesterol cyclopentyl propionate) (Wied and Davis, 1958).*

Progestational activity has also been found in a few other compounds after parenteral administration to women supposedly lacking functioning corpora lutea, pretreated with estrogens. These substances were 20α- and 20β-progesterol (Lauritzen, 1963, 1966) and 17α-methallyl-estrenol (Ferin, unpublished).

A quantitative comparison of potencies is much more difficult. To obtain complete secretory and decidual transformation of the endometrium, certain conditions must be fulfilled. Firstly, the endometrium must have been adequately prepared by estrogens, and, secondly, the progestational compound should be administered together with an estrogen. The ratio between the two is very important. If it is not properly adjusted, the endometrial differentiation becomes atypical. For investigational purposes it is advisable to apply an identical estrogen treatment in the course of every artificial cycle. The sensitivity of the different parts of the genital tract to the hormonal preparations varies from one patient to another (as does sensitivity of the ovary to gonadotrophins). One should, therefore, compare only results obtained in *the same patient*. There have been very few published observations satisfying this requirement. Results are shown in Tables 1 and 2.

Measuring the duration of action seems to be simpler. It would appear that the duration of the so-called *latency period* provides the best criterion.

* 20α- and 20β-progesterol are naturally occurring progestational substances (Zander, 1959).

TABLE 1. COMPARATIVE PROGESTATIONAL ACTIVITY OF VARIOUS LONG-ACTING STEROIDS IN OVARIECTOMIZED WOMEN

End point: endometrial late secretory changes.
Fern abolition (cervix); late luteal vaginal smear.
Estrogenic priming: 1 mg diethylstilbestrol daily, day 1 to day 28/29.
Progestational compound: once, intramuscularly, at the 14th day.
Exploration of the genital tract: performed 14 days thereafter.
Effective doses (ineffective dose in parentheses) in mg.

	Endometrium	Cervix	Vaginal smear	Authors
17α-Hydroxyprogesterone caproate in oily solution	350 (250) 375 (375)	350 (250)	350 (250) 375 (250)	Wied and Davis (1958) Davis and Wied (1957) Wied et al. (1958)
17α-Hydroxyprogesterone acetate in aqueous suspension	350 (250)	250 (150)	250 (150)	Wied and Davis (1958) Davis and Wied (1957)
17α-Ethynyl-19-nortestosterone enanthate in oily solution	150 (100)	100 (75)	150 (100)	Wied and Davis (1958) Davis and Wied (1957)
4-Pregnene-3-one-20α-ol cyclopentylpropionate in oily solution	(300)			Wied and Davis (1958)
6α-Methyl-17α-acetoxy-progesterone in aqueous suspension	50 (25)	50 (25)	50 (25)	Wied and Davis (1961)

TABLE 2. COMPARATIVE PROGESTATIONAL ACTIVITIES OF VARIOUS LONG-ACTING STEROIDS IN OVARIECTOMIZED WOMEN

End point: endometrial late secretory changes.
Estrogenic priming: 7 × 5 mg estradiol benzoate in oily solution, intramuscularly, from day 1 to day 22.
Progestational compound: intramuscularly, once at the 15th day or twice at the 15th and the 22nd days.
Endometrial biopsy: performed generally at the 28th day.
(Boschann and Drews, 1961.)

	Dose	Total dose
(Progesterone)	20 mg ten times	200 mg
17α-Hydroxyprogesterone caproate in oily solution	100 mg twice	200 mg
	250 mg once	250 mg
17α-Ethynyl-nortestosterone enanthate in oily solution	100–150 mg once	100–150 mg
6α-Methyl-17α-acetoxy-progesterone in aqueous suspension	50 mg once	50 mg

This is defined as the time intervening between administration of the progestational compound (one single intramuscular injection) and the beginning of the withdrawal bleeding, provided that estrogen treatment is continued without interruption or decrease of dose.

Published data (Table 3) show considerable variations. This may be due to a number of factors: the dose employed, variations in estrogen treatment, sensitivity of individual patients, possible loss of active substance during administration, the taking of biopsies from the endometrium which seems to precipitate the onset of withdrawal bleeding and associated effects.

In certain cases when plasma levels of active substances decrease very slowly and stay at a certain critical level for a long time, there may be local endometrial necrosis and sloughing, which spreads slowly and may cause abnormally prolonged bleeding (Ober, 1957).

The duration of a rise in body temperature ("plateau hyperthermique") provides a valuable parameter (Table 4), though it need not necessarily be correlated with the effect on the endometrium, since metabolites of the active compound might have a hyperthermic action without being progestational in the strict sense.

Interesting data concerning progestational activity and duration of action have also been obtained by inducing decidualization and maintaining it for 2 to 3 months (pseudopregnancy) and by postponing menstruation (Tables 5 and 6).

TABLE 3. DURATION OF THE PROGESTATIONAL ACTION

Time interval (days) between a single injection of the progestational compound and the onset of withdrawal bleeding in continuously estrogenized ovariectomized women (A), in cases of dysfunctional bleeding (B) or in continuously estrogenized amenorrheic women (C).

	Dose (mg)	Interval	Reference
A. *In ovariectomized women*			
Progesterone			
1. in oily solution	200	2 d	Boschann (1958)
	350	5–6 d	Davis and Wied (1955)
2. in aqueous crystalline suspension (size of the crystals 0.02–0.1 mm)	100 200 300	7 d 10 d 10 d	Ober *et al.* (1954)
17α-Hydroxyprogesterone caproate in oily solution	200 250 350	8 d 7–8 d 13–18 d	Boschann (1958) Boschann (1955) Davis and Wied (1955)
17α-Hydroxyprogesterone acetate in aqueous suspension	150 350	9–16 d 14–15 d	Davis and Wied (1957)
17α-Hydroxy-19-nor-progesterone caproate in oily solution	25 50	 10–13 d	Nevinny-Stickel (1962)
6α-Methyl-17α-acetoxy progesterone, in aqueous suspension	50 50	30–43 d 16 d	Wied and Davis (1961) Boschann (1958) Boschann and Drews (1961)
17α-Ethynyl-nortestosterone enanthate in oily solution	100 100 150 200 200	21–23 d 16 d 25–28 d 28 d 32 d	Boschann (1958) Boschann and Drews (1961) Davis and Wied (1957) Wied and Davis (1958) Ferin and Schlikker (unpublished results)
17α-Ethynyl-estrenol-phenyl-propionate in oily solution	100	21–25 d	Ferin and Schlikker (unpublished results)

TABLE 3—cont.

	Dose (mg)	Interval	Reference
B. *In cases of dysfunctional bleeding**			
Progesterone in aqueous crystalline suspension (size of the crystals: 25% 0.02 mm and 75% 0.05 to 0.1 mm)	200	mean: 12.65 d (401 cases)	Ober (1957)
	200	11.3 d mean: (109 cases)	Herrmann (1958)
	200	10–14 d	Paschen and Schild (1958)
17α-Hydroxyprogesterone caproate in oily solution	500	9–14 d	Gold and Cohen (1958)
	250	mean: 12 d	
	125	mean: 9 d	
	65	mean: 7 d	Pots (1955)
	125	7–9 d (37 cases)	Boschann (1958)
	125	8–16 d mean: 11.5 d (110 cases)	Rauscher and Kofler (1958)
	125 ⎫ 250 ⎬ 375 ⎭	9–16 d mean: 12.5 d (161 cases)	Thomas (1958)
6α-Methyl-17α-acetoxyprogesterone, in aqueous suspension	50 150	3–6 wks	Barfield and Greenblatt (1961)
17α-Ethynyl-19-nortesterone enanthate, in oily solution	67	mean: 17.4 d (71 cases)	Staemmler and Lauritzen (1958)
	50 ⎫ 100 ⎬ 200 ⎭	23–31 d	Pots (1958)
	200	11–22 d	Boschann and Kur (1957) Boschann (1958)
C. *In amenorrheic women*			
16α,17α-dihydroxyprogesterone acetophenide in oily solution	100	14–32 d mean: 19.7 d	Taymor *et al.* (1964)
16α-ethyl-progesterone in oily solution	100	5–10 d	
	200	7–23 d mean: 13.4 d (27 cycles, 10 patients)	
	300	9–10 d	Ferin (unpublished results)

* An estrogen is often injected intramuscularly at the same time.

TABLE 3—cont.

	Dose (mg)	Interval	Reference
C. *In amenorrheic women—cont.*			
20β_F-hydroxy-19-nor-pregnene-3-one 20β phenyl propionate (oxogestone) in oily solution	100	19–20 d	Ferin (unpublished results)
17α-Ethynyl-estrenol phenyl propionate in oily solution	100	17–30 d	Ferin (unpublished results)
Methallyl-estrenol in oily solution	100 200	10–30 d 22 d	Ferin (unpublished results)
9β,10α-Pregna-4,6-diene-3,20-dione (dydrogesterone) in aqueous suspension	100	16–38 d	Ferin (unpublished results)

TABLE 4. DURATION OF THE PROGESTATIONAL ACTION
Duration of temperature rise following a single injection.

	Dose (mg)	Interval	Reference
17α-Hydroxyprogesterone caproate, in oily solution	250 500	7 d 9 to 21 d	Cohen *et al.* (1956)
	125 250 375	5 to 7 d	Seidl *et al.* (1958)
6α-Methyl-17α-acetoxy-progesterone, in aqueous suspension	50 100	until 50 d	Barfield and Greenblatt (1961)
17α-Ethynyl-19-nor-testosterone enanthate, in oily solution	50 100 200	25 to 35 d	Pots (1958)
	100 200	30 to 52 d	Rauscher (1960)
17α-Ethynyl-estrenol-phenyl-propionate or acetate, in oily solution	50	14–21 d	Borglin (1966)
17α-Ethyl-progesterone	200	10 d	Ferin (unpublished results)

TABLE 5. INDUCING AND MAINTAINING DECIDUA FOR 2 TO 3 MONTHS (PSEUDOPREGNANCY)

	Dose	Reference
Progesterone in aqueous crystalline suspension (size of the crystals: 25% up to 20 μ 75% 50–100 μ) +estradiol benzoate, in aqueous crystalline suspension, 10 mg weekly	200 mg weekly	Ferin (unpublished results)
17α-Hydroxyprogesterone caproate, in oily solution +estradiol valerate in oily solution, 10 mg weekly	375 mg weekly	Gold and Cohen (1958)
17α-Hydroxyprogesterone caproate, in oily solution +estradiol valerate in oily solution, 20 mg weekly	375 mg weekly	Durham (1961)
17α-Hydroxyprogesterone caproate, in oily solution +diethylstilbestrol 1 mg daily	375 mg weekly	Durham (1961)
17α-Hydroxyprogesterone caproate, in oily solution +estradiol valerate in oily solution, 10 or 20 mg weekly	500 mg weekly	Ferin (unpublished results)
6α-Methyl-17α-acetoxy-progesterone in aqueous suspension + diethylstilbestrol 1 mg daily or estradiol valerate 10 or 20 mg weekly	100–150 mg weekly	Durham (1961)

METABOLISM AND EXCRETION

Metabolic studies have been performed with only a few injectable progestational compounds.

1. 17α-hydroxyprogesterone-17 caproate (hydroxyprogesterone caproate) in oily solution. The most important urinary metabolites are reported to be different from those of progesterone and of 17α-hydroxyprogesterone (Langecker, 1955). The caproic acid moiety has been found to remain attached to some of these metabolites (Plotz, 1962). The long duration of action has been attributed to the slow resorption from the injection site (Plotz, 1960; Davis et al., 1960). After injections of 4-^{14}C-labelled 17α-

TABLE 6. POSTPONEMENT OF MENSTRUATION DURING 10 TO 20 DAYS

	Dose	Reference
Progesterone in oily solution intramuscularly daily	15 mg (+0.5 mg estradiol in oily solution) daily	Ober (1957)
	30 mg (+1.5 mg estradiol)	Kaiser (1959)
Progesterone in aqueous suspension (size of the crystals: 0.02–0.1 mm) once	200 mg (+10 mg estradiol benzoate, in crystalline suspension) once	Ober et al. (1954) Kaiser (1956)
17α-Hydroxyprogesterone caproate in oily solution intramuscularly weekly	125/250 mg (+10/20 mg estradiol valerate) weekly	Kaiser (1956)

hydroxyprogesterone-17 caproate, fatty tissue shows the highest concentration of radioactivity. In the endometrium and myometrium radioactivity is much less but nevertheless higher than that found after the administration of similarly labeled progesterone (Plotz, 1960; Davis et al., 1960). Radioactivity in plasma, feces and urine increases slowly, stays at a higher level for several days and thereafter falls gradually. In contradistinction, after the administration of labeled progesterone the maximum of radioactivity in the plasma is reached much faster and the decline is far more rapid (Plotz, 1960; Davis et al., 1960).

2. 17α-hydroxy-19-nor-progesterone-17 caproate in oily solution. The main urinary metabolite is 19-nor-pregnanediol-20-one (Breuer and Lisboa, 1966).

3. 6α-methyl-17α-acetoxyprogesterone (medroxyprogesterone acetate) in aqueous suspension. After parenteral as well as after oral administration one metabolite has been isolated; this was described as 6β-17α-21 trihydroxy-6α-methyl-pregna-4-ene-3,20 dione 21 acetate (Castegnaro and Sala, 1962). According to others (Helmreich and Huseby, 1962) the compound is the 17-acetate. The 21-acetate could be an artefact formed by transacetylation in the course of its isolation (Petrow, 1966). This steroid is reported to be excreted mainly as a glucosiduronate. Excretion continues for several weeks after termination of the treatment. This was taken as an indication of the very slow resorption of the drug from the injection site

(Helmreich and Huseby, 1965). However, medroxyprogesterone acetate labeled with ^{14}C in 6 has been injected intravenously (Slaunwhite and Sandberg, 1961) and its biological half-life in plasma was found to exceed 200 minutes. High percentages of radioactivity were recovered from the bile, feces and urine. It appeared that the compound is retained in the organism for a very long time.

4. 17α-ethynyl-19 nortestosterone-17-enanthate (norethisterone enanthate) in oily solution.

Norethisterone and its esters are metabolized to some extent to ethynylestradiol; 80 mg of norethisterone enanthate is reported to have yielded 5 mg of ethynyl-estradiol, about 1 % of which was recovered from the urine (Brown and Blair, 1960).

REFERENCES

BARFIELD, W. E. and GREENBLATT, R. B. (1961) 6-Methyl-17-acetoxy-progesterone injectable: clinical experience. In: *Progesterone: Brook Lodge Symposium*, pp 151–160. Barnes, A. C. (Ed.). Brook Lodge Press, Augusta, Michigan.

BORGLIN, N. E. (1966) Östrenolderivate in der Gynäkologie. *Geburtsh. Frauenheilk.* 26: 616–619.

BOSCHANN, H.-W. (1954) Zur Wirkung des 17-alpha-oxy-Progesteron-Kapronats auf das menschliche Endometrium. *Ärtzl. Wchnschr.* 9: 591–593.

BOSCHANN, H.-W. (1955) Klinische Erfahrungen mit 17-alpha-oxy-Progesteron-17-Capronat. *Geburtsh. Frauenheilk.* 15: 1070–1081.

BOSCHANN, H.-W. and KUR, S. (1957) Über die Wirkung des 17-Äthinyl-19-nor-Testosteronönanthats eines neuen Gestagens mit Depotcharakter auf das menschliche Endometrium und das atrophische Vaginalepithel. *Geburtsh. Frauenheilk.* 17: 928–937.

BOSCHANN, H.-W. (1958) Observations on the role of progestational agents in human gynecologic disorders and pregnancy complications. *Ann. N. Y. Acad. Sci.* 71: 727–752.

BOSCHANN, H.-W. and DREWS, R. (1961) The effect of 6-alpha-methyl-17-alpha-acetoxyprogesterone on the endometrium. In: *Progesterone: Brook Lodge Symposium*, pp. 133–145. Barnes, A. C. (Ed.). Brook Lodge Press, Augusta, Michigan.

BREUER, H. and LISBOA, B. P. (1966) Untersuchungen über den Stoffwechsel von 17 alpha-Hydroxy-19-nor-Progesteron Capronat beim Menschen *in vivo* und von 17 alpha-Hydroxy-19-nor-Progesteron bei der Ratte *in vitro*. *Acta Endocr.* 51: 114–130.

BROWN, J. B. and BLAIR, H. A. F. (1960) Urinary oestrogen metabolites of 19-nor-ethisterone and its esters. *Proc. Roy. Soc. Med.* 53: 433.

CASTEGNARO, E. and SALA, G. (1962) Isolation and identification of 6-beta, 17-alpha, 21-trihydroxy-6-alpha-methyl-delta 4-pregnene-3,20-dione (21-acetate) from the urine of human subjects treated with 6α-methyl-17α-acetoxyprogesterone. *J. Endocr.* 24: 445–452.

COHEN, M. R., FRANK, R., DRESNER, M. H. and GOLD, J. J. (1956) The use of a new long acting progestational steroid (17-alpha-hydroxyprogesterone caproate) in the therapy of secondary amenorrhea. A preliminary report. *Amer. J. Obstet. Gynec.* 72: 1103–1115.

DAVIS, M. E. and WIED, G. L. (1955) 17-alpha-Hydroxyprogesterone-caproate: a new substance with prolonged progestational activity. A comparison with chemically pure progesterone. *J. Clin. Endocr. Metab.* **15**: 923–930.
DAVIS, M. E. and WIED, G. L. (1957) Long-acting progestational agents. *Geburtsh. Frauenheilk.* **17**: 916–928.
DAVIS, M. E., PLOTZ, E. J., LUPU, C. I. and EJARQUE, P. M. (1960) The metabolism of progesterone and its related compounds in human pregnancy. *Fertil. Steril.* **11**: 18–48.
DURHAM, W. C. (1961) Progestational steroid requirements for inducing and maintaining decidua in women. *Fertil. Steril.* **12**: 45–54.
FERIN, J. (1950) Les effets de la 11-déhydro-progestérone chez la femme. *An. Endocr.* **11**: 179–182.
FERIN, J. (1957) Progestational activity of certain 19-nor-steroids. Comparative assays in oophorectomized women. *J. Clin. Endocr. Metab.* **17**: 1252–1255.
GOLD, J. J. and COHEN, M. R. (1958) Clinical application of 17-alpha-hydroxyprogesterone-17-n-caproate. *Ann. N. Y. Acad. Sci.* **71**: 691–703.
HELMREICH, M. L. and HUSEBY, R. A. (1962) Identification of a 6,21-dihydroxylated metabolite of Medroxyprogesterone acetate in human urine. *J. Clin. Endocr. Metab.* **22**: 1018–1032.
HELMREICH, M. L. and HUSEBY, R. A. (1965) Factors influencing the absorption of medroxyprogesterone acetate. *Steroids* **6**, Suppl. II, 79–95.
HERRMANN, U. (1958) Abhängigkeit der durch Oestrogen- und Progesteron-Kristalle induzierten Abbruchblutung von der Korngrösse. *Gynaecologia*, **146**: 318–323.
KAISER, R. (1956) Versuche zur klinischen Anwendung einer "Pseudogravidität". *Dt. Med. Wschr.* **81**: 744–748.
KAISER, R. (1959) Die therapeutische Pseudogravidität. *Geburtsh. Frauenheilk.* **19**: 593–604.
LANGECKER, H. (1955) Das Schicksal des 17-alpha-Oxyprogesterons und seines 17-Capronates im menschlichen Organismus. *Arch. Exp. Path. Pharmak.* **225**: 309–313.
LAURITZEN, C. (1963) Biologische Wirkungen des 20β-Hydroxy-pregn-4-en-3-on. *Acta Endocr.* **44**: 225–236.
LAURITZEN, C. (1966) Untersuchungen zur biologischen Aktivität von Progesterol-20α und -20β. *Geburtsh. Frauenheilk.* **26**: 611–616.
NEVINNY-STICKEL, J. (1962) Die gestagene Wirkung von Hydroxy-nor-Progesteronestern bei der Frau. *8. Symposion der Deutschen Gesellschaft für Endokrinologie*, pp. 248–255. Springer, Berlin.
NEVINNY-STICKEL, J. (1963) Die unterschiedliche morphologische Wirkung verschiedener synthetischer Gestagene auf das Endometrium. *9. Symposion der Deutschen Gesellschaft für Endokrinologie*, pp. 177–180. Springer, Berlin.
OBER, K. G., KLEIN, I. and WEBER, M. (1954) Zur Frage einer Progesteronbehandlung. *Archiv. f. Gynäk.* **184**: 543–616.
OBER, K. G. (1957) Das Ovar. In: *Klinik der inneren Sekretion*, pp. 488–586. A. Labhart. Springer, Berlin.
PASCHEN, H. W. and SCHILD, W. (1958) Behandlung der durch ovarielle Dysfunktion bedingten gynäkologischen Blutungen. *Geburtsh. Frauenheilk.* **18**: 760–765.
PETROW, W. (1966) Steroidal oral contraceptive agents. In: *Essays in Biochemistry*, vol. 2, pp. 117–145. Campbell, P. N. and Greville, G. E. (Eds.). Academic Press, London.
PLOTZ, E. J. (1960) Die Anwendung radioaktiver Isotope in der Erforschung des Gestagenstoffwechsels in der Schwangerschaft. *6. Symposion der Deutschen Gesellschaft für Endokrinologie, Kiel, 1959*, pp. 21–29. Springer, Berlin.
PLOTZ, E. J. (1962) Metabolism of progestins. *Acta Cytol.* **6**: 213–215.
POTS, P. (1955) Zur Progesteronbehandlung funktioneller Blutungen. *Zbl. Gynäk.* **77**: 1754–1759.

POTS, P. (1958) Gestagen-Depotwirkung von Aethinylnortestosteronönanthat. *Geburtsh. Frauenheilk.* **18**: 673–676.

RAUSCHER, H. (1958) Zur Substitution der Gelbkörperwirkung durch 17-alpha-Oxyprogesteron-capronat. *Zbl. Gynäk.* **80**: 312–317.

RAUSCHER, H. and KOFLER, E. (1958) Wirkungserwartung, Zeitpunkt des Eintritts und Dauer der Blutung nach Verabreichung des Depotgestagens, 17-alpha-Oxyprogesteron-capronat. *Geburtsh. Frauenheilk.* **18**: 766–770.

RAUSCHER, H. (1960) Therapie mit Depotgestagenen. *6. Symposion der Deutschen Gesellschaft für Endokrinologie, Kiel, 1959*, pp. 87–92. Springer Verlag, Berlin.

SEIDL, J. E., EPSTEIN, J. A. and KUPPERMAN, H. S. (1958) Evaluation of progestational steroids in habitual abortion. *Int. J. Fertil.* **3**: 349–360.

SLAUNWHITE, W. R. and SANDBERG, A. A. (1961) Disposition of radioactive 17-alpha-hydroxy-progesterone, 6-alpha-methyl-17-alpha-acetoxy-progesterone and 6-alpha-methylprednisolone in human subjects. *J. Clin. Endocr. Metab.* **21**: 753–764.

STAEMMLER, H. J. and LAURITZEN, C. (1958) Über die Behandlung funktioneller Uterusblutungen mit einer Kombination von Östradiol- und Aethinyl-Nortestoster-Estern. *Zbl. Gynäk.* **80**: 1193–1197.

TAYMOR, M. L., PLANCK, S. and YAHIA, CL. (1964) Ovulation inhibition with a long acting parenteral progestogen–estrogen combination. *Fertil. Steril.* **15**, 653–660.

THOMAS, H. H. (1958) Dysfunctional uterine bleeding: a simplified one-injection treatment using long-acting ovarian steroids. *South Med. J.* **51**: 1266–1269.

WIED, G. L. and DAVIS, M. E. (1958) Comparative activity of progestational agents on the human endometrium and vaginal epithelium of surgical castrates. *Ann. N.Y. Acad. Sci.* **71**: 599–616.

WIED, G. L., DEL SOL, J. R. and DARGAN, A. M. (1958) Progestational and androgenic substances tested on the highly proliferated vaginal epithelium of surgical castrates. I. Progestational substances. *Amer. J. Obst. Gynec.* **75**: 98–111.

WIED, G. L. and DAVIS, M. E. (1961) The parenteral effectiveness of 6-methyl-17-alpha-OH-progesterone acetate under varying dosages of estrogenic priming of the endometrium of surgical castrates. *Progesterone: Brook Lodge Symposium*, pp. 147–150. Brook Lodge Press, Augusta, Michigan.

ZAÑARTU, J., RICE-WRAY, E. and GOLDZIEHER, J. W. (1966) Fertility control with long-acting injectable steroids. A preliminary report. *Obstet. Gynec.* **28**: 513–515.

ZANDER, J. (1959) In: *Recent Progress in the Endocrinology of Reproduction*, pp. 255–277. Academic Press, New York.

PART 2

ORALLY ACTIVE SUBSTITUTES FOR PROGESTERONE

CHAPTER 27

THE CHEMISTRY OF ORALLY ACTIVE SUBSTITUTES FOR PROGESTERONE AND CLASSIFICATION OF COMPOUNDS IN USE

Fred A. Kincl

Biological Concepts Inc., New York

INTRODUCTION

A great number of progestational agents have been synthesized since the first highly orally active drug—norethindrone—was made in 1952. The history and the chemical development of these drugs have been reviewed by Zderic (1963), Colton and Klimstra (1965) and Djerassi (1966). This presentation is, therefore, limited to a brief discussion of only those agents that have found clinical use.

As is the case with most drugs, details of industrial syntheses are confidential and not generally available.

1. ESTRANE AND ANDROSTANE DERIVATIVES

The synthesis of the first truly potent oral progestational agent, norethindrone—17α-ethynyl-17β-hydroxy-4-estren-3-one (I)—was achieved by Djerassi *et al.* in 1952 and described in detail in 1954. At almost the same time Colton (1953, 1954) reported the synthesis of a closely related compound norethynodrel—17α-ethynyl-17β-hydroxy-5(10)-estren-3-one (II).

3-Methoxy-2,5(10)-estradiene-17β-ol (III), prepared from 3-methoxy-estradiol (IV) by reduction with sodium in liquid ammonia (Birch and Smith, 1951), is the starting material in the synthesis of both compounds (Fig. 1). Djerassi *et al.* (1954) converted (III) into 19-nortestosterone (17β-hydroxy-4-estren-3-one) by strong acid hydrolysis andoxidized the 17-alcohol. The 3-ketone in the resulting 19-nor-androstenedione (V) was protected by the formation of 3-ethylenol ether (VI) which by ethynylation at C-17 followed by hydrolysis with a mineral acid gave norethindrone (I).

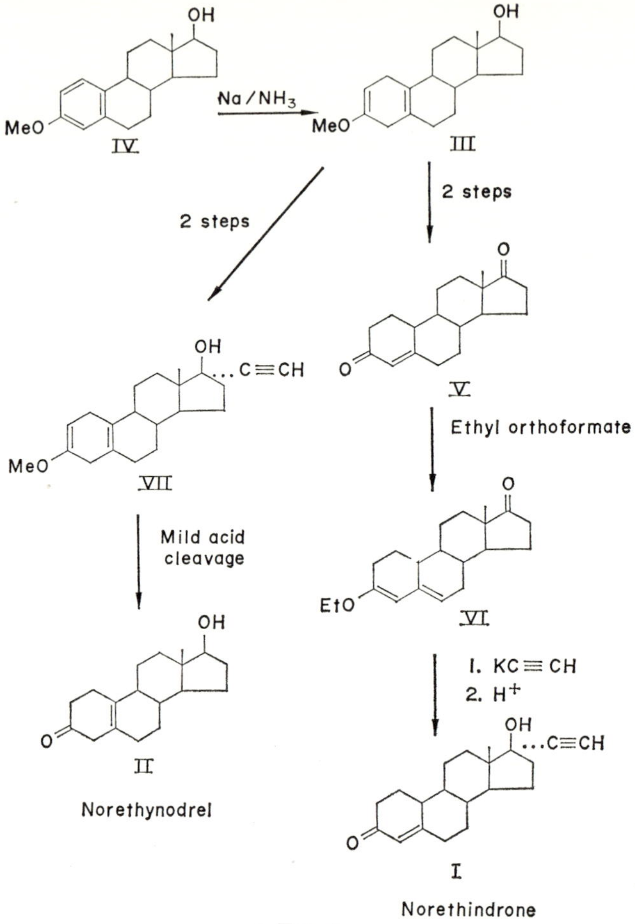

FIG. 1.

By a different procedure (Ringold *et al.*, 1956) the Δ⁴-3-keto function in 19-nortestosterone was protected by the formation of 3-ethylene ketal, the resulting compound being then ethynylated and cleaved to norethindrone.

To prepare (II) the dihydrocompound (III) was oxidized to the corresponding 17-ketone by the Oppenauer oxidation and converted into the 17-ethynyl derivative (VII). Mild acid treatment resulted in the formation of (II) (Colton, 1953, 1954).

Four other closely related compounds are being marketed as antifertility agents at the present. These include norethindrone acetate (VIII), its cyclopentyl enol ether (IX), ethynodiol diacetate (X) and the vinyl analogue of norethynodrel (XI) (Fig. 2).

To prepare norethindrone acetate (VIII), the tertiary 17β-alcohol in (I) was esterified with acetic anhydride in the presence of *p*-toluenesulfonic

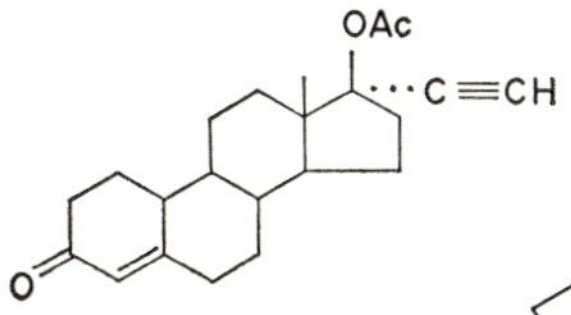

VIII

Norethindrone acetate

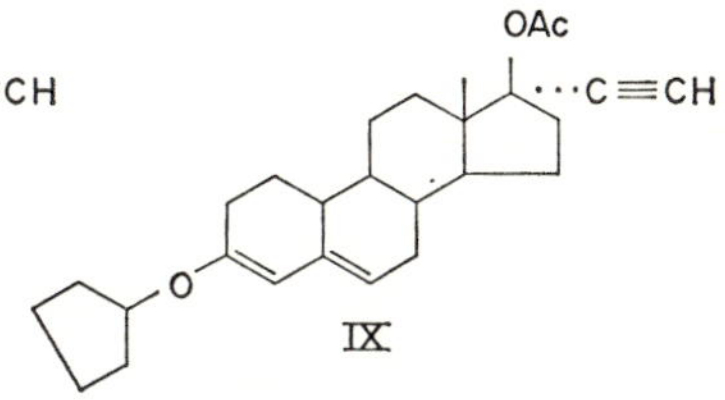

IX

Quingestanol acetate

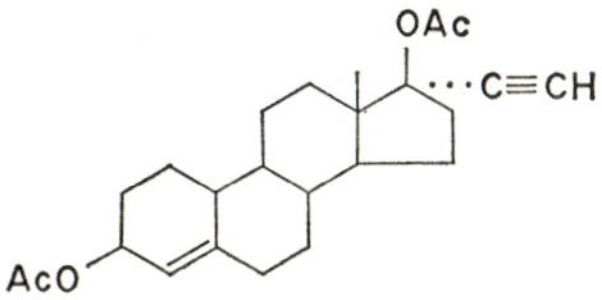

X

Ethynodiol diacetate

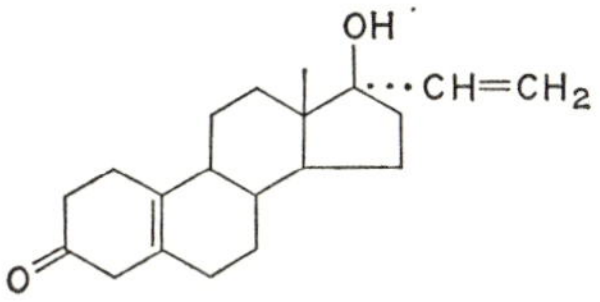

XI

Vinylestrenolone (Norgesterone)

FIG. 2.

acid with concomitant conversion of the Δ^4-3-keto group into the corresponding 3-enol acetate. The resulting 3β,17β-diacetoxy-17α-ethynyl-3,5-estradiene was converted by mild acid, or alkaline treatment to (VIII) (Iriarte *et al.*, 1959; Engelfried *et al.*, 1957; Colton, 1960). Ethynodiol diacetate (17α-ethynyl-3β,17β-diacetoxy-4-estrene) (X) was made by acetylation of the free alcohol with acetic anhydride in pyridine (Colton, 1958). The free alcohol is obtained from norethindrone by reduction with sodium borohydride (Colton, 1958; Sondheimer and Klibansky, 1959). The synthesis of (XI) was achieved by a route similar to that described for norethynodrel (Colton, 1953, 1954). The cyclopentyl enol ether (IX) was prepared from norethindrone acetate enol ether (3β,17β-diacetoxy-17α-ethynyl-3,5-estradiene) by refluxing with cyclopentanol in heptane in presence of *p*-toluenesulfonic acid (Ercoli and Gardi, 1964).

Removal of the oxygen function in (I) at C-3 was another structural

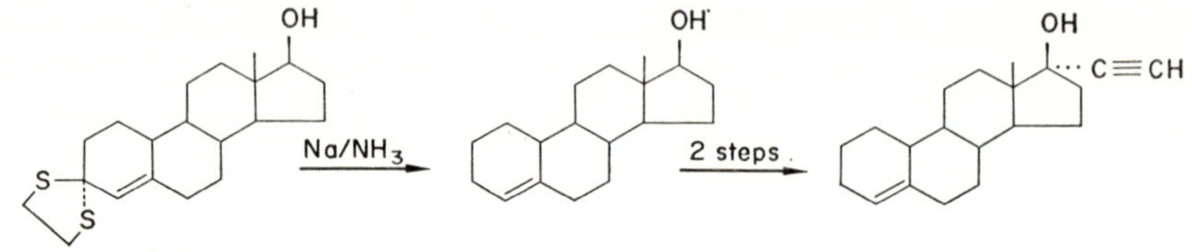

XII XIII XIV

Lynestrenol

XIV a

Allylestrenol

FIG. 3.

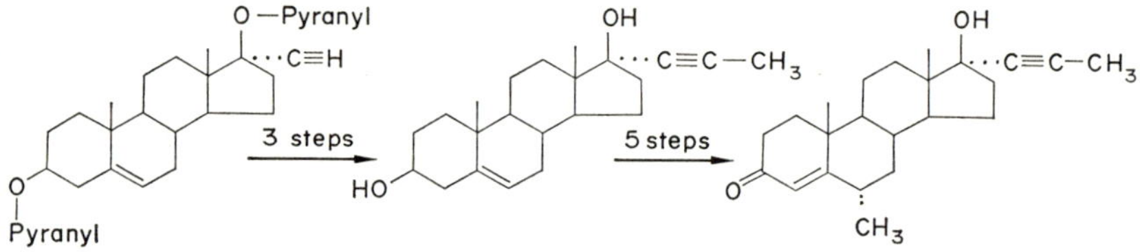

XVI XVII XV

Dimethisterone

FIG. 4.

modification which gave compounds that exhibited a good oral progestational activity. The synthesis of a typical 3-desoxy steroid is shown in Fig. 3 (de Winter *et al.*, 1959).

19-Nortestosterone was converted into 3-ethylene thioketal (XII) by treatment with ethylenedithiol in methanol in the presence of boron trifluoride. Reduction with sodium in liquid ammonia gave 3-deoxy 19-nortestosterone (XIII), which was oxidized and ethynylated at C-17 to provide lynestrenol—17α-ethynyl-4-estren-17β-ol (XIV).

Allylestrenol—17α-allyl-4-estren-17β-ol (XIVa)—used for pregnancy maintenance, has been synthesized by following essentially the same route (de Winter *et al.*, 1959).

6α-Methyl-17α-1-propyne-17β-hydroxy-4-androsten-3-one—dimethisterone (XV)—was synthesized from ethisterone—17α-ethynyl-17β- hydroxy-4-androsten-3-one—by a reaction sequence shown in Fig. 4 (David *et al.*, 1957). The 2′,3′-dihydropyranyl diether (XVI) was alkylated by treating the "21-lithio" derivative with methyl iodide followed by acid treatment (XVII). The 6α-methyl group was introduced by epoxidation of the Δ^5 double bond, followed by treatment with methyl Grignard, oxidation at C-3, removal of 5α-hydroxy group by dehydration and epimerization to give (XV).

2. COMPOUNDS RELATED TO 17α-ACETOXYPROGESTERONE

Five steroids structurally related to 17α-acetoxyprogesterone (17α-acetoxy-4-pregnene-3,20-dione) are of importance. With the exception of one, all are substituted at C-6.

The synthesis of medroxyprogesterone acetate—6α-methyl-17α-acetoxy-4-pregnene-3,20-dione (XVIII)—as shown in Fig. 5, illustrates the method of introducing a substituent at C-6 (Babcock *et al.*, 1958; Ringold *et al.*, 1959). 17α-Hydroxy-4-pregnene-3,20-dione is ketalized at C-3 and C-20 (XIX), the double bond is epoxidized, the epoxide treated with methyl Grignard and the ketal at C-3 cleaved to give the intermediate 5α-hydroxy-6β-methyl compound (XX). Dehydration, C-20-ketal elimination and isomerization of the 6β-methyl group produces the free compound (XXI) which upon acid catalyzed acetylation yields medroxyprogesterone acetate (XVIII).

Chlormadinone acetate—6-chloro-17α-acetoxy-4,6-pregnadiene-3,20-dione (XXII)—was prepared from 6α-chloro-17α-acetoxy-4-pregnene-3,20-dione (XXIII) by refluxing with chloranil in toluene (Fig. 6). Compound (XXIII) was made in a similar manner, as shown in Fig. 5, except that the 5α,6α epoxide was opened out with anhydrous hydrochloric acid (Ringold *et al.*, 1959).

Synthesis of the corresponding 6-methyl derivative, megestrol acetate—6-methyl-17α-acetoxy-4,6-pregnadiene-3,20-dione (XXIV) (Fig. 7)—was achieved in an analogous manner by dehydrogenation of medroxyprogesterone (Ringold *et al.*, 1959; Ellis *et al.*, 1960).

Two 16-substituted 17α-acetoxyprogesterone derivatives are used clinically. The synthesis of 16-methylene-17α-acetoxy-4,6-pregnadiene-3,20-dione (Superlutin (XXV)) was reported independently by three groups of investigators (Syhora, 1960; Mannhardt *et al.*, 1960; Kirk *et al.*, 1961).

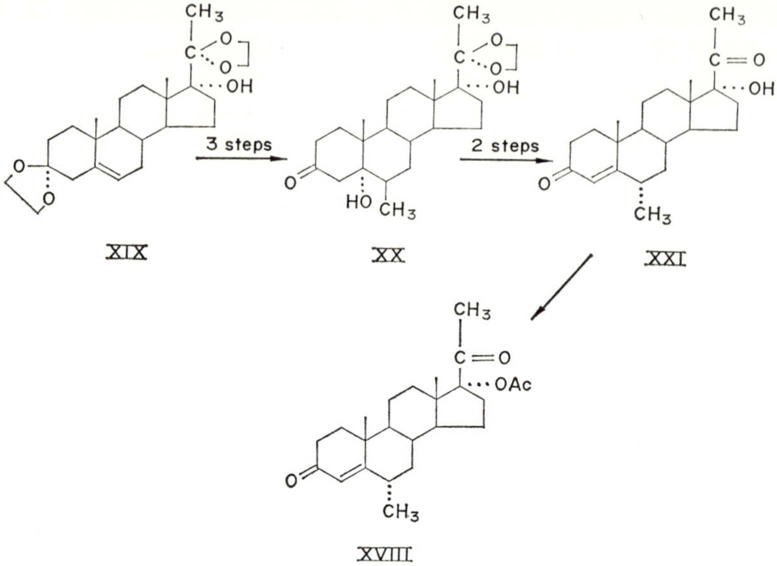

XIX XX XXI

XVIII
Medroxyprogesterone acetate
FIG. 5.

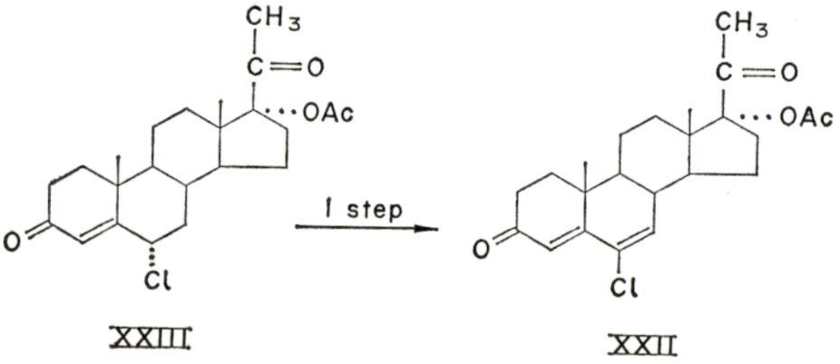

XXIII XXII
Chlormadinone acetate
FIG. 6.

Treatment of 3β-acetoxy-16-methyl-5,16-pregnadiene-20-one (XXVI, Fig. 8) with alkaline hydrogen peroxide gave 16α,17α-oxido derivative which was cleaved with acid to the intermediate 16-methylene-17α-hydroxy derivative (XXVII). Hydrolysis of the 3-acetate, followed by oxidation, acetylation and dehydrogenation at C-6, led to the desired derivative (XXV).

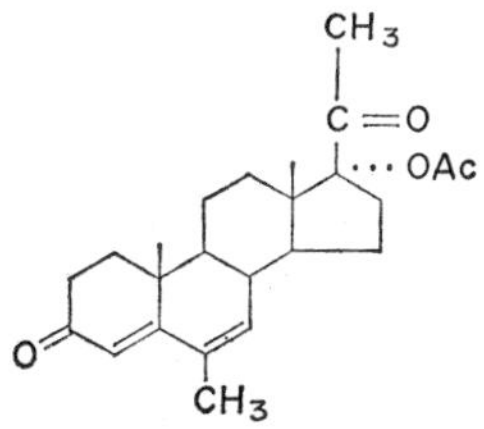

XXIV
Megestrol acetate

FIG. 7.

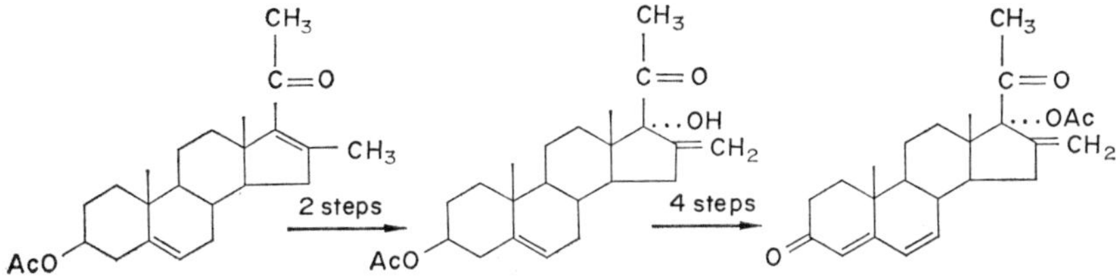

XXVI → (2 steps) XXVII → (4 steps) XXV
Superlutin

FIG. 8.

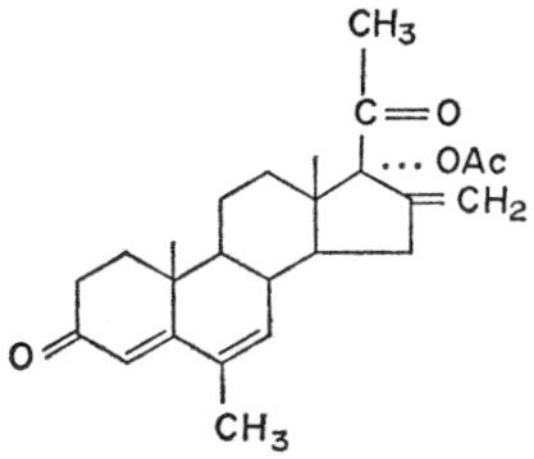

XXVIII
Melengestrol acetate

FIG. 9.

Melengestrol acetate—6-methyl-16-methylene-17α-acetoxy-4,6-pregna-diene-3,20 dione (XXVIII, Fig. 9)—was prepared in an analogous manner except that as the starting material the 6-methyl derivative of (XXVI) was used (Mannhardt et al., 1960; Kirk et al., 1961).

3. GONANES

Synthesis of a novel class of 19-nor steroids was reported in 1963 by Smith and co-workers. The total synthesis used permitted preparation of a wide variety of derivatives, of which the 13-ethyl compounds were of greatest biological interest. The key intermediate in the synthesis (Fig. 10) 3-methoxy-13β-ethyl-1,3,5(10)-gonatriene-17-one (XXIX) was obtained by Michael condensation of 6-*m*-methoxy phenyl-1-hexen-3-one (XXX) with 2-ethylcyclopentane-1,3-dione (XXXI). In the resulting adduct, which under acidic conditions undergoes double cyclohydration, the Δ^{16} double bond was selectively hydrogenated (palladium catalyst on calcium carbonate in benzene), the double bond at C-8 isomerized to C-9(11) and

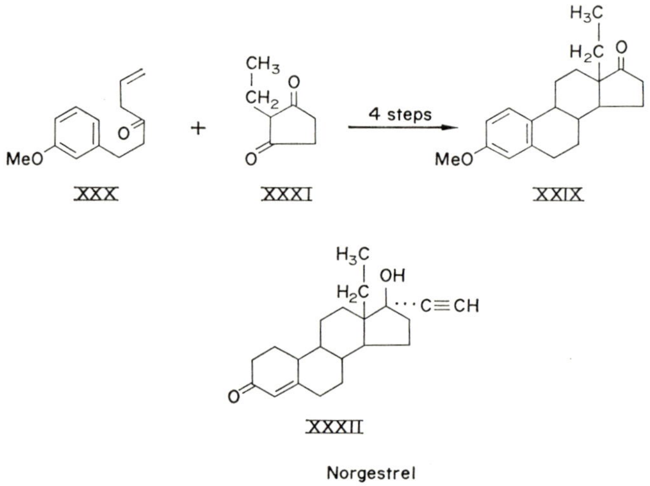

FIG. 10.

catalytically hydrogenated (Pd on carbon in ethanol) to (XXIX). Birch-type reduction, followed by Oppenauer oxidation, reaction of the 17-ketone with lithium acetylide and hydrolysis with ethanolic hydrochloric acid gave (dl)-13β-ethyl-17α-ethynyl-17β-hydroxy-4-gonen-3-one (norgestrel (XXXII)). This compound differs from norethindrone (I) by the presence of an ethyl group, instead of a methyl group, at C-13.

4. 9β,10α-STEROIDS

In the preparation of vitamin-D from plant sterols (ergosterol), irradiation with ultraviolet light of wavelength above 280 mµ gives a mixture rich

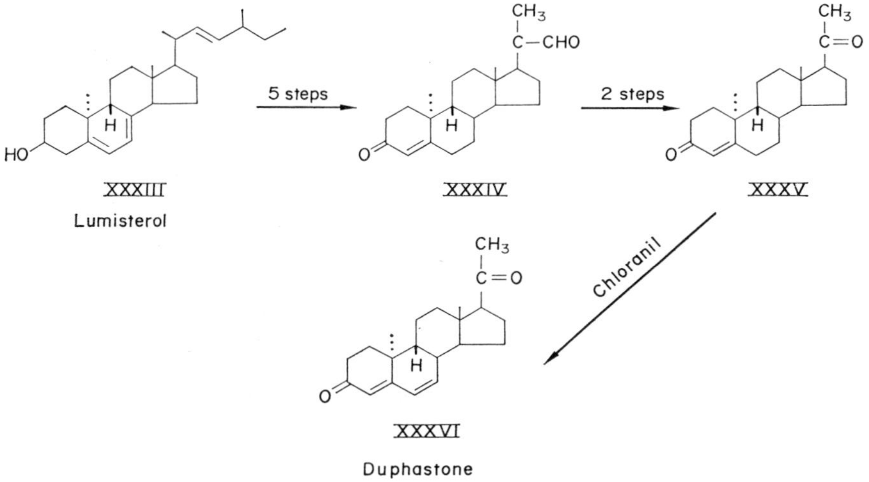

FIG. 11.

in 9β,10α-isomer, lumisterol (XXXIII), which has been used as a starting material for the synthesis of Duphastone® ("6-dehydro-retroprogesterone", 9β,10α-4,6-pregnadiene-3,20-dione (XXXVI)). As the name implies, the C-10 angular methyl group, and the hydrogen at C-9, are isomeric to the normal 9α,10β-configuration of the natural steroids. Figure 11 shows the reaction sequence (Westerhof and Reerink, 1960). Lumisterol was converted in five steps ((i) Oppenauer oxidation, (ii) isomerization with dry hydrochloric acid in isopropanol, (iii) catalytic hydrogenation, (iv) ozonolysis and (v) reductive decomposition with zinc dust in glacial acetic acid) to the aldehyde (XXXIV). Enamine formation with piperidine in benzene–acetic acid mixture gave "retroprogesterone" (9β,10α-4-pregnene-3,20-dione, XXXV) which upon treatment with chloranil (tetrachloro-p-benzoquinone) in boiling butanol gave (XXXVI).

REFERENCES

BABCOCK, J. C., GUTSELL, E. S., HERR, M. E., HOGG, J. A., STUCKI, J. C., BARNES, L. E. and DULIN, W. E. (1958) 6α-Methyl-17α-hydroxy-progesterone 17-acylates; a new class of potent progestins. *J. Amer. Chem. Soc.* **80**: 2904–2905.

BIRCH, A. J. and SMITH, H. (1951) Hydroaromatic steroid hormones, II. Some hydroxychrysene derivatives. *J. Chem. Soc.* 1882–1888.

COLTON, F. B. (1953) Estradienes. U.S. Patent No. 2,655,518 (*Chem. Abst.* **48**: 11503d).

COLTON, F. B. (1954) Estradienes. U.S. Patent No. 2,691,028 (*Chem. Abst.* **49**: 11729h).

COLTON, F. B. (1958) 17-Alkenyl and alkynyl-4-estrene-3 17-dioles. U.S. Patent 2,843,609 (*Chem. Abst.* **53**: 1415c).
COLTON, F. B. (1960) 17α-Alkynyl-17β-acetoxy-4,6-estradien-3-ones. U.S. Patent 2,946,809 (*Chem. Abst.* **54**: 27732c).
COLTON, F. B. and KLIMSTRA, P. D. (1965) Contraceptive drugs. In: *Encyclopedia of Chemical Technology*, Vol. 8, pp. 60–92. Kirk, R. E. and Othmer, D. F. (Eds.). J. Wiley & Sons, New York, N.Y.
DAVID, A., HARTLEY, F., MILLSON, D. R. and PETROV, V. (1957) The preparation and progestational activity of some alkylated ethisterones. *J. Pharm. Pharmac.* **9**: 929–934.
DE WINTER, M. S., SIEGMANN, C. M. and SZPILFOGEL, S. A. (1959) 17-Alkylated 3-deoxo-19-nortestosterone. *Chem. Ind.* (*London*), p. 905.
DJERASSI, C., MIRAMONTES, L. and ROSENKRANZ, G. (1952) Amer. Chem. Soc. Meeting, April 1952. *Div. Med. Chem. Abst.*, p. 18j.
DJERASSI, D., MIRAMONTES, L., ROSENKRANZ, G. and SONDHEIMER, F. (1954) Steroids LIV. Synthesis of 19-nor-17α-ethynyl-testosterone and 19-nor-17α-methyltestosterone. *J. Amer. Chem. Soc.* **76**: 4092–4094.
DJERASSI, C. (1966) Steroid oral contraceptives. *Science* **151**: 1055–1061.
ELLIS, B., KIRK, D. N., PETROV, V., WATERHOUSE, B. and WILLIAMSON, D. M. (1960). Modified steroid hormones, Part XVII. Some 6-methyl-4,6-diene-3-ones. *J. Chem. Soc.* 2828–2833.
ENGELFRIED, O., KASPARE, E., POPPER, A. and SCHENK, M. (1957) 17α-Alkyl-19-nortestosterone acylates. Ger. Patent 1,017,166 (*Chem. Abst.* **53**: 22096e).
ERCOLI, A. and GARDI, P. (1964) 17α-Ethynyl-19-norandostanes. U.S. Patent No. 3,159,620 (*Chem. Abst.* **62**: 6539b).
IRIARTE, J., DJERASSI, C. and RINGOLD, H. J. (1959) Steroids CVII. $\Delta^{5(6)}$-19-norsteroids, a new class of potent anabolic agents. *J. Amer. Chem. Soc.* **81**: 436–438.
KIRK, D. N., PETROV, V. and WILLIAMSON, D. M. (1961) Modified steroid hormones, Part XXII. 6α,16α-Dimethylprogesterone and 17α-acetoxy-6α-methyl-16-methylene progesterone. *J. Chem. Soc.* 2821–2828.
MANNHARDT, H. J., WERDER, F. V., BORK, K. H., METZ, H. and BRUCKNER, K. (1960) Preparation of 16-methylene steroids of the corticoid and progesterone series. *Tetrahedron Letters* **16**: 21–32.
RINGOLD, H. J., ROSENKRANZ, G. and SONDHEIMER, F. (1956) Steroids LXXX. 1-methyl-19-nortestosterone and 1-methyl-17α-ethinyl-19-nortestosterone. *J. Amer. Chem. Soc.* **78**: 2477–2479.
RINGOLD, H. J., PEREZ RUELAS, J., BATRES, E. and DJERASSI, C. (1959). Steroids CXVIII. 6-Methyl derivatives of 17α-hydroxyprogesterone and of Reichstein's substance "S". *J. Amer. Chem. Soc.* **81**: 3712–3716.
SMITH, H., HUGHES, G. A., DOUGLAS, G. J., HARTLEY, D., MCLOUGHLIN, B. J., SIDDALL, J. B., WENDT, G. R., BUZBY, JR., G. C., HERBST, D. R., LEDIG, K. W., MCMENAMIN, J. R., PATTISON, T. W., SUIDA, J., TOKOLICS, J., EDGREN, R. A., JANSEN, A. B. A., GADSBY, B., WATSON, D. H. R. and PHILLIPS, P. C. (1963) Totally synthetic ($\pm$)-13-alkyl-3-hydroxy and methoxygona-1,3,5(10)-trien-17-ones and related compounds. *Experientia* **19**: 394–396.
SONDHEIMER, F. and KLIBANSKY, Y. (1959) Synthesis of 3β-hydroxy analogues of steroidal hormones, a biologically active class of compounds. *Tetrahedron* **5**: 15–26.
SYHORA, K. (1960) Novel type of ring opening of steroidal 16α-17α-epoxides. *Tetrahedron Letters* **17**: 34–38.
WESTERHOF, P. and REERINK, E. H. (1960) Investigation on sterols. XV. The synthesis and properties of 9β,10α-progesterone and 6-dehydro-9β,10α-progesterone. *Rec. Trav. Chim.* **79**: 771–783.
ZDERIC, J. A. (1963) Progestational hormones. In: *Comprehensive Biochemistry* **10**: 166–196. Florkin, M. and Stotz, E. H. (Eds.). Elsevier, Amsterdam.

CHAPTER 28

PHARMACOLOGY OF ORALLY ACTIVE PROGESTATIONAL COMPOUNDS: ANIMAL STUDIES

M. Tausk
Utrecht, The Netherlands
and
J. de Visser
Oss, The Netherlands

CONTENTS

1.	Introduction	36
2.	Effects on the rabbit endometrium	37
3.	The potency of progestational steroids to influence the formation of deciduomas in rodents	48
4.	Induction and delay of nidation	54
5.	The inhibition of ovulation	58
6.	Evidence for inhibition of gonadotrophin secretion by the pituitary	77
7.	Facilitation of ovulation	84
8.	Activation of corpora lutea and induction of pseudopregnancy	87
9.	Other effects on the central nervous system	88
10.	Maintenance of pregnancy	92
11.	Prevention of oxytocin-induced parturition	98
12.	Influence on contractility of the non-pregnant uterus	100
13.	Estrogenic, metrotrophic and antiestrogenic activity	102
14.	Androgenic, myotrophic ("anabolic") and antiandrogenic activities	112
15.	Masculinization of female fetuses	121
16.	"Antifertility action"	132
17.	Interference with established pregnancy	151
18.	Effects of progestational substances on the Fallopian tubes	153
19.	Effects on the mammary gland	158
20.	Effects on the adrenal cortex	160
21.	Various metabolic activities of progestational compounds	168
22.	Effects on liver functions	175
23.	Various biochemical, histochemical and related effects of progestational compounds	175
24.	Effects of progestational compounds on the growth of tumors	182
25.	Miscellaneous observations	187
26.	Concluding remarks	192
	Appendix	193
	References	194

1. INTRODUCTION

The term "orally active progestational compounds" comprises steroids which have at least one effect in common with progesterone: the characteristic progestational transformation ("dentelle") of the rabbit endometrium (see Chapter 2). Unlike progesterone, which is practically inactive on oral administration, they have this effect also when administered by gavage or orally.

A surprising number of such compounds have been synthesized and it would appear that the structural requirements for this effect are not very specific in terms of present-day chemical language. Of course these compounds may have some very specific physical or chemical properties in common that cannot be deduced from their conventional formulas.

In approaching the pharmacology of these substances we have to bear in mind that they have been selected as "hormono-mimetics". It is, therefore, rational to ascertain primarily whether or to what extent they do in fact imitate the effects of progesterone. It is obvious that this should be done in the case of compounds intended for the treatment of proven or assumed progesterone deficiency in women, but it also applies to other uses, particularly oral contraception. This use of drugs is, of course, also one of the results of physiological (endocrine) research, which, as discussed in Chapter 16, has revealed a characteristic pattern in the activities of progesterone. To the extent that progesterone has pre-ovulatory functions, these appear to be synergistic with estrogens and to facilitate conception. After ovulation (the physiological time of fertilization) progesterone assures the development of the ovum, thereby preventing more ova from being released and spermatozoa from reaching them. The contraceptive use of progestational drugs could then be viewed as an extension of the antifertility effects of luteal phase progesterone to the first, normally estrogen-dominated, part of the cycle. Any compound designed for this application should, of course, be tested for its resemblance to progesterone in more than one respect.

In this chapter we focus our attention mainly on the kind of effects that have been ascribed to progesterone. But some of the structures we are dealing with appear to be at least as much related to those of certain estrogens or androgens; animal studies were, therefore, needed to define more precisely the hormone-like activities of such substances. Moreover, some of the progestational drugs would intentionally or sometimes inadvertently be given during pregnancy and their effects on the fetus should be studied.

An effort has been made to present essential data. We have not aimed at a complete survey of the literature, limiting the discussion mainly to progestational compounds used as such in drugs at present commercially available.

We have, therefore, not fully discussed compounds such as norethandrolone or cyproterone acetate, that have a certain progestational activity but which is not the one determining the purpose of their use. The steroids discussed in this chapter are listed in Table 1. The nomenclature used follows mainly the recommendations of WHO. Where no official "Recommended International Non-proprietary Name", (R), is available "Proposed International Non-proprietary Names", (P), are used. Where "USA Established Names" differ from WHO names, they are listed and marked US.

2. EFFECTS ON THE RABBIT ENDOMETRIUM

2.1. THE CLAUBERG TEST

Many authors have undertaken a quantitative comparison of progestational steroids by the Clauberg test (see Chapter 18). The discrepancies found in different laboratories and sometimes in the same place at different times are, at first glance, considerable. They are, of course, due to a number of variables in technique and to some subjective factor in scoring the degree of endometrial glandular changes. A further difficulty is introduced by the reasonable desire to assess the oral activity of synthetic compounds. Since progesterone, the reference standard provided by nature, is practically inactive by this route, activities, even oral ones, are often expressed as percentages of the activity of progesterone given by injection. In view of this situation only *big* differences between activities of different substances should be taken seriously, particularly if found in more than one laboratory. On this basis a ranking of compounds has been attempted as shown in Tables 2 and 3, where they are listed in order of decreasing p.o. activity. As our discussion proceeds it will become clear that the practical usefulness of a compound hardly depends on its activity in the Clauberg test, and the same applies to the recommended clinical dosage.

Table 2 gives data on derivatives of progesterone, all characterized by a very high potency on injection and fair oral activity, which in some cases is stated to amount to some 20–60% of the subcutaneous potency. In discussing structure–activity relationships, Čekan *et al.* (1964) emphasized the potentiating effect on progestational potency, p.o., of 6,7-dehydrogenation, sixfold in the case of 17α-acetoxyprogesterone (even fifteenfold

TABLE 2. ACTIVITIES OF DERIVATIVES OF PROGESTERONE IN THE CLAUBERG TEST

"Doses" and "activities" are usually those which produce endometrial changes graded as 2 or more on McPhail's scale (see Chapter 18)

Compound	Total oral dose (mg)	Oral activity as % of compound's subcut. act. (=100)	Oral activity as % of activity of		Subcut. activity as % of progesterone subcut. (=100)	Reference
			progesterone subcut. (=100)	progesterone oral (=100)		
Megestrol acetate	0.02		5000–10,000			David et al. (1963)
	0.04–0.08	66				Kincl (1961)
			1700		2500	Elton et al. (1960)
			1600		2500	Edgren et al. (1967a)
				33,000	7500	Junkmann (1964)
					7000	McKinney and Braselton (1970)
Medrogestone	0.025		100		400	Revesz and Chappel (1966)
	0.100					Carraro et al. (1967)
Chlormadinone acetate	0.04		5000–10,000			Kincl (1961)
	0.05		2500–5000		7500	Hecht-Lucari et al. (1966)
	0.02	20–30		33,000	10,000–25,000	Čekan (1964)
			700–1200			Junkmann (1963, 1964)
						Brennan and Kraay (1963)
					1500	Edgren et al. (1967a)
						Kincl and Dorfman (1963a)

Compound				References
Medroxy-progesterone acetate	0.025–0.05			Revesz and Chappel (1966)
	0.2–0.4			David et al. (1963)
	0.05			Čekan et al. (1964)
	0.10–0.20	20	1000–2000	Duncan et al. (1964)
			1000	Brennan and Kraay (1963)
	0.3–0.6			Kincl (1961)
			500	Elton et al. (1960)
		20–30	700–1200	Edgren et al. (1967a)
		20	(1)	Miyake and Pincus (1958)
				Desaulles and Krähenbühl (1962)
				Drill (1959)
				Junkmann (1963)
Anagestone acetate	0.1	ca. 10		Barnes et al. (1959)
	0.05[3]			Blye et al. (1965a)
				Junkmann (1963)
Melengestrol acetate	0.025	20–40		Duncan et al. (1964)
				McKinney and Braselton (1970)
Superlutin	0.02–0.05		1000–2500	Čekan et al. (1964)

Notes to Table 2
(1) Oral activity is 50 to 60 times that of ethisterone.
(2) This figure is deduced from the statement that medroxyprogesterone acetate has 6 to 8 times the activity of acetoxyprogesterone, which is 4 to 6 times as active as progesterone.
(3) "An unusual feature of this compound is its ability even in small doses to induce progestational proliferation in the uterus of non-estrogen-primed immature rabbits". Blye et al. (1965a). No documentation.

TABLE 3. ACTIVITY OF VARIOUS PROGESTATIONAL COMPOUNDS IN THE CLAUBERG TEST

"Doses" and "activities" are usually those which produce endometrial changes graded as 2 or more on McPhail's scale (see Chapter 18)

Compound	Total oral dose in mg	Oral activity as % of compound's subcut. act. (= 100)	Oral activity		Subcut. activity as % of progesterone subcut. (= 100)	Reference
			progesterone subcut. = 100	progesterone oral = 100		
Norgestrel	0.110[4]	40			915[4]	Edgren et al. (1966a)
		33	305			Edgren et al. (1967a)
Norethisterone acetate	0.03[1]	100		33,000	2500	Neumann et al. (1964)
				33,000	2500	Junkmann (1963, 1964)
Norethisterone	0.1[1]	60			1200	Neumann et al. (1964)
					1200	Junkmann (1963, 1964)
		10–30			8	Edgren et al. (1967a)
	0.1		200			McGinty and Djerassi (1958)
	0.25	200	100		50	Overbeek et al. (1962)
					100[2]	Drill (1959)
	0.3	550; 140[3]			10;20[3]	Pincus et al. (1956)
						Miyake and Pincus (1958)
						Hertz et al. (1954)
			10		8.5[4]	Kincl (1961)
	0.625–1.25		100[6]	50,000		Edgren et al. (1966a)
	> 5.0[5]					Blye et al. (1965)
						Rudel and Kincl (1966)
					100[13]	Desaulles and Krähenbühl (1964)

Orally Active Progestational Compounds: Animal Studies

Compound					Reference
Normethandrone				100	Overbeek and de Visser (1956)
				100–200	Desaulles and Krähenbühl (1962)
				500	Drill (1959)
				1250	Junkmann (1963)
					Miyake and Pincus (1958)
					Moggian (1959)
					Elton and Nutting (1961)
Ethynodiol acetate	$0.1^{(10)}$ or less	960; $290^{(3)}$	100		Drill (1963)
			100		Junkmann (1964)
			10; $10^{(3)}$	$<100^{(8)}$	Madjerek et al. (1960)
				100–$200^{(10)}$	Kobayashi et al. (1962)
Allylestrenol	0.5			100–200	Desaulles and Krähenbühl (1962)
	3.2			750	Junkmann (1963)
			100	$4000^{(7)}$	Overbeek et al. (1962)
Lynestrenol	0.5			10,000	Rudel and Kincl (1966)
				8	Junkmann (1963, 1964)
			100	75	Kincl and Folch-Pi (1962)
			150		Desaulles and Krähenbühl (1964)
Norgesterone	4	<20	<10	100,000	Ruggieri et al. (1965)
				3000	Drill and Riegel (1958)
				250	Drill and Riegel (1958)
Norvinisterone	0.625	50	250		Schöler (1960)
Dydrogesterone		1.2	40		Junkmann (1963)
				$100^{(13)}$	Kobayashi (1963)
	0.5–1		150	50	Ruiz-Gijon (1962)
	0.9		70	25	Claassen (1968)
Norgestrienone	2.0	28		500	Roussel (1966)
Quingestanol	$2.0^{(14)}$			3400	Giannina et al. (1969)
acetate	2.0/kg/ $day^{(15)}$			250	Mischler et al. (1969)
				3200	Eben-Moussi and Van den Driessche (1970)
				>140	
				120	
				25–50	

TABLE 3.—cont.

Compound	Total oral dose in mg	Oral activity as % of compound's subcut. act. (=100)	Oral activity		Subcut. activity as % of progesterone subcut. (=100)	Reference
			progesterone subcut. =100	progesterone oral =100		
Ethisterone	4.0		12.5			Overbeek et al. (1962)
	1.0					Hertz et al. (1954)
	10.0					Suchowsky and Baldratti (1964)
	10.0	10		100	80	Neumann et al. (1964)
					75	Junkmann (1964)
	3–4					McGinty and Djerassi (1958)
	40.0[11]					David et al. (1963)
Dimethisterone	4.0[11]		200			David et al. (1963)
					250	Junkmann (1963)
					160	McKinney and Braselton (1970)
					100	Pincus et al. (1956)
Norethynodrel	1.0	1–2			<1	Saunders et al. (1957)
	2.5–5	See text		1000–2500	25	Drill and Saunders (1957)
					80	Saunders (1958)
					75	Junkmann (1964)
				1000	?(12)	Junkmann (1963)
					Too low to estimate	Watnick et al. (1965)
						Edgren et al. (1966a)
	1.0	540		12,500		Miyake and Pincus (1958)
					0–25	Rudel and Kincl (1966)
						Drill (1959)

Notes to Table 3

(1) "A transformatory change of the endometrium" is produced. McPhail's score not stated.
(2) With reference to this figure Miyake and Pincus state that "previous data ... were estimated on the basis of minimum effective dose".
(3) The first figure refers to carbonic anhydrase activity, the second to the g/m ratio. See chapter on bioassays.
(4) Compared with McPhail 1.8.
(5) The authors state that with norethisterone given orally no degree of "uterine arborization" higher than 1.1 McPhail can be reached.
(6) This figure refers to a mixture of 10 mg norethisterone with 10 mcg ethynyl estradiol-methyl ether (MEE); *the estrogen increases the progestational activity of norethisterone!*
(7) Oral activity 350 to 400% of ethisterone (= 100).
(8) Potency for low doses equal to that of progesterone; higher doses give much less glandular development than corresponding doses of progesterone.
(9) Oral activity 1600% of ethisterone (= 100).
(10) "Maximal arborization following subcutaneous administration was obtained at a dose of 0.1 mg per day. However as the dose was increased above this level the response of the glandular epithelium in the uterus was reversed and was absent at the 2 and 4 mg dose levels. No such reversal was obtained with progesterone at high dose levels ... when EED was administered buccally no depression of the epithelial response was observed. This suggests differences in absorption and/or metabolism of EED by the 2 routes". (EED stands for ethynyl estrenediol diacetate).
(11) The authors gave a daily dose of 10 mg/kg of ethisterone or of 1 mg of dimethisterone for 4 days to animals weighing 640–1220 g. McPhail score for ethisterone 3.0, for dimethisterone 2.5.
(12) Found inactive at total subcutaneous dose of 12.5 mg. Equally potent as progesterone when given intravenously. Highest mean McPhail 2.1 (highest total intravenous dose 3.0 mg).
(13) Tested in castrated, estrogen-primed adult rabbits at McPhail 3–4.
(14) Clauberg test as modified by McPhail with continuation of estrogen treatment (one-tenth of priming dose) during progestational treatment; McPhail score 3.37.
(15) Animals weighing 800–1000 g.

according to Kincl and Dorfman, 1963b). A further tenfold increase is produced by the introduction of a 16-methylene group.

Table 3 presents a much less homogeneous picture. It comprises a variety of compounds, derived from C_{18} and C_{19} molecules by various substitutions, and includes one substance, dydrogesterone, derived from a progesterone isomer, retroprogesterone. Subcutaneous and oral activities vary within a wide range and show great discrepancies for the same compound.

The group includes norethynodrel, which was singled out by Pincus (1956) for his first human fertility-control studies as a compound related to progesterone and "ten times as active". The basis of comparison was the potency to inhibit ovulation. In the classical endometrium test the compound turned out to be relatively weakly active (but also as an ovulation inhibitor in the rabbit it is now ranking low). Its activity is even much lower on subcutaneous than on oral administration. Thus Drill and Saunders (1957) state that the progestational response following oral administration of norethynodrel in the Clauberg test cannot be distinguished from that of (an approximately equal or lower dose of) progesterone. But "only borderline effects are obtained when the compound is injected subcutaneously". Whether this difference is due to the metabolism of the compound in the body is not known, although we may suspect that that is the case. The histological changes produced by this compound—and by its near relative norethisterone—appear to differ qualitatively from those which progesterone brings about. Thus Elton (1962) found these two compounds to produce *tall* columnar epithelial cells in the rabbit endometrium in contrast with progesterone and all other synthetic progestational substances tested, which all gave *low* columnar cells. Norethynodrel, in a parenteral dose of 2 mg daily, would not produce a degree of arborization higher than 2 (4 being the maximum, attained by the other substances). The behavior of norethynodrel in these studies resembled that of testosterone propionate, which has been known for decades to have weak progestational properties. (For references see Neumann (1968), p. 907.)

Neumann (personal communication)* has pointed out that in his experience the priming dose of estrogen is of decisive influence on the progestational response, particularly in the case of norethynodrel but also, though less conspicuously, in that of norethisterone and its acetate. He found norethynodrel practically inactive after the conventional priming dose of 5 mcg of estradiol, but fully active when only 0.1 mcg of estradiol was used instead. This means that a valid comparison of progestational activities of

* We are grateful to Dr. Neumann for reading this manuscript and for a number of valuable comments.

such compounds (viz. estrane derivatives with inherent estrogenic activity, see subsection 13.2) would really require testing with different levels of the estrogen-priming dose. On the other hand, in the case of compounds which have no "built-in" estrogenic activity, the progestational reaction may be unduly weak when the estrogen-priming dose was too low.

Jones *et al.* (1966) devised a modification of the Clauberg test, whereby steroids are dissolved in DMSO (dimethylsulfoxide) and injected intravenously. The authors compared progesterone with seven other progestational compounds and found "fair correlation between potencies" by the intravenous and the subcutaneous routes, "since rankings of the materials are essentially similar". However, when given intravenously ethynodiol acetate was far less active, which "makes it the most marked exception". It is also exceptional ("a unique steroidal progestin") because it was found to reverse its own progestational effect when given in higher doses subcutaneously, not buccally (Elton and Nutting, 1961).

The *duration* of the effects produced by several synthetic progestational compounds was compared with those of progesterone by Sulman *et al.* (1959). This group set out to analyze a puzzling phenomenon described by the present reviewer's group (de Fremery *et al.*) in 1932. We found that notwithstanding continued injections of corpus luteum extracts the progestational state of the rabbit endometrium could not be maintained beyond 17 days. Sulman *et al.* made the surprising discovery that the progestational characteristics do in fact disappear, as the endometrium breaks down after about 17 days, but reappear when treatment is continued. Such cycles can be indefinitely maintained. This applied to progesterone as well as to 17α-hydroxyprogesterone caproate, norethisterone and methallyl nortestosterone in daily doses of 0.5 mg. Revesz and Chappel (1966) found that one single subcutaneous dose in the rabbit of 10 mg of medrogestone had a progestational effect that lasted for 17 days and in this respect equalled that of 17-hydroxyprogesterone caproate. For duration of action of megestrol acetate in a silastic tube see subsection 25.6, p. 191.

2.2. THE ALLEN–CORNER TEST

Some compounds were also tested in the Allen–Corner test in spayed adult rabbits as shown in Table 4.

2.3. LOCAL EFFECTS OF STEROIDS (MCGINTY TEST)

It is of great pharmacological interest that many substances which, when given systemically, will modify the rabbit endometrium essentially in the same way as progesterone, do *not* do so when applied to the endometrium directly. Substances which are active topically, as demonstrated by the McGinty test, are listed in Table 5. With respect to the high activity of medroxyprogesterone acetate, Salhanick and Swanson (1960) pointed out that it is more potent in the "local assay in the rabbit" than the substances having only one of the two substituents (at either C 6 or C 17).

TABLE 4. ENDOMETRIAL ACTIVITY FOUND IN ALLEN–CORNER TEST (SPAYED ADULT RABBITS)

Compound	Total oral dose (mg) producing McPhail 2	Subcut. activity as percentage of progesterone judged by McPhail 3–4	Reference
Allylestrenol	10.0		Madjerek et al. (1960)
Dydrogesterone	10.0[1]		Marois (1962a)
Lynestrenol	2.5		Overbeek et al. (1962)
		100	Desaulles and Krähenbühl (1964)
Norethisterone		100	Desaulles and Krähenbühl (1964)
		100[2]	Allen and Wu (1959)
Norethynodrel		12.5	Desaulles and Krähenbühl (1964)

(1) Five days treatment, 2 mg once daily, effect described as "positive endometrial reaction." McPhail score not stated.
(2) Progesterone in daily doses of 0.25 and 0.5 mg caused degrees of proliferation of McPhail 3 and 4 respectively, norethisterone of 2 and 3. However, no dose of norethisterone ever attained full arborization (4).

Table 6 lists a number of compounds, that were tested but found inactive. Drill (1959) pointed out "that only compounds active in the McGinty test maintain pregnancy in rats and rabbits", basing this statement on observations by Saunders and Drill (1958) and Saunders and Elton (1959). In the discussion following the presentation of Drill's paper McGinty (1959) disagreed with the statement just quoted. We revert to this point later, in discussing maintenance of pregnancy. The cyclopentyl-enol ether of 17α-acetoxyprogesterone, according to Falconi et al. (1961), appears to be an exception to this rule, since it is reported to maintain pregnancy in spayed rabbits and to be inactive in the intra-uterine assay. Saunders et al. (1957) have suggested that the lack of activity of norethynodrel in this assay may be due to the intrinsic estrogenicity of this compound (see Table 24), since

TABLE 5. ACTIVITY IN MCGINTY TEST (INTRA-UTERINE ADMINISTRATION) EXPRESSED AS PERCENTAGE OF ACTIVITY OF PROGESTERONE

Compound	Activity (progesterone =100)	Active dose	Reference
Chlormadinone acetate	12,000		Brennan and Kraay (1963)
Medroxyprogesterone acetate	2500		Drill et al. (1949)
	2500		Elton et al. (1960)
	2500	0.02 mcg ED_{50}	Junkmann (1963)
	600		Brennan and Kraay (1963)
		10 mcg active	Revesz and Chappel (1960)
		30 mcg	Sala et al. (1960)
Megestrol acetate	1000		Elton et al. (1960)
Medrogestone		10 mcg active	Revesz and Chappel (1960)
Allylestrenol	50		Desaulles and Krähenbühl (1962)
Norgestrel		1.0 mcg[1]	Edgren et al. (1963, 1967a)
Ethisterone	1		Desaulles and Krähenbühl (1962)
	15	3.0 mcg ED_{50}	Junkmann (1963)
	0		Drill (1959)
Dydrogesterone		100 mcg[2]	Marois (1962a)

(1) In their 1963 paper the authors say that 1 mcg produced a McPhail score of 1.0 (generally not yet accepted as fully active) whereas 3 mcg scored only 0.7. In their 1967 paper the authors simply classify norgestrel as "active" in this test without giving quantitative data.
(2) Only dose tested. Illustration shows very strong effect.

"in the intra-uterine assay the addition of 1 mcg or more of estrone to 5 mcg of progesterone will completely block the endometrial gland response to progesterone". (See also subsection 10, p. 96.)

The only compound in Table 5 showing noteworthy activity, which is not a pregnane derivative, is allylestrenol (a pregnancy-maintaining substance). It may be of interest that the corresponding 3-oxo-compound (17α-allyl-19-nortestosterone) has been reported to have the same activity (Drill and Riegel, 1958). A butenyl or methallyl side chain appears to increase topical intra-uterine activity by a factor of 20, that is to 10 times that of progesterone (Saunders, 1958; Saunders and Drill, 1958).

TABLE 6. COMPOUNDS TESTED AND FOUND INACTIVE IN McGINTY TEST

Compound	Highest dose found inactive	Activity in percentage of progesterone	Reference
Ethisterone	see Table 5		
Ethynodiol acetate	100 mcg		Elton and Nutting (1961)
Norethisterone		< 1	Saunders and Drill (1958)
		< 1	Desaulles and Krähenbühl (1962)
	10.0 mcg		Edgren et al. (1963a)
	0.5 mcg		Junkmann (1963)
		inactive	Chappel et al. (1960)
		< 0.5	Drill and Riegel (1958)
Norethisterone acetate	0.5 mcg		Junkmann (1963)
Norethynodrel	100 mg		Ruggieri et al. (1965)
	100 mcg	< 1	Drill and Saunders (1957)
Normethandrone		< 1	Desaulles and Krähenbühl (1962)
		0	Drill (1959)
	0.5 mcg		Junkmann (1963)
Norgesterone	100 mg		Ruggieri et al. (1965)
		< 0.5	Drill and Riegel (1958)
Norvinisterone		< 0.5	Drill and Riegel (1958)

3. THE POTENCY OF PROGESTATIONAL STEROIDS TO INFLUENCE THE FORMATION OF DECIDUOMAS IN RODENTS

3.1. INDUCTION OF DECIDUOMA-FORMATION

Since progesterone is needed to render nidation and the formation of traumatic deciduomas possible (see Chapter 6) it was of great interest to find out whether certain synthetic progestational compounds share this potency. Compounds found active in rats or mice are listed in Table 7, inactive ones in Table 8. It will be noted that compounds active in this test are also active in the McGinty test, with the exception of normethandrone which was found highly deciduomagenic by Pincus et al. in rats, but practically inactive by Madjerek in mice. Krause (1966) studied deciduoma formation in rats, castrated on the fourth day after strong electrical stimulation of the cervix at estrus. At the time of spaying the right uterine horn was traumatized, whereupon the test substance was administered orally. This treatment was continued over the four succeeding days. Dydrogesterone was found very weakly active in this test at a daily dose of 2 mg, in no way comparable with its "Clauberg activity". Chlormadinone acetate was distinctly more active but its "retro" isomer (9β, 10α), which has the same configurational characteristics as dydrogesterone, was very much *more* active. This same increase of deciduomagenic activity through "retro-isomerization" was also found with a few other steroids, e.g. 17α-methyl progesterone.*

A somewhat different approach was studied by Elton *et al.* (1966) in rabbits without uterine trauma. This group had found that in immature female rabbits decidual cell formation could be produced with combinations of estrone and progesterone, but not with progesterone alone. Ethynodiol diacetate (ED) injected daily in doses of 0.5 mg for 6 days produced a decidual cell response (DCR) in the majority of animals, if 0.05 to 0.3 mg of mestranol (ethynyl estradiol 3-methylether) was given simultaneously. Without added estrogen much higher doses of ED were needed and the percentage of responding animals was smaller. The authors attribute these interesting results to the fact that ED has both progestational and estrogenic properties (as is discussed below, in subsection 13.2). The latter are less pronounced in lower dosages and are therefore amenable to reinforcement by added estrogen. ED alone was able to maintain DCR when given daily for more prolonged periods (15 days) without added estrogen.

Shipley (1965) used deciduoma formation to test compounds for their activity when applied percutaneously in rats. Medroxyprogesterone acetate was the most effective of the compounds in this test; chlormadinone was far less active, "which reflects the lower activity of this compound *in rats* via all routes of administration, and correlates with its subcutaneous activity in rats, in contrast to its marked potency in rabbits".

Interesting information was obtained from studies in the golden hamster. Czyba (1963) found this species particularly sensitive to the "progestomimetic action" of certain steroids. He could show that a combination of testosterone propionate and estradiol benzoate would produce deciduomata in the traumatized uterus of the hamster. Together with Chiris (Czyba and Chiris, 1963) he described such a response to norethandrolone and to desoxycorticosterone, both with or without estradiol benzoate. (That testosterone has weak progestational properties has been mentioned above (subsection 2.1). See Neumann (1968), p. 907.) Deckers and Van

---

* Only a very short abstract appeared in the Proceedings of the congress at which this communication was presented. We are grateful to the author for permitting us to quote results from his manuscript; see also *Exc. Med. ICS* **219,** 872 (1971).

TABLE 7. DECIDUOMAGENIC POTENCY OF STEROIDS FOUND ACTIVE, WHEN GIVEN ORALLY OR SUBCUTANEOUSLY TO MICE OR RATS, AT DOSES INDICATED

Compound	Mice daily dose in mg		Activity as percentage of progesterone subcut. (=100)	Rats daily dose in mg		Reference
	oral	subcut.		oral	subcut.	
Allylestrenol	2.5[1]					Madjerek et al. (1960)
Medroxy-progesterone acetate		2.5				Madjerek (1960)
	1.6 (inact).	0.1[2]	200–400		0.03–0.5[6] percut.	Madjerek et al. (1960) Shipley (1965) Miyake et al. (1963b)
Chlormadinone acetate			1500		2.0[4] 0.1 1.0–3.0[6] percut.	Revesz and Chappel (1966) Sala et al. (1960) Shipley (1965)
	1.6 (inact.)	0.1	200–400			Miyake et al. (1963b)
Medrogestone				3.0 2.0[5]	0.25[3]	Chambon (1965) Krause (1966)
Dydrogesterone				2.0[5] (hardly active)	1.0[4]	Revesz and Chappel (1966) Krause (1966)
Normethandrone					3.0[7]	Pincus et al. (1956)

Notes to Table 7.

(1) Dose given on 4 successive days, producing a deciduoma index of 2 or more.
(2) For technique see Miyake *et al.* (1963a). Daily dose administered to adult castrated estrogen-primed mice for 9 days. Intra-uterine irritation on 5th day of progestational treatment by silk thread or 0.1 ml of sesame oil. Activity judged by difference in weight of treated and untreated horn.
(3) Daily administration to spayed rats for 4 days following castration, active dose producing deciduoma of at least 3 mm diameter in 40% of rats (equalling the response to 0.25 mg of progesterone subcutaneously).
(4) Daily dose given to castrated estrone-primed rats for 9 days. No trauma but injection of histamine dihydrochloride into the left uterine horn and comparing weight of this with untreated horn on the 5th day of treatment: Increase with 1 mg medrogestone from 65.0 ± 5.0 to 924.0 ± 112.0 mg, with 2 mg medroxyprogesterone acetate from 90.0 ± 1.9 to 465.0 ± 70.0.
(5) Adult rats castrated on 4th day after electrical stimulation of cervix. Traumatization of right uterine horn at time of castration followed by oral treatment for 4 days.
(6) Administered in 0.1 ml ethanol solution on skin of neck, daily for 9 days of estrone priming beginning on day of castration. One uterine horn traumatized by scratching on day 5 of "progestin treatment". Activity judged by difference in weight of treated and untreated uterine horn.
(7) Rats castrated 5 days after electrical stimulation of cervix; uterine horn traumatized at time of castration. Test compound injected daily for three days. The effectiveness of normethandrone is described as "at least of the same order as progesterone".

TABLE 8. STEROIDS FOUND INACTIVE IN DECIDUOMA TEST IN MICE OR RATS IN HIGHEST DAILY DOSE (mg) INDICATED
(For techniques see notes to Table 7.)

Compound	Mice		Rats		Reference
	oral	subcut.	oral	subcut.	
Norethisterone	2.5				Madjerek et al. (1960)
	1.6	1.2			Miyake et al. (1963b)
Lynestrenol	2.5				Overbeek et al. (1960)
Ethisterone	2.5	1.2			Madjerek et al. (1960)
	1.6	(doubtful)			Miyake et al. (1963b)
Norethynodrel	1.6	0.4			Miyake et al. (1963b)
				15	Pincus et al. (1956)
Medroxypro-gesterone acetate	2.5				Madjerek et al. (1960)
Dimethisterone	2.5				Madjerek (1960)
	2.5				Madjerek et al. (1960)
Normethandrone	2.0[(1)]				Madjerek (1960)

Note to Table 8
(1) The author found a deciduomagenic index of 1.1, not 0 as with some compounds, but according to Madjerek et al. (1960) a "group-mean of the index $I = 2$ or more" is required to be rated as a "positive effect".

der Vies (1968) used the golden hamster to demonstrate a deciduomagenic activity of lynestrenol (125 mcg subcutaneously or 1250 mcg orally), far more pronounced than what they had found in mice. The explanation seems to lie in the poor sensitivity of the hamster to certain estrogens.

Czyba and Cottinet (1968) produced deciduomata in the traumatized uterus of the golden hamster by eight daily doses of 75 mcg of lynestrenol subcutaneously or 100 mcg orally. The parenterally active dose was the same as that of progesterone.

Comparable results as with lynestrenol were obtained with norethynodrel in the hamster (by subcutaneous treatment, much less so by oral treatment). The authors attribute these results to the fact that in the hamster the inherent estrogenicity of these steroids does not antagonize a progestational effect as it would in the mouse, but only reinforces it synergistically, as they had shown in experiments with progesterone and estradiol in these two species. The difference in behavior may well be connected with a histological difference observed by Czyba's group (Dubois *et al.*, 1964), who believe that in the hamster the deciduomata originate from epithelial cells, not from the stroma. (See also Chapter 6, p. 228.)

3.2. INHIBITION OF DECIDUOMAGENESIS

Some compounds which were found incapable of causing the development of deciduomas have on the contrary been shown to inhibit the deciduomagenic effect of progesterone. Miyake *et al.* (1963b) gave 0.4 mg of progesterone daily for 9 days to mice, and triggered the decidual reaction by the injection of histamine or by a silk thread in one horn. The compound to be tested for inhibitory potency was given together with progesterone, or applied locally in one single dose. The effect was judged by the reduction of the weight increase of the uterus caused by progesterone. By these procedures norethisterone and norethynodrel were found active in daily doses of 0.4 mg (systemically) and single doses of 0.2 mg (locally). A comparable inhibition was brought about by the injection of 0.4 mcg of estradiol. So here again we may be dealing with an estrogenic effect of progestational compounds. (See subsection 3.1.) Ethisterone was inactive systemically but active locally.

The antideciduomagenic activity of norethynodrel was also found by Davis (1963) who could drastically reduce the weight of the deciduomas, produced by one single subcutaneous dose of 10 mg of progesterone in spayed rats, by a dose of 10 mg of norethynodrel given orally or by injection. The latter route gave a stronger effect.

4. INDUCTION AND DELAY OF NIDATION

In the presence of an adequate concentration of estrogens, progesterone will enable a blastocyst to nidate (see Chapter 6). If there is not enough estrogen (or a relative excess of progesterone) nidation will be delayed but the blastocysts will be kept alive and will develop normally later.

The question thus arises: which synthetic progestational substances imitate these effects of progesterone, and to what extent?

4.1. INDUCTION

In *rabbits* Chambon (1965a, 1965b) found chlormadinone 15 to 30 times more active than progesterone in securing nidation of blastocysts. Subcutaneously it acted in a daily dose of 0.1 mg, as compared with 1.5 mg of progesterone. The active oral dose was 1.0 mg per day. (The animals were castrated 2 days after mating and treatment began the day before operation.)

Norethisterone was found by Allen and Wu (1959) not to induce nidation in doses up to 4 mg injected daily into rabbits, castrated 20 to 24 hours after mating, though normal blastocysts were found up to the 6th day after fertilization.

In the *hamster*, an animal which does not require estrogen for implantation (or for maintenance of pregnancy), Shipley (1965) found that a daily subcutaneous dose of 0.6 mg of progesterone, for 7 days, was needed to secure an average of 5.2 implantation sites in eleven females (castrated on "second day of pregnancy"), as compared with 10.2 in normal controls and nil in animals treated with 0.03 mg. Also active in comparable doses were norethisterone, medroxyprogesterone and chlormadinone acetate (in that order of decreasing activity) as shown in Table 9. When the substances were administered percutaneously, progesterone in much higher doses was weakly active, chlormadinone acetate and medroxyprogesterone acetate were inactive but norethisterone was distinctly active (0.6 mg, the same as the subcutaneous dose, gave an average of 4.0 implantation sites and 67% pregnancies on day 9). The impression is gained that the property of a compound to induce implantation in the hamster does not correlate with this activity in the rabbit and it is the latter that correlates with deciduomagenic activity in mice and rats. Failure of *rats* to become pregnant after proven copulation and the deposition of sperm in the vagina has been described in various papers as inhibition of nidation. Unless corroborated by histological evidence such statements cannot be accepted as reliable, since the condition could have been caused by failure of fertilization or by

TABLE 9. INDUCTION OF NIDATION IN THE OVARIECTOMIZED HAMSTER

Adapted from Shipley (1965). Duration of treatment 7 days, beginning on second day of pregnancy, sacrificed on the day after the last day of treatment.

Subcutaneous treatment	Daily dose (mg)	No. of hamsters	Implantation sites		No. of hamsters pregnant on day 9	Percentage of hamsters pregnant on day 9
			total	average per hamster		
Intact	—	11	112	10.2	11	100
Progesterone	0.03	5	0	0.0	0	0
	0.10	10	26	2.6	8	80
	0.20	16	42	2.6	12	75
	0.30	34	160	4.7	27	79
	0.60	11	57	5.2	10	91
Chlormadinone acetate	0.15	6	0	0.0	0	0
	0.30	6	0	0.0	0	0
	0.60	6	9	1.5	4	67
	1.20	6	15	2.5	3	50
Medroxyprogesterone acetate	0.10	5	0	0.0	0	0
	0.20	6	0	0.0	0	0
	0.40	6	8	1.3	1	17
	0.80	6	19	3.2	4	75
Norethisterone	0.15	6	19	3.2	5	83
	0.60	6	38	6.3	6	100

the resorption of implanted eggs. This approach is dealt with below, under the heading *Prevention of pregnancy*.

4.2. DELAY OF NIDATION AND MAINTENANCE OF VIABILITY OF BLASTOCYSTS

Delay of implantation has been described by Barnes and Meyer (1964), who injected medroxyprogesterone acetate into intact rats, beginning on the day of insemination. They found that increasing doses (from 0.5 to 2.4 mg per day) would cause steady increases in (a) the percentage of animals with delayed implantation (from 14 to 100%) and (b) the length of the delay. If no implantation had occurred by day 13 it was artificially induced by the injection of 1 mcg of estrone, notwithstanding continued progestational treatment. Higher doses also caused an increase in fetal mortality under these conditions, as established by autopsy on day 29 of pregnancy. These authors mention earlier experiments, proving that progesterone causes delayed implantation only in castrated rats, not in *intact rats*. The 3-desoxy analogue of medroxyprogesterone acetate, anagestone acetate, was reported *not* to delay nidation in intact pregnant rats (Blye et al., 1965a). Nevinny-Stickel (1960) found that norethisterone acetate in "high doses" delayed nidation in ten out of twenty rats which ultimately were found to have implanted embryos (though most of these were later resorbed). In twenty animals nidation was completely prevented.

In rats ovariectomized on day 3 post-coitum, progesterone was found by Nutting and Meyer (1964) to delay nidation in daily doses of 1 to 4 mg, injected from day 3 through to day 8. There was a dose-dependent number of rats with implantation sites and of sites per animal on day 13, with more than half of the fetuses alive. In this series, which did not include medroxyprogesterone, its fluoro derivative (17α-acetoxy-21-fluoro-6α-methylprogesterone) was the only compound other than progesterone found "capable of causing a delay of nidation with any degree of consistency".

Norethisterone in daily doses of 1 mg delayed nidation in two out of ten animals but there were no live fetuses on day 13. Absence of traces of sites suggested very early embryonic death. Neither normal nor delayed implantation occurred with doses of 4 mg of norethisterone nor with 1 or 4 mg daily of norethynodrel or ethynodiol diacetate.

The authors' interesting conclusion was that the ability to maintain blastocysts in a viable condition during periods of delayed implantation is found only in non-estrogenic compounds and closely agrees with the progestational activity as measured in the Clauberg assay. The 21-fluoro derivative of medroxyprogesterone had been found by Elton *et al.* (1960) to have 40–50 times the activity of progesterone and by Nutting and Meyer to be 47.5 times as active as progesterone in keeping blastocysts alive.

The inactive compounds norethynodrel and ethynodiol diacetate had relatively high estrogenicity. The experiments of the Wisconsin group were confirmed by Nutting and Sollmann (1967) who treated intact rats from day 1 through to day 7 after mating and looked for implantation sites on day 8 and if none were found again on day 15. Eight steroids were tested. The *inactive* ones included progesterone and megestrol acetate, the *active* ones medroxyprogesterone acetate (daily dose causing delay of implantation in 50% of the animals calculated to be 720 mcg). This treatment did not affect the conception rate (100%) nor the number of implantation sites.

Taubert (1967), using the same compound in a crystal suspension (Depo-Provera®), injected into post-coitally ovariectomized rats on day 4 after mating, could produce a delay of implantation of 10 days by one single dose of 5 to 10 mg. Implantation of the blastocyst following estrogen administration was the criterion of success. The effect of these single doses equalled that of *daily* injections of 5 mg of progesterone.

Dickson (1969) studied medroxyprogesterone (as Depo-Provera®) in mice by injecting 1 mg subcutaneously after ovariectomy on day 3 of pregnancy. This was repeated on day 8—after laparotomy—and this injection was combined with one of 0.05 mcg of estradiol benzoate. Autopsy on day 12 showed normal numbers of normal implantation sites. Variations of the technique were less effective.

In contrast with the lack of activity of megestrol acetate in intact rats described by Nutting and Sollman (quoted hereabove), Chang and Kincl (1968) reported that the compound is active in rats ovariectomized on day 3 or day 4 post-coitum and treated thereafter until autopsy on day 13, nidation being induced by injection of an estrogen on day 9. The interesting observation was reported that megestrol acetate showed much greater potency in this test when implanted in DPS capsules (see subsection 25.6, p. 191) than when given s.c. or p.o. The 80 to 100% effective doses were 800 mcg/day s.c., 1600 mcg p.o. and only 60 mcg (estimated release per 24 hours) in capsules.

Bindon (1969) could delay nidation in mice by hypophysectomy on the day of successful mating (presence of vaginal plug: day 1 of pregnancy), which would cause degeneration or disappearance of blastocysts by day 8. One single injection of 0.5 or 2.5 mg medroproxygesterone acetate in its depot form (Depo-Provera®) kept the blastocysts fairly normal so that on day 8 they looked like those found on day 5 of normal pregnancy. When

0.1 mcg of estradiol was injected on day 8, normal implantation and development ensued. (Progesterone in a single dose of 2.5 mg in oily solution injected on day 1 did not maintain viability of blastocysts.) Bindon's experiments are also interesting because of his finding that a neurodepressive drug prevented implantation only when administered on the afternoon of day 3, which together with related observations of others led him to conclude "that implantation and ovulation in the mouse are controlled by separate hypothalamo-pituitary mechanisms".

In summary, delay of nidation of viable blastocysts with subsequent normal development of fetuses has been achieved with medroxyprogesterone acetate and megestrol, the latter especially in implanted capsules.

Anagestone and the estrane derivatives were found inactive.

5. THE INHIBITION OF OVULATION

5.1. INTRODUCTORY REMARKS

Interest in the ovulation-inhibiting properties of progesterone has been tremendously stimulated by the fact that Pincus made it the starting point of his approach to a hormonal control of human fertility (see Pincus, 1965). In his first comprehensive lecture on the subject, delivered at the 5th International Planned Parenthood Conference in Tokyo in October 1955 (see Pincus, 1956), he described how his group started screening a variety of steroids "by a single subcutaneous injection in rabbits at a dosage of 10 mg per rabbit. Compounds which fail, at this dosage level, to inhibit either ovulation, fertilization or implantation are discarded". By this procedure he had at the time discovered fifteen active compounds, twelve of which were found less active than progesterone and two (norethisterone and norethynodrel) distinctly more active. Though structurally unrelated to progesterone, these two substances were covered by the title of the paper: "Some effects of progesterone and related compounds upon reproduction and early development in mammals." As we have pointed out (see subsection 2.1) norethynodrel has been shown to be weakly active by classical standards for progestational potency. This was early recognized by Pincus and his group when they wrote (Pincus *et al.*, 1956): "It is a not very potent progestin compared to other compounds, it is either not at all or only feebly deciduomagenic and appears to be unable to sustain implantation in the dosages thus far employed . . . it might almost be denominated an estrogen." In fact norethynodrel has been described as an "estrogen with progestational effects" (Edgren *et al.*, 1967a).

Of course Pincus was fully aware of the fact that inhibition of ovulation can be brought about by a great variety of steroids, notably estrogens, and in his book on the control of fertility we find (p. 65) this colorful sentence: "It should not be deduced from the rather formidable array of compounds in Tables 5 and 6 that practically all steroids are ovulation inhibitors."

At present it would appear to be clear that any discussion of the pharmacology of orally active progestational substances must include their effects on ovulation.

5.2. INHIBITION OF OVULATION IN THE RABBIT

The activities of a number of compounds in this test are shown in Table 10. Chlormadinone acetate is the most active substance when injected or given orally. Of the estrane derivatives, lynestrenol is classified by Kincl and Dorfman (1963c) amongst the most active ones; norethynodrel, allylestrenol and dydrogesterone have very low activity. The ranking does not differ greatly from that based on Clauberg activity (Tables 2 and 3).

The antiovulatory potency of chlormadinone acetate in the rabbit is greatly increased when it is combined with ethynyl estradiol, which by itself is practically without effect in this test (Chambon and Le Vève, 1966c).

5.3. INHIBITION OF OVULATION IN THE RAT

In most laboratories the rat is by far preferred to the rabbit for routine purposes. Activities of compounds tested are shown in Table 11. Ranking is somewhat different when judged in this species. Chlormadinone appears to be much less effective in rats. This point is discussed below, in the subsection on pituitary inhibition (5.5.2).

Bennett et al. (1968b) gave ovulation-suppressing doses of megestrol acetate (12 mg/kg/day) to adult rats (of 200 to 250 g body weight) orally for 7 days consecutively and found that on the 3rd day after cessation of dosing 50% of the animals had eggs in their tubes and 95% had ovulated by the 4th day, with eggs evenly distributed throughout the length of the oviducts, which was described as synchronization of ovulation.

5.4. INHIBITION OF OVULATION IN THE HAMSTER

Several compounds were studied in the hamster, a spontaneously ovulating, short-cycle species, by Greenwald (1965). Results are shown in Table 12. Medroxyprogesterone, which has the highest activity in the rat and ranks high in the rabbit, is quite inactive in the hamster.

TABLE 10. INHIBITION OF (REFLEX) OVULATION IN RABBITS

Compounds administered in one single dose, followed by mating the next day (unless otherwise indicated). Effective doses as listed cause at least 50% suppression of ovulations that would normally follow copulation.

Compound	Effective dose (mg)		Oral activity as percentage of activity of norethisterone ($=100$)	Subcut. act. as percentage of activity of progesterone ($=100$)	Reference
	subcutaneous unless otherwise indicated	oral			
Chlormadinone acetate	0.01–0.02	0.015	3500 (1000–6000)	4000	Kincl and Dorfman (1963a) Kincl and Dorfman (1963b)
	0.1	0.1–0.25			Chambon and Le Bars (1965) Shipley (1965)
	0.1 percut.[8]				
	0.03 intravag.[8]				Kincl and Dorfman (1966)
Medroxyprogesterone acetate	0.04[3]	0.4[3]		at least 2000	Barnes et al. (1959) Pincus (1965)
	0.2 percut.	0.625		2000[1]	Kincl and Dorfman (1963b) Shipley (1965)
	0.5 intravag.[8]				Kincl and Dorfman (1966)
Megestrol acetate	0.1		500		Kincl and Dorfman (1963b)
Lynestrenol	0.016/kg		300		David et al. (1963)
	0.05–1.25				Kincl and Dorfman (1963a)

Norethisterone	0.075–0.15	0.625		500	Kincl and Dorfman (1963a, b)
	0.1–0.25				Pincus et al. (1956)
	0.25	0.25			Pincus 1965
				330[1]	Kincl and Dorfman (1963a)
	1.0 percut.[8]			330	Junkmann (1964)
Norethynodrel	0.1–1.0	5.0[2]			Shipley (1965)
	0.2	0.1			Pincus et al. (1956)
		0.312–2.5[4]	<25		Pincus (1965)
					Kincl and Dorfman (1963c)
					Pincus (1965)
Normethandrone	0.5[3]	0.4			
		0.1–6.4[4]			
Allylestrenol		0.312–7.5	33		Kincl and Dorfman (1963c)
Dydrogesterone	40–60	0.5–19.0[5]	30		Kincl and Dorfman (1963c)
	32[7]			<15[6]	Claassen (1968)
					Kobayashi et al. (1963)

Notes to Table 10
(1) This figure was calculated by Kincl and Dorfman (1963a) from the data of Pincus, G. (1961). Suppression of ovulation with reference to oral contraceptives. In: *Modern Trends in Endocrinology*, p. 231, Second Series, Butterworth & Co. Ltd., London.
(2) Lowest dose tested.
(3) Minimum effective dose.
(4) The figures are given as "dosage range".
(5) Figures indicate "dosage range". The authors add: "Complete suppression could not be obtained even at doses 10 times the minimum effective dose."
(6) Doses of 2 × 10, 2 × 20 and 2 × 30 mg caused 50–60% inhibition of ovulation whereas progesterone in a dose of 2 × 5 mg gave 75% and 2 × 10 mg 100%; 60 mg dydrogesterone did not prevent ovulation caused by i.v. injection of cupri-acetate as opposed to complete inhibition by 10 mg progesterone.
(7) Ovulation caused by i.v. injection of 9 mg cupri-sulfate.
(8) Ovulation induced by i.v. injection of 0.3 ml per kg of 1% copper acetate solution.
(9) 0.02 mg of chlormadinone acetate combined with 2 mcg of ethynyl estradiol is about equally effective (Chambon and Le Vève, 1966c).

TABLE 11. INHIBITION OF OVULATION IN RATS
Doses are in mg daily per rat, given for 4 days, unless otherwise indicated

Compound	Subcutaneous treatment		Oral treatment		Reference
	ED_{50}	Potency as percentage of potency of progesterone = 100	ED_{50}	ED_{100}	
Medroxyprogesterone acetate	<0.05[1] 0.03	>500 3000	0.1		Shipley and Meyer (1965) Suchowsky et al. (1966)
Megestrol acetate	0.19		0.12 0.4		Suchowsky et al. (1965) Suchowsky et al. (1965)
Norethisterone	0.1 >0.1[1]	2000 3000 900	3.0 0.2	2.4–3 (12/kg for 14 days)	Bennett et al. (1968a) Neumann et al. (1964) Junkmann (1964) Shipley and Meyer (1965) Desaulles and Krähenbühl (1964)
	0.5[5] 0.03 0.1	2000	>4.0 0.1 3.0		Rudel and Kincl (1966) Overbeek et al. (1962) Suchowsky et al. (1965) Neumann et al. (1964)
Norethisterone acetate	0.01	170	0.24		Neumann and Domenico (1964) Suchowsky et al. (1965) Desaulles and Krähenbühl (1964)
Lynestrenol	1.2		1.2 2–4 1.5–4[2]		Suchowsky et al. (1965) Overbeek et al. (1962) Uhlarik et al. (1964)

Norethynodrel	0.2	1.0	Suchowsky et al. (1965) Desaulles and Krähenbühl (1964) Watnick et al. (1965)
		>5 mg/kg/day[3] for 11–18 days	
	>0.2[4] 33–86 days		Holmes and Mandl (1962)
Anagestone acetate	120		
Medrogestone	1.5	4.1	Blye et al. (1965a) Revesz and Chappel (1966) Suchowsky and Baldratti (1964)
Allylestrenol	0.5% of potency of 19-nortestosterone (inactive)	1.0/kg[8]	
Chlormadinone acetate	>0.5[5] 0.3 0.75	0.65	Rudel and Kincl (1966) Suchowsky et al. (1965) Dörner and Döcke (1967) Mischler et al. (1969)
Quingestanol acetate	>2.7[6]	2.0[7]	Eben-Moussi and Van den Driessche (1970)

Notes to Table 11
(1) Treatment is given for 7 days, beginning on the 35th day of life, covering the period of first estrus in most of the animals (kept from the 35th to 42nd day). Effect is judged by counting corpora lutea. It is suggested that absence of corpora lutea is due to prevention of ovulation.
(2) Treatment is given for 21 days. Effect judged by absence of corpora lutea. Doses mentioned causing (much) more than 50% reduction of animals having corpora lutea.
(3) Treatment with pregnancy-preventing dose of compound started either 7 days before or at the time animals were placed with the males, and continued until 24 hours before death (on day 12). Presence of ova ascertained microscopically; 83% of animals treated with norethynodrel ovulated.
(4) Only five of the nineteen norethynodrel-injected animals lacked recognizable corpora lutea.
(5) PMS (15 I.U. in saline) injected subcutaneously to 30-day-old rats, test compound injected on days 31 and 32 of life. Authors gave total dose as 1000 mcg.
(6) This dose, given for 15 days, reduced the number of ovulating rats from 10/10 to 6/7 which is recorded as a reduction from 100 to 85.7%.
(7) Dose stated as 10 mg/kg (body weight of rats 200 g) for 5 days.
(8) Percentage of inhibition, body weight of rats and route of administration not stated.

TABLE 12. INHIBITION OF OVULATION IN THE HAMSTER
Minimum effective and maximum inactive single dose (injected on day 1, metestrus) preventing ovulation on day 2 of next cycle, in mg. From Greenwald (1964 and 1965).

Compound	Lowest effective dose	Highest inactive dose	Remarks	Reference
Progesterone	2.5	1.0	all animals ovulating	Greenwald (1965)
Medroxyprogesterone acetate		2.5	3 out of 5 ovulating	Greenwald (1965)
		10.0	2 out of 5 ovulating	Greenwald (1965)
Norethynodrel	5.0		no animal ovulating	Greenwald (1964)
	10.0			
Norethisterone	2.5		2 out of 5 ovulating	Greenwald (1965)
Ethynodiol[1]	0.5		no animal ovulating	Greenwald (1965)
diacetate	1.0			
Medrogestone	0.5		2 out of 5 ovulating	Greenwald (1965)
Estradiol benzoate	0.1		no animal ovulating	Greenwald (1965)
	0.25			

Note to Table 12
(1) "Ethynodiol diacetate revealed an interesting effect on follicular growth, depending on the dose administered. At doses of 0.5–1 mg large persisting follicles from previous cycle were present. However, after the injection of 2.5 mg, atresia—comparable to that resulting from estrogen treatment—was the primary factor responsible for preventing ovulation." "Norethynodrel does not interfere with follicular development."

5.5. MECHANISMS OF INHIBITION OF OVULATION

Various experimental approaches have been tried to identify the mechanism or mechanisms through which these progestational steroids operate in inhibiting ovulation. Some of the questions to be answered concern the site of action (ovary, pituitary or hypothalamus?) and the gonadotrophic hormones (FSH or LH?) whose production or action would be inhibited.

5.5.1. *Interference with exogenous gonadotrophin*

As a first problem to be tackled one might select the question whether these ovulation inhibitors interfere with the effect of exogenous (injected) gonadotrophins, because if they do, this could indicate that the action takes place at the level of the ovary.

Various gonadotrophic agents have been tried, such as crude pregnancy urine, as used for the Friedman- or the Aschheim–Zondek reaction, purified HCG* or PMS† in varying doses and by different routes of administration (intraperitoneal, subcutaneous). Progestational steroids again were given in various doses, mostly orally, and in various cases were found not to inhibit the effect of exogenous gonadotrophins.

In rabbits. Progesterone (1 or 2 mg s.c.) was found to have no marked effect upon ovulation induced by HCG; norethisterone or norethynodrel, according to Edgren and Carter (1962), injected s.c. in doses up to 2 and 8 mg respectively did *not* consistently depress the ovulatory response to 10 or 12 I.U. HCG. Chlormadinone acetate, which inhibited reflex-induced or copper acetate-induced ovulations in rabbits in one parenteral dose of 0.1 mg, did not diminish the effect of 15 I.U. HCG (Kincl, 1963). The same applies to doses of 0.3 mg given once or on 3 days, by gavage (Rudel and Kincl, 1966).

The combination norethisterone (10 mg) and mestranol (60 mcg) present in Ortho-Novum prevented reflex ovulation in rabbits, when given in a dose of 0.5 mg/kg prior to mating and suppressed the rise of LH in the blood, which could be demonstrated by infusion of the blood into one ovary of a recipient rabbit. The effect of such an infusion of blood from an untreated mated rabbit could not be prevented by prior treatment of the recipient with 0.5 mg/kg of the norethindrone/mestranol combination (Hilliard *et al.*, 1966b).

According to Sas *et al.* (1965), lynestrenol in five daily oral doses of 5 to 25 mg given to rabbits, in which ovulations were induced by the i.v.

---
* HCG: human chorionic gonadotrophin.
† PMS: pregnant mares' serum gonadotrophin.

injection of large quantities (12–15 ml) of pregnancy urine, slightly reduced the ovarian response, though the pregnancy test turned out to be positive in fourteen out of fifteen animals. These authors also found that lynestrenol in oral doses of 25, 100 or 1000 mcg on 6 successive days to a large extent prevented the occurrence of ovulations in mice used for the Aschheim–Zondek reaction. There are, however, several snags in the interpretation of this sort of results. The pituitary produces FSH and LH to bring about ovulation. If FSH production is inhibited by the steroid and LH (or its close relative HCG) is given to induce ovulation, the steroid would wrongly seem to be an active inhibitor, only because there would be no ripe follicles for the LH to act upon. Overbeek and de Visser (1964 a, b) have analysed such an experiment and rejected the tempting conclusion that this inhibition of an exogenous hormone proved an effect of the inhibitor at the level of the target organ.

This pitfall can be avoided by the use of hypophysectomized animals. We therefore separately discuss experiments in intact animals on the one hand and those in which the pituitary has been removed before the hormone treatment on the other hand.

Thus, in *hypophysectomized immature rats*, in which ovulation was induced by subcutaneous injection of 30 I.U. PMS, followed by the i.p. injection of 25 I.U. HCG 56 hours later, norethynodrel given by gavage at the time of HCG injection in a dose as high as 10 mg did *not* interfere with ovulation, whereas 5 mg of norethynodrel (not of norethisterone) reduced the number of ovulations to almost one-half in *intact* immature animals under otherwise identical conditions (France and Pincus, 1964). Using a similar design (intact immature rats, injected with 30 units of PMS and 56 hours later with 10 units of HCG) Revesz and Chappel (1966) likewise found that norethynodrel (s.c., with the PMS, 24 hours before the HCG and with the HCG) in a dose of 3.1 mg reduced by half the mean number of ova per rat. (Norethynodrel, it will be remembered, is more active orally than parenterally.)

Of medrogestone under the same conditions the active subcutaneous dose (ED_{50}) was only 1.5 mg, the orally active dose 4.1 mg. Megestrol acetate, on the other hand, in a daily dose of 10 mg/kg/day (orally to intact mature rats for 14 days), which completely blocked spontaneous ovulation in rats, did *not* interfere with the effect of 10 I.U. HCG (Bennett et al., 1968a), because, it is concluded, the compound inhibits only LH secretion. By a different technique, Suchowsky et al. (1965) found remarkably high "anti-HCG activities". They gave intact immature female rats six daily injections of 1 I.U. HCG. Steroids to be tested were administered s.c. 1 day before gonadotrophic treatment started and then 30 minutes before each HCG injection. The animals were sacrificed the day after the last injection, corpora lutea were counted and the average of each group of ten animals was recorded. Their results are shown in Table 13.

TABLE 13. "ANTI-HCG ACTIVITY" OF PROGESTATIONAL STEROIDS TESTED ACCORDING TO SUCHOWSKY et al. (1965)

Compound	Active dose in mg s.c. ED_{50}
Progesterone	0.64
Medroxyprogesterone acetate	0.17
Megestrol acetate	0.66
Chlormadinone acetate	0.52
Norethisterone	0.14
Norethisterone acetate	0.51
Lynestrenol	0.49
Norethynodrel	1.13

Coppola and Perrine (1965) found norethynodrel in oral doses from 1 to 2 mg/day to cause a reduction of the number of animals (immature, intact rats) ovulating in response to 8 I.U. of PMS and daily doses of 3 or 4 mg per rat to block ovulation completely. ("Examination of the ovaries of rats that did not ovulate revealed only presence of numerous follicles; this attested to their stimulation by the PMS treatment".)

In intact mice, injected with 2 I.U. PMS and 1 I.U. HCG (which caused 97.75% of the animals to shed an average of almost 28 ova), 0.25 mg of progesterone partially and 0.5 mg completely prevented ovulation. Norethynodrel in relatively high doses of 0.15 and 1.5 mg caused significant but not complete inhibition (Purshottam et al., 1961).

Kincl (1966) and Rudel and Kincl (1966) tested their steroids for ovulation-inhibitory potency in *hypophysectomized* (30-day-old) rats, given PMS and HCG in a dosage that produced ovulation in 94% of the animals. Chlormadinone acetate and medroxyprogesterone acetate in total oral doses of 0.2 and 2.0 mg did *not* reduce this effect, the latter compound not even in a dose of 20 mg (in 22-day-old hypophysectomized rats). On the other hand, Harper (1964) recorded the interesting observation that chlormadinone acetate (by gavage in a daily dose of 100 mg/kg bodyweight) did not suppress the gonadotrophic effectiveness of PMS and HCG in hypophysectomized rats (40–75 g) as judged by uterine weight and ovarian histology,

TABLE 14. NON-INHIBITION OF OVULATION IN RABBITS, INDUCED BY EXOGENOUS GONADOTROPHIN
Judged by percentage of animals ovulating

Compound	Stimulating dose of gonadotrophin	Highest inactive dose (mg)	Duration of steroid treatment	Reference
Progesterone	HCG 5–40 I.U.	2.0	2 days s.c.	Edgren and Carter (1962)
Norethisterone	HCG 10 or 12 I.U.	2.0	2 days s.c.	Edgren and Carter (1962)
Norethynodrel	HCG 10 or 12 I.U.	8.0	2 days s.c.	Edgren and Carter (1962)
Chlormadinone acetate	HCG 15 I.U.	0.1 3 × 0.3	1 inject. 3 days gavage	Kincl (1963) Rudel and Kincl (1966)

provided steroid treatment started on the same day as the administration of gonadotrophin. "When, however, treatment with the steroid started 4 days earlier... the follicular response to the gonadotrophins was depressed." The author rightly concludes that this *is* evidence for a depression of ovarian response, probably as a result of a direct action on the ovary.

Saunders and Drill (1958) found that the effect of 10 RU of gonadophysin on ovarian and uterine weight of hypophysectomized rats was *not* inhibited by treatment of the animals with norethynodrel (0.2 mg twice daily for 5 days).

Miyake and Kobayashi (1960) examined the ovaries of hypophysectomized immature rats which had been treated with s.c. injections of 1 mg of norethisterone daily for 12 days. They found retention of fluid under the ovarian capsule, but otherwise the organs did not differ very much from the ovaries of untreated hypophysectomized controls. The sensitivity of these glands towards PMS and HCG (as shown by ovarian weight increase and ovulations) had *not* been altered by 5 days of norethisterone treatment. The fluid cysts were not seen with norethynodrel. Smith and Bradbury (1966) using hypophysectomized immature rats stimulated by gonadotrophins (HMG, 10 U Internat. Ref. Prep. plus 1 mg LH, administered together, and subdivided into five equal doses, in 48 hours) found that injections of norethisterone in single daily doses of 1 mg for 2 days preceding gonadotrophin treatment and together with it had *no* influence on the number of rats ovulating (five out of five). "In addition, the augmenting effect of estrogen on ovarian weight was not modified by addition of progestin."

Similarly, Kraehahn and von Berswordt-Wallrabe (1969) found norethisterone acetate in four daily injections of 0.1 mg not to interfere with ovulations in juvenile hypophysectomized rats treated simultaneously with three consecutive daily injections of 10 I.U. PMS and one of 10 I.U. HCG.

Progesterone injected into immature Rhesus monkeys in daily doses of 2 mg/kg and for 30 days did not inhibit the action of 25 I.U. of PMS, as judged by ovarian and uterine weight and histology (Kar and Chandra, 1965).

In order to minimize confusion, we summarize the decisive experiments on (lack of) inhibition of ovulation induced by exogenous gonadotrophin in Table 14 as far as rabbits are concerned and in Table 15 with regard to hypophysectomized immature rats.

The conclusion would appear to be justified that the inhibition of ovulation by progestational compounds, which has been abundantly observed under a

TABLE 15. No Inhibition of Ovulation in Hypophysectomized Immature Rats, Induced by Exogenous Gonadotrophin
Doses of steroids in mg, total (unless indicated as/day), given orally (or) or subcutaneously (s.c.).

Compound	Stimulating doses of gonadotrophin	Doses of steroid highest inactive (mg)	Duration of steroid treatment in days	Judged by number of ovulations (no), or ovarian weight (ow) or histology (oh)	Reference
Chlormadinone acetate	PMS 30 I.U. HCG 10 I.U.	2 s.c.	2	no, ow	Rudel and Kincl (1966)
	PMS 10 I.U. HCG 25 I.U.	about 2/day s.c. (100/kg/day)	4	ow, oh	Harper (1964)
Medroxyprogesterone acetate	PMS 30 I.U. HCG 10 I.U.	20 s.c.	2	no, ow	Rudel and Kincl (1966)
Norethynodrel	Gonadophysin 10 R.U.	0.2/day s.c.	1	ow	Saunders and Drill (1958)
	PMS 30 I.U. HCG 25 I.U.	10 or.	1	no	France and Pincus (1964)
Norethisterone	PMS 80 I.U.	1/day	12	ow	Miyake and Kobayashi (1960)
	PMS 80 I.U. HCG	1/day	5	no	Miyake and Kobayashi (1960)
	HMG 10 U. LH 1 mg	1/day	5	Number of rats with corpora lutea	Smith and Bradbury (1966)
Norethisterone acetate	PMS 30 I.U. HCG 10 I.U.	0.1 mg/day s.c.	4	no, ow	Kraehahn and von Berswordt-Wallrabe (1969)

variety of conditions, is not due to interference with the action of gonadotrophic hormones at the ovarian level, at least as far chlormadinone, medroxyprogesterone, norethisterone and norethynodrel are concerned. This does not mean that these drugs have no effects at all on the ovary, and under certain experimental conditions such an effect seems to be involved in the inhibition of ovulation.

The conclusions are further fortified by the evidence that progestational steroids do in fact inhibit gonadotrophin secretion by the pituitary under a variety of conditions, as discussed in Section 6.

5.5.2. Mechanism of pituitary inhibition

Having shown that several progestational drugs do in fact inhibit ovulation by an action involving the pituitary, we may wonder how exactly this effect is brought about.

Sawyer (1965) implanted small amounts (0.2 mg) of norethisterone in the basal tuberal posterior median eminence (PME) or in the pituitary of rabbits and was able to show that hypothalamic (not hypophyseal) implants prevented ovulation when the animals were mated during the succeeding 5 weeks. This was further worked out by Kanematsu and Sawyer (1965) and was strong indication that the compound interfered with the hypothalamic LH-releasing mechanism. The group (Hilliard *et al.*, 1966a) then found that ovulation could be blocked by a s.c. injection of Ortho-Novum (equivalent to about 0.5 mg/kg norethisterone and containing 0.6% of mestranol) between 15 and 24 hours prior to mating and in these animals the normal, postcoital discharge of LH could be shown not to have occurred. A dose of 0.1 mg of estradiol benzoate injected s.c. 48 and 24 hours before mating partly overcame the blocking action of norethisterone. Norethisterone did not affect the responsiveness to exogenous or endogenous LH. The work of Schally (Schally and Bowers, 1964) on the LH-releasing factor has enabled Sawyer's group to analyse the mechanism of steroid inhibition still further. They were able (Hilliard *et al.*, 1966b) to show that median eminence extracts (MEE) from rabbits with proven LH-releasing potency would induce ovulations when infused directly into the third ventricle or the pituitary. A combination of norethisterone and mestranol, supplied as Ortho-Novum, injected s.c. in a dose of 0.5 mg/kg, 15 to 24 hours before infusion of MEE, prevented ovulations. This looks like prima facie evidence that the ovulation-inhibiting effect of the drug cannot be solely due to interference with the secretion of LH–RF but must have something to do with the action of the releaser. Large doses of atropine sulfate (300 mg/kg subcutaneously) injected 60 minutes before a MEE infusion into the pituitary did *not* inhibit its effect but considerably reduced the effect of an intraventricular infusion. Now, as Sawyer's group had found earlier, "there is evidence that this pharmacological blocking agent acts at the level of the median eminence to prevent pituitary activation", and this could mean that in order to be effective the brainstem extracts require the normal functioning of the median eminence. Also some doubt is cast on the validity of the assumption that norethisterone did prevent the releaser effect at the terminal site in the pituitary, particularly since the authors introduced their cannulas into the pituitary through the median eminence and could show by means of ferric chloride and ferrocyanide that there was considerable backtracking into the median eminence and third ventricle along the cannula path.

At any rate, what these studies show is that norethisterone inhibits ovulation in the rabbit by preventing LH from being released, not from acting on the ovary, and this effect can be partly antagonized by larger doses of estradiol benzoate.

Hooper (1968) studied the concentration of a peptidase, oxytocinase, in particulate and in soluble fractions (supernatant) of rabbit hypothalami and found that "physiologic conditions under which release of luteinizing hormone is suppressed . . . are accompanied by increased peptidase activity" in the supernatant. This applied to treatment with estradiol monobenzoate for 3 days prior to sacrifice, or with ethynyl estradiol (0.5 mcg i.m.) even in a single dose, 7 to 18 hours before sacrifice (Frith and Hooper, 1968). In a later study Frith and Hooper (1971) gave chlormadinone acetate or norethisterone i.m. 24 hours before mating and killed the rabbits $\frac{1}{2}$ hour or 24 hours later. An increase in supernatant peptidase activity was seen in all cases. Since the doses of the progestational compounds were shown to have antiovulatory effects, the authors suggest that their *results point towards an effect on the availability of the gonadotrophic hormone releasing factor*. This has now been shown by Schally *et al.* (1971) to be a decapeptide whose structure is likely to be attacked by peptidases, a fact which would seem to add interest to Frith and Hooper's hypothesis.

McDonald (1968) found that norethisterone (in single s.c. doses of 0.5 mg) prevented the ovulation-inducing effect of electric stimulation of the preoptic hypothalamus in mature rats, possibly as "the result of the antiestrogenic action of this compound". Further studies by McDonald and Gilmore (1969), with particular attention to the influence of the time in the cycle at which the drug is given and the antagonistic effects of estradiol benzoate and of progesterone, led the authors to the conclusion that norethisterone can act on both the pituitary and the hypothalamus depending on the stage of the cycle at which it is administered.

Another compound, chlormadinone acetate, was studied in the rat by Döcke *et al.* (1966 and 1968). They could show that in the immature female the ovulation-inducing effect of estradiol benzoate (15 mcg s.c.), the so-called Hohlweg effect, could be largely suppressed by the s.c. injection of 1 mg of chlormadinone acetate on 2 successive days *or* by implantation of one-hundredth of this dose (0.01 mg) either into the median eminence or the adenohypophysis (Döcke *et al.*, 1966). A direct ovulation-inhibiting effect on the ovary was quite unlikely, since the effective s.c. dose implanted into *one* ovary (of adult animals) inhibited spontaneous ovulation in *both* ovaries, whereas half of this dose implanted into an ovary had no effect at all.

These and further experiments with variously located hypothalamic or pituitary implants, electric stimulation and pentobarbitone blocking led the authors (Döcke *et al.*, 1968) to the conclusion that, in the adult rat, the site of action of chlormadinone is *the pituitary, not the hypothalamus.*

On the basis of their earlier assumption that estradiol benzoate induces ovulation in the rat by sensitizing the pituitary for the action of the LH-releaser (Dörner and Döcke, 1967), they thus arrive at the hypothesis that the inhibiting effect of "progestogens, acting on the hypothalamo-hypophysial system at low levels of circulating estrogen", may be due to the prevention of "the sensitization of the adenohypophysis to the gonadotrophin-releasing factor" which would "suppress the ovulation-inducing gonadotrophin secretion".

The fact that Döcke *et al.* found mediane minence implants effective in immature animals could be due to some transport of the steroid into the pituitary through the portal vessels, a possibility earlier envisaged by other authors. Another observation to be cited in this connection concerns the antagonistic effect of estrogens against the ovulation-inhibiting action of a progestational compound, medroxyprogesterone acetate (MAP), as described by Banik *et al.* (1970). Very small doses of this compound given in single injections on the day before proestrus in 4 day-cyclic rats prevented ovulation in most rats (0.01 mg) or in all of them (0.1 mg) and this could be reversed by the simultaneous administration p.o. of 0.1 to 1.0 mg of ethynyl estradiol (or a new synthetic estrogen, AY-11483). However, the effect of a bigger dose of MAP, 1.0 mg, could not be overcome by this treatment.

Exley *et al.* (1968) studied the mechanism of action of the same compound, chlormadinone acetate, in the rabbit and found that 0.5 mg given

TABLE 16. INHIBITION OF PITUITARY GONADOTROPHIC FUNCTION IN PARABIOTIC RATS (OR MICE IF INDICATED) AS JUDGED BY PREVENTION OF INCREASE IN WEIGHT OF OVARIES

Effective daily dose in mg

Compound	Oral dose	Subcut. dose	Number of days of treatment	Criterion of effectiveness	Activity as % of activity of testosterone subcut.	Activity as % of compound's act. in Clauberg test (= 100)		Activity as % of act. of progesterone (= 100)		Reference
						oral	subcut.	oral	subcut.	
Norethisterone acetate	0.03–0.10	0.01–0.03	12	50% inhibition		30–100	100–300	10,000–30,000	1000	Neumann et al. (1964)
	0.085		10	approx. 70% inhibition						Falconi and Bruni (1962)
Norethisterone	0.35	0.02	10	ED$_{50}$						Suchowsky et al. (1965)
	0.03–0.10	0.01–0.03	12	50% inhibition		100–300	200–600	10,000–30,000	1000	Neumann et al. (1964)
	0.1	0.1$^{(2)}$	10	approx. 75% inhibition						Miyake (1961)
		0.3/kg (0.1–0.7)	10	ED$_{75}$			110			Desaulles and Krähenbühl (1964)
		0.04	10	approx. 50% inhibition	150					Desaulles and Krähenbühl (1962)
		0.08	10	approx. 75% inhibition						Shipley and Meyer (1965)
	0.31	0.065	10	ED$_{50}$						Suchowsky et al. (1965)
	0.40	0.08	10	50% inhibition	150					Kincl and Dorfman (1965b)
Quingestanol acetate		0.08	10	approx. 50% inhibition						Mischler et al. (1969)
		0.32	10	approx. 80% inhibition						
		0.44	10	50% inhibition						Eben-Moussi and van den Driessche (1970)
Lynestrenol	0.13	0.52	10	ED$_{50}$						Suchowsky et al. (1965)
		0.3/kg (0.1–0.7)	10	ED$_{75}$						Desaulles and Krähenbühl (1964)
		0.125	10	100% inhibition						Overbeek and de Visser (1964)
Lynestrenol	55$^{(1)}$	0.2/kg	10	ED$_{75}$						Bagnati et al. (1964)
Norethynodrel		0.03	10	ED$_{50}$						Desaulles and Krähenbühl (1964)
	<0.03	0.0001$^{(2)}$	10	85% inhibition						Suchowsky et al. (1965)
			10							Miyake (1961)
Normethandrone		0.00001$^{(2)}$	10	48% inhibition	200		1000			Desaulles and Krähenbühl (1962)
			10		300–400		2000			Desaulles and Krähenbühl (1962)

Compound					References
Medroxy-progesterone acetate		0.1	10	87–92% inhibition	Shipley and Meyer (1965)
	1.9	0.01[2]	10	approx. 60% inhibition	Miyake (1961)
		0.001[2]	10		Falconi and Bruni (1962)
Megestrol acetate	0.23	0.05	10	ED_{50}	500	Desaulles and Krähenbühl (1962), Suchowsky et al. (1965)
	1.5	0.25	10	ED_{50}		Suchowsky et al. (1965)
Norgesterone	1.0[3]		7	about 50% inhibition		Ruggieri et al. (1965)
	0.21[4]		7	about 86% inhibition		
Medrogestone	>5.0	1–2	10	about 50% inhibition		Revesz and Chappel (1966)
Chlormadinone acetate	>40	10	10	ED_{50}		Kincl and Dorfman (1963a)
		1.3	10	ED_{75}	50	Kincl and Dorfman (1963b)
Allylestrenol		100/kg (70–180)	10	100% inhibition		Suchowsky et al. (1965)
						Desaulles and Krähenbühl (1962)
						Desaulles and Krähenbühl (1964)
Progesterone		1	10	ED_{50}		Miyake (1961)
	>10	0.1–0.3	12	about 140% inhibition		Neumann et al. (1964)
		3.0	10			Shipley and Meyer (1965)
		0.7	10	ED_{50}		Suchowsky et al. (1965)

Notes to Table 16
(1) Lowest dose tested.
(2) Tested in mice.
(3) Intact female with castrated male.
(4) Intact female with castrated female.

intravenously 24 hours before mating blocks reflex ovulation in about three-quarters of the animals and also prevented the normally occurring rise of 20α-hydroxypregn-4-en-3-one in the ovarian venous blood, when the animals failed to ovulate. The treatment did not prevent the normal ovulatory response to either LH injection or electric stimulation of the posterior part of the median eminence and the authors therefore conclude that under their experimental conditions chlormadinone acetate blocks reflex ovulation in the rabbits, following mating, at a site *above* the median eminence.

In pursuing these studies, Harris and Sherratt (1969) avoided anesthesia and laparotomy—which they felt could have influenced the results of Exley *et al.* (1968)—by stimulating the tuber cinereum of the conscious animal and examining the ovaries 48 hours later.

Drug treatment by i.v. injection of 0.5 or 1.0 mg 24 hours before stimulation did not significantly reduce the number of animals ovulating but did reduce the number of ruptured follicles per animal. When electric stimulation was replaced by the infusion of a releaser (median eminence extract) into the pituitary, the reverse occurred; the percentage of ovulating animals was significantly reduced but not the number of ruptured follicles in each. Hypothetical explanations are offered for this behavior but the conclusion of Exley *et al.* that reflex ovulation is prevented by an effect of the drug at a site located above the median eminence is sustained.

Seven progestational compounds were studied as regards their "ovulation-inhibiting action" in the rat and a purified LRF preparation (active dose 0.4 mcg dry weight or less) was used by Schally *et al.* (1968). The LH levels were determined biologically in the plasma of adult animals both with and without LRF treatment. These were the decisive parameters studied, since the animals were all ovariectomized and ovulation itself could not be observed. The progestational steroids were injected on 5 successive days. Of norethynodrel and dimethisterone the daily dose was 20 mg (of the latter also 2.5 mg), of chlormadinone acetate 10 mg (also 5, 1 and 0.05 mg), of medroxyprogesterone acetate 10 mg, of norethisterone 5 mg, of ethynodiol diacetate 2 and of norgestrel 1 mg. (These studies were supplemented by radio-immuno-assays of LH and FSH in the rat plasma and megestrol acetate as well as lynestrenol were included: Schally *et al.*, 1970.)

All these doses lowered plasma-LH levels. Estrogens (1–20 mcg of mestranol or 200 mcg of ethynyl estradiol) were also active in lowering plasma-LH levels and when given in combination with the progestational steroids often increased their effect remarkably. However, none of these compounds, alone or in combination, was able to inhibit the LH-raising effect of an i.v. injection of LRF, given 15 minutes before bleeding.

The authors therefore conclude that the progestational substances (as well as the estrogens) act by interfering with the secretion of the luteinizing hormone-releasing factor (LRF), not with its effect on the pituitary.

Summarizing, we may state that various progestational compounds have been shown to inhibit ovulation in rabbits and rats through an action on the hypothalamo-pituitary region, probably by inhibiting the secretion (or enhancing the destruction) of the LH-releaser, but perhaps also by changing the sensitivity of the adenohypophysis towards the effect of the releaser.

6. EVIDENCE FOR INHIBITION OF GONADOTROPHIN SECRETION BY THE PITUITARY

There is considerable evidence to show that orally active progestational compounds inhibit the gonadotrophic function of the pituitary.

6.1. PARABIOSIS STUDIES

One of the techniques employed for the purpose is based on the well-known fact that in a female rat connected with a castrated partner by *parabiosis*, the ovaries, exposed to the stimulus of an overactive pituitary, undergo considerable hypertrophy. A number of investigators have successfully attempted to inhibit this overstimulation by the administration of ovulation-inhibiting steroids to the castrated partner. Results are shown in Table 16.

R. K. Meyer and his group in Madison (Wis.) investigated the nature of the gonadotrophic component (FSH or LH) in the pituitary secretion which is inhibited by drug administration in these experiments (Sager *et al.*, 1966). For this purpose they joined by parabiosis one castrated 27-day-old female with a hypophysectomized, otherwise equal, partner. Injection of HCG (20 I.U./day for 6 days) into the hypophysectomized animal greatly increased the weight of its ovaries, which was attributed to synergism with FSH supplied by the castrated partner's pituitary (since HCG alone, given to "single" hypophysectomized females, did not increase ovarian weight to anything near that extent).

Medroxyprogesterone acetate (2 mg daily for 6 days) injected into the castrated partner significantly reduced ovarian weight increase in the hypophysectomized partner (whose ovaries were still 7 times as large as those of single hypophysectomized controls) and an even stronger reduction was brought about by 4 mg of progesterone plus 1 mcg estrone (but not by either hormone alone). When no HCG was given to the hypophysectomized partner, the same steroid treatment of the castrated partner would cause ovarian weights one-sixth to one-seventh of those obtained with HCG. The authors conclude from these interesting studies that the amount of "augmenting substance and therefore presumably FSH secreted from the castrated parabiont's pituitary" is significantly reduced by 2 mg of Provera (medroxyprogesterone acetate) or the one combination of progesterone plus estrone. "However, since the augmentation response is definitely not eliminated, some FSH is present to augment with HCG."

6.2. BLOCKING OF COMPENSATORY OVARIAN HYPERTROPHY

A mechanism similar to the one operating in parabiosis with a castrated partner is seen in those experiments where one ovary of a rat is removed and the normally ensuing *compensatory hypertrophy* of the other ovary is prevented by the administration of a pituitary-inhibiting drug.

When given for 14 days from the day of hemicastration, norethisterone prevented such hypertrophy in a daily dose of about 0.5 mg (Madjerek, 1960; Peterson *et al.*, 1964) whereas normethandrone and allylestrenol were ineffective in twice and 4 times this dose respectively (given orally, Madjerek, 1960). Norgestrel had about 60% of the potency of norethisterone (Edgren *et al.*, 1963). Norethynodrel, on the other hand, was active in a much smaller dose of 72.5 mcg. For comparison the active dose of progesterone was found to be 3.6 mg but that of estrone 17.8 mcg (Peterson *et al.*, 1964). Dydrogesterone was active in a daily dose of 1 mg injected for 18 days (Boris *et al.*, 1966). Superlutin was found active in daily parenteral doses of about 0.5 mg (given 12 times in 2 weeks) by Jelinek *et al.* (1968) which represented about 5 times the activity of progesterone (at the ED_{100} level) in the authors' experiments.

In hemicastrated rats the remaining ovary is known to release as many ova as would have been released by both ovaries together. This phenomenon, known as compensatory superovulation, has been used to demonstrate a pituitary-inhibiting effect of steroids (Weifenbach, 1965). Single injections of progesterone (1.0 or 5.0 mg), ethisterone (0.5 or 5.0 mg) or chlormadinone (1.0 or 5.0 mg) in metestrus were without effect on superovulations but medroxyprogesterone acetate completely suppressed them in a dose of 0.5 mg. Haller developed a test (see Haller, 1968) for pituitary

Orally Active Progestational Compounds: Animal Studies

Daily dose in mg

Compound	Oral treatment			Subcutaneous treatment				Reference
	active	in-active	number of days	active	in-active	number of days	activity as percentage of act. of testosterone propionate	
Norethynodrel	0.5/kg		30					Saunders and Drill (1958)
				1				Ruggieri et al. (1965)
Norethisterone	2.0	0.5	14					Madjerek et al. (1960)
	1.0		7					McGinty and Djerassi (1958)
				1				Matscher and Lupo (1960)
							100	Neumann et al. (1964)
							100	Neumann et al. (1964)
Norethisterone acetate	1.0		21					McGinty and Djerassi (1958)
Normethandrone		1.0	7					Madjerek et al. (1966)
		1.0	14					Sas et al. (1966)
Lynestrenol	5 (only dose tested)		28					
Chlormadinone acetate	5–25	0.5	10	0.5–5.0	0.05	10		Chambon et al. (1966)
				0.2–1.2		21		Kincl et al. (1965a)
					0.5			Matscher and Lupo (1960)
Medroxy-progesterone acetate	1.2		10	0.5[(1)]		20		Glenn et al. (1959)
Allylestrenol				1.0				Duncan et al. (1964)
Norgesterone		2.0	14	1				Matscher and Lupo (1960)
								Madjerek et al. (1960)
Melengestrol acetate	0.8		10					Matscher and Lupo (1960)
								Duncan et al. (1964)

Note to Table 17
(1) Author's remark: "much more active than progesterone".

inhibition based on the principle that an ovary (guinea pig) grafted into the spleen of a spayed animal will become hypertrophic because its estrogens, drained into the liver, will be inactivated and so prevented from reaching the pituitary. The de-inhibited hypophysis can be repressed by certain steroids as judged by measuring the surface of the grafted ovary and its follicles. Compounds to be tested are administered as a subcutaneous depot every 10 days, for a total of 90 days. In this way norethisterone acetate in a depot dose of 10 mg (repeated 9 times) was found to inhibit FSH production partly and ICSH production completely (reduced surface of follicles, no corpora lutea). Cessation of treatment is followed by "tremendous ovarian hypertrophy" (Haller, 1964).

6.3. PITUITARY INHIBITION SHOWN BY EFFECTS ON THE MALE GONAD

Another method of demonstrating inhibition of the gonadotrophic function of the pituitary consists in administering the compounds to be tested to *male* rats and looking for atrophy of the testicles. Results of such tests are shown in Table 17. In rabbits Cominos *et al.* (1962) found norethisterone in daily parenteral doses of 0.5 mg, given during 30 days, to reduce the weight of testicles, seminal vesicles and prostate, and to cause some atrophy of Leydig cells and some reversible reduction of spermatogenesis. Ericsson *et al.* (1964) measured volume of ejaculate and sperm count in rabbits given injections of 10 mg chlormadinone acetate or progesterone every other day and found a decrease in both parameters with either steroid, which progressed during prolonged treatment, the sperm count reaching a minimum after about 20 weeks. Thereafter it rose again notwithstanding continued treatment. There was considerable histological damage to the gonads.

6.4. THE CONTENT OF GONADOTROPHIC HORMONES IN THE PITUITARIES OF STEROID-TREATED ANIMALS

The ICSH content of the pituitaries of intact rats could be lowered by oral (gavage) administration of 1.5 to 4 mg of lynestrenol daily for 21 days as judged by grafting the pituitaries into male recipient rats and weighing their ventral prostate lobes. Fourteen days after the end of the treatment the gonadotrophic activity was increased again almost to the level of untreated controls (Uhlarik *et al.*, 1964). The gonadotrophin content in the pituitary of the castrated rats is increased and can be brought back to normal by the administration of pituitary-inhibiting steroids. Saunders (1964a) studied these regulating effects by spaying adult female rats, treating them with steroids for 30 days, starting on the day of operation, and injecting their homogenized pituitaries into immature intact (recipient) rats. The ovarian and uterine weights of the latter were indicative of the gonadotrophin content of the pituitaries of the donor (whose uterine weights reflected any estrogenic or uterotrophic effects of the injected steroids). In this test progesterone—even in very high daily doses (10 mg)—did not significantly reduce the gonadotrophin content of the donors' pituitaries (in striking contrast with estrogens as well as androgens). Norethynodrel caused some inhibition at very low doses (2 mcg). This became significant at a level of 8 mcg and complete at 200 mcg; 800 mcg reduced the level below normal (Saunders, 1964b).

Norethisterone, which has only one-tenth of the uterotrophic potency of norethynodrel (Saunders, 1964a), was also clearly less potent in suppressing the pituitary gonadotrophin content. In contrast to the estrogens proper (estrone, estradiol and diethylstilbestrol), which produced no pituitary inhibition in doses below levels that raised the donor's uterine weight from the castrate to the intact rat level, norethisterone and norethynodrel showed partial pituitary inhibition in doses that were much less "estrogenic" or uterotrophic.

Somewhat comparable experiments were performed by Kraehahn and von Berswordt-Wallrabe (1969), who injected norethisterone acetate (1 mg/100 g bodyweight) daily for 12 days into adult female rats and determined the FSH and LH content in their pituitaries by extraction and subsequent bio-assay and also by implantation into hypophysectomized immature rats. In addition the serum of the donor rats was assayed for FSH and LH (=ICSH) activity. In these studies they followed those of de Jongh's group in Leyden (Paesi et al., 1957; Paesi and van Rees, 1960), which enabled them to distinguish between the ability of the pituitary to produce, to store and to release gonadotrophin.

Norethisterone was found to increase ICSH and FSH levels in the pituitaries, not in the serum, where ICSH was totally absent and FSH significantly reduced. "The hypophyseal propensity for the release" of these hormones "was also reduced". The steroid prevented the normal ovulatory LH peak, found in the control animals. By direct determination of the LH content in the pituitaries of immature female rats (OAAD test of Parlow) and expressing it in mcg of an NIH reference standard, Labhsetwar (1966a) found that medroxyprogesterone acetate in twice-weekly 12.5 mg doses, by injection, for 5 weeks lowered the LH concentration from 1.93 ± 0.39 to 0.39 ± 0.12 mcg/mg wet pituitary and total LH content from 9.70 to 1.19 mcg/gland/100 g bodyweight. The sensitivity of the ovaries of these animals to exogenous gonadotrophin (PMS + HCG) appeared not to be reduced.

When chlormadinone acetate was used in similar experiments (Labhsetwar, 1968)—daily subcutaneous injections of 0.4 mg for 10 days to intact or unilaterally ovariectomized rats—it caused a very conspicuous rise in pituitary FSH and LH, which together with reduced ovarian and uterine weights was considered as indicating that the release, not the synthesis, of the gonadotrophins was impaired. The author furthermore assumes that LH secretion—viz. the ovulatory surge—is more strongly affected than secretion of FSH. The differences between these results and those obtained earlier with medroxyprogesterone acetate need not be due, or not wholly due, to qualitative differences between the compounds, since dosages and duration of treatment differed considerably.

Summarizing we may state that various progestational compounds have been found to increase the stores of hormones in the pituitaries of rats, due to inhibition of release, in experiments of short duration.

After more prolonged treatment, the hormone content in the pituitaries has repeatedly been found decreased, apparently because of interference with hormone synthesis.

6.5. PITUITARY HISTOLOGY

Further evidence for inhibition is furnished by *histological and weight changes of the pituitary.* Thus *norethynodrel* in daily subcutaneous doses of 0.2 mg/kg, given to rats for 33 to 86 days, was shown by Holmes and Mandl (1962) to cause a decrease in the relative volume of pituitary tissue occupied by basophilic cells (considered to be the source of FSH and LH; see Purves, 1961) and increase of chromophobe cells, the function of which is not quite clear.

A decrease in pituitary weight was also observed by Liu and Lin (1970) after 10 weeks of treatment of female rats with 1250 mcg norethynodrel (or 50 mcg mestranol) p.o., 3 times weekly. The animals so treated also gained significantly less weight than controls and their pituitaries contained less growth hormone than normal ones, which seemed to be due to a reduced rate of synthesis of GH. The effect of norethynodrel may have been due to its estrogenic activity.

Medroxyprogesterone acetate, given to rats daily (dose not stated) for 4 weeks, caused cytological changes indicative of suppression of the secretion of ACTH "and some components of the gonadotrophic complex" (Baker and Clapp, 1964). ACTH depletion after treatment with this steroid, known for its adrenal-inhibiting action, had been earlier recorded by Holub et al. (1961).

Logothetopoulos et al. (1961) injected medroxyprogesterone acetate in daily doses of 1.5 mg per 100 g bodyweight into rats starting on the second to fourth day after birth and continuing for 70 or 110 days. "The pituitaries of the treated animals were decreased in size. The complete absence of gonadotrophs was striking." These are defined as the oval basophils which do not stain with aldehyde-fuchsin, according to Purves and Griesbach (1951); delta cells of Halmi (1950). (The observations of the authors on ACTH and the adrenal are discussed in subsection 20.)

Ectors et al. (1966) have to some extent repeated these studies, in as much as they gave medroxyprogesterone acetate in daily doses of 1 to 4 mg/kg/day during 14 days, but they claim greater specificity for their method of staining. By this they can demonstrate that LH-producing cells in the pituitaries of treated rats show a very strong retention of PAS-positive granules (even more pronounced than in the preovulatory phase of untreated animals), whereas prolactin-producing cells appear to be very much stimulated ("de manière spectaculaire") and thereby have lost their granules. (In accordance with this they see strong mammary hyperplasia.) The authors could prove that the prolactin content of these glands is depleted and they state that the ovulation-inhibiting activity of the compound, accompanied by stimulation of prolactin secretion, is comparable to the effect of high doses of progesterone. Pasteels and Ectors (1967) showed that the potency of extracts from rat hypothalamus to depress prolactin production of rat pituitaries on incubation in vitro is reduced by prior treatment of the hypothalamus donors with medroxyprogesterone acetate.

As a corollary to these studies reference should be made to those of Baker et al. (1965) who found the secretion of prolactin increased and that of LH decreased in young adult female rats injected with norethynodrel, as judged by the activity of the corpora lutea (prolactin is luteotrophic in the rat) and the involution of interstitial tissue, apparently mediated by the pituitary. (See also subsection 19, Effects on the mammary gland, and subsection 8, Activation of corpora lutea.)

In daily oral doses of 30 mg, medroxyprogesterone acetate, administered to baboons for 1 to 6 months, was found by Goisis (1964) to cause "sharp inhibition of the anterior pituitary ... with histofunctional depression of all basophils", but, referring to an earlier report, the author states "progesterone does not inhibit the genital tract through the pituitary gland, the cytology of which remains completely normal".

The effects of norethisterone acetate on the pituitary of *male rats* were studied by Gerard *et al.* (1963). Adult animals received 2 mg daily for periods varying between 24 hours and 10 days. The immediate effect (after 24 hours) was very conspicuous. Hyperemia (congestion of capillaries) and cytological changes in the basophils (pale and vesiculated nuclei); after 48 hours there is progressive cytoplasmic degranulation. These changes become more pronounced in the course of the next days when basophils increase in number and typical castration cells appear. At the end of 10 days these are very numerous and many appear to be in the process of destruction. The picture resembles that after castration but developing at a highly increased rate.

This apparently contrasts to some extent with the studies of Dhom *et al.* (1965) who treated intact adult and castrated male and female rats with norethisterone by gavage, and immature males with injections in doses varying between 0.2 and 1 mg per 100 g bodyweight, and in all categories found "cytological phenomena of secretion and production inhibition. . . . Reduction in size of cells and of nuclear surface." Castration hyperplasia was suppressed and puberal maturation of the gonadotrophic system of the pituitary gland markedly inhibited.

The discrepancy between the two last-mentioned results seems to be entirely due to the difference in dosage. As Neumann pointed out, the high doses employed by Gerard would, on account of the estrogenicity of norethisterone, predominantly stimulate prolactin-producing cells and this would mask the inhibition of the gonadotrophin secretors.

7. FACILITATION OF OVULATION

The conditions under which progesterone can induce ovulation have been fully discussed in Chapter 13. Synthetic compounds have been tested for this ability, often in combination with gonadotrophic hormones, the efficacy of which can be increased by progesterone and some of its substitutes. R. K. Meyer and his group in Wisconsin have shown that "a properly timed injection of progesterone markedly increases the percentage of immature rats which ovulate in response to a single injection of pregnant mare serum gonadotrophin (PMS) . . . ovulation is caused by a release of pituitary ovulating hormone . . . which occurs on the afternoon of the day that progesterone is administered" (McCormack and Meyer, 1965).

In one of these studies PMS alone (15 I.U. subcutaneously on the 22nd day of life) caused ovulations in 25% of the animals, releasing an average number of 9.3 ± 5.5 ova per ovulating rat. One single injection of 0.05 mg of progesterone on day 24 raised these values to 75% and 45.7 ± 8.6 ova; 0.5 mg produced ovulations in all the animals. Comparable results were obtained with the steroids shown in Table 18.

TABLE 18. INDUCTION OF OVULATION IN PMS-TREATED IMMATURE RATS
Adapted from McCormack and Meyer (1965)
Doses are in mg, given in one single injection 2 days after PMS priming.

Compound	No. of rats	Dose	% of rats ovulating
Vehicle (CMC)			25
Progesterone	8	0.05	75
	4	0.5	100
Norethisterone	10	0.05	80
	8	0.5	100
Norethynodrel	9	0.05	33
	12	0.5	91
Medroxyprogesterone acetate	8	0.031	87
	4	0.125	100

By treating immature rats of about 40 to 75 g body weight with chlormadinone acetate orally in a daily dose of 100 mg/kg and with gonadotrophins (10 I.U. PMS or 25 I.U. HCG), Harper (1964) found that the steroid did not affect the ovarian weight response "but undoubtedly facilitated the induction of ovulation". In a subsequent study with chlormadinone given for 8 days and a single dose of HCG on the 8th day, the steroid greatly increased uterine weight, but there was no augmenting effect in hypophysectomized animals. The author suggests that these effects could be explained by assuming that chlormadinone inhibits the release of LH, thus causing its storage in the pituitary whereupon HCG would trigger its release.

Kincl (1964b) gave one single dose of PMS to immature, 22-day-old, rats, and steroids 48 hours later by injection. Ovulation was induced by injecting 75 mcg of progesterone, norethisterone or dydrogesterone. This compound was also tested by means of injection into rats with 5-day cycles, where shortening to 4 days was considered evidence of induction of ovulation and the activity of dydrogesterone (1.5 mg) found equal to that of progesterone. The same effect was seen by overriding the inhibition of ovulation caused by pentobarbital (Claassen, 1968).

TABLE 19. ACTIVITY OF PROGESTATIONAL STEROIDS TO FACILITATE OVULATION IN RATS

Compound	Dose (mg)	Mode of administration	Evidence of effectiveness	Reference
Progesterone	0.05	1 injection, 48 hr after PMS	75% of rats ovulating	McCormack and Meyer (1965)
	0.5	"	100%	"
	0.2	1 injection, 24 hr after PMS	45% of rats ovulating 48 hr after PMS	Gallo and Zarrow (1970)
	0.5	1 injection, 24 hr after PMS	42%	Gallo and Zarrow (1970)
	1.0	1 injection, 24 hr after PMS	72%	Gallo and Zarrow (1970)
	2.0	1 injection, 24 hr after PMS	78%	Gallo and Zarrow (1970)
	0.075	1 injection, 48 hr after PMS	10/12 rats ovulating	Kincl (1964b)
	1.5	1 injection on day 3 of 5-day cycle	Shortening of cycle by 1 day	Claassen (1968)
	0.5	3 hr before pentobarbital on day 3 of cycle	Ovulation on day 4	Claassen (1968)
Dydrogesterone	1.5	1 injection on day 3	Shortening cycle	Claassen (1968)
	0.5	3 hr before pentobarbital	Ovulation on day 4	Claassen (1968)
	0.075	1 injection, 48 hr after PMS	4/6 rats ovulating	Kincl (1964b)
	0.05	1 injection, 48 hr after PMS	80% of rats ovulating	McCormack and Meyer (1965)
Norethisterone	0.5	1 injection, 48 hr after PMS	100%	"
	0.075	1 injection, 48 hr after PMS	3/5 rats ovulating	Kincl (1964b)
	0.5	1 injection, 24 hr after PMS	71% of rats ovulating 48 hr after PMS	Gallo and Zarrow (1970)
Medroxy-progesterone acetate	0.031	1 injection, 48 hr after PMS	87% of rats ovulating	McCormack and Meyer (1965)
	0.125	1 injection, 48 hr after PMS	100%	McCormack and Meyer (1965)
	0.100	1 injection, 24 hr after PMS	88% of rats ovulating 48 hr after PMS	Gallo and Zarrow (1970)
Chlormadinone acetate	100/kg/day (approx. 5 per day)	By gavage for 3 to 4 days together with PMS (3 days) or PMS (3 days) and HCG (1 day)	Presence of corpora lutea or advanced ovulation	Harper (1964)
	0.1	24 hr after PMS	Inactive	Gallo and Zarrow (1970)

Zarrow studied the ovulation-facilitating effect of progesterone in a different way. It was found (Zarrow and Gallo, 1969) that 2 mg of progesterone injected into immature rats 24 hours after an injection of 30 I.U. of PMS *advanced* ovulation by 24 hours (from the otherwise expected time of 72 hours after PMS). This effect could also be obtained (Gallo and Zarrow, 1970) with 0.1 mg of medroxyprogesterone or 0.5 mg of norethisterone, but not with 0.1 mg of chlormadinone acetate. As far as can be seen the doses of the synthetic compounds were the only ones tested and the statement of the authors, that "norethindrone and medroxyprogesterone proved equally as effective as progesterone itself", should therefore not be interpreted literally in a pharmacological sense.

Also inactive were "20α-OH-progesterone" (1 mg), corticosterone (1 mg), "20β-OH-progesterone" (0.5 mg), testosterone propionate (0.5 mg), and estradiol benzoate (1 and 50 mcg).

Data on ovulation-facilitating potency of progestational compounds are summarized in Table 19.

In the Japanese quail (*Coturnix coturnix japonica*) Kincl and Sickles (1969) were able to induce ovulations (increased egg production) by daily p.o. doses of 0.1 mg of chlormadinone acetate, while 10 mg was inhibitory, as was norethisterone in doses of 0.1 or 1.0 mg.

8. ACTIVATION OF CORPORA LUTEA AND INDUCTION OF PSEUDOPREGNANCY

Progesterone has been shown not only to induce ovulation under certain conditions but also to activate corpora lutea, a process which in the rat involves an increased secretion of the luteotrophic hormone LTH or prolactin. Some synthetic compounds have been tested for this potency. Thus norethynodrel in a dose of 1.5 mg/100 g body weight for 2 to 5 days was found to cause enlargement of corpora lutea and lipid depletion, not after hypophysectomy (Baker *et al.*, 1965). There were indications that an increase in prolactin secretion went *pari passu* with a decrease in LH secretion.

Labhsetwar (1966b) gave adult rats two s.c. injections of 0.2 to 0.6 mg of norethynodrel on the day of proestrus and again on the day of estrus and the day thereafter applied a deciduoma test, which led to the conclusion that the treatment had activated the corpora lutea.

An increased prolactin content was found in the pituitary of castrated rats injected with 0.375 or 1.5 mg/100 g norethynodrel daily for 7 days (Kahn and Baker, 1966). It is interesting to note that the same authors had found strong stimulation of mammary development in intact rats treated with the same dose of norethynodrel but for a longer period (28 days). Induction of hypophyseal release of prolactin was invoked to explain the effect (Kahn and Baker, 1964). It will be remembered that the secretion of prolactin—unlike that of the gonadotrophins—is regulated by the hypothalamus, not by means of a releaser but of an inhibitor. Evidence of increased prolactin secretion (brought about by repression of the inhibitor) under the influence of medroxyprogesterone acetate has been discussed in subsection 6.5, Pituitary histology.

A hypothalamic effect, causing increased prolactin secretion, is also suggested by the studies of Richards (1966) who was able to prolong pseudopregnancy (induced by sterile mating) in golden hamsters by the injection of 2×5 mg progesterone (in aqueous suspension) or of 1×2.5 mg medroxyprogesterone acetate (Depo-Provera®). A daily dose of 1.25–2.5 mg of this compound given orally 7 days to adult rats caused "delaying the reappearance of estrus comparable to that seen in pseudopregnancy (11.0–16.0 days)", as reported by Velardo and Fedden (1964).

9. OTHER EFFECTS ON THE CENTRAL NERVOUS SYSTEM

Sawyer and his group (Sawyer, 1965) studied the effects of electric stimuli on sharply defined hypothalamic areas in the rabbit. As discussed in Chapter 17, they distinguished between an "EEG arousal" and an "EEG after-reaction". The thresholds for both responses had been found to drop sharply after the injection of progesterone during estrus and to rise to high levels during the ensuing progesterone-dominated anestrus. Medroxyprogesterone acetate, like progesterone, showed this biphasic effect on EEG arousal but only a rise in the EEG after-reaction. Norethindrone also raised the EEG after-reaction curve during the period of effective blockade of ovulation.

The group (Kawakami and Sawyer, 1967) studied the effects of several synthetic steroids on these reactions. Their conclusions are very interesting. The compounds were all injected into adult female rabbits after 2 days of estrogen priming. The animals had electrodes permanently implanted in cortical and subcortical regions of the brain and the electroencephalic reactions were induced by high-frequency stimulation of the medial reticular formation (arousal) or low-frequency stimulation of the mamillary peduncle (after-reaction). Progesterone (2 mg) caused a lowering of these thresholds, reaching a nadir after about 5 to 8 hours and thereafter a rise, starting about 12 hours after injection, reaching a peak at about 24 hours.

Chlormadinone acetate (2 mg) "gave threshold curves very similar to those of progesterone itself at the same dosage", which surprised the authors since they had expected higher activity on the basis of antiovulatory activity ratios (as assessed by Kincl and Dorfman, 1963a). ("On the other hand, the more active 19-norprogesterone was four times as potent as chlormadinone both on thresholds and on antiovulatory capacity.")

"Medroxyprogesterone gave unusual results in as much as dosages which induced biphasic influences on the EEG arousal threshold and behavior in the estrogen-primed doe failed to lower the EEG after-reaction threshold."

Norethynodrel and norethisterone, on the other hand, "in ovulation-blocking dosages in the rabbit (1 and 5 mg) gave threshold curves fundamentally different from those of the progesterone derivatives." They influenced arousal threshold very little if at all, but differentially elevated the EEG after-reaction threshold curve with no prior depression. With norethynodrel (given orally)... the curves remained elevated more than 24 hours, and 1 mg/day norethynodrel kept the threshold up. This was not true of norethindrone; it raised the after-reaction threshold for a few hours, but by 24 hours, at which time it still blocked copulation-induced ovulation, the threshold had dropped to preinjection levels. It is suggested that this may be a further indication of the assumed direct effect on the pituitary, in conformity with the results of Hilliard et al. (1966b) discussed by us in subsection 5.5.2, Mechanism of pituitary inhibition. See also subsection 16.3 (p. 133) for influences on mating behavior and anesthetic effects.

Anticonvulsant effects of steroids have become a subject of interest since Spiegel and Wycis (1945) showed that some such compounds, including testosterone and progesterone under certain conditions, increase the threshold of production of convulsions by electric stimulation of the brain (through an electrode in the conjunctival sac) in female rats. 6-(α)Acetoxyprogesterone acetate is recorded as inactive in doses of 5 and 10 mg per 100 g bodyweight.

Woolley and Timiras (1962 showed—though by a more elaborate technique and with far more data—that progesterone, administered in daily doses of 250–375 mcg per 100 g bodyweight to immature, ovariectomized rats and in doses of 500 mcg/100 g to mature ovariectomized females, decreased excitability, i.e. increased the seizure threshold for

TABLE 20. Compounds Active in Maintaining Pregnancy in Rabbits, Castrated on Day of Pregnancy Indicated in Column 2, by Daily Dose of Compounds, in mg, Given in Column 3, Resulting in Percentage of Fetal Survival in Column 5

Compound	Day of castration	Daily dose giving maximum effect		First and last day of treatment	Percentage of survival (for explanation of FSI see p. 92)	Ineffective dose		Activity as percentage of act. of progesterone (progesterone subcut. =100)		Reference
		oral	subcut.			oral	subcut.	oral	subcut.	
Progesterone	14		1 mg/kg	14–32	FSI 58					Brennan and Kraay (1963)
	10		1 mg/kg	10–17	16/18$^{(3)}$					Saunders and Drill (1958)
Chlormadinone acetate	14		0.25–1 mg/kg	14–32	FSI 52–70					Brennan and Kraay (1963)
		0.5–1 mg/kg		14–32	FSI 150–60	0.25				Brennan and Kraay (1963)
Medroxy-progesterone acetate	14	1 mg/kg	0.025–0.5 mg/kg	14–32	FSI 48–52					Brennan and Kraay (1963)
				14–32	FSI 85				400	Desaulles and Krähenbühl (1962)

Compound								Reference
Norgestrienone	13	5	10-40(1)	14-27 11 or 14-31	80-100		50	Roussel (1966) Wu (1962)
Allylestrenol	14	20-40	(1)	11 or 14-31	100	5-10		Wu (1962)
Dimethisterone	8	25(2) plus 5 mcg ethynyl estradiol		8-31	2 of 11 rabbits produced normal litters(2)			Aydar and Greenblatt (1961)
Normethandrone	10		1 mg/kg	10-17	1 out of 5 rabbits protected			Saunders and Drill (1958)
							50-100	Desaulles and Krähenbühl (1962)
Dydrogesterone	11-14	5		6, 7 or 15 days after castration	83	5	12.5	Jost (1963)
		200		,, ,,	95			

Notes to Table 20
(1) Total daily doses, subdivided into two, three or more daily administrations.
(2) Compound in "aqueous solution . . . was administered as part of the daily fluid intake". "Nine rabbits were overdue and autopsies revealed whole or partial reabsorption of all the fetuses."
(3) "Number of rabbits protected": 16 out of 18. Autopsy 7 days after spaying.

20 days, after which the effect was reversed. Estradiol lowered the threshold and this effect was delayed by the concomitant action of progesterone. No synthetic analogues were tested. Stitt and Kinnard (1968) confirmed that estradiol lowers the seizure threshold when injected into rats (4 mcg/day/100 g bw) daily for 7 days, whereas progesterone (0.5 mg daily per 100 g bw) for 7 days had practically no effect. Medroxyprogesterone acetate, either alone (1 mg/100 g/day, 7 times) or in combination with ethynyl estradiol, caused a very slight *lowering* of the threshold, a lowering significant only with the combination. Norethynodrel with or without mestranol behaved similarly. The latter drugs also caused a significant fall in seizure threshold when applied topically to the cerebral cortex of cats.

According to Overbeek *et al.* (1962) lynestrenol in very high doses "considerably reduced" exploratory behavior (Bonta, 1958) 1 hour after oral administration, not after 48 hours, a fact which is described by the investigators as "not surprising, since this test is more suitable for the study of central nervous system inhibitors than for stimulators".

Suchowsky *et al.* (1969) report that the aggressive behavior of male mice, kept in isolation and permitted to encounter a non-isolated smaller partner every 5th day, was completely inhibited by treatment with estradiol (1 mcg daily) and partly with progesterone (1.0 mg) or medroxyprogesterone acetate (MAP, 1.0 mg) daily for 15 days. In castrated isolated mice aggressive behavior was readily induced by testosterone propionate, moderately by progesterone, never by MAP. In these animals norethisterone or norethynodrel (1.0 mg/day) induced aggressive behavior which became manifest only after the termination of treatment, as is also seen with combination of testosterone propionate and estradiol.

10. MAINTENANCE OF PREGNANCY

Only a limited group of orally active synthetic progestational compounds can replace progesterone in maintaining pregnancy in animals, ovariectomized after conception (see Chapter 10). The effect may be dose-dependent, the higher dose safeguarding the survival of a greater percentage of fetuses. Rabbits and rats differ in their response to replacement therapy and are dealt with separately below.

Some authors use numerical values to indicate the efficacy of a compound, such as a "fetal survival index (FSI)" in rabbits (Brennan and Kraay, 1963), expressing the number of fetuses found on day 32 of pregnancy as a percentage of those present on day 14 when the animals were castrated. These authors also count dead and resorbing fetuses, multiplying the number of the first by 0.5 and of the latter by 0.25. The justification for this sort of arithmetic is found in the fact that "placebo treatment following ovariectomy on day 14 consistently results in complete obliteration of fetal material by the end of gestation". The presence of fetuses dead or in the process of being resorbed does, therefore, after all reflect a certain degree of hormonal protection. A "net success index", NSI, was introduced for work with rats (Stucki, 1958). It is calculated by the formula

$$\text{NSI} = \frac{\text{Living young/group}}{\text{No. of mothers/group} \times 11 \text{ implantation sites}} \times 100.$$

Table 20 lists compounds found active in maintaining pregnancy in rabbits, Table 21 lists inactive ones.

Compounds active in rats are listed in Table 22 and inactive ones in Table 23.

TABLE 21. COMPOUNDS FOUND NOT TO MAINTAIN PREGNANCY IN THE CASTRATED RABBIT

Compound	Day of castration	First and last day of treatment	Highest daily dose found inactive		Reference
			subcut.	oral	
Norethisterone	14	14–21	8 mg		Allen and Wu (1959)
		12–31	21 mg[1]		
Norethynodrel	10	10–17	1 mg/kg		Saunders and Drill (1958)

(1) After injecting 1 mg daily from day 12 to day 31 after mating followed by cesarian section on day 32, there were twenty fetuses near term in size but dead and macerated. With higher doses (4 and 8 mg) there was no evidence that pregnancy had survived much beyond the day of castration.

The rat requires much higher doses of progesterone or of synthetic substitutes than the rabbit. Whereas in rabbits doses of 1 to 2 mg of progesterone per kg bodyweight injected daily will normally suffice to preserve pregnancy after ovariectomy, the rat, with only one-tenth of the bodyweight, needs 5 to 10 mg daily or as much as 50 mg/kg daily (see Chapter 10).

Similar ratios were found for some synthetic compounds that were tested in both species. Thus medroxyprogesterone acetate was found to give at least partial protection in doses of 0.025–0.5 mg/kg in rabbits (Brennan and

TABLE 22. COMPOUNDS MAINTAINING PREGNANCY IN RATS CASTRATED ON DAY OF FIRST TREATMENT OR ONE DAY LATER, WHEN GIVEN IN DAILY DOSES INDICATED IN COLUMN 3

Rate of success (column 4) indicated as percentage of fetuses present on day of castration. NSI means net success index (p. 93). Doses of estrogens in mcg, EE stands for ethynyl estradiol.

Compound	First and last day of treatment	Effective dose in mg		Normal fetuses at end of treatment		Percentage of animals pregnant at the end of treatment	Subcutaneous activity expressed as percentage of activity of progesterone (subcut. = 100)	Reference
		oral	subcut.	percentage	mean number			
Progesterone	8–21		25 mg/kg		3.1(1)	70		David et al. (1963)
	8–20		3.0			90		Kobayashi (1962)
			5	ED$_{50}$	4(3)	100		Suchowsky (1963)
			8	NSI:36	6.8	100		Stucki (1958)
			4 + 1 estrone(4)	NSI:62				Stucki (1958)
Normethandrone			0.3	ED$_{50}$	5.3	33		Suchowsky (1963)
			10.0	16.3			100–200	Madjerek et al. (1960)
								Desaulles and Krähenbühl (1962)
Norgestrel	8–17	10.0	1.0		8.7	87.5		Edgren et al. (1966a)
	8–17		1 + 10 EE		8.6	62.5		Edgren et al. (1966a)
					0.0	0.0		Edgren et al. (1966a)
Dydrogesterone	14–20	10.0(4)	1.250	86				Marois (1962b)
	10–21	10.0 + 10 EE(5)	0.080 + 1 estradiol benzoate	70		80		Marois (1962b)
								Schöler (1964)
								Schöler (1964)
		0.312(2)		75			ca. 100	Schöler (1964)
		+2 EE						
		0.625(2)		100				Schöler (1964)
		+4 EE						
Allylestrenol	9–21	6.0	1.6	ED$_{50}$	8	55		Suchowsky (1963)
	10–16	10.0		40.9				Madjerek et al. (1960)
								Desaulles and Krähenbühl (1962)
Melengestrol acetate	8–20	10.0	5.0 + 0.5 EE	NSI:89		25		Kobayashi et al. (1962)
			0.05 + 0.1 estradiol			20		Kobayashi et al. (1962)
			0.10 + 0.1 estradiol	NSI:61		100		Duncan et al. (1964)
						100		Duncan et al. (1964)

Orally Active Progestational Compounds: Animal Studies

Compound	Days	Dose	ED$_{50}$			References
Medroxy-progesterone acetate	8-21	0.2				Suchowsky (1963); David et al. (1963)
	9-20	7.5-10/kg$^{(2)}$	14.4	5.2-5.9	90-100	Madjerek et al. (1960)
	8-20	10.0	NSI:82	9	22	Stucki (1958)
	8-20	5.0$^{(2)}$	NSI:70		100	
	8-20	2.5	NSI:64			Duncan et al. (1964)
		0.625	NSI:55	4.3	50-100	Duncan et al. (1964); Revesz and Chappel (1966); Revesz and Chappel (1966)
	9-20	0.1 + 0.1 estradiol	NSI:82			
	9 (single dose)	0.15 + 0.1 estradiol	14.4			
	9 (single dose)	10.0	80		2500	Desaulles and Krähenbühl (1962)
Medro-gestone	9-20	2.0	54.7	7.6	66	Revesz and Chappel (1966)
		5.0	100	10.6	100	Revesz and Chappel (1966)
	9 (single dose)	10.0	25	6.4	50	Revesz and Chappel (1966)
	9 (single dose)	12.0	60.8			Revesz and Chappel (1966)
			84.3			
Megestrol acetate	8-21	10.0/kg		2.3	70	David et al. (1963)
	8-21	10.0/kg + 0.5 EE		3.4	70	David et al. (1963)
	8-21	10.0/kg + 4.0 EE per kg		4.1	100	David et al. (1963)
Chlormadi-none acetate	8-21	18.0	45.6			Chambon and Le Vève (1966a)
	8-21	6	57.7			Chambon and Le Vève (1966a)
	8-21	2 + 0.05 EE				Chambon and Le Vève (1966b)

Notes to Table 22
(1) Figure for intact (sham-operated) controls: 9.3.
(2) Drug administered in the diet.
(3) Figure for intact controls 11.
(4) Figures given are not comparable with other figures in this table. Many dead or deformed fetuses were seen.
(5) With oral ethynyl estradiol many more live fetuses and no deformities.

TABLE 23. COMPOUNDS FOUND NOT TO MAINTAIN PREGNANCY IN SPAYED RATS IN DAILY DOSE INDICATED

Compound	Highest inactive daily dose (mg)		Reference
	oral	subcut.	
Ethisterone	10.0		Madjerek et al. (1960)
		25.0[1]	Stucki (1958)
Norethisterone	10.0		Madjerek et al. (1960)
		3.0	Edgren et al. (1966a)
		50.0[1]	Stucki (1958)
	10.0		Schneider and Rauscher (1959)
Dimethisterone	10.0		Madjerek et al. (1960)
Lynestrenol	10.0		Overbeek et al. (1962)
Norethynodrel		10.0[1]	Stucki (1958)
Quingestanol acetate	10.0		Mischler et al. (1969)

(1) Also inactive when combined with 1 mcg estrone/rat/day

Kraay, 1963) whereas in rats the lowest value for 50% protection is that of Suchowsky (1963) which amounts to 0.2 mg *per animal* and other authors gave higher doses. On the other hand, according to Desaulles and Krähenbühl this compound has 25 times the activity of progesterone in rats as against 4 times in rabbits. As with other biological effects of progestational compounds, quantitative comparisons are difficult and may easily give quite unreliable impressions. Qualitatively, however, the same compound will be either active or inactive in both species.

The mode of administration may be of major influence on the effect of treatment. With particular reference to the *mouse*, McGinty (1959) pointed out that normethandrone, norethandrone (17α-ethyl-19-nortestosterone) or norethisterone do not maintain pregnancy in the spayed female when given p.o. or s.c. once daily, even in doses as high as 5 mg, but they have this effect when mixed with the food at a daily intake between 0.6 and 2.0 mg and norethisterone also becomes effective when injected as a long-acting ester. Similar observations were made with respect to medroxyprogesterone acetate: when mixed with the food this compound had the same potency as norethisterone in this test.

An interesting question is raised by the different ways in which the addition of estrogens modifies the effects of progestational substances in the maintenance of pregnancy. Several authors (see Chapter 9, p. 280 and

Chapter 10, p. 296) say that very small amounts of estrogens markedly improve the protective effect of progesterone in the pregnant spayed rat. The same applies to some of the synthetic compounds. Stucki (1958) remarked: "With the exception of 17α-hydroxyprogesterone acetate, all compounds which maintained pregnancy when administered concomitantly with estrone also maintained pregnancy when administered alone. Higher doses were required, however, for comparable results." Dydrogesterone is reported as not maintaining pregnancy on oral administration unless combined with an estrogen. Schöler (1964) showed that the same percentage of live fetuses could be salvaged in spayed rats when decreasing doses of dydrogesterone were p.o. combined with increasing doses of ethynyl estradiol up to a certain limit. Larger quantities of ethynyl estradiol diminished the pregnancy-maintaining effect of dydrogesterone. Overbeek, referring to similar observations with respect to allylestrenol, has remarked (personally) that these facts might explain, why some progestational compounds, like lynestrenol and norethisterone, which are by themselves estrogenic, do not maintain pregnancy in spayed rats. In the case of norgestrel, which is markedly active in a subcutaneous daily dose of 1 mg, a much less active dose of 0.3 mg would show an increase in effectivity when combined with 0.1 to 1.0 mcg of ethynyl estradiol, but this is completely lost when the dose of the estrogen is raised to 10 mcg, so, like with progesterone, a certain ratio of progestational and estrogenic activities is required for optimum efficacy.

As has been pointed out (see subsection 2.3, p. 46) activity in the McGinty test in general seems to go with pregnancy-maintaining potency. This is apparently also paralleled—at least qualitatively—by deciduomagenic potency. A compound which cannot nidate a blastocyst in a spayed animal would appear not to maintain pregnancy if the animal is spayed a few days after *natural* nidation.

If the McGinty test is somehow related to the potency in maintaining pregnancy, this would almost of necessity have to be due to the fact that the compound concerned is active as such, without any prior metabolic changes, and could influence the myometrium locally as required by Csapo's theory. Csapo and Wiest (1969) have shown that rats ovariectomized between the 14th and 22nd days of pregnancy and given sustained progesterone treatment display distinct placental hypertrophy. This could be suppressed by the concomitant administration of 2–4 mcg per day of an estrogen (estradiol dipropionate). It is interesting, in this respect, that a somewhat similar effect has been observed in studies with injections of progesterone or allylestrenol given orally (van der Vies and Feenstra, 1967) to spayed—not to intact—rats during pregnancy. Placental weight increase was prevented by simultaneous administration of estradiol.

10.1. RELAXATION OF THE SYMPHYSIS PUBIS IN THE GUINEA PIG

The possible relationship between progesterone and relaxin has been discussed in Chapter 16, p. 370. This polypeptide hormone, characterized by its property of causing a relaxation of the symphyseal connective tissue and widening the gap between the pubic bones (in guinea pigs and other species), is believed to be produced in the uterus under the influence of progesterone.

Madjerek (1961) studied the effect of four synthetic progestational compounds on the symphysis of spayed female guinea pigs and compared it with that of progesterone. All the experimental animals received 2.5 mcg of estradiol benzoate (EB) daily for the duration of the treatment (15 days). (Progesterone without EB was entirely inactive, EB alone gave some dilatation (from 1.1 to 3.0 mm).) Together with EB, norethisterone and normethandrone in daily oral doses of 5.0 mg widened the symphysis to 3.6 and 3.8 mm respectively (considered by the author as doubtful), but progesterone (2.5 mg s.c. daily), allylestrenol and medroxyprogesterone acetate (5.0 mg orally per day) caused pubic distances of 7.5, 7.2 and 6.5 mm respectively. The author suggests that this property is associated with the ability to maintain pregnancy.

Casaglia and Gualandi (1961) equally found norethisterone and normethandrone inactive but medroxyprogesterone acetate highly active in this test. The presence of the uterus was essential.

Marois (1962c) treated guinea pigs with dydrogesterone (2.5 mg daily for 20 days, orally or s.c., together with 10 mcg of estradiol) and found this to cause progressive widening of the symphysis, which started to regress (at a dose of 10 mg per day) when the animals were hysterectomized on the 15th day of treatment. The drug was very effective when administered (at the same dose level) *in* the uterus. The author concludes that the mechanism of action of dydrogesterone on the symphysis pubis in the guinea pig is identical with that of progesterone.

11. PREVENTION OF OXYTOCIN-INDUCED PARTURITION

Just how some compounds exert their pregnancy-maintaining effect is only partly known. In all probability an action on uterine contractility is involved. On the other hand, the ability of a compound to maintain pregnancy in a castrated rodent is not necessarily reflected by its potency in counteracting the effect of oxytocin on the rabbit uterus at term and to prolong pregnancy beyond it.

Fuchs and Koch (1963) found that the effect of 10 mg progesterone, given by injection, could in this test be reproduced by the parenteral administration of 1 mg of medroxyprogesterone or 10 mg of dydrogesterone, but not by the same quantity of normethandrone nor of allylestrenol. These two steroids which were active when injected intramuscularly had essentially the same effect when injected into the amniotic sacs (5 mg of progesterone or 1 mg of medroxyprogesterone acetate, 3–6 hours prior to oxytocin induction).

Neumann and Hempel (1965) studied the prevention of oxytocin-induced labor in rabbits and found progesterone (subcutaneously, in oily solution) 100% active in a dose of 1.0 mg. The same activity was found for chlormadinone acetate. Norethisterone acetate in the same dose gave only 75% protection and the free alcohol 40%. Of allylestrenol 10 mg were needed for 83% protection.

The authors also found that chlormadinone acetate in oily solution needed 6 hours to become effective; as a microcrystalline suspension (intramuscularly or intravenously) it produced some effect after 3 hours, even in a much smaller dose (0.1 mg). A number of water-soluble esters of 17α-hydroxyprogesterone derivatives were shown to prevent induction of delivery when given intravenously as late as 1 hour before the oxytocin injection.

In the guinea pig Schofield (1964) could not delay spontaneous or oxytocin-induced delivery by injections of either progesterone or medroxyprogesterone acetate in doses of 2.5 mg 12-hourly intramuscularly or 10 mg daily subcutaneously. Similar results had been obtained by Zarrow et al. (1963).

In rats Edgren and Peterson (1966) found parturition could be delayed by daily steroid administration beginning on day 15 of pregnancy and continued until parturition or until autopsy (usually on day 25). For progesterone the ED_{50} dose was approximately 1 mg. For norgestrel it was 0.1 mg, for medroxyprogesterone acetate 0.3, and for norethisterone 1 mg. The corresponding Clauberg activities (expressed as percentage of progesterone = 100) are given for norgestrel as 900, for medroxyprogesterone acetate 3500, and for norethisterone 8.

12. INFLUENCE ON CONTRACTILITY OF THE NON-PREGNANT UTERUS

The suppression of the response of the uterus to oxytocin was one of the first biological effects of corpus luteum extracts to be discovered and there is ample evidence that it is inherent in progesterone.

Luraschi (1958) studied the effects of progesterone, ethisterone, normethandrone, norethisterone and norethynodrel on the spontaneous activity and oxytocin response of the uterus of castrated rats *in vitro* after priming the animals *in vivo* with one dose of estradiol valerianate and administering the progestational compounds (beginning 6 days later) orally. One dose level only (0.1 mg/day) was studied of each compound. Of progesterone this dose was given orally and parenterally. All these doses inhibited spontaneous contractile activity and oxytocin response, the estran derivatives apparently more than progesterone, but quantitative comparison would hardly appear to be permissible.

König and Haller (1965) studied the influence of several orally active progestational compounds on the response of the rat uterus to oxytocin and acetylcholine *in vitro* and compared it with that of progesterone. As a solvent they used Lutrol 9, an "ethylated polymer of propylene glycol".

Progesterone, added to the medium in a concentration of 3 mcg/ml, reduced the height of oxytocin contractions 60 seconds later by 50%. Of the synthetic compounds ethynodiol acetate was active in a dose of 16 mcg, followed in order of decreasing activity by norethisterone acetate (18 mcg), chlormadinone acetate (20 mcg), allylestrenol (32 mcg) and finally lynestrenol (53 mcg). Five times these doses were required to bring about the same degree of inhibition of contractions elicited by acetylcholine.

The authors describe the effect of progesterone as "completely reversible", unlike that of the synthetic substitutes. By this they mean that the effect of progesterone is visible only immediately at the end of the 60-second period of action (when the drug was apparently washed out). There was no residual effect on contractions, elicited by oxytocin 5 minutes after the addition of progesterone, and no cumulative effect when this experiment was repeated 8 times in the course of 80 minutes. Allylestrenol, on the other hand, under the same conditions, caused progressive inhibition, leading to complete absence of response after 80 minutes and the same held, with slight variations for the other compounds investigated. 30–120 minutes later, oxytocin sensitivity returned. Dutta and Sanyal (1969) studied the effect of norethisterone added *in vitro* to a bath containing the uteri of spayed rats or mice, pretreated *in vivo* with estradiol benzoate for 3 days

(2 mcg or 0.2 mcg, respectively, per day), and found that in rats the drug, in concentrations of at least 1.25 mcg/ml, reversibly reduced the tone and spontaneous contractions and suppressed the response to oxytocin. The influence on contractions and oxytocin sensitivity (not on tone) was comparable with that of progesterone. Norethisterone acted on the uterus of mice in a similar way as in rats but at somewhat higher doses. By contrast medroxyprogesterone acetate had no such effects in either rats or mice.

Allylestrenol was studied by Willems and de Schaepdrijver (1966) in ovariectomized rabbits, primed with daily injections of 30 mcg estradiol for 7 days and thereafter treated with 1 mcg estradiol with or without 5 mg allylestrenol s.c. daily for 3 days. Uterus contractions were measured isometrically *in situ* in the anesthetized animal and found to be considerably reduced (from a force of 36.6 to 22.7 g) by allylestrenol. Pharmacological studies revealed a preponderance of α-receptors in the estradiol as well as in the progesterone-dominated uterus, but a preponderance of β-receptors under the influence of allylestrenol (as is found in the progesterone-dominated uterus at the end of gestation). Epinephrine under these conditions inhibited spontaneous motility. The guinea-pig uterus was studied after addition of a variety of steroids *in vitro* by Gazzaniga *et al.* (1962), with a view to determining their influence on oxytocin contractions. Of the progestational substances progesterone had the strongest inhibitory effect, followed by medroxyprogesterone acetate and lynestrenol in that order.

Neumann and Hempel (1965) in *in vitro* studies found high doses of water-soluble 17α-hydroxyprogesterone derivatives to produce some inhibition of the oxytocin response of the non-pregnant rat uterus. Medroxyprogesterone acetate (MAP) administered orally (50 mcg daily for 6 days) was found by Matscher and Lupo (1959) to have a strong inhibiting effect on spontaneous and oxytocin-induced uterine contractions of rats pretreated with estradiol benzoate. At this dosage MAP was superior to 100 mcg of progesterone (subcutaneously) but inferior to 1 mg of 17α-acetoxyprogesterone (orally) given daily for the same period. These dosages corresponded to the "Clauberg activities" found earlier.

Norgesterone (also called vinylestrenolone) was examined by Lupo and Poggi (1964) for its effect on spontaneous and oxytocin-induced contractions of the uterus of adult, spayed rats treated with 5 mcg of estradiol benzoate (s.c.) for 3 days and thereafter for 6 days with daily oral doses of 50 or 100 mcg of the progestational compound.

This treatment practically abolished the effect of the estrogens and reduced the spontaneous and oxytocin-induced contractions to the low amplitudes of castrated controls. The effect was far more pronounced than that of 6 daily injections of 100 mcg progesterone.

In summary, several progestational compounds have been found to have a depressing effect on spontaneous or pharmacologically induced uterine motility, when administered "in vivo" or added to the uterus "in vitro".

13. ESTROGENIC, METROTROPHIC AND ANTIESTROGENIC ACTIVITY

13.1. INTRODUCTORY REMARKS

In assessing the estrogenic activity of progestational compounds the conventional methods, the Allen–Doisy test and the uterine weight method present certain difficulties.

In the vaginal cycle progesterone modifies the structure of the epithelium. It has been argued (de Jongh, 1968) that this effect of progesterone should not be called *antiestrogenic*, but on the other hand it does, of course, terminate estrus. Also, since the appearance or disappearance of estrous smears depends on the *ratio* of estrogen to progesterone, as has been known for a long time (see Chapter 9), it makes sense to call the effect of progesterone antiestrogenic (as is indeed customary), as long as one realizes that the condition induced is not identical with that due simply to the absence of estrogen.

If uterine growth is used as the yardstick it is again a matter of terminology whether or not one calls all "metrotrophic" actions estrogenic. Edgren (1958) found that compounds that have steep dose-response curve slopes are true estrogens because they also produce vaginal cornification in spayed rats, "whereas those with impeded slopes may be estrogens, androgens, or progestins". Quantitative differences may certainly be found in the assessment of "estrogenicity", depending on the method, viz. vaginal smears or uterine growth.

Attention should be called to the fact that at a relatively early period a number of investigators certainly used progestational compounds of the estrane series that contained appreciable quantities of estrogens (such as ethynyl estradiol or mestranol). It was only at about the mid-sixties that the difficulties in removing these contaminations were fully recognized.

13.2. ESTROGENIC ACTIVITY

Progestational compounds in which some estrogenic potency has been found are listed in Table 24, inactive ones in Table 25. It will be seen that norethynodrel has the most pronounced estrogenic activity and, as Pincus *et al.* showed as early as 1956, its dose-response curve (mouse uterine weight) is much steeper than that of norethisterone.

The latter compound was found inactive when injected in acute experiments, but when given orally for 2 weeks, showed some activity. It was suggested that this might be due to its conversion into a more active compound (Edgren, 1966a, 1967a). Also Junkmann (1964) and Neumann *et al.* (1964) found norethisterone (and its acetate) more active when given orally than when injected. Norethynodrel, on the other hand, when given intragastrically had only 35% of its subcutaneous activity but both methods of administration yielded log dose-response curves with the same slope ($b = 21.30$ and 21.94 for subcutaneous and intragastrical respectively) as against 24 for estrone (subcut.) and 6.25 for norethisterone (intragastr.) (Edgren, 1958).

Ethynodiol acetate has relatively high estrogenicity but has a "shallow curve" when tested for uterine growth (not for cornified smears) which seems to be curiously connected with the fact that the compound also has antiestrogenic effects.

Lynestrenol has some estrogenic activity. Most of the other compounds discussed by us were found inactive. Dydrogesterone was found inactive in the rat vagina test but had a very weak uterotrophic effect and was for this reason listed in Tables 24 and 25.

13.3. ANTIESTROGENIC ACTIVITY

13.3.1. *Tests using vaginal cornification and uterine growth*

Several tests have been devised to assess the antiestrogenic potency of progestational compounds. Some of them are based on the suppression of vaginal cornification in spayed rodents injected with estrogens, others on the inhibition of uterine weight increase. For the latter assay mice are usually preferred, while for vaginal smears mice or rats have been used.

Results obtained in mice are listed in Table 26, in rats in Table 27. Norgestrel and normethandrone are by far the most active compounds.

The intravaginal administration of estrogens and of estrogen-inhibitors offers interesting possibilities of gaining insight in their mode of action, as has been thoroughly discussed by Emmens *et al.* (1960), Emmens (1962) and by Emmens and Martin (1964).

It should be emphasized that antiestrogenicity is by no means restricted to progestational compounds and that the most potent antiestrogens were

TABLE 24. ESTROGENIC AND METROTROPHIC ACTIVITY (IN THE RAT, UNLESS STATED OTHERWISE)

Compound	Subcutaneous assay activity expressed as percentage of that of		Oral assay activity expressed as percentage of that of		Reference
	estradiol = 100	estrone = 100	estradiol = 100	estrone = 100	
Norethynodrel		3–5 (vagina) 7 (uterus, mouse) 7			Saunders and Drill (1958), Drill (1959) Saunders and Drill (1958) Edgren et al. (1967a) Junkmann (1964) Pincus et al. (1956)
Ethynodiol acetate	3.3 0.48$^{(2)}$ (vagina)	1.25–2.5$^{(1)}$ (mouse uterine weight) 4–5 4 ("shallow curve" for uterine growth)			Drill (1965) Elton and Nutting (1961)
Norethisterone	0.03 0.03	0 (vagina) 0.01 (uterine weight) 0.015–0.01$^{(1)}$ (mouse uterine weight) inactive (acute expt.) 0.3$^{(8)}$ shallow curve	0.1 1.0		Junkmann (1964) Neumann et al. (1964) Drill (1959) Drill (1959) Pincus et al. (1956)
Norethisterone acetate	0.1 0.1		0.33 3.0	1$^{(3)}$ (two weeks treatment) 0.3$^{(8)}$	Edgren (1966a) Edgren (1967a) Kincl and Dorfman (1965) Junkmann et al. (1964) Neumann et al. (1964) Drill (1965)
Lynestrenol	0.1	0		0.5–1 (vagina)$^{(4)}$ 0.1 (uterine weight)	Junkmann (1964) Overbeek et al. (1962) Overbeek et al. (1962)

	(uterus) 1–2[5]			
Norgestrienone Norvinodrel		0.1[7]		Roussel (1966) Ruggieri et al. (1965)
Dydrogesterone	<0.01 6) 6) 6)			Kobayashi (1963) Boris et al. (1966) Claassen (1968) Kobayashi (1963)
Medroxy-progesterone acetate	<0.1 (uterine weight)[9] <0.01[10]		inactive	Brennan and Kraay (1963) Velardo and Fedden (1964)

Notes to Table 24

(1) The dose-response curves of norethisterone and of norethynodrel are not parallel with those of estrone nor with each other. The figures given are rough estimates.
(2) Note 1 applies with respect to estradiol.
(3) Supposed to be due to conversion into an estrogen.
(4) Compared *not* with estrone but with ethynyl estradiol (= 100).
(5) Rough calculation based on table, showing effect on uterine weight in comparison with effects of estradiol monobenzoate. The authors estimate the compound's activity to be about one-third of that of norethisterone.
(6) Boris et al. (1966) report that dydrogesterone given subcutaneously to intact infantile rats in doses of 1 to 4 mg daily for 3 days caused a distinct weight increase of the uterus but this was not compared with the effect of estradiol or any other hormone. Similar results by Claassen (1968) in mice. No effect when given orally. Kobayashi (1963) found the growth response of the infantile rat uterus to 8 mg of dydrogesterone comparable to that caused by 10 to 20 mg progesterone.
(7) More active in oily solution than in aqueous suspension. Much less active in producing weight increase of the uterus than vaginal cornification.
(8) Figures apply to "estrogen-free norethindrone", obtained by a process which excludes ring A aromatic compounds as starting material.
(9) Subcutaneous doses of 100 mcg produced an increase in uterine weight smaller than that produced by 0.1 mcg of estrone. Increase of dose to 2000 mcg produced no further increase in uterine weight.
(10) 2.5 mg daily for 3 days produced uterine weights of 24% over aqueous-treated controls whereas 0.1 mcg estrone more than doubled control weights.

TABLE 25. COMPOUNDS IN WHICH NO ESTROGENIC ACTIVITY HAS BEEN DETECTED

Compound	Dose found inactive, if stated	Route of administration	Reference
Allylestrenol	3 mg total dose (rat, vagina) 0.3 total dose[1] (uterine weight, rat)	p.o.	Madjerek et al. (1960)
Anagestone acetate		s.c.	Kobayashi et al. (1962) Blye et al. (1965a) Junkmann (1964)
Chlormadinone acetate	25 mg/100 g (rat, vagina) 5 mg (infantile rat vagina opening, uterus) 0.5 mg (infantile rat vagina opening, uterus)	s.c. p.o. p.o. s.c.	Hecht-Lucari et al. (1965) Chambon and Picard (1966)
Dimethisterone	32 mcg/20 g (mouse, vagina)	s.c.	David et al. (1959)
Dydrogesterone	10 mg (rat, vagina) (see also Table 24)	s.c. & p.o.	Marois (1962d)
Ethisterone	10 mg total dose (rat, vagina) (See also Table 24)	s.c. & p.o.	Neumann et al. (1964) Edgren et al. (1967a)
Medroxyprogesterone acetate			
Megestrol acetate	5 mg/kg mouse (vagina)	p.o.	David et al. (1963)
Norgestrel	5 mg/kg rat (uterine weight)	p.o.	David et al. (1963) Edgren et al. (1966a)
Normethandrone	1 mg/day for 2 weeks		Drill (1959)
Quingestanol acetate	0.1 mg/kg for 3 days	p.o.	Eben-Moussi and van den Driessche (1970)

Note to Table 25
(1) This represents less than 0.1% of the activity of estradiol benzoate.

found amongst the androgens and certain non-steroid substances, particularly dimethylstilbestrol (DMS) which, unlike all steroids tested, when given intravaginally antagonized some *early* vaginal reactions to estrogen, viz. cell division and tetrazolium reduction, and "at any rate antagonizes the natural estrogens more effectively than it does its own analog, diethylstilbestrol" (Emmens and Martin, 1964). It was assumed that the action of steroid antiestrogens tested (which in contrast to DMS are also active when given systemically) must be directed at "decidedly later events of a more physiological nature", not at the primary binding at the receptor sites.

We call attention to these phenomena in order to caution the reader against some tempting simplifications. It will not do to interpret antiestrogenic activity of a compound as being due to its progestational or its androgenic activity, and antiestrogenicity is not even incompatible with estrogenicity. This may be illustrated by the example of ethynodiol acetate, described by Elton and Nutting (1961) as "a unique steroidal 'progestin' ". The compound is "estrogenic as measured in both the mouse uterine growth assay and the rat vaginal smear assay, yet when administered in conjunction with estrone (it) acts as an estrogen antagonist".

Another observation worth recording is one by Maekawa (1960) which concerns norethisterone. When it was injected into adult spayed female rats (30 days after castration) in a daily dose of 2 mg for 5 days, the vaginal estrogenic index increased, reaching a maximum on day 4, thereafter decreased again (minimum on day 6) and then increased again (maximum on day 8). These same fluctuations had been observed with a combination of 0.125 mg of estrone and 2.0 mg of progesterone. In other words, norethisterone behaved as if it combined the effects of both those hormones.

Edgren *et al.* (1967b, 1968) devoted a special study to the interactions of norgestrel with ethynyl estradiol, since the two substances are used in combination in commercial preparations. Edgren's group found that ethynyl estradiol had by itself some progestational activity, since it produces some arborization of the endometrium in the Clauberg test. When given together with norgestrel in doses of 1 to 10 mcg subcutaneously or 10 mcg orally it depressed the progestational effect of norgestrel over a wide range of doses. While this does not strictly come under the heading of antiestrogenic effects, it nevertheless shows some antagonism between the two compounds.

In the mouse vaginal smear test, doses of 10 or 30 mcg norgestrel suppressed or reduced the effect of 0.1 to 0.4 mcg ethynyl estradiol when both compounds were injected subcutaneously; 30 to 100 mcg of norgestrel gave comparable results on gavage administration, though the relative

TABLE 26. ANTIESTROGENIC ACTIVITY, AS ASSESSED BY SUPPRESSION OF VAGINAL CORNIFICATION AND OF UTERINE GROWTH IN MICE
All doses in mcg

Compound	Subcut. dose of estrone to be antagonized	Cornification active dose subcut.	Cornification active dose oral	activity as percentage of progesterone subcut. (=100)	Uterine growth active dose subcut.	Uterine growth active dose oral	progesterone subcutaneous = 100	Reference
Norgestrel	2	5.4 (ED_{50})		7400			>3300	Edgren et al. (1966b, 1967a)
Norethisterone	0.5 for 4 days	40 (ED_{50})		14,600[2]			800	Edgren et al. (1966b, 1967a)
	2[3]			1000				
	0.4				16	32	ca. 3000	Dorfman et al. (1961a)
	0.4				3[9]	9[9]		Dorfman et al. (1961b) Kincl and Dorfman (1965b)
	0.06 estradiol 0.5 for 4 days	500						Emmens et al. (1960)
Normethandrone	2			730[1]			880	Edgren (1966)
	0.4			1800			ca. 1500	Edgren (1960) Dorfman et al. (1961a)
	0.4				32	40		Dorfman et al. (1961b)
Chlormadinone acetate	0.3			130			300	Edgren et al. (1957a) Hecht-Lucari et al. (1965)
	0.4				50	100	500 subcut. 250 oral	Dorfman and Kincl (1963)
	0.4					100	500	
	0.3				20–100	100–500		Brennan and Kraay (1963)
Allylestrenol Dydrogesterone	0.3[7]					<100		Brennan and Kraay (1963) Hecht-Lucari (1966)[8] Boris et al. (1966) Claassen (1968)
Dimethisterone	0.3				3000			McKinney and Braselton (1970)
Anagestone acetate	0.3				100[10]			
					mod.	active[11]		Blye et al. (1965)

Compound					Reference
Melengestrol acetate	0.3			approx. 2000	McKinney and Braselton (1970)
	0.3	4.3[10]	500	290	Edgren et al. (1967a, b)
Medroxy-progesterone acetate	0.4			approx. 300 subcut. 50 oral	Dorfman and Kincl (1963)
	0.3	150		100	Brennan and Kraay (1963)
		100	500	500	Edgren et al. (1967a)
				60	Lee and Williams (1964)
Megestrol acetate	0.3[5]	approx. 137			David et al. (1963)
	49±10 ED$_{50}$		10	ca. 50	
	40/kg abt.				Dorfman and Kincl (1963)
	0.4/mouse				McKinney and Braselton (1970)
	0.4	1000		25	
	0.3	80[10]	500	100	Edgren et al. (1967a)
Norethynodrel		inactive		inactive	Edgren (1958)
				inactive	Hecht-Lucari (1966)
				inactive[8]	Elton and Nutting (1961)
	0.3	100	100		Edgren et al. (1967a)
Ethynodiol acetate	0.3	100[4]	1000		Dorfman et al. (1961b)
	2	500	4000[6]	100	Dorfman et al. (1961)
Ethisterone	0.4		27		

P.E.S.R.D.—E

Notes to Table 26
(1) Ratio of antiestrogenic to progestational potency (Clauberg, McPhail 2) given 85.9.
(2) Potency adjusted (doubled) from data obtained with racemates. Antiestrogenic: progestational ratio 8.
(3) The dose of estrone used in the uterine weight test appears to have been 0.3 mcg.
(4) Doses above 100 mcg failed to antagonize estrone-induced uterine growth since the uterine weights produced with these doses approach the asymptote in the curve obtained with the compound alone.
(5) Estrone given in drinking water in a concentration of 40 mcg/l, producing a state of constant estrus. Antiestrogenic compound reduces number of estrous smears on the 3rd or 4th day after injection.
(6) Maximum doses giving only 20% inhibition as opposed to 40 for norethisterone 32 mcg or normethandrone 40 mcg.
(7) The estrogen was estradiol benzoate, 0.1 mcg per day for 3 days s.c. Dydrogesterone, daily dose 1-4 mg, was also given for 3 days.
(8) Hecht-Lucari quotes Kraft and Kieser from the endocrinological department of E. Merck A.G., Darmstadt, as his source.
(9) Figures apply to "estrogen-free norethindrone". See Table 24, note 8.
(10) Estimated ED$_{50}$.
(11) Species, dose, and route of administration not stated.

TABLE 27. ANTIESTROGENIC ACTIVITY AS ASSESSED IN RATS BY VAGINAL SMEARS, UNLESS OTHERWISE INDICATED

Compound	Estrogen to be antagonized	Effective dose (mg)		Activity as percentage of progesterone (subcut.) = 100	Reference
		subcut.	oral		
Chlormadinone acetate	Estrone s.c. 0.5 mcg daily	0.05–0.5 uterine weight		500	Chambon and Picard (1966)
	,,		0.5–5.0 uterine weight		
Norethisterone	Estradiol benzoate s.c. 1 mcg daily		10		Schneider and Rauscher (1959)
	Estradiol undecylate s.c. 25 mcg one injection	3		approx. 100	Neumann et al. (1964)
Norethisterone acetate	Estradiol undecylate s.c. 25 mcg one injection	0.3			Neumann et al. (1964)
Allylestrenol	Ethynylestradiol p.o. 10 mcg		2		Madjerek et al. (1960)
Ethisterone	Estradiol undecylate s.c. 25 mcg one injection	>10		inactive	Neumann et al. (1964)
Dydrogesterone	Estradiol s.c. 10 mcg daily	10[1]	10[1]	100	Marois (1962d)

(1) These are daily doses, given for 10 days, together with estradiol. There was mucification, the same that would be produced by an equal combination of progesterone and estradiol.

antiestrogenic efficacy of norgestrel diminished with increasing dosage by gavage.

Norgestrel blocked the effects of ethynyl estradiol on uterine growth in mice, but not in rats where its action was additive or at low doses of the estrogen even potentiating.

13.3.2. *Other parameters of antiestrogenic activity*

Of possible practical interest are studies on the interaction with estrogens in the *inhibition of pituitary gonadotrophic function*. It is of course essential that the ovulation-inhibiting properties of estrogens and progestational substances should not antagonize each other when they are combined in a single contraceptive drug. Edgren *et al.* (1967b) in their ("not entirely satisfactory") study found that a low dose of 40 mcg norgestrel would completely suppress compensatory ovarian hypertrophy in hemicastrated rats, that this effect is definitely prevented by the administration of high doses of ethynyl estradiol, but "that no dose of norgestrel antagonized the pituitary blocking effects of the low dosages of ethynyl estradiol". Neumann (personal communication) considers the possibility that a stimulating effect of the estrogen on prolactin secretion might well be involved in these experiments, since prolactin is known to be luteotrophic in the rat.

A new method of testing progestational compounds for antiestrogenic activity has recently been developed by Nishino and Neumann (1971). It measures the increase in sialic acid in the vagina of spayed, estrogen treated mice (see also Chapter 31, Section 7, p. 286) and enables both estrogenic and antiestrogenic properties to be assayed. In lower doses the latter prevail, in higher doses the former. Norethynodrel proved to be the only compound that did not show antiestrogenic activity at any dose level.

Norethisterone in low doses (0.1 mg daily for 11 days) in the experiments of Ramirez and Sawyer (1965) together with an estrogen suppressed the precocious initiation of puberty produced by estrogen alone but not the inhibitory effect of the latter on LH release and formation of corpora lutea. In this connection the work of Eisenfeld and Axelrod (1965) deserves attention who studied the influence of a "progestin" on the distribution of radioactive (tritium-labeled) estradiol in organs of the rat. The compound studied was norethynodrel which, when given intravenously 15 minutes before the injection of ^{3}H-estradiol, markedly reduced its accumulation in the hypothalamus, anterior pituitary, uterus and vagina, but 15 minutes after the estrogen reduced its uptake only in the uterus and vagina. Quantitative studies led to the assumption of competitive inhibition.

Now norethynodrel occupies a special place amongst the progestational compounds and, as shown in Table 26, has no antiestrogenic activity judged by conventional standards. It is, on the other hand, distinctly estrogenic. While these studies may therefore not immediately bear on the problem of the mechanism of antiestrogenic action of other compounds, they do show that competitive binding may require different concentrations at different sites and this has to be kept in mind when one considers the differential antiestrogenic effects of progestational drugs at various sites.

Kraay and Black (1970) administered norethynodrel and norethisterone to immature female mice at various times before a tracer dose of radioactive estradiol, which was given 1 hour before sacrifice. At low doses the two compounds enhanced accumulation of estrogen in the uterus but they inhibited it at higher doses. They also significantly reduced estrogen binding to estrogen receptors in rat uterine cytoplasm. By contrast chlormadinone acetate does not bind to estrogen receptors. It was found to have little or no effect on the uptake of estradiol, given 2 hours later, but by 6 hours the uterus accumulated significantly *more* estradiol. The response was dose-related up to 100 mcg of chlormadinone acetate per mouse. This would certainly fit in with Emmens' and Martin's statement quoted under subsection 13.3.1 (p. 107). And, as Kraay and Black point out, "competitive inhibition of estrogen for the binding receptor is not essential for the anti-uterotrophic action of a progestin".

Since certain estrogen antagonisms have been demonstrated *in vitro* by means of the placental dehydrogenase system, a statement made by Dorfman (1963) would appear to be relevant, i.e. that in this system estriol inhibits estradiol but "other substances, such as progesterone and cortisone,* which are classified as antiestrogens on the basis of *in vivo* studies, neither stimulate the placental isocitric acid dehydrogenase system nor inhibit the action of 17β-estradiol".

14. ANDROGENIC, MYOTROPHIC ("ANABOLIC") AND ANTI-ANDROGENIC ACTIVITIES

14.1. INTRODUCTORY REMARKS

The androgenic activity of steroids is usually measured by means of the weight of accessory male sex organs in castrated rats, which include the seminal vesicles, the (ventral) prostate and the levator ani muscle. These

---

* See Lerner (1964).

three parameters are not entirely interchangeable. The seminal vesicles have been known for decades to respond to estrogens by an increase of their muscular sheath and thereby their weight. Responsiveness of the levator ani muscle (MLA) to various steroids does not parellel that of the two glandular organs mentioned and it is often referred to as myotrophic activity. It has been suggested that this is correlated with the protein-anabolic effect of steroids more closely than with their potency of increasing prostate weight. The MLA is therefore widely used as an indicator of "anabolic"—as distinguished from "androgenic"—activity. A discussion of the validity and merits of this distinction is outside the scope of this chapter. Van der Vies (1965) has shown that retarded resorption of a steroid from the injection site suffices to bring about a shift in the ratio of "anabolic" and "androgenic" activities.

14.2. ANDROGENIC AND MYOTROPHIC ACTIVITIES

Compounds which have been shown to have at least some activity are listed in Table 28, others in Table 29. The most active are normethandrone, norgestrel, norethisterone and lynestrenol. Norethisterone and norgestrel are described by Edgren et al. (1966b) as "conventional androgens with normal, linear, dose-response curves", the latter being about 5 times more potent than the former, but having much greater progestional potency and thus "a ratio of effects greatly in (its) favor".

Quingestanol, the cyclopentylenol ether of norethisterone, is described as distinctly androgenic and a comparison with such enol ethers of other related steroids leads to the conclusion "that the nature of the parent ketone and not enol etherification *per se* governs the biological behavior of these compounds" (Mischler et al., 1969).

The effect of progestational steroids on the fructose concentration of seminal vesicles and the anterior lobes of the prostate in intact and castrated mice was studied by Thomas and Strauss (1965). Castration causes a rapid decrease of fructose values and these can be practically normalized again by treatment with testosterone or methyltestosterone (50, 400 or 800 mcg per day for 10 days). Ethisterone and norethisterone in equal doses caused a far less complete restoration of fructose values and norethynodrel was inactive, as was progesterone.

While androgenic properties may at first glance be considered to be a source of undesirable side effects, they need not necessarily be so. They may contribute to the antiestrogenic effects and their contraceptive action. In view of the low doses of these compounds used for oral contraception

TABLE 28. COMPOUNDS SHOWING SOME ANDROGENIC AND MYOTROPHIC ("ANABOLIC") ACTIVITY IN THE CASTRATED MALE RAT

Given in doses (mg) × days, indicated in columns 1, 3, 5, 7, 9 and 11. When possible, activities are expressed as percentages of those of testosterone propionate (% TEP) on injection and of 17α-methyltestosterone (% MET) given orally. These figures represent crude approximations. i = inactive.

Compound	Seminal vesicle				Ventral prostate				Musc. levator ani.				Reference
	subc.	% TEP	oral	% MET	subc.	% TEP	oral	% MET	subc.	% TEP	oral	% MET	
Normethandrone (methylestrenone)			0.5 × 7	100							0.5 × 7	400	Overbeek and de Visser (1956) Schneider and Rauscher (1959)
			2 × 7	(2)			2 × 7					(2)	
	0.01 × 7(3)	37(5) MET 100	0.1 × 7 0.3 × 14	100	0.001 × 7(3)	37(5) MET	0.1 × 7 0.3 × 14	100	0.010 × 7(3)	400–600 MET	(0.1–1.0) × 7 0.3 × 14	>100	Desaulles and Krähenbühl (1962) Segaloff (1963)
Norgestrel		6			(0.5–1) × 7	6 7.5 NE(5) 470				100			McGinty and Djerassi (1958) Drill (1959) Edgren et al. (1967a) Edgren et al. (1963a)
Medroxy-progesterone acetate	(0.5–2) × 7 5/100 g × 15				(0.5–2) × 7 5/100 g × 15				(0.5–2) × 7				Revesz and Chappel (1966)
Ethisterone	(1–10) × 14	1	10 × 14	i	5/kg × 15 ED25				3 × 14	1	10 × 14	i	Carraro et al. (1967) Neumann et al. ('64)
Norethisterone	(1–10) × 14	2	10 × 14	10	10/kg × 15 ED25			2	(1–10) × 14	10–20	3 × 14	<10	Desaulles and Krähenbühl (1964) Neumann et al. (1964)
		2.2								18 1			Junkmann (1964) Drill (1965) Desaulles and Krähenbühl (1964)

Orally Active Progestational Compounds: Animal Studies

									References
Norethisterone		2 × 7(1) 0.3 × 14(1)				2 × 7(1) 0.3 × 14(1)			Schneider and Rauscher (1959) McGinty and Djerassi (1958) Edgren et al. (1967a) Neumann et al. (1964)
Norethisterone acetate	(1–10) ×14	10 × 14	10	1.6			11	10 × 14	i	Junkmann (1964) Drill (1965)
Quingestanol acetate	1.5 25(6)	0.8 × 15		2.5 25(6)		0.8 × 15	11 4	0.8 × 15	i	Eben-Mousse and van den Driessche (1970) Mischler et al. (1969)
Medrogestone		(0.2–0.8) ×7 (0.2–0.8) ×7	30		50	(0.2–0.8) ×7				Giannina et al. (1969)
Lynestrenol	2.5/100g ×15(7) 2 × 7		25		30					Carraro et al. (1967)
Norgesterone	1 × 7	2.5/100g ×15	2.5/100g ×15							de Visser (unpublished)
		1 × 7		i	6	1 × 7	almost "i"		12.5	Ruggieri et al. (1964) Ruggieri and Matscher 1959
Allylestrenol				10(4)			10(4)			Desaulles and Krähenbühl (1962) Madjerek et al. (1960)
Ethynodiol diacetate	10(4)	4 × 7	i	1				4 × 7	i	Drill (1965)

Notes to Table 28
(1) Very little effect.
(2) Effect much more pronounced than after treatment with norethisterone.
(3) Immature castrated rats, weighing 45 to 55 g, as described by Segaloff and Gabbard (1962).
(4) Compared with testosterone. Also tested on capon's comb, 0.8% of testosterone by subcutaneous and 0.3% by topical administration.
(5) Compared with norethisterone "roughly five times more potent".
(6) Compared with testosterone, p.o.
(7) See also Table 29.

TABLE 29. COMPOUNDS WHICH WHEN TESTED IN CASTRATED RATS WERE FOUND NOT TO HAVE ANDROGENIC OR MYOTROPHIC ("ANABOLIC") ACTIVITY

Highest inactive doses given, in mg/day, followed by number of days of administration. Criterion: increase of weight of target organ

Compound	Seminal vesicle	Ventral prostate	Musc. lev. ani	Reference
Anagestone acetate[2]				Blye et al. (1965a)
Chlormadinone acetate	5 × 10, s.c. and p.o.	5 × 10, s.c. and p.o.	5 × 10, s.c. and p.o.	Chambon et al. (1966)
Megestrol acetate	100/kg × 7, p.o.		100/kg × 7, p.o.	David et al. (1963)
Medrogestone[1]	5 × 7, s.c. and p.o.	5 × 7, s.c. and p.o.	5 × 7, s.c. and p.o.	Revesz and Chappel (1966)
Dydrogesterone	4 × 7, s.c. and p.o.	4 × 7, s.c. and p.o.	4 × 7, s.c. and p.o.	Boris et al. (1966)
	8 × 7, s.c.	8 × 7, s.c.	8 × 7, s.c.	Kobayashi (1963)
	4 × 6, s.c.	4 × 6, s.c.	4 × 6, s.c.	Claassen (1968)
	10 × 7, s.c. and p.o.	10 × 7, s.c. and p.o.	10 × 7, s.c. and .p.o.	Marois (1962a)
Norethynodrel		inactive	inactive	Drill (1962, 1965)
		inactive		Edgren et al. (1967a)
	"almost negligible"	"almost negligible"	"almost negligible"	Miyake (1961)
Dimethisterone	64/kg × 7, s.c.		64/kg × 7, s.c.	David et al. (1959)

(1) See also Table 28.
(2) Devoid of frank "androgenic activity".

undesirable clinical effects of androgenicity will only rarely manifest themselves.

Of the compounds listed in Table 28 only one, allylestrenol, is recommended for use in pregnancy and was found to be devoid of androgenic activity by Overbeek's group, who introduced it. Besides, masculinizing effects on the female fetus do not simply depend on androgenic activity, as it can be demonstrated in the castrated male animal. This is discussed below in Section 15.

In this connection it should be noted that progesterone has been found to be definitely androgenic in "relatively enormous quantities" by Greene et al. (1939c). The authors gave daily doses of 2.0 to 3.0 mg to intact immature rats for 5 days, 3.0 to 6.0 mg to castrated immature rats for 10 to 20 days and 2.0 to 35.0 mg for 7 days to adult castrates. They observed significant increases in prostate weight in most experiments (in adult castrates only with the highest doses) and histological signs of secretion. The changes in the seminal vesicles were less conspicuous and "secretory granules" were not found. In a few new-born females enlargement of the clitoris was achieved with gradually increasing doses totalling 45.0 to 73.0 mg until the 30th day of life. The authors believe they have settled a controversial question regarding the androgenicity of progesterone.

The so-called *early androgen syndrome* (see Chapter 11), characterized by female sterility due to steroid treatment within the first 5 days of postnatal life, has been produced by Shipley and Meyer (1965) by injecting a single dose of 1 mg of norethisterone. Animals so treated had ovaries of greatly reduced weight and no corpora lutea, when inspected at the age of 44–46 days. Progesterone (4.0 mg) and medroxyprogesterone acetate (MAP) (1 mg) did not have this effect (but did reverse the damaging effect of an injection of estradiol on the 5th day of life). MAP was also found to be ineffective in a dose of 2.5 mg by Gorski (1966). Kincl et al. (1965), at variance with Shipley and Meyer, found norethisterone inactive over a dose range 0.1 to 1.0 mg (and chlormadinone acetate inactive at the same dose levels in *male* newborn rats as judged by testicular development at the age of 45 days).

Seven of the orally active progestational compounds generally dealt with in this chapter have recently been examined by Cupceancu et al. (1971) by early postnatal administration with a view to possible influences on subsequent gonadotrophic pituitary function and fertility. Of these chlormadinone acetate was the only compound which, in the only dose tested (3.0 mg), given s.c. on the first day of life, did not impair estrous cycles or fertility in any of the four animals treated. Megestrol acetate, norgestrel (in

1.0 mg single dose) and medroxyprogesterone acetate (3.0 mg), in that order, increasingly reduced fertility. The first of these compounds had no influence on estrus cycles; with norgestrel there was inhibition of vaginal development in more than half (of seven) animals; medroxyprogesterone acetate somewhat reduced the total length of diestrous periods and increased that of estrus.

Three estrane derivatives, ethynodiol diacetate (1 mg, ten animals), norethisterone acetate (1.0 mg, twenty-four animals), and allylestrenol (10.0 mg, ten animals), strongly interfered with estrous cycles (effects comparable with those of 5 mcg estradiol benzoate or 10 mcg testosterone propionate) and completely abolished fertility. In this group ovarian weights were reduced by more than 50%, corpora lutea being present or lacking. Whether these effects are due to estrogenic, androgenic or other properties of the steroids cannot be stated in general.

The effect of this treatment on subsequent mating behavior was studied by Steinbeck *et al.* (1971). Norethisterone acetate and ethynodiol diacetate (1 mg each) permanently reduced female behavior (lordosis) under estradiol-progesterone stimulation, the former also inducing a certain shift towards male behavior on testosterone stimulation. Allylestrenol and medroxyprogesterone acetate (10 and 3 mg respectively) had the first but not the second effect. Other steroids were inactive in this respect.

14.3. ANTIANDROGENIC ACTIVITIES

The property possessed by certain progestational steroids of antagonizing the actions of (exogenous or endogenous) testosterone has become a subject of major—at least theoretical—interest, since a group of investigators in the laboratories of Schering in Berlin (Hamada *et al.*, 1963), while testing a new compound for possible fetal virilization, found it to have antimasculinizing effects. This steroid, now known as cyproterone acetate, is 6-chloro-1,2α-methylene-$\Delta^{4,6}$-pregnadien-17α-ol-3,20-dione-17 acetate; it could also be described as the 1,2-methylene derivative of chlormadinone acetate. The structure is shown in Fig. 1.

Since then the pharmacology of this substance and of its parent compound, the free alcohol, has been studied most thoroughly by the Schering group (see for reviews Neumann *et al.*, 1967, 1970) and has yielded results bearing on a number of important endocrinological problems.

With regard to our subject we call attention to the fact that, while both the free alcohol and the acetate are antiandrogenic, only the acetate has

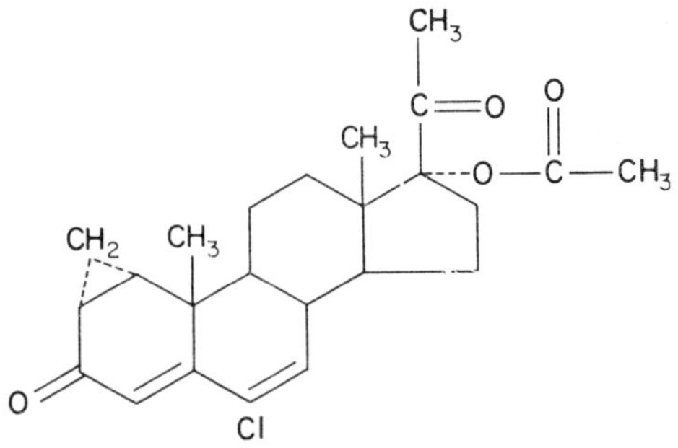

FIG. 1. Cyproterone acetate.

progestational activity, even to a very high degree (250 times that of progesterone s.c., 1000 times p.o.) (Hamada et al., 1963). The free alcohol has negligible progestational potency (Neumann et al., 1967). The analogy with 17α-hydroxyprogesterone is striking and poses a problem of structure–activity relationship.

Antiandrogenic potency was measured by the Schering group in castrated rats (about 80–100 g), treated for 7 days with daily doses of 0.1 mg of testosterone, by assessing the reduction in weight increase of seminal vesicles and prostate caused by varying doses of the compounds to be tested.

The ED_{50} in this test according to Junkmann and Neumann (1964) was 0.25 mg for cyproterone acetate as against 3.5 mg of progesterone (judged by seminal vesicles). Judged by prostate weight the difference is still greater and cyproterone acetate was reported to have 45 times the activity of progesterone.

Assigning to cyproterone acetate the value 100, chlormadinone acetate has about 40% s.c. and 50 p.o., judged by prostate weight, and about 30% by either route, judged by seminal vesicles, according to Neumann et al. (1967), who found progesterone to be "very weakly active" by these standards.

The same groups of authors give data on the dose-dependence of the antiandrogenic effect of cyproterone acetate in castrated mice treated with 0.03 mg of testosterone proprionate daily (for 7 days) and find a steep curve between a minimum effective dose of 30 mcg and almost total inhibition at 1.0 mg/day. Using the same protocol, Revesz and Chappel

(1966) found 2.0 to 5.0 mg medrogestone p.o. or s.c. more active than 25 mg of progesterone (on ventral prostate).

These figures lie in a very different range from those of Dorfman (1963b), who had to give a total dose of 40 mg chlormadinone acetate (that is 5.7 mg per day) to reduce by about 40% the weight of the seminal vesicles (mg/g bw) and by about one-third that of the prostate of mice, stimulated by daily injections of 0.8 mg methyltestosterone. Progesterone in these studies was "as active an antiandrogen" as any of the compounds reported. In a later paper Dorfman (1968) found chlormadinone acetate (tested in mice against testosterone) 2.1 times as active as progesterone, although the slopes of the dose-response curves were not parallel.

Using Dorfman's method, except that testosterone was given in daily doses of 100 mcg/mouse for 7 days, McKinney and Braselton compared dimethisterone, megestrol acetate and melengestrol acetate with progesterone and found that dimethisterone "had essentially three times the antiandrogenic potency of progesterone in the male mouse" (ED_{50} 1.16 and 3.30 respectively, s.c.) whereas both megestrol acetate and melengestrol acetate, in spite of their much greater progestational potency, were only slightly more antiandrogenic than progesterone.

Kraft and Harting (1968) tested their compounds in immature rats in six daily doses, immediately following castration, against one single dose of 0.5 mg of testosterone enanthate, judging the result by the weight of seminal vesicles or that of the prostate. They find progesterone to cause roughly 55–60% inhibition of seminal vesicles or prostate in daily subcutaneous doses of 70.0 mg. Chlormadinone acetate was about 10 times as active when given parenterally (a little less orally) and cyproterone acetate had roughly 100 times the activity of progesterone, but all the dose-response curves, from the data supplied, would seem to be rather shallow. Notwithstanding the differences in technique these data seem to approach those of Neumann and his group.

The data of Hecht-Lucari (1966), though from the same laboratory, are not quite comparable with those of Kraft and Harting, but it should be recorded that the authors finds ethisterone and norethisterone inactive (orally) and allylestrenol approaching the activity of progesterone.

Dydrogesterone was tested for antiandrogenicity in castrated rats receiving 25 mcg of testosterone propionate daily for 7 days and showed a weak, barely dose-dependent, inhibition in doses of 1–4 mg subcutaneously and 2–4 mg orally (Boris et al., 1966).

Cyproterone acetate does not belong to the compounds more generally dealt with in this chapter (see p. 37). Of the progestational compounds used as such, chlormadinone acetate is the one in which so far the strongest antiandrogenic activity has been demonstrated.

This was recently confirmed by Neri (1970) (Schering Corporation, Bloomfield, N.J.), who stated that some of the most potent antiandrogenic agents reported thus far were those which also possess progestational properties, and included cyproterone acetate, chlormadinone acetate, and its 16-methylene analogue, Sch 12600. These compounds also reduced the androgen-dependent canine hyperplastic prostate. This effect was accompanied by a marked diminution in epithelial cell heights with loss of acid phosphatase, an increase of fibrous tissue elements relative to smooth muscle and the disappearance of the granular endoplasmic reticulum, the Golgi apparatus and secretory granules. It is suggested that these agents may be useful in the management of human prostatic hyperplasia.

For certain "antiandrogenic" effects of medroxyprogesterone acetate in rats see Chapter 31, Section 9 (p. 290).

15. MASCULINIZATION OF FEMALE FETUSES

15.1. INTRODUCTION

It became highly desirable to test progestational (and other) drugs for possible masculinizing effects on the fetus, when clinicians in the late 1950s reported the birth of baby girls with abnormal external genitalia, whose mothers had been treated with a variety of hormone-related drugs during pregnancy. In the beginning these drug-effects were often ascribed to classic androgenic properties, and testing of compounds for these became an urgent requirement, although as early as 1959 Bongiovanni et al. had indicted estrogenic therapy (diethylstilbestrol) as the culprit in at least four cases of masculinization of female infants. While androgenicity is normally assessed in castrated male animals—adult or prepuberal—methods for studies in the fetus were soon developed. It is only imperfectly known whether, or to what extent, these studies allow predictions regarding possible harmful effects in the human.

Some authors gave the compounds to be tested to pregnant animals (usually rats) during a number of days, varying from one institute to another, either orally or subcutaneously. Others combined these studies with experiments concerning the pregnancy-maintaining activity of progestational substances and therefore had to ovariectomize the animals. The fetuses which were then kept alive were examined for possible genital anomalies. Results obtained in intact and in spayed pregnant females are not necessarily comparable. Neumann and his group (Neumann et al., 1968b, 1969, 1970) have introduced the use of an antiandrogen, cyproterone acetate, to analyze the role of androgens in normal sexual development (in the rat fetus) and of androgenic drugs in its disturbances.

15.2. SIGNS OF MASCULINIZATION IN RATS

Parameters studied include:
(1) the length of the anogenital distance (AGD) in the newborn animals (less than 2 mm in the normal female, more than 3 mm in the normal male, in between in partially masculinized females);
(2) the histological appearance of the internal genitalia; and
(3) other signs of masculinization, in particular enlargement or phallus-like appearance of the clitoris. There is an increasing tendency not to rely on any single parameter alone. This was strongly emphasized by authorities such as Jost (1963). Applicable methods have been described by Mey (1963b), Neumann and Junkmann (1963), Suchowsky (1964), Neumann and Kramer (1964) and Neumann (1968).

The anogenital distance (AGD) may or may not be affected by compounds which in comparable doses already disturb to some degree the differentiation of the female genital tract.

Histological studies have covered the development of the vagina and the urethro-vaginal septum, the presence, and number, or absence, of prostatic buds and proliferation of the *anlage* of the seminal vesicles, the detection of persistent remnants of the Wolffian ducts and the development of the urethra.

In earlier studies some authors appear to have overlooked the fact that the caudal part of the rat vagina at the time of birth is a solid structure without a lumen and this was quite erroneously described as vaginal aplasia. Such results were challenged (Overbeek, 1962; Mey, 1963a; Neumann and Junkmann, 1963). This mistake is avoided when the animals are sectioned sagittally, as recommended by Suchowsky (1964) and Neumann and Junkmann (1963), not tranversally. These authors have introduced a classification of stages of masculinization, mainly based on the progressive shortening of the urethro-vaginal septum, which in turn is due to progressive inhibition of development of the caudal (non-Müllerian) segment of the vagina. Neumann et al. (1969) state that "the greatest sensitivity to androgens is shown by the epithelium of the dorsal sinus wall, from which the caudal segment of the vagina develops. Consequently the virilization of female fetuses will be marked initially by a partial inhibition of (this) vaginal segment. ..."

It is not advisable to rely on this parameter alone because, as Turolla *et al.* (1963) and Suchowsky *et al.* (1967) have pointed out, a shortening of the septum can also be produced by the administration of *ethynyl estradiol*. In that case it is accompanied by thickening of the caudal segment of the vagina and dilatation of the Müllerian segment, as well as by suppression of the prostatic buds (see also Greene *et al.*, 1939b).

Overbeek and his group have repeatedly emphasized the desirability of checking the fertility of the offspring of rats treated with potentially masculinizing drugs during pregnancy. This would be of far greater importance than histological studies at birth which may reveal changes of a reversible (not permanent) kind.

15.3. PHARMACOLOGICAL EFFECTS

Data on activity or inactivity of progestational compounds are given in Table 30. No activity has been reported for dydrogesterone (three studies), medrogestone (one) or chlormadinone acetate (four studies), though with the highest dose one author (Mey, 1963b) saw a slight increase in the number of prostatic buds (three to four instead of one or two).

There was some controversy in the literature regarding the reported lack of masculinizing activity in *allylestrenol* (Madjerek *et al.*, 1960). However, reports on the occurrence of such activity as shown by histological appearance (Schöler and de Wachter, 1961; Suchowsky and Junkmann, 1961) were refuted as being due to inadequate technique (Overbeek, 1962; Mey, 1963a) and one of the authors, who originally had described masculinizing effects of allylestrenol, found practically none at all in the course of a later study, even with much higher doses (Suchowsky, 1967). Mey (1963a) found no increase in the very sensitive prostatic buds and only a few animals with remnants of the cranial (most sensitive) parts of the Wolffian ducts on very high oral doses.

Jost and Moreau (1963) obtained certain morphological changes in the female fetuses when intact (not castrated) rats were given very high doses (20–30 mg per day) of allylestrenol from day 13 to day 21 of pregnancy. These changes included part persistence of Wolffian ducts. Madjerek (unpublished work) repeated these experiments under identical conditions and found the young born after maternal treatment with still higher doses (30–60 mg/day) of normal fertility (see Tausk, 1967). Jost and Moreau described the effects observed as not identical with those of androgens

TABLE 30. FETAL MASCULINIZATION

All doses in mg/rat/day, unless indicated otherwise. Figures in brackets indicate period of pregnancy (first and last days) during which compound was administered. Criteria of activity are indicated as follows: AGD = anogenital distance. EC = enlarged clitoris. IDV = impaired development of vagina. PPW = part persistence of Wolffian ducts. PB = prostatic buds.

Compound	Oral administration				Parenteral administration				Reference
	lowest active dose	criteria	activity as percentage of methyl-testosterone (=100)	highest dose found inactive	lowest active dose	criteria	activity as percentage of test. propionate (=100)	highest dose found inactive	
Allylestrenol		AGD		10 (9–21) (1)	5 (15–21)	AGD			Madjerek et al. (1960)
						IDV(2)	1		Schöler and de Wachter (1961)
	20 (13–21)	PPW			10 (16–19)	IDV(2)	1	(20 13–21)	Suchowsky and Junkmann (1961)
	10 (16–19)	PPW			1	AGD		30 (16–19)	Jost and Moreau (1963)
									Mey (1963a)
									Jost and Moreau-Stinnakre (1970)
									Suchowsky et al. (1967)
									Marois (1968)
Chlormadinone acetate	10.0 (14–19)	AGD IDV PPW PB		7.5 (15–20) 10.0 (16–19)	50 (14–21)	IDV PPW IDV AGD		10 (14–20)	Kraay and Brennan (1963)
									Kincl and Dorfman (1962)
					10.0 (15–20)	AGD IDV AGD PB		10 (16–19) 10 (14–21)	Mey (1963b)
									Mey (1963b)
									Maqueo and Kincl (1965)
									Suchowsky et al. (1967)
									Marois (1968)
									Marois (1968)
Dimethisterone					10 (14–21) 5 (15–21)	AGD IDV EC	5		Schöler and de Wachter (1961)
					1–3 (16–19)	AGD			Suchowsky and Junkmann (1961)
					1 (14–21)	IDV PB PPW IDV AGD AGD		25 (14–21) 125 (15–21)	Marois (1968)
					5 (14–21)				Marois (1968)
									Marois (1968)
									Marois (1968)
						IDV			Schöler and de Wachter (1961)
						EC			Schöler and de Wachter (1961)

Orally Active Progestational Compounds: Animal Studies

Compound	Dose (days)	Effect	Dose (days)	Effect	Ratio	Dose (days)	Reference
Dydrogesterone		IDV				10 (14–20)	Marois (1962d)
Ethisterone			0.3 (16–19)	IDV		10 (14–20)	Suchowsky et al. (1967)
				IDV		10 (16–19)	Suchowsky and Junkmann (1961)
				IDV	ca. 30	10 (15–20)	Revesz and Chappel (1966)
Medrogestone			1.0 (14–19)	AGD			Lerner et al. (1962)
Medroxy-progesterone acetate			0.5 (15,20)	AGD			Revesz and Chappel (1966)
			0.25–1.0	AGD			Revesz et al. (1960)
			(15–20)	AGD			
			2.5	IDV			Kraay and Brennan (1963)
			(14–20)	AGD			
			0.3	AGD			Suchowsky and Junkmann (1961)
	1.5 mg/kg	AGD	1.0	IDV			Schöler and de Wachter (1961)
	(15–20)			AGD			
	0.15 (15–20)	(3)		EC			
	1.5 (15–20)	IDV					David et al. (1963)
	7.5 (15–20)	AGD					Kincl and Dorfman (1962)
			0.18	IDV[7]	250		Suchowsky et al. (1967)
			(16–19)				
			0.2 (14–21)	IDV			
				PPW			Marois (1968)
Megestrol acetate	1.5 (15–20)	AGD	0.5 (14–21)	AGD			Marois (1968)
			0.3 (17–20)	IDV[8]			Cupceancu and Neumann (1969a)
			1.0 (17–20)	AGD[8]			
			1.0 (17–20)	PB[8]			David et al. (1963)
do. containing 1.15% ethynyl estradiol			1.0 (14–21)	PPW			Marois (1968)
				PB			
			3.0 (14–21)	IDV			Marois (1968)
				AGD			Marois (1968)
Melengestrol acetate			0.25 (15–20)	AGD			Duncan et al. (1964)
			>50	IDV			
Norethisterone			2.5 (14–19)	AGD		5 (14–21)	Lerner et al. (1962)
			3.0 (16–19)	AGD		5.0 (15–20)	Suchowsky and Junkmann (1961)
				IDV			
			0.5 (15–21)	AGD	ca. 30		Schöler and de Wachter (1961)
	5.0 (15–20)	(4)		EC			
			2.5 (14–20)	AGD			Kraay and Brennan (1963)
				AGD			Kincl and Dorfman (1962)
			1.0 (15–20)	EC			Revesz et al. (1960)
			0.3 (16–19)	IDV[6]	ca. 100		Neumann et al. (1964)
	0.1–10	IDV[6]	1.0 (16–19)	IDV[7]	45		Suchowsky et al. (1967)
	(16–19)		2.5 (14–21)	PB			Marois (1968)
				IDV			
		ca. 100	10.0 (14–21)	PPW			Marois (1968)

TABLE 30—cont.

Compound	Oral administration				Parenteral administration				Reference
	lowest active dose	criteria	activity as percentage of methyl-testosterone (=100)	highest dose found inactive	lowest active dose	criteria	activity as percentage of test. propionate (=100)	highest dose found inactive	
Norethisterone acetate	0.1–1.0 (16–19)	IDV[6]	ca. 20		3.0 (16–19)	AGD IDV[6]	ca. 30		Suchowsky and Junkmann (1961) Neumann et al. (1964) Lerner et al. (1962) Cupceancu and Neumann (1969a)
					0.3 (16–19) 1.0 (14–19) 1.0 (17–20) 1.0 (17–20) 3.0 (17–20) 10.0 (17–20)	AGD IDV[8] AGD[8] PB[8]	ca. 50		
Norethynodrel	12.5 (15–20)	IDV			2.5 (15–21)	AGD IDV			Kincl and Dorfman (1962) Schöler and de Wachter (1961) David et al. (1963)
	1.5 mg/kg (15–20)	AGD IDV							
	(5) 10 (9–21)	AGD			1.0 (16–19) 3.0 (16–19)	IDV AGD	10		Suchowsky and Junkmann (1961) Madjerek et al. (1960) Schöler and de Wachter (1961)
					0.5 (15–21)	AGD IDV EC			
					0.1 (16–19) 0.9 (16–19)	AGD IDV IDV[7]	50		Suchowsky and Junkmann (1961) Suchowsky et al. (1967)
Norethynodrel containing 1.5% mestranol Norgestrel					10.0 (14–21)	PPW			Marois (1968)
Quingestanol	0.1 (15–21)	AGD					"active"		Edgren et al. (1967a) Giannina et al. (1969)

Notes to Table 30
(1) According to a verbal statement of the first author, quoted by Overbeek (1962), he has never observed any histological changes after oral administration of allylestrenol to pregnant rats.
(2) The validity of these histological results has been questioned by Mey (1963a).
(3) Criterion: enlarged prostate and decreased distance between vaginal orifice and urinary papilla in genetic females.
(4) Criterion: decreased distance between vaginal orifice and urinary papilla in females.
(5) +Indicates activity. Dose and route of administration not stated.
(6) Stages of impairment of vaginal development (masculinization) are defined according to progressive shortening of the urovaginal septum. Highest stage include strong external masculinization. Method described by Neumann and Junkmann (1963).
(7) Dose represents ED_{50}.
(8) Effects antagonized by the simultaneous administration of 20 mg of cyproterone acetate.

nor with those of estrogens, though somewhat resembling the latter. The group has now extended these studies (Jost and Moreau-Stinnakre, 1970). In daily s.c. or p.o. doses of 10–30 mg, given to normal or castrated rats from day 13 to day 20 or 21 of pregnancy, allylestrenol caused a slight but significant increase of the ano-genital distance. Partial or complete persistence of Wolffian ducts was, however, observed only after *oral* administration (of 20 to 30 mg/day) of the compound, and mainly in intact animals. Very slight changes were seen in a few castrated females. These changes disappeared more or less completely within the first 21 days of postnatal life and the authors conclude that the persistence of Wolffian ducts until birth, in certain animals, represents a delay in regression, not a permanent stabilization of these ducts. Certain morphological changes were seen in the vaginae of orally treated animals, even at a postnatal age of 21 days but these resembled those occurring after estrogen treatment during pregnancy. Seven females were examined for their estrous cycles, which were found normal. Among these there were only three pregnancies, none of which yielded live litters.

The authors stress the fact that anomalies were not seen after injection of the drug and that the presence of the ovaries is an important factor in the development of the abnormalities observed, for which a metabolic conversion of the drug may therefore be responsible. It is, however, unlikely that the metabolite would be an estrogen proper, since no abnormalities were seen in male fetuses.

Relatively high masculinizing properties were reported for *ethisterone*, *norethisterone* and *medroxyprogesterone acetate* by Suchowsky *et al.* (1967). Their interpretations of the anomalies observed are subject to criticism and are in some respects in disagreement with older findings reported in the literature (on estrogen-androgen antagonism). The statement by Neumann *et al.* (1969) that medroxyprogesterone acetate stimulated the Wolffian ducts more than norethisterone acetate, according to verbal information from Dr. Neumann was made in error. The opposite is correct. (Incidentally these authors record the remarkable fact that the right Wolffian duct requires more androgen than the left, which is more sensitive to androgen, in accordance with older observations by Greene *et al.* (1939a).)

In a study concerning the effects of seven progestational steroids on the sexual differentiation of the rat, Marois (1968) paid attention not only to masculinizing effects on the female fetus (these data have been incorporated in Table 30) but also to any feminizing effects in the males, including a shortening of anogenital distances, inhibition of development of the penis and prostate buds. Such feminizing effects were observed with high doses of norethisterone (2.5 mg), medroxyprogesterone acetate (5 mg), chlormadinone acetate (10 mg) and allylestrenol (50 mg). Dimethisterone, apart from being masculinizing (in doses of 1 to 5 mg), is also feminizing (in doses of 1 to 25 mg).

A number of steroids were studied for fetal-masculinizing effects in guinea pigs by Foote et al. (1968). They included progesterone, testosterone and two orally active progestational compounds, viz. medroxyprogesterone acetate (MAP) and norethisterone (Norlutin). Doses of 1 mg were injected daily, starting on day 18 postcoitum and continued through today 60.

MAP caused a totally misleading male appearance in the female newborn on external inspection, but internally these animals had normal vaginae, completely separated from the urethra. The Wolffian ducts were largely retained, histologically somewhat resembling the ductus deferens of untreated males.

Norethisterone caused clitoral enlargements in the females resembling those produced by testosterone treatment but no other external or internal masculinizing changes were induced by these two steroids. ("Paradoxically testosterone has a greater masculinizing influence than MAP on the adult female", at a dose level of 5 mg.)

15.4. THE PREDICTIVE VALUE OF ANIMAL STUDIES

Most of the studies reported on were performed by pharmaceutical manufacturers with the obvious purpose of assessing possible risks involved in the practical use of the drugs concerned. It is therefore fair to ask what predictions these animal experiments would justify. The answer must be given with caution, not only because of the considerations applying to the transfer of animal experiments to the human in general, but also because of the discrepancies which would appear to have already been observed.

Masculinization of genetically female babies has been described following the treatment of the mother with classical androgens like testosterone or methylandrostenediol (Zander, 1953; Grumbach and Ducharme, 1960); furthermore with ethisterone, norethynodrel (Grumbach et al., 1959; Wilkins et al., 1958), stilbestrol (Bongiovanni et al., 1959), progesterone (Hayles and Nolan, 1958) and without any "hormonal" treatment.

Table 31 lists a number of reported drug effects, but it should be emphasized that in some cases there is very little evidence for a cause–effect relationship. This applies, for instance, to the one case treated with norethynodrel (Enovid), in which the mother had also produced signs of virilization and which should be viewed against the background of large series of women—pregnant and non-pregnant—treated with sometimes very high doses of the drug for prolonged periods, without any virilization of the woman or a baby. (For a review see Drill, 1966.) Not enough is known about the spontaneous incidence of masculinization in infants with normal adrenal function, though according to Wilkins *et al.* (1958) the condition is very rare. His group had seen a total of seventeen cases between 1950 and 1958, of which only three had been born to mothers who had not had a progestational drug (plus, very often, stilbestrol).

Most gynecologists seem to be ready to accept a causal role attributed to notoriously androgenic drugs, such as ethisterone, particularly since this was given in very high doses before 1958, and without much hesitation, to pregnant women. On the other hand, some compounds which are known to cause genital disturbances in female fetuses have so far not been found guilty of masculinization in the human.

As regards the intriguing experience of Bongiovanni *et al.* (1959) with stilbestrol, the authors state that the effects must be regarded as unusual since "at the Joslin clinic 950 diabetic pregnant women have been treated with female sex hormones without any apparent influence on the genitalia of the offspring". Seven hundred were given stilbestrol in high doses, beginning at a very early period in gestation and continuing until delivery. The authors think, therefore, that a special susceptibility of the fetus might have played a role in their cases.

In a later study Goldman and Bongiovanni (1967) were able to make a noteworthy contribution to the solution of these problems. Their paper contains a report on a case of a male infant born with third degree hypospadia whose mother had taken medroxyprogesterone acetate 10 mg b.i.d. from the seventh week to the sixth month of gestation. Three other cases of feminization of male fetuses had been ascribed to maternal administration of diethylstilbestrol, progesterone or acetoxyprogesterone. When it was found that hypospadias could be produced in rats by treating pregnant females with cyproterone acetate (see subsection 14.3) Goldman and Bongiovanni were struck by the similarity between these deformities and those seen in the rare form of the adrenogenital syndrome due to the inborn deficiency of 3β-hydroxysteroid dehydrogenase. They assumed, and could prove (see subsection 23.3, p. 181), that estrogens and certain progestational compounds can inhibit this enzyme and, as a result, would (amongst other things) bring about a deficiency of testosterone and a surplus of

TABLE 31. CASES OF INTRAUTERINE MASCULINIZATION OF FEMALE BABIES OCCURRING IN WOMEN TREATED WITH HORMONE-LIKE DRUGS DURING PREGNANCY

Doses in mg per day unless otherwise indicated

Drug or drugs used	Period of pregnancy treatment		Range of dosage	Number of virilized babies	Number of mothers with signs of virilization	Reference
	begun	terminated				
Ethisterone	8–21 w	21 w–9 mo	10–320	3		Wilkins et al. (1958)
	4–16 w	12–38 w[(1)]	30–100	6		Grumbach et al. (1959)
Ethisterone + Progesterone i.m.	4–6 w	8–9 mo	50–200	2		Wilkins et al. (1958)
	8–15 w	9–17 w	25–100			
Ethisterone + [a]	4 w	20 w–6 mo	200		1	Wilkins et al. (1958)
17α-OH-P-capr. i.m. [b]	4 w	4–12 w	50–250/week	2		
[a]	15 w	31 w[(1)]	10	1		Grumbach et al. (1959)
[b]	7 w	32 w	250/500–week	7	1	
Ethisterone + Stilbestrol [a]	4–8 w	8 mo-term	20–200			Wilkins et al. (1958)
	2–4 w	22–36 w[(1)]	30–120	2	1	Grumbach et al. (1959)
[b]	6–7 w	36–38 w	100–250			
Ethisterone + [a]	1–10 w	4 mo-term	25–175			Wilkins et al. (1958)
Ethynyl estradiol [b]	1–10 w	4 mo-term	30–40	2		
Norethisterone	6–10 w	34–36 w[(1)]	0.04–0.10	4		Grumbach et al. (1959)
Norethisterone acetate	5 w	34 w	10–40			Thomsen and Napp (1960)
			25			

Compound					Reference
Norethisterone + Stilbestrol	7-19 w 8-13 w	28-29 w[1] 28-29 w	5-15 50-175	3	Grumbach et al. (1959)
Norethisterone + Premarin	5 w	35 w[1]	15-40	1	Grumbach et al. (1959)
Norethynodrel containing 1.5% mestranol	5 w 6 w	35 w 38 w[1]	3.75-10 10	1	Grumbach et al. (1959)
Normethandrone	12 w	23 w	10	1	Carpentier (1958)
Progesterone i.m.	10 w	10 w[3]	3 × 10	1	Hayles and Nolan (1958)
Progesterone oral + Premarin	6 w	38 w[4]	2 × 10– 3 × 20	1	Hayles and Nolan (1958)
Progesterone i.m. a +Stilbestrol b	9 w 5 m	11 w[2] term[2]	100 q. 2 d. 10		Wilkins et al. (1958)
Stilbestrol	4-14 w	9-25 w	5-75	4	Bongiovanni et al. (1959)

Notes to Table 31
(1) Pregnancy dated from 2 weeks after last menstrual period.
(2) Dosage and period of treatment not stated in one case.
(3) The total dose was 30 mg i.m. and "the mother related that the injections were followed by an increase in libido and a growth of long hairs under the chin and about the breasts". (Post aut propter? M.T. and J. de V.).
(4) In this case progesterone was given as "linguets" in doses of 10 mg daily from November 3 until late March, when the patient was hospitalized for threatened abortion and the dose increased to 3 × 20 mg per 24 hr until June 1 (thereafter 10 mg 4 times daily until June 14).

dehydroandrosterone. The latter could be responsible for clitoral hyperplasia in genetic females without displacement of the urethral orifice.

With increasing awareness of both the manufacturers and the medical profession, incidents of fetal masculinization in the human would appear to have become exceedingly rare. Obviously manufacturers will have to avoid launching new compounds, destined for use in pregnancy, which are known to cause fetal masculinization in animals, although the predictive value of such tests may be relatively low. After all, only gross external changes in a new-born baby will be recorded and the thought that certain other anomalies might not become manifest until many years later is enough to sharpen the conscience of all those who are concerned with the development of new drugs.

16. "ANTIFERTILITY ACTION"

16.1. INTRODUCTORY REMARKS

Numerous studies have been made with the purpose of suppressing the fertility of experimental animals by treatment with progestational compounds. Sometimes such tests consist in the more or less continuous administration of the compound to females caged with males, absence of pregnancy being the sole criterion of efficacy. In that case further studies are needed to decide whether the drug has interfered with mating behavior, ovulation, transport (of gametes or zygotes) or nidation. Timing of drug administration (with regard to phase of the cycle or presence of vaginal plugs, etc.) will be among the simpler means of analysis of the mechanism of fertility blockage. For a global antifertility action of steroids, Petrow (1960) proposed the term *claudogenic*, derived from the Latin word (*claudere*) for locking or barring.

We do not propose to deal systematically with all the possible mechanisms in this section, since this would cause considerable redundancy. Ovulation, nidation, tubal function have of course all separate sections. The emphasis in the present one will mainly be on certain methodological aspects, particularly where more than one mechanism may be involved. The grouping of facts may not always appear to be very systematic, because it was adapted to some fortuitous circumstances, such as the greater or lesser amount of data from the literature available to cover particular subjects.

16.2. STUDIES INVOLVING CONTINUOUS DRUG ADMINISTRATION

Table 32 lists results obtained by daily administration of compounds, by injection or stomach tube, mixed with the feed or as implanted depot. In general, female animals were treated for a few days before being exposed to males and thereafter the treatment was continued. In some studies it was shown that addition of an estrogen may increase the efficacy of progestational compounds in preventing pregnancy (as it does in maintaining it).

In one experiment Ruggieri et al. (1965) gave the compounds to be tested, norgesterone (also called norvinodrel) or norethynodrel with 1.5% of mestranol, in a single injection and found that 1 mg of either drug considerably prolonged the time between cohabitation and conception (from 6 days in controls to 17 days) as determined by the date of delivery.

As early as 1956 Pincus described that norethisterone and norethynodrel, in single or multiple, oral or subcutaneous doses (2–25 mg of the former, 1 to 5 of the latter) considerably prolonged the time between "cohabitation and successful mating".

From the point of view of the structure-activity relationship the following observation by Falconi and Ercoli (1961) deserves attention. They compared the influence of cyclopentylenol etherification (at C-3) on the activities of norethisterone acetate and medroxyprogesterone acetate (MAP). Clauberg activity and maintenance of pregnancy were left unchanged by this chemical operation, which reduced the estrus-inhibiting and contraceptive potency of MAP and increased that of norethisterone acetate. Thus, the authors conclude, "enol etherification produces a striking dissociation in the contraceptive and progestational activities".

16.3. INFLUENCE ON MATING BEHAVIOR

Interference with mating behavior is a possible factor contributing to the overall antifertility effect.

In a detailed analysis Saunders (1958b) found that one injection of progesterone (5 mg/kg) or of 0.5 mg/kg of methallyl-19-nortestosterone in late diestrus prevented the animals (rats) from progressing into full estrus and mating, but norethynodrel (in a dose of 0.5 mg/kg) did not interfere with acceptance of the male. Therefore the antifertility effect of this compound when given in smaller doses for longer periods (see Table 32) must be due to another mechanism.

TABLE 32. Prevention of Pregnancy by Prolonged Continuous Administration of Drug
Doses in mg per animal per day unless otherwise indicated. EE stands for ethynyl estradiol.

Compound	Species	Route of admin.	Duration of treatment (days)		Lowest active dose resulting in		Highest inactive dose	Reference
			before caging with males	after caging with males	no pregnancy	reduced percent pregnant (%)		
Medrogestone	rat	s.c.	7	14	0.5	0.25 (20%)		Revesz and Chappel (1966)
with 4 mcg premarin	rat	s.c.	7	14	0.25			Revesz and Chappel (1966)
Megestrol acetate	rat	p.o.	5	365		0.0015[(1)] (50%)		Sanwal et al. (1970)
Norgestrel	rat	s.c.	5	30			1.0	Peterson and Edgren (1965)
	rat	p.o.				3.0 (50%)	0.3	Edgren et al. (1966a)
with 6 mcg EE	rat	p.o.	7	15	0.3			Allen et al. (1964)
Norethisterone with mestranol as Ortho-Novum	rat	p.o.			2/kg			
Norethisterone acetate	rat	p.o.	5	30		1.0 (25%)	0.1	Peterson and Edgren (1965)
	mouse	p.o.	7	21			8/kg/week	Doolittle (1963)
with EE as Norlutin	mouse	p.o.	7	21	2/kg/week			
	rat	p.o.	15	16	1.362			Falconi and Ercoli (1961)
Norgesterone	rat	p.o.		7	1.0			Ruggieri et al. (1965)

Orally Active Progestational Compounds: Animal Studies

Compound	Species	Route			Dose	Result	References
Norethynodrel	rat	p.o.	5	30	1.0		Peterson and Edgren (1965)
	rat	s.c.	5	30	0.2/kg		Saunders (1958a)
with mestranol as Enovid	mouse	p.o.	7	21		1.5/kg/week (17%)	Doolittle (1963)
	rat	s.c.		48	0.2/kg		Holmes and Mandl (1962)
	rat	s.c.	5	30	0.2/kg		Munshi (1964)
	mouse	s.c.	5	30	0.2/kg		Munshi (1964)
	rat	s.c.	3–7	15–19 (total period 22 days)	0.5–1.0	0.2 (see text)	Wakeling (1965)
with mestranol	rat	p.o.	7	7		0.5 (63%)	Ruggieri et al. (1965)
Norgestrienone	rat	p.o.		—		1.0 (34%)	Roussel (1966)
Quingestanol acetate	rat	p.o.	15	16	0.409		Falconi and Ercoli (1961)
Chlormadinone	mouse	impl.	2	50		6.0 (20%)	Folch-Pi et al. (1965)
acetate							
Medroxypro-	rat	p.o.	7	15	4.5/kg		Allen et al. (1964)
gesterone acetate	rat	p.o.	15	16	0.387		Falconi and Ercoli (1961)
	mouse	diet	4	7–10	(no mating) 0.6–1.0		Dziuk (1960)
	mouse		1 (single inj.)		(no mating)	2 (50%) conception delayed for 30 days	Sala et al. (1960)
Progesterone	rat	s.c.	5	30	5/kg		Saunders (1958a)

(1) Number of normal litters 3 from 16 females, as against 16/22 controls. See also subsection 23.2.

Wakeling (1965) approached the mechanism of the antifertility effect of norethynodrel in rats by injecting it daily in a dose of 0.2 mg for 22 days, into females that were exposed to males from the 3rd day or the 7th day of treatment (during the night only). Animals that mated were killed on the 1st, 2nd, 3rd or 4th day postcoitum (p.c.). Forty-eight out of seventy females mated (but only one out of eighteen which were only exposed to the male after 7 days of treatment). As is well known, the rat normally mates a few hours before ovulation. Wakeling found that only twenty-one treated animals copulated at the "correct" time with respect to ovulation, as judged by the size of the most recent set of corpora lutea and in these—if killed on the 1st day p.c.—nearly all the expected eggs were found in the oviducts (though not all were fertilized). In animals killed on day 2 or 3 p.c. far fewer eggs were located in the oviducts and all were degenerating.

The remaining rats that mated had either corpora lutea of atypical size, no recent corpora lutea or corpora resembling those such as one would find 1 to 3 days after p.c. in normal controls.

The author concludes that with the dosage schedule used, norethynodrel did not consistently inhibit ovulation or lead to refusal of the male. Acceptance of the male, however, was not always *synchronized* with follicular rupture. (Tubal transport of ova may be more susceptible to the action of norethynodrel than are the processes of ovulation or fertilization.)

In fact Salloch *et al.* (1971) could show that norethynodrel accelerates tubal transport of ova in rats qualitatively in the same way as caused by estradiol.

Soderwall *et al.* (1966) gave small doses of Enovid (0.2 mg/100 g) daily to young adult female hamsters for periods of 14 weeks and found that it lengthened the intervals between behavioral estrus periods from 4.1 days in controls to 15.0 days. (There was pronounced increase in developing follicles, none reaching the Graafian stage.)

A number of data on the suppression of estrus and mating behavior are listed in Table 33.

Related to the subject of suppressing or "desynchronizing" mating behavior—though *not* in the context of preventing pregnancy—is that of *inducing* it, as progesterone has been shown to be able to do.

This potency of steroids was studied by means of the copulatory reflex in spayed estrogen-primed guinea pigs by Kincl and Dorfman (1961) who found progesterone active in single doses (s.c.) of 50–100 mcg. Chlormadinone acetate, though about 50 times as active in the McPhail test, was inactive, at least with 4 times the dose of progesterone (19-norprogesterone had 20 times the potency of progesterone, and two dichloroprogesterone

TABLE 33. INTERFERENCE WITH MATING BEHAVIOR
Lowest dose of compound preventing percentage of females indicated in column 7 from mating, when administered as shown in columns 3–5. Doses per animal per day unless otherwise stated.

Compound	Species	Route of adm.	Number of doses	Time of adm. (day 0 = proestrus)	Lowest active dose (mg)	Per cent females refusing	Highest inactive dose (mg)	Reference
Norethynodrel	rat	s.c.	1×	−1			0.5/kg	Saunders (1958b)
	rat	p.o.	35×	cont.	1.0	50 (4/8)	0.1	Peterson and Edgren (1965)
Norethisterone acetate	rat	p.o.	35×				1.0	Peterson and Edgren (1965)
	rat	p.o.	25×	cont.			2.724	Falconi and Ercoli (1961)
Norgestrel	rat	s.c.	35×			37 (3/8)	1.0	Peterson and Edgren (1965)
	rat	p.o.	35×		3.0			
Quingestanol acetate	rat	p.o.	25×				3.268	Falconi and Ercoli (1961)
Medroxyprogest- erone acetate	mouse	diet	4–15×	cont.	0.6	100		Dziuk (1960)
	rat	p.o.	25×	cont.	0.387	100		Falconi and Ercoli (1961)
Megestrol acetate	rat	s.c.	14×	cont. from 0	0.4	37 (3/8)		Chang a Kincl (1968)
		p.o. implant (capsule)	14×	cont. from 0	0.8[(1)] 0.06[(2)]	46 (6/13) 25 (2/8)		
		p.o.	365×	cont.	0.0015	50		Sanwal et al. (1970)

(1) Twice and four times this dose inactive!
(2) Estimated release per 24 hours.

derivatives were 13 and 16 times more active than the parent compound). For a somewhat more elaborate discussion see Kincl (1964a).

Meyerson (1967) studied estrous-behavior-inducing activity of steroids in castrated rats, 48 hours after estrogen priming, judging the effect by a "clear-cut lordosis reflex to mounting by a vigorous male on at least 2 occasions or on the last test" (which is 8 hours after injection). With the submaximal priming dose used the dose of progesterone needed for a 45% response was 4 mg per animal.

Medroxyprogesterone acetate was found to have 3.75 times this potency, dydrogesterone 2.07 (*sic*) and allylestrenol 0.25 times the activity of progesterone.

Norethisterone gave a weak response in doses up to 10 mg; norethynodrel, lynestrenol and normethandrone (methylestrenolone) were inactive.

Of the compounds which induced mating behavior, only one, medroxyprogesterone acetate, caused clear-cut anesthesia (as judged by loss of righting reflex) on i.v. injection (15 mg). (The author finds a positive correlation of the ability of a compound to maintain pregnancy with its potency to induce mating behavior (not general anesthesia).) Earlier Meyerson (1966) had found that the effect of progesterone of activitating estrous behavior in castrated rats is inhibited by imipramine and related antidepressive drugs. This was interpreted as supporting the assumption, that an increased activity of serotoninergic synapses is involved in the inhibition of estrous behaviour.

Interesting studies concerning the influence of hormonally active steroids on mating behavior in primates were reported by Michael (1968). He observed male and female sexual behavior in Rhesus monkeys and often found a maximum of activity around the middle of the 28-day cycle in the female, as judged by frequency of mounting and grooming, attractiveness of the female ("female success ratio") or her readiness to refuse the partner ("male success ratio"). When ovariectomized females where given estradiol (5 mcg) mounting activity was high, but this could be significantly depressed by the concomitant injection of 25 (not 10) mg of progesterone. The number of ejaculations per test fell equally "dramatically". Both mechanisms—loss of female attractiveness, thus loss of male interest and increase of female refusals—were found to operate.

A synthetic progestational compound, ethynodiol acetate mixed with 5% of mestranol, was administered in two daily doses of 1 mg to two intact female Rhesus monkeys (each paired with two males) for 21 days and intervals of 7 days between two cycle treatments, thus closely imitating a human contraceptive regimen. The results were at the time described as complex, but the most conspicuous feature was a progressive fall in the number of ejaculations per test. Marked variations did not permit any reliable conclusions to be drawn.

In a subsequent study Michael (1969) investigated two progestational compounds, ethynodiol acetate and chlormadinone acetate, by subcutaneous injection (1 mg and 0.75 mg respectively), the former in a standard combination with mestranol, the latter according to a sequential schedule (mestranol alone (0.05 mg daily) for 11 days and thereafter mixed with chlormadinone acetate for 10 days). Apart from the parameters mentioned earlier, the numbers of "intromitted thrusts occurring prior to ejaculation" were recorded, these being lowest at the time of greatest female receptivity (when the male has to "work less hard"). There was an increase in the number of "thrusts to ejaculation" in all (four) pairs while the females were receiving contraceptive agents. This was more marked during the combined than during sequential treatment. (These reviewers regret that different drugs were used in the two different schedules, but this was apparently done to imitate recommended usage in the human.)

"With mestranol ethynodiol both the depression of ejaculation and the increase in thrusting changed progressively with successive cycles of treatment, and in one pair during the seventh month of treatment, ejaculation occurred only once in twelve tests while the number of thrusts required to achieve it had trebled. With mestranol chlormadinone, in contrast, the impairment of ejaculation was not obviously progressive and thrusting remained virtually unchanged."

The author cautions the reader against extrapolation across species boundaries, especially when human sexual behavior is concerned, but he feels sure that the data reported by himself are clear-cut and point to the possibility "that prolonged medication with these powerful steroids may in time modify human sexual behavior".

Another interesting warning should be cited. Lindsay and Scaramuzzi (1969) who studied estrous behavior in ewes under the influence of fourteen different steroids, found eight of these, including norethisterone, to inhibit behavioral response and four (not including norethisterone) to inhibit the vaginal response. "Vaginal and behavioural responses were not necessarily related and responses obtained in the ewe to particular steroids were not identical with those obtained in laboratory animals by other workers using similar tests."

16.4. OTHER MECHANISMS INVOLVED IN ANTIFERTILITY EFFECTS IN RATS OR MICE

16.4.1. *Studies concerning the effects of norethynodrel*

Available literature seems to justify a separate discussion of the various antifertility effects of norethynodrel in rats—including some work done with mice.

The claudogenic action of norethynodrel was lucidly analyzed by Saunders. He showed (1958b) that norethynodrel, given on day 2 or 3 *after* mating (day 1: sperm plug), drastically reduces the number of fetuses per rat found on day 15. Since in this case inhibition of ovulation cannot be involved, nidation must have failed (but this could also have been due to an effect on transport of the fertilized ovum through the oviduct). Even so, according to later studies of Saunders (1964), this can still not be the main mechanism responsible for the antifertility action of norethynodrel since the daily dose needed for a practically complete inhibition of conception (nidation), given on days 2, 3 and 4 *post coitum*, was "approximately 5 times as large as that adequate to prevent fertility when treatment was begun well *before* ovulation". Therefore, the author concludes, "The antifertility effect observed with continuous administration must be pre-ovulatory". These very low doses are, according to further studies, sufficient to depress the level of pituitary gonadotrophin needed for follicular maturation in the ovary—and *this* would appear to be the most likely mechanism, also in view of the absence of large ($>55\mu$) follicles observed by Holmes and Mandl (1962). What these studies show again is *inter alia* the fact that *the same drug may interfere with normal fertility by more than one mechanism*. Results obtained with prolonged, continuous administration need not be due to the same mechanism as those following treatment for short periods, sharply defined with respect to phase of cycle or time of mating.

Saunders (1965) injected rats with norethynodrel (with 1.5% of mestranol, Enovid) on days 2, 3 and 4 p.c. which reduced the total number of implantation sites, counted in groups of 10 rats on day 15 p.c., by about 98, when the dose was 0.5 mg/kg. The fertility index FI (ratio of total number of normal-sized fetuses to total number of females mated) was thereby reduced from 10.2 for normal controls to zero. That the estrogen contributed a good deal to this postcoital effect is shown by the fact that the same result could be obtained by injection of 0.05 mg of estrone and almost the same (FI 0.9) with 0.02 mg of mestranol or 1.0 mg (FI 0.1) of pure norethynodrel. "Norethynodrel, which has 3–7% the estrogenicity of estrone, was approximately 2% as effective in inhibiting nidation in rats."

As we have remarked above, failure of blastocysts to nidate could be due to a disturbance of transport.

Davis (1963a) injected norethynodrel into rats either on 1 or on 3 successive days after mating and before the 6th day p.c. and found that a dose of 0.9 mg (on day 2) was needed and sufficient to reduce to zero the number of fetuses, found at autopsy on day 10–12 p.c. The result of Saunders (1965) is in close agreement with this. Further studies by Davis (1963b), in mice, ovariectomized on day 2 p.c., led him to the conclusion that inhibition of the occurrence of nidation and induction of fetal resorption were apparently brought about by norethynodrel by a direct action on the uterus, particularly because the "ability of recovered blastocysts to implant following transplantation into pseudopregnant ovariectomized mice was impaired by treatment of the donor with norethynodrel to only a minor degree in one of two experiments" *but* "administration of 0.6 mg norethynodrel to the host elicited a response that almost completely inhibited nidation". On the other hand, Watnick *et al.* (1965, 1966) have reasons to believe that the postcoital contraceptive effect of norethynodrel (at the lowest effective dose of 5 mg/kg/day) in rats is to a large extent due to inhibition of nidation but also to a change in tubal transport of ova.

16.4.2. *Other compounds*

Kincl and Dorfman (1965a) began the administration of drugs to be tested on the morning of proestrus and on the same day the females were caged with fertile males for 2 days in succession. Treatment was either by subcutaneous injection or by gavage for a total of 7 days. This procedure was likely to interfere with ovulation or transport of sperm or ovum. Two compounds of high activity in the human and in other animal tests, norethisterone and chlormadinone acetate, given orally in daily doses up to 2.4 and 5 mg respectively were *inactive* in this test. So was progesterone, subcutaneously in daily doses up to 15 mg. The most active neutral steroid compound was 17α-ethynyl-5α-androst-2 en-17β-ol, but this was by far surpassed by estradiol subcutaneously—ED_{100} 0.45 mcg —and mestranol orally (45 mcg). In most cases, the authors conclude, antifertility (as shown by this test) was correlated with estrogenicity.

Chlormadinone acetate, in doses of 1.0 mg/100 g, was also of little effect when given orally to rats on days 1–3 "of pregnancy" (day 1: sperm plug) and quite inactive on days 4–6, as demonstrated by Hecht-Lucari *et al.* (1966).

Norgestrel administered to rats for 7 days after mating (day 1: sperm plug) in doses up to 62.5 mcg alone or in combination with 6.25 mcg ethynyl estradiol was found by Edgren *et al.* (1968) not to decrease the numbers of normal pregnancies significantly. (These low doses were chosen in order to mimic the effects of the pharmaceutical preparation Ovral on a mg/kg bodyweight basis, assuming an average weight of about 50 kg in a woman, for whom the dose would represent approximately 10 mcg norgestrel and 1 mcg EE per kg.)

Quingestanol administered orally in daily doses of 0.5 mg/animal from day 1 to day 11 after mating was found by Giannina *et al.* (1969) *not* to prevent pregnancy in rats, but a daily dose of 5 mg during the preimplantation period "interfered with the nidation processes". Given on the day of implantation (day 4 after mating) or for the following 7 days it prevented normal development of conceptus (see Section 17 below).

16.5. ANTIFERTILITY MECHANISMS IN THE RABBIT

The rabbit with a sexual organization so different from that of the rat has in many ways provided information on the pharmacological mechanisms of actions of steroids. Ovulation can be exactly timed by injection of HCG and this procedure has been used in antifertility studies.

Medroxyprogesterone acetate in a single subcutaneous dose of 2 or 10 mg delayed mating in 70% of treated rabbits for 10 days and drastically reduced the number of conceptions according to Sala *et al.* (1960). The mechanisms of this effect was not further analysed.

Hungarian investigators (Sas *et al.*, 1967) reported that a single dose of Lyndiol (5 mg lynestrenol plus 150 mcg mestranol) given by gavage made the does refuse the male the next day (no control or placebo treatment reported) and administered between 0 and 30 hours after mating prevented pregnancy as ascertained on day 15. Ovulation was reported not to have occurred in the animals treated before the 28th hour after mating (absence of corpora lutea after 72 hours). In two animals treated between 28 and 30 hours p.c., there were corpora lutea but no pregnancy, and when the drug was administered still later (30–60 hours) there was an increasing percentage of pregnant animals (100% after 72 hours). The progestational component alone had essentially the same effect; mestranol was reported to have caused somewhat comparable results within 24 hours p.c. The authors introduce the term "postovulatory inhibitory effect" without being able to elucidate the mechanisms involved. Much more insight was gained through the studies of Bennett *et al.* (1967b), in which rabbits were given various steroids for 3 days (by gavage). On the 4th day they were subjected to artificial insemination (AI), immediately followed by an intravenous injection of 25 I.U. HCG. The rabbits were autopsied about 30 hours after AI and the Fallopian tubes and uteri flushed out to recover the ova shed and to determine their number in various parts of the genital tract in relation to the number of corpora lutea in the ovaries. The percentage of unfertilized (single-cell stage) and fertilized (two- and four-cell stages) ova was determined and when fertilization was found to be inhibited, sperm migration was studied in animals having undergone the same treatment but without induction of ovulation (since the presence of eggs in the oviduct influences the number of sperms to be found there).

In these studies the cervix proved to be the most important barrier to fertilization. Three progestational pregnane derivatives were compared. Megestrol acetate and chlormadinone acetate in three preovulatory daily doses of 0.1 mg/kg considerably reduced the number of fertilized eggs, 1.0 mg/kg completely prevented fertilization while not affecting the excellent total recovery of ova. Of melengestrol, a 10 times higher dose (10.0 mg/kg) was needed for total suppression, though at the ED_{50} level it seemed to be as potent as chlormadinone acetate. The latter, curiously enough, seemed to be less effective at a dose of 10.0 than at one of 1.0 mg. It seems to us to be difficult to establish ratios of activities on the basis of these figures. The effect on sperm migration is illustrated in Table 34, adapted from Bennett *et al.* (1967b). The authors conclude "that these progestagens probably acted by preventing the access of sufficient numbers of spermatozoa to the site of fertilization" and they assume that they did this by "producing a hostile cervical mucus". As expected, an estrogen, ethynyl estradiol, did not interfere either with fertilization, or with sperm transport to the uterus, which was even increased by higher doses. One would thus be inclined to put the barrier effect of the progestational steroids down to an antiestrogenic effect. It is, therefore, interesting and surprising to see that a highly potent antiestrogen, dimethyl stilbestrol in the experiments here described *increased* sperm transport through the cervix, which shows that estrogen antagonism at various sites of the organism may be brought about by quite different mechanisms.

The mode of action of megestrol in preventing pregnancy in ovulating rabbits was again studied by Kendle and Telford (1970). The compound was given orally in daily doses varying between 12.5 and 200 mcg/kg to rabbits on three successive days (-2, -1 and 0) before artificial insemination (AI) and induction of ovulation by means of 25 I.U. of HCG (on day 0). It was found that a daily dose of 100 mcg/kg completely prevented pregnancy and 50 mcg/kg in nine out of ten animals, as shown by autopsy on day 16. The latter dose was chosen because it was more in agreement with

TABLE 34. INFLUENCE OF STEROID TREATMENT FOR 3 DAYS BEFORE ARTIFICIAL INSEMINATION (AI) IN RABBITS, ADAPTED FROM BENNETT et al. (1967)

Doses are expressed in mg/kg/day. Percentages of eggs fertilized were determined in animals with induced ovulation by HCG injection at the time of AI, sperm counts in animals similarly treated but without ovulation induction.

Compound	Dose	% of eggs fertilized	Mean no. of spermatozoa inseminated ($\times 10^6$)	Mean number of spermatozoa ($\times 10^3$) and percentage of sperm cells inseminated found in uterus and numbers in tubes		
				uterus		Fallopian tubes
				no.	%	no.
Megestrol acetate	0.001	74				
	0.01	56	300	138	0.046	2.5
	0.1	2.5	159	8	0.005	0.2
	1.0	0	284	14	0.004	0.3
	10.0	0				
Melengestrol acetate	0.001	85				
	0.01	72	314	46	0.014	2.4
	0.1	47	276	56	0.020	1.1
	1.0	7.5	448	12	0.003	0.2
	10.0	0				
Chlormadinone acetate	0.001	80				
	0.01	45	456	143	0.031	0.25
	0.1	40	338	63	0.018	0.42
	1.0	0	236	18	0.007	0.42
	10.0	20				

the incomplete contraceptive effect of the continuous low-dose progestational regimen in the human, the mechanism of which the authors wanted to elucidate. Sperm penetration (recovery from uterine flushing 3, 6, 12 and 24 hours after AI) was reduced by about 50% but the maximum was reached at the same time as in controls, which in the author's judgment indicated "no change in the rate of cervical transport". Also there was some overlap between controls and treated animals.

By contrast, there was a consistent acceleration of egg transport through the oviduct, since all recovered ova were found in the uterus on day 2, that is 2 days too soon. In addition, experiments involving the transfer of 4-day-old ova from untreated animals to the uteri of megestrol acetate-treated rabbits on day 4 of pseudopregnancy showed a reduced number of implantations and a great increase in fetal resorption, whereas more normal results were obtained when these ova were transferred to 2-day-pseudopregnant uteri. Thus it looks as if these uteri advanced more rapidly in progestational development when the animals were given the drug and this increased the disparity in developmental stage between the ova that arrived too soon and the endometria that were in a far advanced phase. This was confirmed by histological examination.

One of the present authors (de Visser) has developed a pharmacological test for contraceptive effects of progestational steroids in ovulating rabbits. This has not yet been published *in extenso*; only a short communication was made at a federation meeting in the Netherlands (de Visser, 1969).

The test is based on the well-known fact that in a rabbit, which has been pseudopregnant (progesterone-dominated) for at least 5 days, ovulations can be induced by means of gonadotrophic hormones but that the ova so released cannot be fertilized through artificial intravaginal insemination (Wislocki and Snijder, 1933; Boyarski *et al.*, 1947).

We synchronized estrus in our rabbits by having them mated with a vasectomized male. This would be followed by a state of pseudopregnancy for about 16 days and a period of regression of corpora lutea lasting for 5 days. On the 21st day after sterile mating (SM) all the animals were in full estrus and ovulations were induced by an intravenous injection of 25 I.U. HCG, immediately thereafter followed by artificial intravaginal insemination as described by Adams (1961). Under these conditions fertilized eggs were regularly found in the oviducts.

Progesterone, given in daily doses of 2 to 4 mg for 8 days, beginning on the 16th day after SM, with HCG–AI treatment on the 22nd and autopsy on the 24th day, prevented fertilization of 50% and 99% of eggs, respectively. When steroid treatment was started 4 days later and lasted for 4 days only (20–23 after SM), other conditions remaining the same, a daily dose of only 1 or 2 mg prevented fertilization of all ova. We then developed a routine procedure, in which the steroids to be tested are administered for 8 days, beginning on the 21st day after SM, with HCG–AI treatment on day 27 and autopsy on day 29. Antifertilizing activity was judged by flushing the oviducts and uterus and determining the percentage of unfertilized ova amongst those recovered. Recovery itself, as expressed as percentage of ruptured follicles, was used to judge loss of eggs (fertilized or unfertilized) through disturbances of transport. Compounds were rated as *active* in preventing fertilization when more than 70% of the ova recovered were unfertilized, as inactive with less than 40%, and weakly active in between. In applying these criteria, the active daily dose of progesterone (s.c.) was 1 mg, of chlormadinone acetate 0.125, of megestrol acetate 0.25 and of medroxyprogesterone acetate 2 mg. Dydrogesterone was inactive at 4 mg. Of the estrane derivatives, norethynodrel and norethisterone were inactive (4 mg), lynestrenol was active at 4 mg, but of methandrolone only 1 mg was needed. These data are also shown in Table 35.

TABLE 35. POTENCY OF STEROIDS IN PREVENTING FERTILIZATION OF AT LEAST 70% OF OVA, RECOVERED AT AUTOPSY IN RABBITS 48 HOURS AFTER INDUCTION OF OVULATION BY MEANS OF HCG AND ARTIFICIAL INTRAVAGINAL INSEMINATION (AI)
Compounds adminstered orally for 8 days, including day of AI (day 7) and day thereafter (de Visser, unpublished).

Compound	Minimum effective dose (mg per day)
Chlormadinone acetate	0.125
Megestrol acetate	0.25
Normethandrone	1
Medroxyprogesterone acetate	2
Allylestrenol	1–4
Lynestrenol	4
Norethisterone	>4 (inactive)
Dydrogesterone	>4 (inactive)

In order to elucidate the mechanisms involved, we studied sperm transport and found that 5–6 hours after intravaginal AI, as practiced in our test, 1.5% of spermatozoa were found in the cervix (6 millions out of 400×10^6 deposited in the vagina), 0.3% (1.2×10^6) in the uterus and 0.025% (10,500) in the tubes, when the animal was in estrus. By contrast, in animals on the 8th day of pseudopregnancy, smaller percentages (0.1–0.2%) were found in the cervix, none or few in the uterus and *none* in the tubes. Progesterone (1 mg/day, s.c. for 8 days) and chlormadinone acetate (0.5 mg/day, orally for 8 days) produced shifts in the same direction but were less effective in barring passage through the cervix than were the animals' own *corpora lutea*.

Our conclusion that in these experiments this was the main factor responsible for the antifertilizing effects observed was strengthened by the observation that these disappeared completely, both in pseudopregnant and in progesterone-treated animals, when insemination was performed in the uterus instead of intravaginally, even though the number of sperm cells was only 1% of those used in routine intravaginal AI, which is about equal to the physiological number of sperms entering the uterus after normal mating. These experiments also show that under these conditions an impairment of capacitation of sperm was not involved in the antifertilizing action of progesterone. They furthermore point to the similarity in the hormonal conditioning of the cervix in the rabbit and the human. This is borne out by the observation that an estrogen, mestranol, in eight daily doses from 7.5 to 120 mcg was practically without antifertilizing effect.

There are certain other analogies between the rabbit and the human cervix. The mucus found in the estrous rabbit vagina near the cervix shows estrus-dependent "spinnbarkeit" and ferning. This mucus is actually produced in the cervix. Mucus-secreting (goblet) cells, visible during estrus (PAS staining), are inactive (regenerating) during the luteal phase. Ciliated cells are present in the rabbit and, as shown by Stegner and Beltermann (1969), in human cervical epithelium.

It would not be justifiable to draw firm conclusions from these observations with respect to steroid effects to be expected in the human cervix. Our observations may be summarized by the statement that in rabbits with synchronized estrus and ovulation, administration of progesterone or certain progestational compounds, at least four days before and one day after induced ovulation, produces antifertility effects, visible 48 hours after ovulation and probably entirely accounted for by changes in the cervix.

In this experimental set-up, chlormadinone acetate has been the most active compound so far. Petrow's term *claudogenic* would seem to be particularly apposite here. Chang (1966) also used rabbits with artificial induction of ovulation and insemination but gave higher doses of HCG (45–90 I.U.), restricted steroid administration to three oral doses, before and on the day of insemination, and examined the ova only 6 days later.

Apart from progesterone (2 mg s.c.), medroxyprogesterone acetate (MAP) and ethynyl estradiol (EE) were the only compounds studied. With progesterone treatment recovery of eggs was poor (21% of the number of corpora lutea) and no normal blastocysts were found in the uterus. The same result was obtained with 2 mg MAP, while decreasing doses (1, 0.5, 0.2, and 0.1 mg) gave increasing yields of normal blastocysts. Fifty mcg of EE had little effect when given alone before insemination but caused complete loss of blastocysts when given on 3 successive days after AI.

Further studies led to the conclusion that administration of progesterone before ovulation or of estrogen after ovulation speeds the transport of eggs and causes their degeneration or expulsion from the uterus. This is discussed below (Section 18, Influence on oviducts).

Both factors—prevention of fertilization and disturbance of transport of ova—were considered by Vickery and Bennett (1969) in their studies involving the oral administration of three, four and eleven small doses of chlormadinone acetate, beginning 2 or 3 days before AI + HCG treatment and continuing for periods between 0 and 8 days thereafter. At varying periods after AI the animals were sacrificed and the number of ova, fertilized or unfertilized, in the tubes or uterus and the development of blastocysts were recorded. A daily dose of 0.1 mg/kg (definitely more than our dose of 0.125 mg per animal) prevented fertilization of about 80% of ova; 1 mg/kg prevented it completely. But at doses of 3 mcg to 100 mcg/kg some 25–30% of ova were already found in the uterus about 30 hours after insemination which proves a considerably increased speed of transport. In fact a dose of 0.09 mg/kg/day for 3 days, before and on the day of insemination, which was still compatible with the fertilization of a high percentage of ova, completely inhibited the development of pregnancy. No viable fetuses were found on day 15. The authors conclude that it makes no difference, whether chlormadinone acetate is given only before, or before and after, ovulation and that the compound "was at least 10 × more effective in terminating pregnancy than in inhibiting fertilization". "Terminating" in the context does, of course, mean the prevention of normal development because of initial disturbance of the rate of transport through the tubes required for normal nidation.

A more recent investigation by Nutting and Mares (1970) deserves attention in this connection, though no orally active synthetic compounds were used, because it contributes to our understanding of the antifertility effect of progesterone in rabbits. These authors induced ovulation with 100–200 I.U. HCG after periods of 1 to 7 days of progesterone treatment immediately followed by artificial intravaginal insemination and one more

TABLE 36. The Effect of Progesterone on the Number of Spermatozoa Recovered from Various Segments of the Rabbit Genital Tract 4–24 Hr After Artificial Insemination with 10×10^6 to 40×10^6 Spermatozoa[a]
From Nutting and Mares (1970)

Segment of genital tract	Control no. of hours after insemination				Progesterone no. of hours after insemination			
	4	8	16	24	4	8	16	24
Cervix	147,600	122,500	28,630	25,070	191,600	180,000	17,290	29,980
Uterus-posterior	54,040	34,590	12,390	34,590	41,830	24,470	2993	8796
Uterus-middle	105,200	5724	5445	19,330	6462	838	2693	7060
Uterus-anterior	49,430	11,670	15,560	86,830	3231	180	3531	4847
Oviduct-posterior	2454	3711	3860	6822	0	180	718	180
Oviduct-middle	300	4847	2154	957	0	0	120	120
Oviduct-anterior	0	3531	2244	838	0	0	0	0
Uterus-complete	208,670	51,984	33,395	140,750	51,523	25,488	9217	20,703
Oviduct-complete	2754	12,089	8258	8617	0	180	838	300

[a] Animals were treated daily with 1 mg progesterone in 0.2 ml corn oil or with corn oil only injected subcutaneously for 7 days and inseminated on the 7th day. Each value is the mean from three rabbits.

day of progesterone. Their first remarkable finding was that the effect of a daily dose of 1 mg was by far the greatest, when treatment had been started 3 days before AI (total dose, therefore, 4 × 1 mg).

With this schedule *no* fertilized ova were found, as against 97% with AI on first day and 13% on the 7th day. Also total recovery of ova was smallest with AI on 3rd day of treatment. (It will be recalled that we too found an increased efficacy of progesterone with 4 days' treatment.) Nutting and Mares interpret their observation by saying that "rabbits under the influence of progesterone apparently pass through two distinct periods of lowered fertility. The first period occurs on the 3rd day of treatment and is short in duration." They therefore settled for a standard treatment of 8 days (−6 to +1), AI on D 0 and autopsy on D +2 (48 hours after AI). With this schedule the lowest daily dose reducing the percentage of fertilized ova significantly ($p \leq 0.05$) below control levels was 0.2 mg. Four milligrams (highest dose tested) yielded 2% of ova fertilized (versus 93% average of controls). As in our studies, described above, *intra-uterine* insemination produced a *normal*, undiminished, percentage of fertilized ova, thus implicating the cervix as a major barrier and eliminating faulty capacitation as a probable antifertility factor.

Increased speed of transport of ova must have occurred when AI was performed on day 3 of treatment. However, effects on sperm transport beyond the cervix were also found. Figures for sperm counts in the cervix, in three successive uterine and three tubal segments in controls and progesterone-treated animals are shown in Nutting and Mares' table 5 (our Table 36). Moreover, the inhibitory effect of progesterone on sperm transport was partly reversed by the injections of large doses (50 USP U) of oxytocin (see Chapter 8, p. 266). The authors believe that, particularly in view of the changes in sperm transport observed, the rabbit would be a useful model for the testing of potential contraceptive agents, an opinion which we fully share.

16.6. OBSERVATIONS IN FERRETS

Chang (1967) studied the effect of medroxyprogesterone acetate (MAP) administered to ferrets in daily doses of 2 mg p.o. for 3 days before an ovulation-inducing intraperitoneal injection of 90 I.U. HCG. *Uterine* insemination of epididymal spermatozoa was performed (day 0) at the same time or 12 hours later. From eight animals so treated sixty-four eggs were recovered on day 4; 77% of these were in the uterus (as against *one* control animal with eggs in uterus), but only 1.6% were fertilized (as against 68% in controls).

On days 13 to 18 another four animals were examined and no embryo was found (as against twenty in the controls). Since the eggs had reached the uterus 4 to $4\frac{1}{2}$ days after the ovulation-inducing injection of HCG—as contrasted with 6 days after normal mating (the interval between this and ovulation being the same as after HCG injection, viz. about 30 hours)—the author concludes that in the ferret the preovulatory administration of MAP increased the rate of transport of the ova through the oviducts. It also prevented fertilization (which it does not do in the rabbit prior to ovulation) and this could have been due to disturbed transport of gametes or to failure of capacitation.

17. INTERFERENCE WITH ESTABLISHED PREGNANCY
(Including some data on lactation)

In Section 16 we have dealt with the adverse effects of progestational compounds on preludes to pregnancy. In some of the studies there was clear evidence of damage to nidating blastocysts. Without going into the question of the time when pregnancy begins, which is considered of great importance in some discussions on the ethical or legal aspects of certain birth-control methods, we are trying to separate those early phases, covering ovulation, fertilization, transport of gametes and of fertilized ova, including their nidation in the endometrium, from later phases, when an established pregnancy which otherwise would most probably have yielded a normal litter is disturbed.

When treatment with progestational steroids disturbs an established pregnancy, the observed effect is usually death and more or less advanced resorption of embryos. Malformations (teratogenicity) have in general not been recorded, apart from those genital abnormalities we have discussed in Section 15, Masculinization of female fetuses. Some authors compared the damaging effects of progestational compounds with those of estrogens. Thus Overbeek *et al.* (1962) found that lynestrenol, a clearly estrogenic compound, had about the same damaging effect on rat fetuses as "equivalent doses of estrogen", viz. one-hundredth the dose of ethynyl estradiol.

Saunders (1967) used his studies on possible impairment of pregnancy to show that a daily dose of 0.1 mg/kg of mestranol caused more damage to the fetuses than 0.2 mg/kg of Enovid-E (containing 8 mcg of mestranol). He also continued to treat the rats during the ensuing period of *lactation* and found doses of Enovid-E up to 0.5 mg/kg apparently innocuous but of eight females treated with 1 mg/kg only four raised young to weaning. There was no impairment of fertility in the offspring of rats treated with a dose of 0.05 mg/kg of Enovid during pregnancy *and* lactation; but only eleven of twenty pairs from the 0.1 mg/kg group, and none treated with larger doses, were fertile. The effects are mainly considered as estrogen damage, including early post-natal steroid damage (see Chapter 11). Similarly Edgren and Peterson Clancy (1968) gave norgestrel alone or combined with ethynyl estradiol in doses meant to correspond with human doses of the oral contraceptive drug Ovral® (10 mcg/kg plus 1 mcg/kg EE) or 5 times and 25 times this dose. This had no effect on the fetus when given to the mothers from days 8 to 21 inclusive, and there were no abnormalities in the young at the age of 29 days. Fertility of the F_1 generation was normal "although the data suggest some decrease in fertility in offspring that received the high dose of estrogen".

When a similar treatment was given to lactating rats (by gavage), as described by Peterson Clancy and Edgren (1968), there was no discernible effect on either the mothers or the offspring.

Table 37 shows the results of a number of studies. It includes one investigation of Rhesus monkeys (Wharton and Scott, 1964), in which norethisterone was given in a high dose of 25 mg, subcutaneously, beginning on or about the 31st day of pregnancy and continued until delivery. Only two out of ten females so treated progressed to at least the 160th day of pregnancy or to term (normal 160–165 days) and only one additional "term-sized fetus" was delivered at 133 days. The duration of the other seven pregnancies varied between 96 and 143 days. Only two newborn were alive. The five newborn females were all visibly masculinized, though there was no virilization in the mothers. The ovary in the fetuses "at times appears to be disproportionately retarded in its maturation process". Progesterone in double the dose (50 mg daily) had no adverse effects.

Relatively few studies have been published that were undertaken with the purpose of demonstrating the occurrence of this sort of effect. From some papers it can be inferred that in the study reported—though directed at a different object—no damaging effect, such as discussed here, incompatible with fetal life had been observed. This can, for example, be said of the paper by Kraay and Brennan (1963) dealing with the lack of a fetal-masculinizing property in chlormadinone acetate and its occurrence in medroxyprogesterone acetate and norethisterone.

In view of this situation we can by no means claim to have completely covered the reports in the literature.

18. EFFECTS OF PROGESTATIONAL SUBSTANCES ON THE FALLOPIAN TUBES

Our discussion on antifertility effects (especially in subsections 16.5 and 16.6) has already yielded a number of experimental results indicating an influence of progestational compounds on the rate of egg transport through the oviducts. In the present section we attempt to group available data systematically as is, in our judgment, required for a pharmacological approach to the subject.

In Chapter 7 we elaborated on the various factors, particularly estrogen and progesterone concentrations, on which the rate of transport through the oviduct depends. We pointed out that it is not muscular activity alone that determines the final result, particularly because this activity is not merely propulsive. Both peristaltic and antiperistaltic movements and muscular locking all play a part, in addition to ciliary action, volume of secretion, and fluid currents. A recent analysis of this process, based on original observations, has been given by Humphrey (1970). Since most observations reported here are limited to recording the overall effect and to locating ova—fertilized or unfertilized—in various parts of the female genital tract at certain times after ovulation, it will not be surprising that in most cases it is not possible to give a more precise description of the factors involved.

A number of data are shown in Table 38. Attention is again called to the work of Chang (1966), already referred to on p. 150. This investigator has studied not only the influence of medroxyprogesterone acetate (MAP) given p.o. at various times before (or after) the induction of ovulation in the rabbit but also its effect on the transport of ova transplanted into the Fallopian tubes of estrous, "non-ovulated", rabbits. Whereas estrogens (ethynyl estradiol) always increase the speed of egg transport, progesterone or MAP did so only when given before ovulation or transplantation. The author's hypothetical explanation of this unexpected phenomenon is that progesterone has the ability to counteract the action of estrogen for only 3 days and the ensuing acceleration would be a kind of rebound effect of the (endogenous) estrogen. Opposed to this view is the finding of Bennett, Vickery and Dorfman (1969), quoted by Bennett (1970), "that if progestin dosing is initiated before ovulation in the rabbit and continued after ovulation for a further 8 days, an accelerated rate of egg transport still occurs".

Kendle and Telford (1970), who found that megestrol acetate, given *before* ovulation, increases the rate of transport through the oviduct (see

TABLE 37. INTERFERENCE WITH ESTABLISHED PREGNANCY

Doses are in mg per day per animal unless otherwise indicated. Period of treatment is indicated in days of pregnancy or postcoitum. Reduced numbers of litters and incidence of resorption are given in parentheses over numbers of animals treated. Reduced numbers or percentages of fetuses are given in parentheses over numbers found earlier on inspection. i.p. stands for intraperitoneal.

Compound	Species	Route of admin.	Period of treatment	Highest dose found inactive	Active dose resulting in:				Day of autopsy	Reference
					no litter	reduced number of litters	reduced number of fetuses	incidence of resorption		
Norethynodrel	rat	p.o.	9–13		10			10 (5/5)	21–27	Davis (1963a)
with 4% mestranol as Enovid-E	mouse	i.p.	10–12		2	10 (3/5)		10 (5/5)	21–27	Davis (1963b)
	rat	p.o.	8–10	0.5/kg		1/kg (9/10)		100%	15	Saunders (1967)
Lynestrenol	rat	p.o.	7–21				2.5 (40%/119)		inspected at birth	Overbeek et al. (1962)
	rat	p.o.	9–20				5 (15%/111)		21	Overbeek et al. (1962)
	rat	p.o.	9–20				10 (26.8%/109)		21	Overbeek et al. (1962)
Allylestrenol	rat	p.o.	9–20	20					21	Madjerek et al. (1960)
	rat	s.c.	6–15	20					21	Richter (1963)
	rat	s.c.	14–21	20					21	Jost and Moreau-Stinnakre (1970)
	rat	p.o.	14–21	10–30						
Dydrogesterone	rat	p.o.	14–21	10		5 every 5th day (1/5)				Marois (1962b)
Norethisterone	macaca mulatta	s.c.	31-delivery				25 (see text)			Wharton and Scott (1964)
	rat	s.c.	14–21							Montuori et al. (1960)

Compound	Animal	Route	Days	Dose	Dose	Number	Reference
Norethisterone acetate	rat	s.c.	14–21	5 every 5th day			Montuori et al. (1960)
Melengestrol acetate	rat	s.c.	15–20		1.0 (31/4 mothers) 5.0 (11/3 mothers) 16 dead fetuses		Duncan et al. (1964)
Megestrol acetate	rat	s.c.	14–20	10			David et al. (1963)
	rat	p.o.	15–20	15/kg			
Medroxyprogesterone acetate	rat	s.c.	6–21		5 every 5th day (3/6)	22	Montuori et al. (1960)
Normethandrone	rat	s.c.	14–21	5 every 5th day	1 every 5th day (3/6)		Montuori et al. (1960)
Norvinisterone	rat	s.c.	14–21		5 every 5th day (3/4)	22	Montuori et al. (1960)
Norgestrel	rat	s.c.(?)	8–21	0.0625			Edgren and Peterson Clancy (1968)

subsection 16.5, p. 143 could show that this treatment (50 mcg/kg orally per day for 3 successive days) had no influence on oviduct opening pressure, i.e. the pressure under which a saline solution has to be injected, through the ovarian end of the tube in order to initiate and maintain a regular flow. "Similarly, examination of the recordings failed to reveal any consistent change in any other parameter of muscular activity such as pressure wave amplitude or frequency." The only other change observed concerned the volume of tubal secretion, which in normal animals falls by about 30% on days 3 and 4 of pregnancy but as early as days 1 and 2 (after ovulation on day 0) in rabbits that had received preovulatory megestrol treatment. This was also reflected in an accelerated decline (by 48 hours) of distension of oviducts ligated at the ovarian end during the first days of pregnancy.

Although this chapter deals with animal studies we include some data concerning the human oviduct. As reported in Chapter 7 (p. 257), Erb found that the threshold dose of acetylcholine to induce contractions of the excised human Fallopian tube rises from a low level in the proliferative phase (ED_{50} 0.9 mcg) to about 10 times that value (ED_{50} 9.2 mcg) in the progesterone-dominated secretory phase. The sensitivity of the tube could equally be lowered by three daily injections of 100 mg of progesterone (Erb and Wenner, 1967). In the same year Erb (1967) reported that under the influence of oral contraceptives of the combination type in five women there were no cyclic changes of tubal acetylcholine sensitivity, which remained high. Chlormadinone acetate in a non-ovulation-suppressing dose of 0.5 mg daily caused a reduced postovulatory decrease in tubal sensitivity (ED_{50} of acetylcholine 3.9 mcg) (Erb, 1969). Lynestrenol in a very low daily dose, 0.15 mg, which did *not* suppress ovulation as shown by LH-peak in urine and pregnanediol excretion, caused a decrease of tubal sensitivity (acetylcholine ED_{50} 5 mcg) already in the preovulatory phase of the cycle, which was further depressed after ovulation (ED_{50} 10 mcg) (Erb 1970). This contrasts with the accelerating effects of lynestrenol on tubal transport observed in rats by Overbeek *et al.* (1962) as shown in Table 38. It also demonstrates the variety of pharmacological patterns encountered amongst compounds bearing the common name *progestational*.

Terragno *et al.* (1968) studied the effects of two ovulation-inhibiting drugs (norethynodrel with mestranol as Enovid® and ethynodiol acetate with mestranol as Ovulen® and Metrulen®) on the isolated human oviduct *in vitro*. Spontaneous rhythmic contractions of these surviving organs were inhibited in every case after the addition of the drugs (30–35 mcg added to a cup containing 50 ml Locke–Ringer solution). Motility became immediately normal again after washing.

TABLE 38. INFLUENCE OF PROGESTATIONAL COMPOUNDS ON THE RATE OF EGG TRANSPORT THROUGH THE FALLOPIAN TUBES

Doses in mg/day unless otherwise indicated. Period of administration is given in days before induction of ovulation by HCG or mating (negative numericals), on day of induction (0) and thereafter (+). An accelerating effect is marked as + in column 6, retarding as −.

Compound	Species	Route of admin.	Period of admin.	Dose	Effect	Criteria for judging effect	Reference
Medroxyprogesterone acetate	rabbit	oral	−1	2	+	71% of ova in uterus on +2	Chang (1966)
	rabbit	oral	−2, −1, 0	2	+	97% of ova in uterus on +3	Chang (1966)
	rabbit	oral	0	2	−	100% of ova in tubes on +4	Chang (1966)
	rabbit	oral	−2, −1, 0 transpl.[1]	2	+	94% of ova in uterus after 40–42 hr	Chang (1966)
	rabbit	oral	0, +1, +2[1]	2	−	100% of ova in tubes 64 hr later	Chang (1966)
Chlormadinone acetate	rabbit	oral	−2, −1, 0	0.003/kg	+	12% of ova in uterus on +1	Vickery and Bennett (1969)
	rabbit	oral	−2, −1, 0	0.01	none		Vickery and Bennett (1969)
	rabbit	oral	−2, −1, 0	0.03	+	13% of ova in uterus on +1	Vickery and Bennett (1969)
Norethynodrel	rabbit	oral	+1	20	+	27% of ova in uterus on +2	Chang (1964)
Lynestrenol	rat	oral	+1, +2, +3, +4[2]	0.5–1.0	+[3]	subnormal number or no ova or embryos in uterus on day +5 or +9	Overbeek et al. (1962)

Notes to Table 38
(1) Day 0 in this case is not the day of ovulation but that of transplantation of 1-day-old ova into the Fallopian tubes of non-ovulated females having received the steroid treatment indicated.
(2) Day 0 = day of conception.
(3) In original paper interpreted as retardation. Acceleration had to be assumed when later work (de Visser, unpublished) failed to detect ova in tubes (which must have been expelled).

Similar results were described by Jakobovits *et al.* (1970) obtained with Enovid,® Anovlar,® Ovulen, lynestrenol and its combination with mestranol.

Since effects on the oviducts may be an important factor in the contraceptive action of drugs which do not inhibit ovulation, a further and more profound analysis is certainly desirable. One wonders whether changes in progesterone secretion by the corpora lutea should not be looked for.

19. EFFECTS ON THE MAMMARY GLAND

The role of progesterone among the many factors determining the structure of the mammary gland has been fully discussed in Chapter 3. Several synthetic progestational compounds have been studied in this respect.

Griffith *et al.* (1963) fed medroxyprogesterone acetate (MAP), chlormadinone acetate and norethisterone or its acetate to ovariectomized virgin rats for 19 days and in most experiments additionally gave them daily injections of 1 mcg of estradiol benzoate (EB). The animals were autopsied on the day following the last treatment and the six abdominal-inguinal mammary glands were dissected and used for determinations of dry fat-free tissue (DFFT) and DNA content (mcg per mg DFFT). This value as found on the 18th to 20th day of pregnancy (viz. 33.2 ± 0.8 mcg) could practically be reproduced in spayed animals by the daily injection of 1 mcg of EB + 3 mg of progesterone for 19 days (31.5 ± 1.0). The same result was obtained with daily oral doses of 1 mg of MAP or chlormadinone acetate (with 1 mcg of EB parenterally), whereas norethisterone was inactive. Table 39, adapted from table 1 of Griffith *et al.* (1963), shows the data bearing this out.

A remarkable finding is the fact that a long-acting ester, norethisterone enanthate, whose parent compound was described as ineffective, strongly stimulated mammary-gland development when injected (with 1 mcg of EB) in nineteen daily doses of 3 mg, yielding a DFFT value of 522 mg with 38.7 ± 1.0 mcg/mg DNA.

In chronic toxicity studies of chlormadinone acetate involving administration of the drug to dogs for periods up to 5 years (see p. 174) Mary J. Tucker observed extensive hyperplasia of mammary tissue but *no* discrete nodules and no evidence of neoplasia. The same has been reported by Fairweather (1968) with respect to 2 years' study of norgestrel, given in daily doses of 0.1 to 1.0 mg/kg p.o. ("The toxicological findings at high dose levels in dogs showed evidence of hyperplastic disease of the breast, but there was no evidence of malignancy.") See also subsection 24.2, p. 183.

TABLE 39. INFLUENCE OF FOUR ORALLY ACTIVE PROGESTATIONAL COMPOUNDS ON WEIGHT OF DRY FAT-FREE TISSUE (DFFT) AND DNA CONTENT OF MAMMARY GLANDS OF OVARIECTOMIZED RATS, TREATED FOR 19 DAYS

Doses in mg per day. EB estradiol benzoate given concomitantly (parenterally), mcg per day. Adapted from Griffith et al. (1963), table 1. Figures in columns 4 and 5 are means from numbers of animals given in column 6.

Compound	Dose	Dose of EB	DFFT mg	DNA mc/mg DFFT	No. of animals
Norethisterone	2.8	1	328	27.4 ± 1.5	10
	2.16	—	225	20.4 ± 1.3	5
Norethisterone acetate	2.7	1	315	27.8 ± 0.7	8
	2.22	—	267	18.2 ± 0.9	5
Chlormadinone acetate	1.0	1	478	35.3 ± 1.5	10
	2.98	1	638	28.1 ± 1.2	7
Medroxy-progesterone acetate	1.0	1	598	33.7 ± 2.8	10
	3.0	1	611	29.8 ± 1.2	10
Controls pregnancy 18–20 day	—	—	749	33.2 ± 0.8	19
EB, 1 mcg, once (ovariect.)			340	25.4 ± 1.5	20

Norethynodrel was studied by Kahn and Baker (1964), who gave it s.c. to intact virgin rats, either alone or in combination with mestranol for periods of 28 days. On the day following the last injection the animals were killed and the mammary glands were examined histologically for duct growth, lobulo-alveolar development and secretion, which were scored as 1.0 to 4.0. Whole mounts of the glands and sections were inspected but the scores do not differ materially; 1.5 mg per 100 g body-weight of norethynodrel with or without mestranol (0.02 mg) gave strong alveolar development, with signs of secretion (4.0 versus controls 1.3). As the authors remark, norethynodrel fulfils part of the hormonal requirements of mammary development in late pregnancy "since its progestational activity is synergized by an intrinsic estrogenic activity".

In a subsequent paper (Kahn et al., 1965) the authors showed that this activity of norethynodrel is completely abolished by hypophysectomy, which points to the role of prolactin in producing the effect described. In fact Kahn and Baker (1966) showed that norethynodrel in daily s.c. doses of 0.375 to 1.5 mg per 100 g bodyweight for 7 days significantly increased the prolactin content of the pituitaries of the rats so treated.

As mentioned in Section 17 (pp. 151–152) the effects of norethynodrel on the suckling offspring of rats was studied by Saunders (1967). Oral administration of 0.05, 0.1, or 0.2 mg/kg during pregnancy, and for 21 days after parturition, had no effect on lactation. All litters survived and at weaning age the average weight of the young was 43.8 g (as against 43.1 g in controls). Higher doses did affect the young, presumably by suppressing lactation, since at a 1.0 mg dose only two of three litters survived, comprising a total of only seven young of average weight only 22.3 g.

The effect of four progestational compounds on fetal development of the *anlage* of mammary glands and nipples in rats was studied by Cupceancu and Neumann (1969). These compounds were medroxyprogesterone acetate, norethisterone, allylestrenol and the caproic ester of 17α-hydroxy-19-norprogesterone (Gestonoron caproate). The steroids were given subcutaneously from the 13th to the 21st day of pregnancy. The first two compounds in daily doses of 3 mg inhibited the mammary and nipple *anlage* in female fetuses, the two others were inactive in much higher doses (allylestrenol 10 mg, Gestonoron caproate 30 mg per day).

Norethisterone was more inhibiting than medroxyprogesterone. The authors ascribed these activities to the masculinizing effects produced by these compounds as demonstrated in the genital organs. They describe the *anlage* of mammary glands and nipples in the rat as particularly androgen-sensitive (which would not apply to other species, including the rabbit, cow, monkeys and man).

20. EFFECTS ON THE ADRENAL CORTEX

20.1. COMPOUNDS INHIBITING ADRENAL FUNCTION

It has been repeatedly shown that certain progestational compounds will cause a reduction of adrenal size and inhibition of adrenal function when given in adequate dosage to intact animals. A number of pertinent data are presented in Table 40.

One of the first compounds shown to suppress adrenocortical size and function was medroxyprogesterone acetate (MAP). Since this substance has by itself some corticosteroid-like (anti-inflammatory) activity, it is not surprising that it inhibits ACTH secretion to some extent.

This is even more pronounced with the chemically related compound melengestrol but less with megestrol. McKinney and Weikel (1965) studied the effect of stress ("etherization or exposure to cold") in rats after having fed them the various steroids in "20–300 times the human dosage", judging an inhibitory effect from plasma levels of corticosterone and adrenal weight. The following steroids were found inhibitory in order of increasing potency: megestrol acetate < dimethisterone < medroxyprogesterone acetate < melengestrol acetate. Norethisterone was not suppressive. The adrenal-weight-inhibiting effect of MAP has been clearly shown to be due to suppression of pituitary ACTH secretion. It did not occur in hypophysectomized animals and the effect of exogenous ACTH was not antagonized (Glenn et al., 1959). The ACTH content of the pituitary of rats treated with 1 mg MAP daily for 7 or 14 days was reduced to about half the values of controls (Holub et al., 1961). MAP-treated rats responded with a significantly reduced rise in plasma-free corticosteroid levels to the injection of ACTH (Steinetz et al., 1965).

Fekete and Szeberényi (1965) found that, when injected into male rats for 6 days in daily doses of 0.2 to 3.0 mg, MAP not only produced a dose-dependent decrease of adrenal weight but also reduced the quantity of corticosterone (mcg/hr/100 mg tissue) which these adrenals would produce when incubated *in vitro*. This inhibition disappeared completely when ACTH was added to the incubation medium. The depressing effect of MAP was quantitatively comparable to that of prednisolone, though the latter continued its inhibiting action in the presence of ACTH. The same difference was found when these two steroids, instead of being administered to the animals *in vivo*, were directly added to the incubation medium, when 15 mcg of prednisolone would already have a significant depressing effect whereas even 180 mcg of MAP remained inactive. MAP reduced the weight of the fetal adrenals when given to pregnant guinea pigs (Foote et al., 1968).

The compound has a remarkably strong anti-inflammatory effect when injected topically into a granuloma pouch. Its glycogenic activity is in a way comparable to that of cortisol; it produces much less liver glycogen than half the dose of cortisol when determined 7 hours after injection, but much more when determined after 24 hours.

By contrast, megestrol acetate, which was found by David (1963) not to be anti-inflammatory, did reduce adrenal weight in hypophysectomized rats (Arends, 1963) and also in intact rabbits and rats, but not in mice or guinea pigs.

An acceleration of adrenal atrophy after hypophysectomy was still observed with doses of MAP of 1 mg for 7 days by Holub et al. (1961) who therefore assume the possibility of an (additional) extra-pituitary effect. The influence of MAP on pituitary cytology in rats was studied by Baker and Clapp (1964) after treatment for 4 weeks with adrenal-weight-reducing

TABLE 40. INHIBITION OF THE ADRENAL CORTEX

Effect judged by: reduction of adrenal weight (aw), adrenal histology (ah), reduction of corticosteroid production in vitro after treatment of animal in vivo (incub.)
(a) only dose tested. EE: ethynyl estradiol. TD: Total dose.

Compound	Species	Route of admin.	Daily dose (mg)	Duration of treatment (days)	Criterion of activity	Notes	Highest dose when found inactive	Reference
Medroxyprogesterone acetate	rat	s.c.	0.5	6	32% red. aw			Glenn et al. (1959)
	rat	s.c.	4.0	6	50% red. aw			Glenn et al. (1959)
	rat	i.m.	1.0	30	aw			Tokuda et al. (1963)
	rat	s.c.	1.0	10	corticosterone rise after stress incub.			Possanza et al. (1964)
	rat	s.c.	5.0	1 inj. depot		> megestrol acetate		Possanza et al. (1964)
	rat	s.c.(?)	0.3	14	aw	ovariectomized females		Brennan and Kraay (1963)
	rat	s.c.(?)	0.3	14	aw	intact males		Brennan and Kraay (1963)
	rat	p.o.	5/100 g(a)	15	aw blood corticosterone			Carraro et al. (1967)
	rat	s.c.	1.0(a)	14	aw	spayed females almost 70% red. intact females red. 55%		Edgren et al. (1959b)
	rat	p.o.	1.48	14	aw			Edgren et al. (1959)
	rat	p.o.	2.05(a)	14	aw	males 4/7 dead controls 0/10		Edgren et al. (1959)
	mouse	s.c.	0.5	14	cold resist.			Edgren et al. (1959)
	rat	?	0.3	14	aw	spayed females abt. 30% red. males		Elton et al. (1960)
	rat	s.c.	0.2–3.0	6	aw, incub.			Fekete and Szeberényi (1965)
	rat	p.o.	0.5–2.0	14	aw, ah, corticosterone rise after ACTH	females		Steinetz et al. (1965)
	rat	p.o.	2.0–10.0	14	aw, ah, corticosterone rise after ACTH	males		Steinetz et al. (1965)

Orally Active Progestational Compounds: Animal Studies

Compound	Animal	Route	Dose	Days	Effect	Notes	Ref dose	Reference
Chlormadinone acetate	rat	s.c.(?)	1.0	14	aw	ovariect. females		Brennan and Kraay (1963)
	rat	s.c.(?)				in intact males it increases weight		Brennan and Kraay (1963)
	rabbit	?	1.0	60	aw	intact females effect increased by EE	3.0	Chambon and Le Bars (1966)
Megestrol acetate	rat	i.m.	1.0	30	aw	< medroxyprog.		Tokuda et al. (1963)
	rat	s.c.	2.5	8 weeks	aw			Arends (1963)
	rat	s.c.	10.0/kg TD	7	aw			Arends (1963)
	rabbit	s.c.	8.9/kg TD	7	aw			Arends (1963)
	guinea pig	s.c.		7				Arends (1963)
	mouse	s.c.	1.0(a)	7		spayed females abt. 50% red.	10.0/kg TD	Arends (1963)
	rat			14	aw		54/kg TD	Elton et al. (1960)
Medrogestone	rat	p.o.		15	aw blood corticosterone incub.		5/100g(a)	Carraro et al. (1967)
Normethandrone	rat	s.c.	2.0(a)	10	aw	spayed females abt. 20% red.		van der Vies (1960)
Progesterone	rat	s.c.	1.0(a)	14				Edgren et al. (1959b)
	rat			14	aw		1(a)	Elton et al. (1960)

doses. Relative numbers of so-called α_2 and α_3 cells were reduced, α_1 cells and chromophobes were increased. The authors suggest that their results "point to the alpha cells and possibly chromophobes as being the sources" of ACTH and some components of the gonadotropic complex. When injected for prolonged periods (1.5 mg daily for 70 or 110 days from the 2nd, 3rd or 4th day after birth) it caused a pronounced reduction in weight of the pituitaries and adrenals at the time of autopsy. In the former "the complete absence of gonadotrophs was striking", the chromophobes "were of decreased size and showed narrow cytoplasmic rims". The adrenals reached only one-sixth of the weight of the control groups. "The columnar pattern of the fasciculata could not be recognized." The cells of this zone and the reticularis contained no stainable lipid (but those of the glomerulosa were perfectly normal). The hypoplastic adrenals were promptly stimulated by a short treatment of ACTH, irrespective of continued MAP treatment.

After treatment for 6 and 12 months with doses of 0.9 or 3.4 mg of MAP s.c. per day Leonora and Crane (1970) saw comparable changes in organ weight and histology but they did find atrophy of the zona glomerulosa. Medrogestone in the dose tested (5 mg/100 g bodyweight orally to rats of 200 g for 2 weeks) caused no reduction in adrenal weight nor blood corticosterone levels (Carraro et al., 1967).

An interesting observation concerns chlormadinone acetate. It was found by Brennan and Kraay (1963) to reduce adrenal weight in ovariectomized females but to increase it in males. It had no corticoid activity (thymolysis). The adrenal-weight-reducing effect of chlormadinone acetate is enhanced by the concomitant administration of ethynylestradiol in the female rabbit as shown by Chambon and Le Bars (1966).

Since a certain correlation between adrenal inhibition and corticosteroid-like (anti-inflammatory thymolytic or glycogenic) activity is to be expected, data on the latter are given in Table 41 to assist study of the correlation.

20.2. COMPOUNDS STIMULATING THE ADRENAL

The substances listed in Table 42—all estrane derivatives—behave differently from the pregnane derivatives listed in Table 40.

Norethynodrel was not found to inhibit adrenal size or function; on the contrary it stimulates them under certain conditions. This has been related to comparable effects of estrogens. Baker (1965) described that very small doses (11 mcg/100 g) given for 10 days (s.c. or p.o.) caused lipid depletion

TABLE 41. CORTICOSTEROID-LIKE (ANTI-INFLAMMATORY AND GLYCOGENIC) ACTIVITY
Doses in mg per day unless otherwise indicated. IEGP: Inhibition of exudate (volume) in granuloma pouch.

Compound	Species	Route of admin.	Duration of treatment	Lowest active dose	Highest inactive dose	Criterion	Reference
Megestrol acetate	rat	p.o.	5 days		50/kg	turpentine-agar pellets	David (1963)
Medroxyprogesterone	rat	i.m.	3 days	1.0		<Medroxyprogesterone	Tokuda et al. (1963)
	rat	s.c.	7 days	0.2		12% IEGP	Glenn et al. (1959)
				2.0		47% (=0.1 cortisol)	Glenn et al. (1959)
	rat	topic. (in pouch)	7 days	0.5		99% (=0.3 cortisol)	Glenn et al. (1959)
	rat	s.c.	one inj.	2.0		see text	Glenn et al. (1959)
	rat	s.c.	7 days	1.0		56% IEGP (>0.5 cortisol)	Duncan et al. (1964)
	rat	i.m.	3 days	1.0		one-tenth of act. of prednisolone	Tokuda et al. (1963)
	rat	s.c.(?)	14 days	0.3		weight of thymus	Brennan and Kraay (1963)
Melengestrol acetate	rat	s.c.	7 days	0.5		71% IEGP (>0.5 cortisol)	Duncan et al. (1964)
Chlormadinone acetate	rat	s.c.(?)	14 days		3.0	thymus weight	Brennan and Kraay (1963)
Dydrogesterone	rat	s.c.			10.0	liver glycogen in adrenalect. animals anti-inflammatory	Claassen (1968)
Norgestrel	rat	s.c.	2 days		1–4	thymus weight	Claassen (1968)
	mouse	s.c.	6 days		5.0	carrageenin granuloma weight	Edgren et al. (1968)
					0.250		Edgren et al. (1968)
	rat		6 days		0.250	IEGP	Edgren et al. (1968)

TABLE 42. COMPOUNDS FOUND NOT TO INHIBIT THE ADRENAL CORTEX AS JUDGED BY: REDUCTION OF ADRENAL WEIGHT (AW), ADRENAL HISTOLOGY (AH), REDUCTION OF CORTICOSTEROID PRODUCTION *in vitro* AFTER TREATMENT OF ANIMALS *in vivo* (INCUB.) (a) only dose tested.

Compound	Species	Route of adm.	Duration of treatment (days)	Criterion	Highest dose found inactive (mg per day)	Reference
Allylestrenol	rat	s.c.	10	incub.	2	van der Vies (1960)
	rat	s.c.	1 single injection		60/kg	van der Vies (1960)
Norethisterone	rat	p.o.	180	aw, ah	5	Blaquier (1964)
	rat	s.c.	14	aw	1	Edgren et al. (1959b)
	rat	p.o.	14	aw	5	Steinetz et al. (1965)
Lynestrenol	rat	p.o.	21	aw, ah	4	Uhlarik (1964)
Norethynodrel	rat	s.c.	27–34	ah	1.5/100 g	Baker (1965)
	rat	p.o.	180	aw, ah	5	Blaquier (1964)
	rat	s.c.	14	aw	1[a]	Edgren et al. (1959b)
	rat	p.o.	14	aw	5	Steinetz et al. (1965)
Norgestrel					inactive	Edgren et al. (1967a)
Quingestanol acetate	rat	p.o.	14	aw, see text	5	Giannina et al. (1969)

of the adrenal cortex (a sign of activation) in intact, not in hypophysectomized, rats. Norethynodrel resembled estrogen in the histological alterations which it induced in the adrenal cortex, except for failure to induce adrenocortical hypertrophy and hyperplasia. For this reason Baker *et al.* (1965) doubted whether the lipid depletion observed is really due to increased ACTH secretion (though the pituitary is obviously involved). Further studies (Baker *et al.*, 1966) then showed that larger doses (1.5–3.0 mg of norethynodrel per 100 g bw) given daily for not more than 5 days to intact females do in fact cause an increase in adrenal weight (but block the afternoon rise in corticosterone levels in the adrenals and plasma). In ovariectomized rats only, low doses of norethynodrel (0.09 mg/100 g) did increase plasma corticosterone levels. In order to explain the absence of a more generalized increase of corticosterone secretion the possibility is invoked of an interference with corticosteroidogenesis at the adrenal level as it has been observed with estrogens. Norethynodrel and norethisterone (5 mg p.o.) daily for 14 days increased the weight of the adrenals but not their corticosterone output after ACTH injection. On the contrary plasma-free corticosteroid levels were distinctly lower than in controls, at least in female rats (Steinetz *et al.*, 1965).

Blaquier (1964) gave large doses of norethynodrel (up to 5 mg daily) for periods between 15 and 180 days (orally) and these invariably caused considerable weight increase of the adrenals and histological changes, interpreted as showing strong stimulation. Essentially comparable changes, though less marked, were seen with (somewhat lower doses of) norethisterone. Holmes and Mandl (1962) gave norethynodrel by daily injection in high or low doses (0.1 and 0.02 mg per 100 g bw respectively) for periods varying between 22 and 86 days. It is stated that the adrenal glands tended to be heavier in the experimental than in the control animals, the difference being significant in one group (low dose, 3 weeks). Pituitary weight was also generally greater in treated animals, but with considerable variation, the increase apparently being due to the chromophobes.

After periods varying from 6 to 21 months during which mice were injected with 0.125 mg norethynodrel twice weekly, Kahn (1966) saw general *atrophy* of the adrenals (glomerulosa and fasciculata). In long-term experiments with golden hamsters Sichuk *et al.* (1967) saw no influence on adrenal size or structure from the daily administration of relatively large doses of norethynodrel and mestranol (see subsection 24.4, Other tumors).

A conspicuous increase in weight of the adrenals was observed after treatment with quingestanol acetate (Giannina *et al.*, 1965) but these enlarged glands did not produce more hormone than normal-sized controls as judged from the level of free plasma corticosterone, determined by the method of van der Vies *et al.* (1960), after stimulation with ACTH.

Daily doses of 2 mg of norethisterone and normethandrone are reported to overcome the adrenal atrophy caused by administration of prednisone in rats (Matscher, 1958).

Norethisterone injected into pregnant guinea pigs in doses of 1 mg per day from day 18 to day 60 postcoitum increased the weight of the fetal adrenals (Foote *et al.*, 1968).

In a much smaller dose of 66 mcg and combined with 1 mcg of mestranol, norethisterone, given daily orally for 1 month (as Ortho-Novum), produced significant ovarian, adrenal and pituitary weight losses. However, norethisterone without mestranol and rigorously freed from estrogen contaminations (as present in the commercial grade substance) no longer depressed organ weights. No changes occurred in plasma corticosterone. We refrain from any attempt at interpreting these findings.

The general impression is gained that progestational steroids which tend to increase adrenal weight do not consistently enhance adrenal hormone secretion.

21. VARIOUS METABOLIC ACTIVITIES OF PROGESTATIONAL COMPOUNDS

Many metabolic changes have been found in women taking oral contraceptives. Although the majority of these changes have so far not been considered as having clinical significance they certainly deserve pharmacological analysis. This chapter deals with metabolic effects of the progestational components of those drugs, as revealed by animal studies.

21.1. BODYWEIGHT AND COMPOSITION OF BODY MASS

In Chapter 15 some effects of progesterone on bodyweight and the composition of body mass have been discussed. The same group of authors (Hervey *et al.*) have also investigated a number of synthetic compounds. Their data, as far as they can be derived from the papers cited (Hervey *et al.*, 1967, 1968), are tabulated in Table 43. Of the compounds tested only medrogestone and dydrogesterone produced gains in weight (lean body mass and fat) comparable with those caused by equal doses of progesterone. All the others were less active and norethisterone even caused weight loss.

Chlormadinone acetate, which in the experiments just cited caused

TABLE 43. INFLUENCE OF PROGESTATIONAL COMPOUNDS ON BODYWEIGHT IN FEMALE RATS, DERIVED FROM HERVEY et al. (1967, 1968) Doses indicated are in mg per day per animal, given by injection for 26 days.

Compound	Dose	Weight increase compared with effect of equal dose of progesterone		Notes
		less	equal	
Medrogestone	5.0		=	gain of bodyweight similar in amount and composition to that caused by progesterone; at lower doses relatively more effective (flatter dose-response curve)
Megestrol	0.5 1.6 5.0	∨ ∨ ∨ ∨ ∨ 		some weight gain, not regularly dose-dependent, fat only; similar to chlormadinone acetate
Dydrogesterone	0.4 1.25 4.0		= = =	dose-response curve almost coincident with that of progesterone
Chlormadinone acetate	0.5 1.6 5.0	∨ ∨ ∨ ∨ ∨ ∨ ∨ 		weight gain less at all doses and including a higher proportion of fat
Norethisterone acetate	0.5 1.6 5.0	∨ ∨ ∨ ∨ ∨ 		lowest doses net weight gain (lean tissue and water) highest doses net weight loss

smaller weight gains, including more fat when compared with the action of progesterone, was studied by Shimizu and Okazaki (1967), also with a shorter period of treatment (10 days, 5 mg/day, s.c.) and a longer period of observation (until 60 days after treatment). Chlormadinone acetate at first caused slightly less weight gain than progesterone (both compared with untreated or vehicle-injected controls) but the duration of the effect was longer.

Medroxyprogesterone acetate was studied in rats by Crane and Leonora in daily s.c. doses of 2.0 mg for 3 weeks, in combination with high sodium intake (1 % saline *ad lib.*). This treatment was reported to cause a decrease in bodyweight (over saline controls) in males only.

Norethynodrel mixed with mestranol as in Enovid-E was given orally in daily doses of 1 mg for 4 days only to female rats in a study by Aftergood and Alfin-Slater (1969) and found to cause weight loss of 10 to 11 g, as against a 16-g gain in controls. The animals had gained weight when examined 30 days after the final dose but lost more when administration was resumed for another 4 days.

Bodyweight changes caused by norethynodrel treatment were also recorded by Holmes and Mandl (1962) in experiments involving daily s.c. administration of 0.02 or 0.1 mg/100 g or 0.2 mg for 48 to 86 days. The treatment reduced the growth of young rats (aged 55–66 days) and caused a slight reduction in the weight of fully grown animals (aged 148 days).

Kahn *et al.* (1965), who injected norethynodrel in doses varying between 0.011 and 1.5 mg/100 g for periods of 5 to 10 days, expressed some concern about the loss in bodyweight of the animals treated with higher doses and for longer periods, which "may represent a toxic effect".

21.1.1. *Weight changes in long-term* (*chronic toxicity*) *studies*

A number of authors studied the influence of compounds on bodyweight in experiments of much longer duration.

Thus norethisterone and norethynodrel were found to reduce weight gain in female rats in daily oral doses of 4 mg and 5 mg respectively for periods of 6 months (Blaquier, 1964).

Dogs appear to be particularly sensitive to the progestational effect of chlormadinone acetate. This compound was given in daily doses of 0.06 and 0.6 mg/kg p.o. for successive periods varying from 5 to 39 months up to a total duration of 5 years by Tucker (1971).* At the higher dose the treated dogs gained weight much faster than the controls.

* I am indebted to Miss Mary J. Tucker for permission to quote from her manuscript.

Melengestrol too was found to cause obesity (and adrenal depression) in chronic toxicity studies in dogs, while dimethisterone caused little change; but this substance depressed growth and caused fat deposits in rats, while melengestrol was well tolerated (Weikel and Wheeler, 1965).

In some studies, where steroids were given mixed with the feed, smaller weight increase was observed and attributed to reduced food intake because of the less attractive taste of the diet.

The following papers contain data on chronic toxicity studies. Salient points are quoted briefly.

Allylestrenol
Madjerek et al. (1960). Rats, 25 mg/kg, 4 months; slight inhibition of gonads.
Tóth (1964). Rats, 0.1 mg/100 g twice weekly, 15 weeks.
No hepatic or renal changes.

Anagestone
Lubansky and King (1965). Dogs, 20 mg/kg/day p.o., 20 months. Elevations in SGOT, SGPT, alkaline phosphatase; Reduction in size of adrenals.

Ethynodiol diacetate
Self (1965). Rats, highest dose 1.9 mg mixed with 0.1 mg mestranol s.c., 2 years. Pituitary cytology. (No influence on incidence of tumors.)

Lynestrenol
Overbeek et al. (1962). Rats, 25 mg/kg p.o., 5 months; slight changes in growth and organ weights as expected from hormonal activities. Dogs, 25 mg daily p.o., 6 months. Expected gonadal inhibition only.
Tóth (1964, 1966). Rats, 0.1 mg/100 g p.o., 60 days. No changes in liver and kidneys.

Medroxyprogesterone acetate
Logothetopoulos et al. (1961). Rats, 1.5 mg/100 g/day s.c., 16 weeks. Depression of growth of males to female levels, weight changes in adrenals and gonads due to pituitary inhibition.
Leonora and Crane (1970). Rats, 3.4 mg daily s.c., 6 months. Decrease in weight of pituitaries, adrenals and spleen in females; adrenal weight decrease in males.

Megestrol acetate
David et al. (1963). Rats, 20 mg/kg/day p.o., 12 weeks. Decreased adrenal weight in females.

Norethisterone
King and Lubansky (1963). Rats, 2 mg/kg/day *combined with mestranol*, 12 mcg p.o., 2 years. Increase in organ/body weight ratios for liver, uterus, thymus and pituitaries. No deleterious drug effects.

Norethisterone acetate
Schardein et al. (1969). Rats, fed a mixture of 98% norethisterone acetate and 2% ethynylestradiol in the diet at about 10- and 100-fold recommended human dose for 2 years. Dose related growth retardation, hair loss, mastopathy, liver hyperplasia. Increased survival rate compared to controls.

Norethynodrel
Kahn and Baker (1969). Mice, 0.125 mg/20 g s.c., twice weekly. Mammary changes and tumors (see subsection 24.2). Depression in bodyweight curves.

Norgestrel
   Fairweather (1968). Dogs, 0.01 mg/kg p.o., 104 weeks. Rats, 0.01% in diet 88½ weeks. Also combinations with ethynyl estradiol tested. Non-malignant mammary hyperplasia in dogs. No other histopathological anomalies.

Normethandrone
   Tóth (1964, 1966). Rats, 0.1 mg/100 g day, 80 days. No hepatic or renal damage.

21.2. CARBOHYDRATE METABOLISM

Beck (1969a, b) reported on studies concerning the influence of progesterone and several synthetic analogues on glucose metabolism and insulin secretion in female Rhesus monkeys.

Three weeks of treatment with progesterone in daily s.c. doses of 20 mg "produced no consistent changes in either the mean fasting serum glucose or insulin concentrations, even though the mean serum progesterone level (17 ng/ml) 16 hours after the last progesterone injection was 12 times greater than the control value and four times that reported by Neill, Johansson and Knobil in pregnant Rhesus monkeys" (Beck, 1969a). Much to the author's surprise, however, progesterone treatment produced a marked *increase* in the plasma insulin response to intravenous glucose or tolbutamide, without significant alterations in the glucose disappearance rates. (It did, however, antagonize the depression of this disappearance rate; in other words "the deterioration of glucose tolerance" caused by cortisol.) In accordance with these observations progesterone was found to reduce the sensitivity of the animals to the hypoglycemic action of small doses of insulin. "Thus, the administration of pure progesterone clearly enhanced insulin release following glucose and tolbutamide stimulation in the Rhesus monkey and produced a mild but significant amount of peripheral resistance to the hypoglycemic action of insulin."

Of the synthetic compounds tested, each in one dose in four to ten monkeys, all except ethynodiol acetate increased the insulin response to glucose as can be seen from Table 44. Chlormadinone acetate, as distinguished from progesterone, also increased glucose disappearance rate (utilization) and fasting insulin levels.

Of the estrogens studied, estriol, ethynyl estradiol and mestranol (in doses of 0.5, 1.0 and 2.0 mg respectively) injected daily for 2 weeks all depressed the glucose disappearance after injection of insulin, in other words the efficacy of this drug, but only mestranol increased the plasma-insulin response to glucose.

The anti-insulin effects of the progestational drugs appear not to be mediated by increased secretion of growth hormone, but otherwise many questions regarding the mechanisms involved remain open.

TABLE 44. INFLUENCE OF PROGESTERONE AND SOME PROGESTATIONAL COMPOUNDS ON PLASMA CONCENTRATION IN RESPONSE TO INTRAVENOUS GLUCOSE (INTEGRATED RESPONSES ΣI), DISAPPEARANCE RATE OF GLUCOSE (K) AND SENSITIVITY TO EXOGENOUS INSULIN (ΔG: MEAN GLUCOSE DISAPPEARANCE PER 10 MINUTES AFTER INTRAVENOUS INSULIN) IN RHESUS MONKEYS AFTER TREATMENT FOR 3 WEEKS WITH DAILY SUBCUTANEOUS DOSES INDICATED
Adapted from Beck (1969a)

Compound	Daily dose (mg)	Σ (μu/min) $\pm$SEM	Different from control p	K (mg % min) $\pm$SEM	ΔG (mg %) $\pm$SEM	Different from control p
Controls (olive oil)		5349 ± 1049		6.16 ± 0.57	26.9 ± 2.6	
Progesterone	20	15,433 ± 937	<0.005	6.35 ± 0.58	18.4 ± 2.8	<0.05
Norethisterone	2.5	15,561 ± 2237		5.77 ± 0.46		
Chlormadinone acetate	0.75	11,128 ± 613	<0.005	7.27 ± 0.71		
Norethynodrel	5.0	9828 ± 1078	<0.05	4.91 ± 0.52	14.0 ± 1.9	<0.05
Ethynodiol acetate	1.0	6013 ± 808		6.34 ± 0.83		

The presence of a "partial positive charge at the C5 carbon" seems to be a structural requirement for increasing the plasma insulin response to glucose.

Introduction of a double bond at C6—as present in chlormadinone acetate—had been reported by others as significantly reducing the gluconeogenic effect of cortisol (Fried *et al.*, 1955), and Beck (1969a) ventures the prediction that no decrease of glucose utilization ("diabetogenic" action) would be found in man after administration of chlormadinone or megestrol acetate, which seems to have been at least partly confirmed in human studies.

On the other hand, in long-term studies Tucker (1971) found a very clear diabetogenic effect of chlormadinone acetate in dogs. One out of four treated females (0.06 mg/kg p.o. daily for 5 months, thereafter 0.6 for 7 and again 0.06 mg for 39 months) developed overt diabetes in the 34th month and had to be killed at 41 months: of the seven surviving dogs (three females, four males) two males and two females had impaired glucose tolerance. In the two abnormal males the drug was withdrawn on three occasions. This caused a gradual return of glucose tolerance to normal but 10 days after resumption of dosing it was again grossly abnormal in both animals. Insulin levels in the two abnormal males were abnormally high and correlated clearly with the blood-sugar levels.

The response of steroid-treated rats to the injection of 0.1 mg/kg of glucagon was studied by Thomas (1963), who found that estrogens (estradiol benzoate and diethylstilbestrol) apparently depressed the hyperglycemic reaction, if blood-sugar rises were expressed as percentages of preinjection levels and this was due, at least in part, to rise in the fasting blood glucose. Norethynodrel (1 mg daily for 5 days, s.c.) behaved similarly, but its effects were less pronounced. Norethisterone was far less active in these tests.

21.3. LIPID METABOLISM

A mixture of 2.5 mg of norethynodrel and 0.1 mg of mestranol, as present in Enovid-E, was used by Aftergood and Alfin-Slater in studies regarding its influence on lipid metabolism in female rats. A daily dose of 1 mg was administered orally for periods of 4 or 7 days. This treatment caused a decrease of cholesterol concentration and of polyunsaturated fatty acids, particularly arachidonic acid, in cholesterol ester fractions in the plasma and the adrenals, but an increase of cholesterol in the liver. The excretion of cholesterol in the feces and its biosynthesis in the liver fell, but biosynthesis in the adrenals and ovary rose. It is, of course, impossible to decide what was the contribution of each of the two components of the drug to these metabolic changes.

Cholesterol levels were abnormally high in dogs during long-term treatments with chlormadinone acetate, as reported by Tucker (1971). For dosage see subsection 21.2, p. 174.

22. EFFECTS ON LIVER FUNCTIONS

In contrast with numerous studies of liver functions in women taking oral contraceptives and also in animals subjected to chronic toxicity studies, relatively little seems to have been published on pharmacological studies concerning an influence of synthetic progestational compounds on liver functions in animals. Thus Palmer et al. (1969) mention norethisterone and norethynodrel (amongst a variety of forty-two steroids) as inactive in inducing BSP retention in rats.

Lennon (1966) gave steroids buccally to rabbits for 4 days and compared BSP retention tests before and after the treatment. The uniform daily dose was 10 mg/kg and at this level allylestrenol, ethisterone and lynestrenol were inactive, norethisterone, norvinisterone and norethynodrel were significantly active ($P < 0.05$), and normethandrone even more so ($P < 0.01$).

Heikel and Lathe (1970), who had found earlier that ethynyl estradiol decreased the bile flow of rats much more than estradiol and had thought of the possibility that the influence of the ethynyl group might be due to an effect on cation transport, studied the effect of a number of 17α-ethyl substituted steroids (including norethisterone and lynestrenol) on liver membranes obtained from rat livers by fractionation and ultracentrifugation. The parameter examined was ATPase (adenosine triphosphatase) activity, subdivided into the fraction stimulated by Na + K + Mg and that stimulated by Mg alone. The difference between the two, i.e. $Na^+ - K^+$-sensitive ATPase, was more or less reduced by several ethynyl-substituted steroids, most markedly by norethisterone acetate (to the same degree as by stilbestrol) but not by lynestrenol. The results do not show a simple parallel between inhibition of bile flow *in vivo* and capacity to inhibit Na + K-stimulated ATPase *in vitro*.

23. VARIOUS BIOCHEMICAL, HISTOCHEMICAL AND RELATED EFFECTS OF PROGESTATIONAL COMPOUNDS

Under this heading we discuss a number of effects produced by progestational compounds, which, we are afraid, will not be considered as a homogeneous group. Some of these items could (or perhaps should) have been dealt with elsewhere in this chapter.

23.1. EFFECTS ON THE OVARY

Changes in enzyme activities in the ovaries of rats after treatment with lynestrenol or ethynyl estradiol (EE) were investigated by Dastugue et al. (1966). The animals received either 100 mcg of EE or 4 mg of lynestrenol orally per day for 11 days, in order to block ovulation. The ovaries were removed on the 12th day and homogenized. The following enzymes were studied (by means of the substrates indicated): arylesterases and lipases (β-naphthyl-caprylate with or without sodium taurocholate, which inhibits esterases and activates lipase); phosphatases (p-nitro-phenyl-phosphate); β-glucuronidase (phenolphthaleine-glucuronide).

Lynestrenol-treated ovaries had about half the weight of controls, and contained 19% less protein (per g of fresh tissue). Enzyme activities (as percentage of metabolized substrate) were strongly increased in the case of alkaline phosphatase and lipase; β-glucuronidase was slightly diminished; there were little changes in the other enzymes. Ethynyl estradiol decreased ovarian weight by only 18%, caused no reduction of protein content, decreased lipase and arylesterase and, very clearly, β-glucuronidase (32%).

Lacroix et al. (1968) found that treatment of rats with daily oral or parenteral doses of 2 mg lynestrenol reduced estradiol synthesis and also the conversion of testosterone to estradiol, when the ovaries of the animals were incubated in vitro. This was clearly due to the preceding gonadotrophin deprivation in vivo, since it was abolished by the concomitant administration of PMS gonadotrophin.

Callantine et al. (1967) studied "estrogen-induced ovarian growth" (an increase in ovarian weight and in RNA + DNA content), brought about by daily injections of 1 mg of diethylstilbestrol (DES) into immature hypophysectomized rats, for 2 weeks. That estrogens have a site of action inside the ovary had been known for a long time and the authors wondered whether progesterone or its synthetic analogues would modify this effect synergistically or antagonistically. The progestational steroids (1 mg/rat/day) were injected concomitantly during the second week of DES treatment.

Progesterone was without significant effect, whereas norethisterone, its acetate, and medroxyprogesterone acetate, were found to inhibit the stimulatory action of DES on ovarian growth (weight and DNA + RNA content). These progestational compounds did not counteract the increase in RNA:DNA ratio produced by DES. Norethynodrel—apparently by virtue of its own estrogenicity—augmented the effect of DES on ovarian growth. Callantine *et al.* also studied the uptake of ^{14}C-labeled DES and found that norethisterone, administered simultaneously, significantly reduced ovarian dry weight and total radioactivity without affecting ^{14}C uptake per unit of dry weight of ovarian tissue.

The effects of melengestrol acetate (MGA) were studied by optical and electron microscopy as well as by histochemical examination of rats ovaries by Priedkalns (1969). He injected mature rats for 1 to 4 weeks daily with 50 mcg of the progestational compound and 0.2 mcg of estradiol benzoate, though the impression is gained that the observed effects were attributed to MGA alone. These consisted in an arrest of follicular maturation and maintenance of corpora lutea beyond their normal life span, which would be accounted for by an inhibition of LH release (which is luteolytic in the rat), and a stimulation of prolactin (=LTH) secretion (see also subsection 6.5, Pituitary histology).

Appelgren (1969a) developed a technique for demonstrating the presence of Δ^5-3β-hydroxysteroid dehydrogenase in whole body sections of mice, using pregnenolone as a substrate, in the presence of a tetrazolium salt, which is changed to blue formazan crystals and precipitated at the site of the enzyme reaction. He used this method to test various drugs for possible interference with this biochemical step in the production of progesterone, by either adding them to the incubation medium or injecting them into the animals before freezing and sectioning. In this way Appelgren (1969b) showed that medroxyprogesterone acetate interfered with progesterone biosynthesis in the corpora lutea of mice, cows, sows and ewes. Norethisterone, on the other hand, showed this activity in corpora lutea obtained from swine but not consistently in those from mice, cows and ewes. He concludes that these findings suggest that the substances tested "besides their inhibitory effect on the pituitary also interfere with the synthesis of progesterone in functioning corpora lutea". Aakvaag (1969) studied the biosynthesis of progesterone in porcine ovaries *in vitro* and found that the addition of chlormadinone acetate to the incubation medium inhibited the conversion of pregnenolone to progesterone by a 10,000-g supernatant of ovarian homogenate at concentrations low enough to indicate that the drug may possibly play a role at the ovarian level *in vivo*. In guinea pigs with splenic ovarian grafts Haller (1970) showed that medroxyprogesterone acetate (MAP) significantly depressed corpus luteum function, possibly by a direct effect on ovarian enzymes. MAP did not interfere with either endogenous or exogenous FSH.

23.2. EFFECTS ON THE UTERUS

Since alkaline and acid phosphatases are known to be cycle-dependent in the endometrium of women and monkeys, Manning et al. (1969) studied the influence of an oral contraceptive, quingestanol (Q) plus ethynyl estradiol (EE), on these enzymes in Rhesus monkeys.

These steroids were administered in a ratio of 10:1 (multiples of 10 mcg/kg of Q and 1 mcg/kg of EE) by gavage, according to a cyclical schedule (21 days on drug, 7 days off) for 6 months. A low-dose group received 40 mcg/kg of Q, a middle-dose group 200 mcg/kg and a high-dose group 1000 mcg/kg, all with the corresponding quantity of EE, except four animals, treated with 1000 mcg/kg of Q and 50 mcg/kg of EE.

The histochemically demonstrated alkaline and acid phosphatases in the control animals corresponded with the menstrual cycles, rising towards a maximum at the late follicular stage and decreasing in the luteal phase in both the basal and the functional layers. The group had reported earlier that these conditions could be imitated in castrated females by administration of estradiol, estriol and progesterone. (The alkaline phosphatase changes closely mimic those in the stratum functionale of the human endometrium, not quite so in the stratum basale. Acid phosphatase behaves differently in the two species.)

When treated with low or middle doses of the drug combination, seven out of eight monkeys, killed 8 days after the final treatment, were histologically graded in the follicular phase. These animals also had had consistently normal vaginal bleedings throughout the experiment. The enzyme findings, however, were not normal, since the stratum basale had only a trace reaction of alkaline phosphatase; the stratum functionale showed weak to good activity. Acid phosphatase was normal in the low-dose group but the middle-dose "follicular stage" group resembled midluteal stage controls. By contrast five of six high-dose monkeys "were in the luteal stage and showed an enzyme reaction which, although variable, was closer to the expected activity for this phase. ... Thus quingestanol may have an 'overriding' effect at the higher doses of the combined regimen."

One must conclude from these interesting observations that pharmacological effects on the primate endometrium may be subject to different assessments when judged by different criteria.

Another, though not strictly comparable, example of this can be found in an early study of Tullner and Hertz (1957) who compared progesterone, 19-norprogesterone, ethisterone and norethisterone with respect to their potency to delay estrogen-withdrawal bleeding in ovariectomized Rhesus monkeys. Such a delay was achieved with daily s.c. injections of 1 mg of progesterone or 0.125 mg of norprogesterone, which was found to be in accordance with "Clauberg activities". Norethisterone also prevented bleeding in a daily oral dose of 5 mg daily, for the duration of treatment and there was an excellent histological response. Ethisterone, on the other hand, in doses varying between 5 and 200 mg daily, "failed to effect a significant delay in estrogen–withdrawal bleeding". The authors do not report on the histology of the endometria of the animals so treated but they do express surprise "in view of the demonstration of progestational activity in women of an oral dose of ethisterone, 6 to 8 times that of the effective intramuscular dose of progesterone" or a quarter of the human progestational dose of norethisterone.

Histological and histochemical studies of rat endometria under the influence of medroxyprogesterone acetate (MAP) were performed by Turolla (1960). Doses (s.c.) varied between 0.1 mg daily for 6 to 40 days and 0.5 or 2.0 mg for 10 days. Low-dose short-term treatment produced typical progestational changes. However, after 40 days of treatment other pictures appeared. There was conspicuous development of surface epithelium as one layer of cylindrical cells, the cytoplasm containing alcian-blue material near the cellular surface, where alkaline phosphatase activity as well as lipase was often though not always demonstrable in moderate quantities. Glands were sparse, with vacuolated cells and apical PAS-positive granules, low phosphatase and lipase and high esterase activity. Stromal cells contained no demonstrable acid mucopolysaccharides, with alkaline phosphatase exclusively localized near the walls of vessels, in particular precapillaries. In his conclusion the author stresses the fact that the progestational changes in the stroma do not correspond to those in the glandular epithelium, which leaves open the question whether this is due to a specific effect of the compound used (MAP) or to a change in the reactivity of the uterus due to the changes induced in the ovaries and the adrenals.

Information on the distribution of megestrol and of progesterone between epithelial and other structures in the rat uterus was obtained by Rogers and John (1970) by tritiating these steroids, injecting them into ovariectomized rats and studying the uteri autoradiographically. There was much less radioactivity in the epithelial cells than in the stromal or muscle cells and no preference for the nuclei. This investigation started from the observation that both progesterone and megestrol stimulate the uptake of *iodine* to several times plasma levels as it also occurs on the third and fourth day of pregnancy.

Low-dose continuous treatment with megestrol acetate, viz. 1.5 mcg per rat daily p.o. for 12 months, as reported by Sanwal et al. (1970), which did not inhibit ovulation or disturb the estrous cycle, produced the following biochemical changes in the endometria; a significant decrease of alkaline phosphatases, and of glycogen but an increase in G6P- and lactic acid-dehydrogenase, suggesting a shift from the Krebs cycle to the pentose phosphate cycle and to glycolysis. Apart from the observed inhibition of mating behavior (see Table 33) the metabolic changes in the endometrium, in the authors' opinion, "may be crucially involved in the anti-implantation and fetal effects" of this drug regimen, which made "a substantial proportion of the fetuses undergo resorption" (see also Table 32).

An enzyme (protease) inhibitor has been discovered in the uterine secretion of the rabbit, just before implantation (i.e. on day 6 postcoitum). It was studied by Beier (1970). Administration of estradiol (50–100 mcg from day 1 before, up to and including day 1 after coitus) either alone or followed by 5 days of progesterone treatment (5 mg per day) increased this antitrypsin activity. It also retarded blastocyst development. We are not aware of analogous studies using synthetic progestational compounds.

Suppression of a plasminogen activator in mouse uterine fluid by norethynodrel has been reported by Harpel et al. (1968). They found that in the fluid accumulating in the uterus in the course of 90 days after cervical ligature an activator of fibrinolysis, a soluble plasminogen activator, appears. This is reduced when the animals are given daily injections of 20 mcg of "Enovid", i.e. 20 mcg of norethynodrel plus 0.3 mcg of mestranol, or either component alone, which is, however, less effective than the combination. Acid phosphatase *rose* under the same conditions, except with mestranol alone.

Highly interesting observations were made by Smith and Henzl (1969) who studied the influence of estradiol and of chlormadinone acetate on mucopolysaccharides and lysosomal enzymes in the endometrium of spayed rabbits. The animals were treated from the 20th day after ovariectomy with injections of 1 mcg/kg of estradiol for 9 to 15 days and in a number of experiments concomitantly with chlormadinone acetate, 25 mcg/kg orally for 3 days only (days 7, 8 and 9 of treatment). Histochemical and electron-microscopic methods revealed that mucopolysaccharides accumulated during estradiol treatment, mainly along the luminal surface of the epithelial cells and the microvilli but also in the stromal ground substance and along the bands of collagen fibers. Chlormadinone acetate applied simultaneously caused a slight but definite decrease of this material and after the termination of hormone treatment there was further progressive depletion of it.

Acid phosphatase was studied as representing lysosomal hydrolases and it was found to increase markedly under the influence of estradiol, principally in epithelial cells. "Densely labeled lysosomes, multi-vesicular bodies, and Golgi vesicles were characteristic features of an estrogen responsive epithelial cell." Chlormadinone acetate induced a distinct increase in acid phosphatase activity in the epithelium, particularly in Golgi cisternae, and also in stromal cells. "The most dynamic changes in enzyme activity occurred during the period 48 hours to six days after both hormones had been withdrawn" and the authors interpret this as meaning "that while the endometrium undergoes proliferation and differentiation, the tissue is already accumulating destructive potential, which will eventually set into motion a chain of reactions leading to tissue regression. . . . Acid phosphatase bound in lysosomes and in Golgi vesicles becomes rapidly, within 48 hours, engaged in autophagic activities exercising a degrading function on different intracellular material and structures." They quote Weissmann (1964) as having shown that progesterone *in vitro* is a strong (lysosome) membrane labilizer and they conclude that "it now seems reasonable to suggest that progestins play several profound roles in the regression of the endometrium". The variety of progestational substances encountered makes one wary of succumbing too easily to such highly attractive generalizations. (We refer to the work of Sulman quoted under subsection 2.1 on p. 45.)

23.3. OTHER RELATED OBSERVATIONS

In their studies concerning the pathogenesis of certain genital anomalies, developing during fetal life, Goldman and Bongiovanni (1967) focused their attention on the 3β-hydroxysteroid dehydrogenase ("3β-enzyme") which was found to be implicated in certain rare cases of inborn errors. It was assumed that progestational and estrogenic agents may cause congenital disorders of sexual development by inhibiting this enzyme. This was tested using a bacterial enzyme, the testosterone-induced 3β-enzyme of *Pseudomonas testosteroni*. In an *in vitro* system the amounts of steroids needed to inhibit 70 units of the enzyme by 50% were determined. A synthetic androstene derivative (2α-cyano-4,4,17α-trimethyl-androst-5-en-17β-ol-3-one), which had earlier been described as a 3β-enzyme-inhibitor, had the greatest potency in this test (dose needed, 0.2 mcg), followed by estradiol (5 mcg). Medroxyprogesterone acetate (10 mcg) and norethisterone (12 mcg) were about equally active, whereas of progesterone a dose of 50 mcg was required. (See also subsection 23.1, Appelgren (1969) p. 177 and subsection 15.4, p. 129.)

The influence of medroxyprogesterone acetate (MAP) on the oxidation of reduced TPN (TPN-2H) in the presence of certain fractions (S 57.000) of rat liver was studied by Glenn et al. (1959) and found to be inhibitory, by contrast with that of progesterone, which stimulated the oxidation of this co-enzyme. "These results are construed to mean that in some unknown fashion a 6α-methyl group in this type of steroid prevents it from accepting hydrogen from the reduced co-enzyme—an action which prevents subsequent inactivation of the steroid." This was assumed to be an explanation for the prolonged duration of action of MAP, in particular in inhibiting the adrenals.

Feuer and Granda (1970) became interested in the factors "responsible for the delayed development of drug metabolizing capacity in the fetus". Suspecting that maternal steroids may be amongst them, they tested a variety of steroid hormones for their effect on the induction of hydroxylating enzymes needed for the purpose, by giving the steroids to rats *in vivo* or adding them to concentrates of liver microsomes *in vitro* (0.5–100 mcg per mg of protein). The substrates were coumarin or 4-methyl coumarin. Inhibiting effects were found with β-estradiol, mestranol and norethynodrel (*in vivo* and *in vitro*). No effect was seen from estriol, progesterone or medroxyprogesterone acetate. Increased activity was found with quingestanol acetate and, to a slight extent, medroxyprogesterone acetate (*sic*). Testosterone was amongst the strong inhibitors.

24. EFFECTS OF PROGESTATIONAL COMPOUNDS ON THE GROWTH OF TUMORS

Relatively old studies concerning an inhibitory effect on certain fibromas in rodents and the more recently awakened interest in the use of progestational substances in the treatment of endometrial carcinoma would, apart from other considerations, seem to justify a discussion of the literature on the effects of synthetic progestational compounds on a variety of tumors in animals.

24.1. ABDOMINAL FIBROIDS

As early as 1956 the group of Lipschütz which had found that estrogen-induced abdominal fibroids could be counteracted by progesterone (see

Lipschütz, 1950) investigated the effect of ethisterone and norethisterone on these neoplasmas in guinea pigs (Jadrijević et al., 1956). The animals were spayed and had implants of estradiol pellets. These were to be antagonized by pellets of ethisterone, implanted subcutaneously, releasing 71 (35–127) mcg, or of norethisterone, releasing 80 (49–126) mcg of steroid per day. Norethisterone, as distinguished from ethisterone, greatly diminished fibroid growth (but was still far less active than 19-nor-progesterone or even progesterone). The antitumoral effects of ethisterone and norethisterone paralleled their antiestrogenic effects as judged by the weights of the uteri of the animals.

24.2. MAMMARY TUMORS

Huggins et al. (1956) described a transplantable mammary fibro-adenoma, which was found to grow in 95% of intact adult female rats. The growth of this tumor was retarded by ovariectomy and still more when this was combined with adrenalectomy. Its growth was stimulated by phenolic estrogens and this increase was *enhanced* when progesterone was added. Norethisterone (1 mg/day injected for 50 days), without added estrogen, also accelerated the growth of this tumor, which had some of the functional properties of a normal mammary gland and neoplastic traits as well. In its response to hormones, it was said, it had characteristics which set it apart from all other endocrine targets of the rat.

A benign transplantable mammary fibro-adenoma, studied in rats by Glenn et al. (1959), was enormously stimulated by estradiol (in daily doses of 0.2 to 3.0 mcg/kg, less by higher doses, and also, though much less, by progesterone in doses of 1 or 2 mg/day). The action of medroxyprogesterone acetate (MAP) was peculiar. It inhibited the growth of this tumor in its first generation, when the tumor was very sensitive to testosterone propionate (TEP). With successive transplantations this tumor became increasingly resistant to TEP and, in the fourth generation, to MAP, in the same dosage range as before (1–8 mg/day, s.c.) appeared now to stimulate tumor growth very markedly. A tentative, hypothetical explanation is offered, based on observations of Huggins, to the effect that pituitary removal retards the growth rate of testosterone-sensitive mammary fibro-adenomas but does not interfere with testosterone-resistant tumors. Glenn et al. assume that the pituitary-depressing effect of MAP inhibited the growth of the mammary tumor while it was still testosterone-sensitive, after which the progestational activity of the compound enhanced it.

A mammary carcinoma, induced by a single feeding of 7,12-dimethylbenzanthracene (DMBA) as described by Huggins *et al.* (1959, 1961), was used by Griswold *et al.* (1966) as a model that could be developed into a system for routine evaluation of potential anticancer agents destined for application in women. Amongst the steroids found to inhibit tumor growth, when injected daily or 3 times weekly for 2 months, were testosterone propionate in doses of 25 mg and less per day, normethandrone, a distinctly androgenic progestational compound, in doses of 1.7 and 17 mg/kg daily (in lower doses it stimulated tumor growth) and medroxyprogesterone acetate, which appeared to inhibit in high and in very low doses, with irregular and questionable dose-dependence.

Continuing along the same lines, Weisburger *et al.* (1968) induced DMBA mammary tumors in rats (aged 40–45 days) and at the same time treated experimental groups with 3.0 or 0.3 mg of "crystalline Enovid" (norethynodrel containing 1.5% of mestranol) daily, by gavage for 45 days. Rats treated with carcinogen and the higher doses of the steroids "showed a reduced incidence of mammary tumors and a lower multiplicity of the tumors as compared to controls on carcinogen, in a period of observation of 9 months".

DMBA-induced mammary carcinomas were stimulated by lower doses (0.25 mg) of Enovid® (norethynodrel with mestranol) or Norlestrin® (norethisterone with ethynyl estradiol) but not with higher doses (1.0 mg) (McCarthy, 1965).

Two strains of mice, one with high spontaneous incidence of mammary carcinoma (C_3H/HeJ) and one with very low incidence (A/J), were treated with norethynodrel (s.c.) for long periods (about 2 years) by Kahn and Baker (1969).

The initial doses of 0.5 mg/20 g bodyweight twice weekly were later reduced to 0.25 and then to 0.125 mg/20 g. The number of mammary tumors occurring in both strains of mice was significantly increased by this treatment. (The influence of estrogenicity of the compound and effects on prolactin secretion are considered.)

In a transplantable mammary carcinoma in C_3H mice norethisterone in doses of at least 0.3 mg reduced the growth (Suchowsky, 1960).

In 1970 the question whether chlormadinone acetate could cause the development of mammary tumors in the human caused considerable excitement, after a certain type of nodules had been observed in dogs (beagles) during long-term treatment with the compound. (See also Chapter 34, Section B9, p. 449.) The U.S. Food and Drug Administration recommended that clinical trials with chlormadinone acetate be discontinued and as a result several companies withdrew such preparations from the market in a number of countries. Remarkably little has been published so far about the findings, which were apparently made in several industrial laboratories, but the impression is gained that nodules, found in beagles under long-term treatment with chlormadinone acetate (CAP) and also with medroxyprogesterone acetate (MAP), are drug-related, dose-dependent and predominantly benign.

In view of the highly important question regarding the applicability to the human of conclusions drawn from these observations in dogs, Hill *et al.* (1970) have compared the sensitivity of different species to the effects of CAP and of norethisterone (NET). In estrogen-primed infantile dogs, according to these authors, the two progestational compounds cause a very conspicuous increase in uterine weight (mg dryweight per 100 g body weight) and in this respect CAP was 225 times as potent as NET, whereas the ratio on the basis of histological endometrium changes appeared to be much smaller, more in the neighborhood of ratios found in rabbits. Basing themselves on the uterine weight changes and on the small differences in activity found for the two compounds in women (*ca.* 5:1) Hill *et al.* conclude that the beagle dog, unlike the human, is relatively far more sensitive to CAP than to NET and that therefore the doses used in the toxicity studies, supposed to be 2, 10 and 25 times the human doses on a weight for weight basis, are in fact far in excess when regarded as pharmacologically analogous doses, for which the new abbreviation PAD is introduced.

24.3. TUMORS IN THE UTERUS

Lipschütz *et al.* (1967) compared the activity of long-term administration of progesterone, norethisterone and norethynodrel to induce neoplastic changes in the uterus of mice. The steroids were subcutaneously implanted in the form of pellets and daily doses varying between 5.5 and 900 mcg were released for periods of 13 to 19 months. Progesterone in these circumstances caused a great increase in uterine weight and, particularly in higher doses, a myometrial endometriosis with cystic glands appearing on the serosal surface. Norethisterone and norethynodrel, which were tested in much lower doses (7.7 and 5.5 mcg/day respectively), also caused endometriosis but to a lesser extent. In addition stromal tumors were found, diagnosed as *sarcoma*. The incidence depended on the dose and the duration of treatment. The same tumor was found in four out of twenty-five animals receiving 8–16 mcg/day of norethisterone, but never with norethynodrel which, by contrast, produced some metaplasia in the endometrial surface epithelium and glandular cells.

Blanzat-Reboud and Russfield (1969) studied the induction of cervical carcinomas in mice by means of an intracervical silk thread impregnated with about 1 mg of 20-methylcholanthrene, according to a technique of Murphy (1961), and the influence of norethynodrel and of mestranol (jointly and separately) on this effect. The doses of these steroids were 15 and 0.5 mg respectively, by subcutaneous implantation, per mouse, at 3-week intervals. They were compared with 15 mg pellets of progesterone (alone or with 0.5 mg of mestranol).

The following tumors were found: adeno-acanthoma of the uterus, squamous carcinoma of the cervix and of the vagina. *All* the steroids—except mestranol alone—significantly increased the total number of tumors induced (relative to the number of mice at risk). Mestranol alone or in combination specifically increased the percentage of adeno-acanthomata in the uterus.

24.4. OTHER TUMORS

Schermund and Napp (1962) found that daily s.c. injections of norethisterone acetate (3.3 mg/kg) inhibited the growth of five different kinds of transplantable tumors in mice and rats, without increasing the survival time of the animals. Since none of these tumors were known to be hormone-dependent, a direct inhibitory effect on the growth of the tumor cells was assumed to be involved.

Four different transplantable tumors (sarcomas) were reported to have been inhibited by lynestrenol, administered to rats in daily oral doses of 5–10 mg, whereas melengestrol was inactive in these studies (Karady and Hooton Frayn, 1967).

Chemically-induced sarcomas, one transplantable (Yoshida) sarcoma (rats) and one ascites sarcoma (mouse), were inhibited by oral administration of Lyndiol® (lynestrenol + mestranol) in doses of 0.1 mg per 100 g bodyweight twice weekly for 7 months (Tóth and Szónyi, 1966).

Growth of the Yoshida sarcoma in rats was inhibited by injections of norethisterone acetate (1.5 mg every other day) as reported by Kaiser and Mohr (1961).

Using a life-table technique (adaptation of actuarial principles to the estimation of both the "effective number" of rats in a group throughout the duration of a test and the probability of the occurrence of a tumor in any group) McKinney et al. (1968) could show that a sequential treatment with ethynyl estradiol (average daily dose 53 mcg/kg) and megestrol acetate (average daily dose 2.63 mg/kg) significantly reduced the spontaneous incidence of "any tumor, a mammary tumor and any malignant tumor".

Spontaneous tumors occurring in Syrian (golden) hamsters (in a great variety) in 80% of normal males and 60% of females, as influenced by norethynodrel with 1.5% of mestranol, were studied by Sichuk et al. (1967). The steroids were administered s.c. 3 times a week at a dose level of 4.0 mg (34.0 mg/kg) from day 529 of life to the age of 658 days, thereafter 2.0 mg until the age of 728 days and 1.0 mg for the remainder of their life. "The test agents had no influence on the incidence or metastastic propensity of a wide variety of spontaneous tumors, including adenomatous polyps and adenocarcinoma of the intestine, adrenal nodular hyperplasia or adenoma, islet cell adenoma, melanoma or adenocarcinoma of Cowper's gland."

Norethynodrel (with mestranol) and norethisterone (with ethynyl estradiol) fed by gavage to 13-week-old mice were found by Poel (1966) to enhance the development of pituitary tumors in C57 Leaden (C57L) mice. Two dose levels (7 and 70 mcg 5 times weekly) were studied. After 84 weeks of exposure one out of eight vehicle-treated controls had a pituitary tumor, as against 7/7 high-dose norethynodrel- and 5/8 high-dose norethisterone-treated animals. These pituitary tumors in the steroid-treated animals were grossly mammotrophic (as judged from the appearance of the mammary glands, though there were no mammary carcinomas). The pituitary tumors invaded the surrounding tissue ("locally malignant").

As can be seen, the progestational compounds tested (often in combination with estrogens) have greatly varying effects on a diversity of experimental tumors; any generalizations seem hardly to be justified.

25. MISCELLANEOUS OBSERVATIONS

25.1. EFFECTS ON IMMUNOLOGICAL REACTIONS

Hungarian investigators, Szontagh et al. (1964), sensitized rats by injecting them with horse serum and provoking an anaphylactic reaction 13 days later by reinjecting the same material. This reaction was negligible, unless the animals had been (orally) treated for the last 7 days before the second injection with 2.5 mg/day of lynestrenol (the only compound and the only dose tested in this study). Of the rats treated with the steroid, nine out of eighteen died in anaphylactic shock (against none out of thirteen controls). Hypothetical explanations are offered.

By contrast Hulka et al. (1965) could delay the rejection of allografts on the ears of castrated rabbits by injecting them with norethynodrel (2.5 mg/day), norethisterone or medroxyprogesterone (5.0 mg/day) or cortisone acetate (50.0 mg twice weekly). In animals treated with norethynodrel there was a tendency towards a decrease of antibovine-serum-albumin antibodies, which was more pronounced and more consistent after treatment with progesterone, medroxyprogesterone acetate and cortisone.

25.2. EFFECTS ON THE KIDNEY

After prolonged treatment of golden hamsters with norethynodrel plus mestranol, Sichuk et al. (1967) (see subsection 24.4) saw renal hypertrophy in the male animals, in the absence of any remarkable change in tissue architecture, which, in the authors' opinion, "appears to be a response which is unique to the combination of synthetic oestrogen and progestin used in the current study".

25.3. BLOOD VESSELS

Danforth et al. (1964) described changes in the aorta and certain other vessels occurring in rabbits during pregnancy, which could be imitated by the injection of an ovulation-inhibiting dose of Enovid® (0.2 mg of norethynodrel with 1.5% of mestranol) daily for 6 days. The changes consisted in an increase of muscle, a decrease in the proportion of collagen, marked fragmentation of the reticulum and a marked loss of acid mucopolysaccharides. In the norethynodrel-treated animals reticular fragmentation and loss of acid mucopolysaccharides were conspicuous and indistinguishable from those in pregnancy. As shown in a subsequent paper (Manalo-Estrella et al. (1965)) these changes disappear rapidly after termination of treatment (mucopolysaccharides become normal almost immediately, other affected structures within 10 to 15 days).

An effect of progestational (and other) steroids on the bone marrow of rabbits was observed under special experimental conditions by Little (1970). The animals were given injections of high doses of cortisone acetate (10 or 15 mg/kg for 2 weeks) and thereafter a combination of cortisone acetate with 5 mg/kg of another steroid for 2 weeks. Steroids used in conjunction with cortisone included testosterone, three anabolic steroids and three progestational compounds, viz. lynestrenol, norethynodrel and norethisterone. In the bone marrow of these rabbits abnormally numerous large megakaryocytes were seen, sometimes in the process of liberating thrombocytes, whose numbers in the peripheral blood showed great fluctuations. Thrombi were frequently observed, particularly in the liver. The author states that increased cortisone (or cortisol) levels are a prerequisite for the production of thrombi and he suggests that these may be different when different steroids (such as testosterone or progestational compounds) are added to the regimen, but this has not been documented.

25.4. EFFECTS OF NORETHYNODREL AS INFLUENCED BY THYROID STATE

Ward and De Prospo (1968) investigated the influence of thyro-parathyroidectomy in rats and conversely that of thyroxine administration to intact animals on a number of known effects of norethynodrel. They administered this steroid subcutaneously in a dose of 1.5 mg/100 g daily for 10 days, thereby following Kahn and Baker (1964) and Kahn et al. (1965). The proliferation of the mammary glands described by these authors was found to be significantly, though slightly, *enhanced* by "hypo- and hyperthyroidism" as induced by Ward and De Prospo. On the other hand, the hypothyroid group showed a distinct increase of ovarian weight and increased diameters of corpora lutea, whereas in other groups norethynodrel reduced ovarian weight. There was no difference between norethynodrel-induced adrenal weight increase in hypo- or hyperthyroid animals.

25.5. PERCUTANEOUS ABSORPTION

As early as 1934 the German investigator R. Fussgänger (whose method of demonstrating androgenic activity by applying testicular extracts topically to the comb of capons has become very widely known) showed that corpus luteum extracts would be absorbed and show target organ activity after application in oily solution to the shaven skin of rabbits. For a Clauberg test, performed in this way, the required dose was 10 times the s.c. dose. Shipley (1965), after a comprehensive review of the history of the percutaneous activity of progesterone, presented her own data obtained by this application of synthetic progestational steroids and of progesterone as measured by different parameters. (See also subsection 3.1, Induction of deciduoma-formation, p. 49.) In general she applied the compounds in ethanol solution to an area of skin of the neck. A number of Shipley's results have been put together in our Table 45.

It was not intended to determine exact ratios of potencies for percutaneous and other routes of administration. It is nevertheless striking that progesterone is apparently much more active percutaneously in the rabbit

TABLE 45. PERCUTANEOUS ACTIVITY OF PROGESTATIONAL COMPOUNDS

Adapted from Shipley (1965). Doses—total or daily as indicated—are in mg per animal.

Compound	Clauberg test. Total dose causing score of McPhail 2 or more	Inhibition of copper acetate-induced ovulation (rabbit) (total dose preventing ovulation in at least 70% of animals)	Deciduoma formation (rat). Daily dose (9 days) causing more than 300% weight increase of traumatized horn	Facilitation of PMS-induced ovulation (rat) (total dose causing ovulation in at least 50% of animals)
Progesterone	4.0	4.0	inactive (8.0)	5.0
Medroxyprogesterone acetate	0.025	0.4	0.03	0.1
Chlormadinone acetate	0.025	0.2	1.0	0.125
Normethandrone	0.25	—	—	—
Norethisterone	0.4	2.0	—	—

Compound	Implantation and maintenance of pregnancy in ovariectomized hamsters (Daily dose in mg)		Inhibition of ovulation (antiluteinization) in prepuberal rats. Daily dose causing at least 50% inhibition
	Percutaneously	Subcutaneously for comparison	
Progesterone	6.0 (50% pregn.)	0.1 (80% pregn.)	inactive (3.0 causing 14% inhib.)
Medroxyprogesterone acetate	4.0 (inactive)	0.8 (75% pregn.)	0.2
Chlormadinone acetate	4.0 (inactive)	0.6 (67% pregn.)	0.125
Normethandrone	—	—	—
Norethisterone	0.3 (67% pregn.)	0.15 (83% pregn.)	—

than in the rat, and very poorly in the hamster. This last species does not respond to the percutaneous administration of two other pregnane derivatives either but it does respond very readily to norethisterone (in an implantation and pregnancy-maintenance test).

In a study limited to two effects (endometrial response and inhibition of copper-induced ovulation) in the rabbit, Ringler (1966) showed that medroxyprogesterone acetate, chlormadinone acetate, norethisterone and norethynodrel (amongst other steroids) all gave maximum responses when applied in a 1-mg dose (the only dose tested) in ethanol to the skin. The first two compounds were equally active, the other less active when given in a cream. A maximal duration of action (as judged from the condition of the endometrium 5 days after a single dose) was found for chlormadinone acetate (0.125–1.0 mg) in a cream base. When administered percutaneously every day for 5 days, only one-third to one-sixth of the oral dose of this steroid (and of medroxyprogesterone acetate) was needed for a comparable endometrial response.

Norethynodrel (5 mg/kg) and ethynodiol acetate (2.5 mg/kg) were found by Kar et al. (1968) to be effective in preventing the establishment of pregnancy when administered to rats on day 1 to day 3 postcoitum, in an ethanol solution on the shaved skin. Estrogens on day 1 were effective in much lower doses.

25.6. ABSORPTION OF PROGESTATIONAL COMPOUNDS FROM IMPLANTED CAPSULES

Kincl's group (Folch-Pi et al., 1965; Chang and Kincl, 1968, 1970; Benagiano et al., 1970) studied the possibilities of providing progestational compounds in a pharmaceutical form that would allow a regular 24-hours release of the drug for long periods. Dimethylpolysiloxane (DPS) membranes seemed to offer a solution to the problem since crystalline steroids were shown to diffuse from such capsules (into distilled water) with remarkable constancy. Chang and Kincl (1968) could show that megestrol acetate, implanted in DPS capsules, delayed nidation in rats and suppressed copper-acetate-induced ovulations in rabbits, in doses that were calculated to be much lower than the required oral or subcutaneous doses. The same applied to inhibition of fertility in rats and hamsters.

The groups then set out to study the regularity of drug release in long-term *in vivo* studies (Benagiano et al., 1970), using radioactively labeled megestrol acetate in hamsters, rabbits and rats and determining radioactivity in urine and feces. Disappointingly diffusion rates became irregular after a few weeks. The reasons for this have not yet been elucidated but the authors believe that the principle of DPS implants remains promising.

In view of what has been said about the duration of action of progesterone and of some synthetic compounds in the rabbit (subsection 2.1, p. 45) it is remarkable that Kincl and Rudel (1970) found that megestrol acetate, implanted in rabbits in DPS capsules (releasing 30 mcg/24 h *in vitro*), produced a progestational effect still demonstrable after 270 days (McPhail score 2.0 (0.5–2.5)).

It was shown by Kincl *et al.* (1970) that biologically comparable doses of $6\text{-}^{14}C$ megestrol acetate as DPS implants (60 mcg, thirty implants) or given p.o. (1.6. mg/day) caused quite different plasma levels of the drug, judged by radioactivity in the plasma. Implants in male rats produced plasma levels of about 10 mcg/100 ml after about 4 days, which remained constant for at least 14 days, whereas the corresponding oral dose produced peak levels up to 50 mcg/100 ml after 8 hours; the radioactivity had almost completely disappeared after 24 hours. Administration by the latter route caused much higher retention of radioactivity in various organs, in particular in the liver and in the kidney, than by DPS implantation (40 and 60 times respectively).

25.7. ABSORPTION FROM THE VAGINA

Some data on the absorption of progestational compounds after vaginal deposition in rabbits have been included in Table 10.

25.8. INFLUENCE ON FUNCTION OF THE LUNGS

Aviado and McKinney (1969) described a technique of producing pulmonary emphysema in rats by letting them inhale cigarette smoke through a tracheal cannula or by i.v. injections of nicotine or lobeline. The development of emphysema was prevented by s.c. injections of progesterone (10 mg/kg), dimethisterone (10 mg/kg) or megestrol acetate (0.2 mg/kg) 3 times a week for 4 weeks or by p.o. administration of 5 times greater doses of either dimethesterone or megestrol acetate. The mechanism of this action is not completely understood.

26. CONCLUDING REMARKS

At the end of a chapter like this the reader might well feel entitled to a brief summary but we have preferred to incorporate this in the general summary in Chapter 35, where we attempt to group some basic data not according to actions but by compounds so that a concise characterization of each compound may emerge. That chapter will have to be a summary of the two volumes of this section, which gives us an opportunity of focusing attention again on progesterone, and perhaps of bringing in some essentially new facts or some that may have escaped the attention of authors in the first instance.

The present chapter has grown under our hands to unforeseen dimensions and we have been wondering more than once whether we have not been rushing in where angels fear to tread.

APPENDIX

An Outline of Desirable Routine Tests for the Preclinical Evaluation of Progestational Compounds.

The present appendix has been written following a suggestion from one of the Executive Editors of this Encyclopaedia, Professor G. Peters in Lausanne, who thought that recommendations with respect to methods and species would be useful for industrial or government pharmacologists or toxicologists who have to investigate progestational compounds. Clearly such tests are only needed for compounds whose properties have not yet been fully established. Normally this work will be done with the purpose of selecting compounds for clinical evaluation.

As a first hormone screening test the following has been found useful. A standard dose of 1 mg/day is given s.c. to immature male and female rats daily for one week. By checking vaginal smears if vaginal opening takes place and determining organ weights at the end of the test, the following activities can be detected: estrogenicity (vaginal cornification, uterine weight), androgenicity (seminal vesicles, ventral prostate), anabolic (myotrophic) activity (levator ani muscle), gonad inhibition (testicles, ovaries and secondary sex characters), glucocorticoid activity (adrenals and thymus).

Reference preparations of known potencies must always be run concomitantly in more specific assays. The preferred test for progestational activity is the Clauberg test in the estrogen-primed immature rabbit, as described in Chapter 18 (see also remarks by Neumann, p. 44).

More specific tests for progestational activities are used if the Clauberg test is found positive. These include the formation of deciduomata (Chapter 18, p. 397) and maintenance of pregnancy in spayed rats (Chapter 10, p. 298). Irrespective of the outcome of this test, progestational compounds should be tested for possible interference with an established pregnancy in rats and for adverse effects on the fetus, more particularly as regards disturbances of genital development (see subsection 15.2, p. 122) and fertility of the F_1 generation (p. 123)

If a compound is considered *for contraceptive use* it should be tested for inhibition of ovulation at least in rats (subsection 5.3, p. 59) though some laboratories prefer an antifertility test as a first orientation (subsection 16.2, p. 132).

Subchronic and Chronic Toxicity Studies

Requirements for these studies are particularly severe when oral contraceptives are concerned, since these will normally be taken by healthy women for prolonged periods. In most laboratories—even outside the U.S.—the guidelines of the Food and Drug Administration will be followed (see "Current Views on Safety Evaluation of Drugs" by Edwin I. Goldenthal, FDA Papers, May 1968, pp. 1–8).

Serious objections have been raised against the use of dogs for judging the effects of steroids on the mammary gland and extrapolation of the findings to the human, because of the high incidence of spontaneous tumors in many strains of dogs and their exceedingly high sensitivity to some progestational compounds (see subsection 24.2, p. 184).

REFERENCES

AAKVAAG, A. (1969) Formation of steroid hormones in the porcine ovary *in vitro*. *J. Endocr.* **43**: xxv-xxvi.

ADAMS, C. E. (1961) *Artificial Insemination in the Rabbit*. Technical Bulletin No. 1. Commercial Rabbit Association, Farnborough (Hants).

AFTERGOOD, L. and ALFIN-SLATER, R. B. (1969) Effect of an oral contraceptive steroid mixture on some aspects of lipid metabolism in the rat. In: *Metabolic Effects of Gonadal Hormones and Contraceptive Steroids*, pp. 265–274. Salhanick, H. A., Kipnis, D. M. and van de Wiele, R. L. (Eds.). Plenum Press, New York and London.

ALLEN, JR. G. O., KING, T. O. and MILLMAN, N. (1964) DMAP (6α-methyl-4-pregnene-17-ol-20 one acetate) a new progestational contraceptive agent. *Fed. Proc.* **23**: 361.

ALLEN, W. M. and WU, D. H. (1959) Effects of 17α-ethynyl-19-nortestosterone on pregnancy in rabbits. *Fertil. Steril.* **10**: 424–438.

APPELGREN, L. E. (1969a) Histochemical demonstration of drug interference with progesterone synthesis. *J. Reprod. Fert.* **19**: 185–186.

APPELGREN, L. E. (1969b) Interference with progesterone synthesis of some antifertility compounds as shown by histochemistry. In: *Second European Congress on Sterility, Dubrovnik, October 1969*, p. 6. Drobnjak, P. (Ed.). Tiskara izdavačkog zavoda Jugoslavenske akademije, Zagreb.

ARENDS, J. (1963) Undersogelse over binyreatrofi hos forskellige dyreartei efter indgift af gestagene steroiden. (Study of adrenal atrophy in various animal species following administration of gestagenic steroids). *Archiv. for Pharmaci og Chemi* **70**: 907–913.

AVIADO, D. M. and MCKINNEY, G. R. (1969) Oral progestagens and experimental pulmonary emphysema. *Pharmac. Res. Comm.* **1**: 283–287.

AYDAR, C. K. and GREENBLATT, R. B. (1961) Clinical and experimental studies with a new progestogen—Dimethisterone. *J. Med. Assoc. State of Alabama* **31**: 53–59.

BAGNATI, E. P., ZAPATI, A. C., BUR, G. F., GURUCHARRI, C. A. and COLILLAS, O. J. (1964) Acción antigonadotrófica de la 3-desoxi-17 alfa-etinil-19 nor-testosterona. *Rev. Soc. Obstet. Ginec. B. Aires* **43**: 26–29.

BAKER, B. L. (1965) The influence of norethynodrel on the adrenal cortex of rats. *Anat. Record* **151**: 320.

BAKER, B. L. and CLAPP, H. W. (1964) The cytology of the hypophyseal pars distalis following treatment with the progestin, 6α-methyl-17α-hydroxyprogesterone. *Anat. Record* **148**: 257.

BAKER, B. L., KAHN, R. H. and BESEMER, D. (1965) Ovarian histology after treatment of rats with norethynodrel. *Proc. Soc. Exp. Biol. Med.* **119**: 527–531.

BAKER, B. L., KAHN, R. H. and ZANOTTI, D. B. (1965) Influence of norethynodrel on the adrenal cortex of rats. *Endocrinology* **77**: 155–161.

BAKER, B. L., KAHN, R. H., ZANOTTI, D. B. and HEADINGS, M. (1966) Influence of norethynodrel on the level of corticosterone in the adrenal glands and blood of rats. *Endocrinology* **79**: 1095–1099.

BANIK, U. K., HALTRECHT, I. and HERR, F. (1970) Induction of ovulation in progestin-treated adult rats. *Acta Endocr. (Kbh.)* **63**: 747–752.

BARNES, L. E. and MEYER, R. K. (1964) Delayed implantation in intact rats treated with medroxyprogesterone acetate. *J. Reprod. Fertil.* **7**: 139–143.

BARNES, L. E., SCHMIDT, F. L. and DULIN, W. F. (1959) Progestational activity of 6α-methyl-17α-acetoxyprogesterone. *Proc. Soc. Exp. Biol. Med.* **100**: 820–822.

BECK, P. (1969a) Effects of gonadal hormones and contraceptive steroids on glucose and insulin metabolism. In: *Metabolic Effects of Gonadal Hormones and Contraceptive Steroids*, pp. 97–125. Salhanick, H. A., Kipnis, D. M. and van der Wiele, R. L. (Eds.). Plenum Press, New York–London.

BECK, P. (1969b) Progestin enhancement of the plasma insulin response to glucose in Rhesus monkeys. *Diabetes* **18**: 146–152.

BEIER, H. M. (1970) Hormonal stimulation of protease inhibitor activity in endometrial secretion in early pregnancy. *Acta Endocr. (Kbh.)* **63**: 141–149.

BENAGIANO, G., ERMINI, M., CHANG, C. C., SUNDARAM, K., and KINCL, F. A. (1970) Sustained release hormonal preparations. 5. Absorption of 6-methyl-17α-acetoxy-pregna-4,6-diene-3,20-dione from polydimethylsiloxane implants *in vivo*. *Acta Endocr. (Kbh.)* **63**: 29–38.

BENNETT, J. P. (1970) The effect of drugs on egg transport. In: *Advances in the Biosciences* vol. 4, pp. 165–180. Schering Symposium on Mechanisms Involved In Conception. Pergamon–Vieweg, Oxford–Braunschweig.

BENNETT, J. P., VALLANCE, D. K. and VICKERY, B. H. (1967a) A method for the direct observation of ovulation inhibition in the mature rat. *J. Reprod. Fert.* **13**: 567–569.

BENNETT, J. P., VALLANCE, D. K. and VICKERY, B. H. (1967b) Inhibition of gamete migration and fertilization in the rabbit. *Postgraduate Med. J.* December Supplement, pp. 39–43.

BENNETT, J. P., VALLANCE, D. K. and VICKERY, B. H. (1968a) Investigation of block to gonadotrophin release in mature female rat. *J. Reprod. Fertil.* **15**: 233–237.

BENNETT, J. P., VALLANCE, D. K. and VICKERY, B. H. (1968b) The synchronization of ovulation in the adult female rat by oral administration of megestrol acetate. *J. Reprod. Fertil.* **16**: 159–163.

BINDON, B. M. (1969) The role of the pituitary gland in implantation in the mouse: delay of implantation by hypophysectomy and neuro-depressive drugs. *J. Endocr.* **43**: 225–235.

BLANZAT-REBOUD, S. and RUSSFIELD, A. B. (1969) Effect of parenteral steroids on induction of genital tumors in mice by 20-methylcholanthrene. *Amer. J. Obstet. Gynec.* **103**: 96–101.

BLAQUIER, J. A. (1964) Effects of prolonged oral administration of progestational steroids in the female rat. *Acta Physiol. Latinoam.* **14**: 255–263.

BLYE, R. P., BERLINER, V. R. and HOMM, R. E. (1965a) Endocrine profile of a new oral contraceptive: 3-desoxy-6α-methyl-17α-acetoxyprogesterone. *Fed. Proc.* **24**: 701.

BLYE, R. P., HOMM, R. E. and KING, T. O. (1965b) Biological characterization of norethindrone and norethynodrel alone and in combination with ethynylestradiol-3-methyl ether. *VI. Panam. Congress of Endocrinology*, page E 143, Abstract 317. Internat. Congress Series 99, Excerpta Medica, Amsterdam.

BONGIOVANNI, A. M., DI GEORGE, A. M. and GRUMBACH, M. M. (1959) Masculinization of the female infant associated with estrogenic therapy alone during gestation: four cases. *J. Clin. Endocr.* **19**: 1004–1011.

BONTA, I. L. (1958) New application of the motility test in screening tranquillizing drugs. *Acta Physiol. Pharmac. Neerl.* **7**: 519–522.

BORIS, A., STEVENSON, R. H. and TRMAL, TH. (1966) Some studies of the endocrine properties of dydrogesterone. *Steroids* **7**: 1–10.

BOYARSKI, L. H., BAYLIESS, H., CASIDA, L. E. and MEYER, R. K. (1947) Influence of progesterone upon the fertility of gonadotrophin-treated female rabbit. *Endocrinology* **41**: 312–321.

BRENNAN, D. M. and KRAAY, R. J. (1963) Chlormadinone acetate, a new highly active gestation-supporting agent. *Acta Endocr.* (*Kbh.*) **44**: 367–379.

CALLANTINE, M. R., LEE, S.-L., and HUMPHREY, R. R. (1967) Action of progesterone and synthetic progestogens on estrogen-induced ovarian growth. *Proc. Soc. Exp. Biol. Med.* **124**: 1001–1005.

CARPENTIER, P. J. (1958) Malformation génitale du foetus féminin après administration d'un nouveau stéroide de synthèse pendant la grossesse. *Bull. Soc. Roy. Belge Gynéc. Obstét.* **28**: 137–148.

CARRARO, A., KLINGER, R. and MOTTA, M. (1967) Studi sull'attivitá farmacologica di un nuovo progestativo di sintesi. *Boll. della Soc. It. di Biol. Sper.* **43**: 427–431.

CASAGLIA, C. and GUALANDI, L. (1961) Steroidi progestativi e fenomeno di diastasi della sinfisi pubica. (Progestational steroids and relaxation of symphysis pubis). *Folia Endocr.* (*Pisa*) **14**: 272–285 (*Chem. Abstr.* **55**: 22625a, 1961).

ČEKAN, Z., ŠEDA, M., MIKULÁŠKOVÁ, J. and SYHORA, K. (1964) Steroid derivatives XXXIV. On the progestational activity of 6-dehydro-16-methylene-17α-acetoxyprogesterone. *Steroids* **4**: 415–421.

CHAMBON, Y. (1965a) Action progestagène de la Δ-6,6-chloro-17α-acétoxyprogestérone chez la lapine et la ratte castrées. *Ann. Endocr.* **26**: 327–332.

CHAMBON, Y. (1965b) Action de trois dérivés de la 17α-acétoxyprogestérone sur l'installation de la gestation chez la lapine castrée. *C.R. Acad. Sci.* (*Paris*) **260**: 690–693.

CHAMBON, Y. and LE BARS, S. (1965) Activités antiovulatoire et antigonadotrope de la chlormadinone chez le lapin et chez le rat. *C.R. Soc. Biol.* **159**: 2479–2483.

CHAMBON, Y. and LE BARS, S. (1966) Effects of 6-dehydro-6-chloro-17α-acetoxyprogesterone and ethynylestradiol alone and together on the adrenal in rabbits and rats. In: *Second Internat. Congress on Hormonal Steroids*, p. 343. Internat. Congress Series no. 111, Excerpta Medica, Amsterdam–New York.

CHAMBON, Y. and LE VÈVE, Y. (1966a) Importance des conditions expérimentales dans

l'évaluation de l'activité des gestogènes. *C.R. Acad. Sci. (Paris)*, Série D, **263**: 1255-1257.
CHAMBON, Y. and LE VÈVE, Y. (1966b) The synergistic action of 6-dehydro-6-chloro-17αacetoxy-progesterone and ethynylestradiol on maintenance of pregnancy in rabbits and rats. In: *Second Internat. Congress on Hormonal Steroids*, p. 343. International Congress Series. Excerpta Medica, Amsterdam-New York.
CHAMBON, Y. and LE VÈVE, Y. (1966c) Effets antiovulatoires de l'éthynyloestradiol et du mestranol, isolément ou en association avec la chlormadinone chez le lapin et chez le rat. *C.R. Soc. Biol.* **160**: 2411-2415.
CHAMBON, Y. and PICARD, F. (1966) Activités oestrogénique et anti-oestrogénique de la chlormadinone chez le rat. *C.R. Soc. Biol.* **160**: 376-379.
CHAMBON, Y., LE VÈVE, Y. and GOURVÈS, M. (1966) Activités androgénique et antigonadique de la chlormadinone chez le rat. *C.R. Soc. Biol.* **160**: 1720-1724.
CHANG, C. C. and KINCL, F. A. (1968) Sustained release hormonal preparations: 3. Biological effectiveness of 6-methyl-17α-acetoxy-pregna-4,6-diene-3,20-dione. *Steroids* **12**: 689-696.
CHANG, C. C. and KINCL, F. A. (1970) Sustained release hormonal preparations: 4. Biologic effectiveness of steroid hormones. *Fertil. Steril.* **21**: 134-139.
CHANG, M. C. (1957) Effects of medroxyprogesterone acetate and of ethynyl oestradiol on the fertilization and transportation of ferret eggs. *J. Reprod. Fertil.* **13**: 173-174.
CHANG, M. C. (1964) Effects of certain antifertility agents on the development of rabbit ova. *Fertil. Steril.* **15**: 97-106.
CHANG, M. C (1966) Effects of oral administration of medroxyprogesterone acetate and ethinyl estradiol on the transportation and development of rabbit-eggs. *Endocrinology* **79**: 939-948.
CHAPPEL, C. I., REVESZ, C. and GAUDRY, R. (1960) Biological studies on new orally active 6,17-halogenated progesterones. *Acta Endocr. (Kbh.)*, Suppl. **51**: 915.
CLAASSEN, V. (1968) Personal communication on experiments performed in Philips-Duphar Research Laboratories in 1967.
COMINOS, A. C., PAPATHEODOROU, B. and CHALKIADAKIS, J. (1962) Der Einfluss des 17α-Äthinyl-19-Nortestosterons (Norethisteron) auf die Spermatogenese der Kaninchen. *Geburtsh. Frauenheilk.* **22**: 887-891.
COPPOLA, J. A. and PERRINE, J. W. (1965) Inhibition of gonadotrophin induced ovulation by norethynodrel in immature rats. *J. Reprod. Fertil.* **9**: 109-110.
COPPOLA, J. A., LEONARDI, R. G. and RINGLER, I. (1966) Reversal of the effects of antioestrogens and norethynodrel on gonadotrophin-induced ovulation in rats. *J. Reprod. Fertil.* **11**: 65-71.
CRANE, M. G. and LEONORA, J. (1970) Effect of medroxyprogesterone acetate (MPA) and other steroids in combination with high sodium intake in the rat. *Clin. Res.* **18**: 167.
CSAPO, A. I. and WIEST, W. G. (1969) An examination of the quantitative relationship between progesterone and the maintenance of pregnancy. *Endocrinology* **85**: 735-746.
CUPCEANCU, B. and NEUMANN, F. (1969a) Sensibilitätsunterschiede der verschiedenen Strukturen des Genitaltraktes von weiblichen Rattenfoeten unter dem Einfluss von Medroxyprogesteronacetat oder Norethisteronacetat. *Endokrinologie* **54**: 66-80.
CUPCEANCU, B. and NEUMANN, F. (1969b) Der Einfluss verschiedener Gestagene auf die Entwicklung der Milchdrüse von Ratten. *Endokrinologie* **54**: 423-432.
CUPCEANCU, B., NEUMANN, F. and STEINBECK, H. (1971) Beeinflussung der Ovarialfunktion erwachsener weibliche Ratten durch neonatale Behandlung mit verschiedenen Sterioden mit bekannter Gestagen-Wirkung. *Acta Endocr. (Kbh.)* **67**: 337-344.

CZYBA, J. C. (1963) Sur l'action "progestomimetique" du propionate du testosterone chez le hamster doré ovariectomisé. *C.R. Acad. Sci.* **256**: 2242.

CZYBA, J. C. and CHIRIS, M. (1963) Sur l'action de quelques stéroides au niveau de l'endomètre chez le hamster doré. *C.R. Soc. Biol.* **157**: 1587–1588.

CZYBA, J. C. and COTTINET, D. (1968) Action comparée du lynestrénol et de la progestérone sur la formation du déciduome expérimental chez le hamster doré. *C.R. Soc. Biol.* **162**: 95–96.

DANFORTH, D. N., MANALO-ESTRELLA, P. and BUCKINGHAM, J. D. (1964) The effect of pregnancy and of Enovid on the rabbit vasculature. *Amer. J. Obst. Gynec.* **88**: 952–962.

DASTUGUE, G., BASTIDE, P. and RENARD, M. P. (1966) Variations des activités arylestérasiques-lipasiques, phosphatasiques et β-glucuronidasique dans les ovaires des rattes pubères, traitées comparativement à l'éthynil-oestradiol et au lynestrénol. *C.R. Soc. Biol.* **160**: 2318–2321.

DAVID, A., EDWARDS, K., FELLOWES, K. P. and PLUMMER, J. M. (1963) Anti-ovulatory and other biological properties of megestrol acetate. 17α-acetoxy-6 methyl pregna: 4: 6–diene-3:20 dione (BHD 1298). *J. Reprod. Fertil.* **5**: 331–346.

DAVID, A., FELLOWES, K. P. and MILLSON, D. R. (1959) Some biological properties of dimethisterone "Secrosteron" a new orally active progestational agent. *J. Pharm. Pharmac.* **11**: 491–495.

DAVID, A., HARTLEY, F., MILLSON, D. R. and PETROW, V. (1957) The preparation and progestational activity of some alkylated ethisterones. *J. Pharm. Pharmac.* **9**, 929–934.

DAVIS, B. K. (1963a) Termination of pregnancy in the rat with norethynodrel. *Nature (London)* **197**: 308–309.

DAVIS, B. K. (1963b) Studies on the termination of pregnancy with norethynodrel. *J. Endocrin.* **27**: 99–106.

DECKERS, G. H. and VIES, J. VAN DER (1968) Deciduoomvorming bij hamsters als test voor progestatieve activiteit. Paper presented at the ninth meeting of the federation of medical-biological Societies, Nijmegen, April 18 and 19. To be published.

DE FREMERY, P., LUCHS, A. and TAUSK, M. (1932) Untersuchungen über die innere Sekretion des corpus-luteum. *Pflüg. Arch. ges. Physiol.* **231**: 341–359.

DESAULLES, P. A. and KRÄHENBÜHL, C. (1962) Comparaison du spectre d'activité de certains gestagènes de synthèse. *Acta Endocr. (Kbh.)* **40**: 217–231.

DESAULLES, P. A. and KRÄHENBÜHL, C. (1964) Comparison of the anti-fertility and sex hormonal activities of sex hormones and their derivatives. *Acta Endocr. (Kbh.)* **47**: 444–456.

DE VISSER, J. (1969) Development of an antifertilization test in rabbits. *Arch. Int. Pharmocodyn.* **182**: 407–408.

DHOM, G., KRULL, P., MÄUSLE, E. and STRUBE, R. (1965) Der Einfluss eines Ovulationshemmers (17α-Äthinyl-19-nortestosteron) auf die gonadotropen Zellen der Rattenhypophyse. *Beitr. Path. Anat.* **132**: 1–24.

DICKSON, A. D. (1969) Effectiveness of 6α-methyl-17-acetoxyprogesterone, in combination with oestradiol benzoate, in inducing delayed implantation in the mouse. *J. Reprod. Fertil.* **18**: 227–233.

DÖCKE, F., DÖRNER, G. and VOIGT, K.-H. (1966) Ovulationshemmung bei Ratten durch Implantation von Chlormadinonazetat in den Hypothalamus und in die Hypophyse. *Acta Biol. Med. german.* **17**: 557–559.

DÖCKE, F., DÖRNER, G. and VOIGT, K.-H. (1968) A possible mechanism of the ovulation-inhibiting effect of chlormadinone acetate in the rat. *J. Endocr.* **41**: 353–362.

DOOLITTLE, D. P. (1963) The contraceptive level of certain drugs in the house mouse. *Steroids* **2**: 355–371.

DORFMAN, R. I. (1963a) Inhibitors of steroid actions and cholesterol and steroid biosynthesis. In: *Metabolic Inhibitors*, Vol. I, pp. 567–583. Hochster, R. M. and Quastel, J. H. (Eds.), Academic Press, New York and London.
DORFMAN, R. I. (1963b) Anti-androgens in a castrated mouse test. *Steroids* 2: 185–193.
DORFMAN, R. I. (1968) Anti-androgens. In: *Testosterone. Proceedings of the Workshop Conference held from April 20th to 22nd 1967 at Tremsbüttel*, pp. 130–132. Tamm, J. (Ed.), Georg Thieme Verlag, Stuttgart.
DORFMAN, R. I. and KINCL, F. A. (1963) Steroid anti-estrogens. *Steroids* 1: 185–209.
DORFMAN, R. I., KINCL, F. A. and RINGOLD, H. J. (1961a) Anti-estrogen assay of neutral steroids administered by subcutaneous injection. *Endocrinology* 68: 17–24.
DORFMAN, R. I., KINCL, F. A. and RINGOLD, H. J. (1961b) Anti-estrogen assay of neutral steroids administered by gavage. *Endocrinology* 68: 43–49.
DÖRNER, G. and DÖCKE, F. (1967) The influence of intrahypothalamic and intrahypophyseal implantation of estrogen or progestogen on gonadotrophin release. *Endocr. Exper.* 2: 65–71.
DRILL, V. A. (1959) Biological effects of some steroids with progestational activity. *Federation Proceedings* 18: 1040–1048.
DRILL, V. A. (1962) Endocrine properties of norethynodrel and related steroids. *J. Endocr.* 24: xvii–xviii.
DRILL, V. A. (1963) Contraceptive effect of oral progestins: properties of compound SC-11800, a new oral inhibitor. *J. Reprod. Fertil.* 5: 462.
DRILL, V. A. (1965) Endocrine properties and long-term safety of oral contraceptives. *Metabolism* 14: 295–310.
DRILL, V. A. (1966) *Oral Contraceptives*. McGraw-Hill Book Co., New York.
DRILL, V. A. and RIEGEL, B. (1958) Structural and hormonal activity of some new steroids. In: *Recent Progress in Hormone Research*, vol. 14, pp. 29–67. Pincus, G. (Ed.). Academic Press, New York and London.
DRILL, V. A. and SAUNDERS, F. J. (1957) Biological activity of norethynodrel. In: *Proceedings of a Symposium on* 19-*norprogestational Steroids, Chicago*, Searle Research Laboratories, pp. 1–13.
DUBOIS, P., CZYBA, J. C. and DUMONT, L. (1964) Les premiers stades de la décidualisation de l'endomètre chez le hamster doré. *C.R. Soc. Biol.* 158: 745–748.
DUNCAN, G. W., LYSTER, S. C., HENDRIX, J. W., CLARK, J. J. and WEBSTER, H. D. (1964) Biologic effects of melengestrol acetate. *Fertil. Steril.* 15: 419–432.
DUTTA, N. S. and SANYAL, R. K. (1969) Effects of some synthetic progestational steroids on uterine contractions. *Indian J. Med. Sci.* 23: 11–13.
DZIUK, P. J. (1960) Inhibition and synchronization of mating in the mouse by oral administration of Progestins. *Endocrinology* 66: 898–900.
EBEN-MOUSSI, E. and VAN DEN DRIESSCHE, J. (1970) Evaluation de l'activité d'un nouveau progestagène: l'acétate de quingestanol. *Thérapie* 25: 181–190.
ECKSTEIN, P., and MANDL, A. M. Effect of Norethynodrel on the ovarian response of the immature rat to gonadotrophic stimulation. *Endocrinology* 71: 965–971.
ECTORS, F., PASTEELS, J. L., and HERLANT, M. (1966) Action de la médroxyprogestérone (Provera) sur l'hypophyse, les glandes mammaires et les ovaires chez la ratte. *C.R. Acad. Sci. (Paris)* Serie D 263: (25) 1588–1991.
EDGREN, R. A. (1958) The uterine growth-stimulating activities of 17α-ethynyl-17 hydroxy-5(10)-estren-3-one (Norethynodrel) and 17α-ethynyl-19-nortestosterone. *Endocrinology* 62: 689–693.
EDGREN, R. A. (1960) Estrogen antagonisms: Effects of a series of 19-nortestosterone derivatives on vaginal changes induced by estrone. *Proc. Soc. Exp. Biol. Med.* 105: 252–254.
EDGREN, R. A. (1966) Estrogen antagonism: relationship between estrogen antagonistic

and progestational potencies of Δ^4-3-oxosteroids. *Proc. Soc. Exp. Biol. Med.* **123**: 788–790.

EDGREN, R. A. and CARTER, D. L. (1962) Failure of various steroids to block gonadotrophin induced ovulation in rabbits. *J. Endocr.* **24**: 525–526.

EDGREN, R. A. and PETERSON, D. L. (1966) Delay of parturition in rats by various progestational steroids. *Proc. Soc. Exp. Biol. Med.* **123**: 867–869.

EDGREN, R. A. and PETERSON CLANCY, D. (1968) The effects of norgestrel, ethynylestradiol and their combination (Ovral) on the young of female rats treated during pregnancy. *Internat. J. Fertil.* **13**: 208–214.

EDGREN, R. A., CALHOUN, D. W., ELTON, R. L. and COLTON, F. B. (1959a) Estrogen antagonisms: the effects of a series of relatives of 19-nortestosterone on estrone induced uterine growth. *Endocrinology* **65**: 265–272.

EDGREN, R. A., HAMBOURGER, W. E. and CALHOUN, D. W. (1959b) Production of adrenal atrophy by 6-methyl-17-acetoxy-progesterone, with remarks on the adrenal effects of other progestational agents. *Endocrinology* **65**: 505–507.

EDGREN, R. A., JONES, R. C. and PETERSON, D. L. (1967a) A biological classification of progestational agents. *Fertil. Steril.* **18**: 238–256.

EDGREN, R. A., JONES, R. C., PETERSON, D. L. and GILLEN, A. L., (1967b) Studies on the interactions of ethynyl oestradiol and norgestrel. *Acta Endocr.* (*Kbh.*), Suppl. 115.

EDGREN, R. A., JONES, R. C., PETERSON CLANCY, D. and NAGRA, C. L. (1968) The biological effects of norgestrel alone and in combination with ethynyl oestradiol. *J. Reprod. Fert. Suppl.* **5**: 13–45.

EDGREN, R. A., PETERSON, D. L. and JONES, R. C. (1966a) Some progestational and antifertility effects of norgestrel. *Internat. J. Fertil.* **11**: 389–400.

EDGREN, R. A., PETERSON, D. L., JONES, R. C., NAGRA, C. L., SMITH, H. and HUGHES, G. A. (1966b) Biological effects of synthetic gonanes. In: *Recent Progress in Hormone Research*, Vol. 22, p. 305. Pincus, G. (Ed.). Academic Press Inc., New York.

EDGREN, R. A., SMITH, H., PETERSON, D. L. and CARTER, D. L. (1963a) The biological effects of a series of 13β-substituted gonanes related to norethisterone (17α-ethynyl-19 nortestosterone). *Steroids* **2**: 319–335.

EDGREN, R. A., WEINBERG, I. P. and COCHRAN, T. G. B. (1963b) Estrogen antagonism: a comparison of the effects of various anti-estrogens administered separately and as mixtures with the estrogen. *Endocrinology* **72**: 665–666.

EISENFELD, A. J. and AXELROD, J. (1965) Selectivity of estrogen distribution in tissues. *J. Pharmacol* **150**: 469–475.

ELTON, R. L. (1962) Morphological changes in the glandular epithelium of rabbit endometrium due to hormonal treatment. *Anat. Rec.* **142**: 469–477.

ELTON, R. L. and NUTTING, E. F. (1961) 17-Ethynyl-4-estrene-3,17-diol diacetate: a unique steroidal "Progestin". *Proc. Soc. Exp. Biol. Med.* **107**: 991–994.

ELTON, R. L., EDGREN, R. A. and CALHOUN, D. (1960) Biological activities of some 6-methylated progesterones. *Proc. Soc. Exp. Biol. Med.* **103**: 175–177.

ELTON, R. L., KLIMSTRA, P. D. and COLTON, F. B. (1966) Induction of deciduoma in rabbits without uterine trauma by treatment with ethynodiol diacetate: a synthetic progestogen. *Proc. Soc. Exp. Biol. Med.* **121**: 1194–1196.

ELTON, R. L., NUTTING, E. F. and SAUNDERS, F. J. (1962) Effects of reduction of the 3-ketone of 17α-ethynyl-19-nortestosterone on its endocrine properties. *Acta Endocr.* (*Kbh.*) **41**: 381–390.

EMMENS, C. W. (1962) Estrogens. In: *Methods in Hormone Research*, vol. II, pp. 59–111. Dorfman, R. I. (Ed.). Academic Press, New York.

EMMENS, C. W. and MARTIN, L. (1964) Anti-estrogens, In: *Methods in Hormone Research*, Vol. III, pp. 81–125. Dorfman, R. I. (Ed.). Academic Press, New York.

EMMENS, C. W., COX, R. I. and MARTIN, L. (1960) Oestrogen inhibition by steroids and other substances. *J. Endocrin.* **20**: 198–209.

ERB, H. (1967) Bedeutung der Corpus-luteum-Aktivität für die Tubenmotilität. In: *Investigations on Sterility: Proceedings of the First European Congress on Sterility*, pp. 166–172. Published by Clinica Ostetrica e ginecologica dell'Università di Genova.

ERB, H. (1969) Zur Wirkung niedrig dosierter Progestagene auf die Motilität der menschlichen Tube. *Geburtsh. Frauenheilk.* **3**: 255–260.

ERB, H. (1970) Tubenmotilität unter Low-dose-progestin treatment. *Schweiz. Z. Gynäk. Geburtsh.* **1**: 53–59.

ERB, H. and WENNER, R. (1967) Influence of progesterone on motility of fallopian tubes in menopause (*in vitro* experiments on human fallopian tubes). In: *Fertility and Sterility*, pp. 286–289. Westin B. and Wiqvist, N. (Eds.). Internat. Congress Series no. 133, Excerpta Medica, Amsterdam–New York.

ERICSSON, R. I., DUTT, R. H. and ARCHDEACON, J. W. (1964) Progesterone and 6-chloro-Δ^6-17-acetoxy-progesterone as inhibitors of spermatogenesis in the rabbit. *Nature* **204**: 261–263.

EXLEY, D., GELLERT, R. J., HARRIS, G. W. and NADLER, R. D. (1968) The site of action of "chlormadinone acetate" (6-chloro-Δ^6-dehydro-17α-acetoxyprogesterone) in blocking ovulation in the mated rabbit. *J. Physiol.* **195**: 697–714.

FAIRWEATHER, F. A. (1968) Toxicological requirement of oral contraceptives. *J. Reprod. Fert. Suppl.* **5**: 47–49.

FALCONI, G. and BRUNI, G. (1962) Studies on steroidal enol ethers: anti-gonadotrophic activity of cyclopentyl derivatives of some orally active progestins. *J. Endocr.* **25**: 169–173.

FALCONI, G. and ERCOLI, A. (1961) Effect of enol etherification on antiestrual and contraceptive activity of some progestins in rats. *Proc. Soc. Exp. Biol. Med.* **108**: 3–6.

FALCONI, G., GARDI, R., BRUNI, G. and ERCOLI, A. (1961) Studies on steroidal enol ethers: an attempt to dissociate progestational from contraceptive activity in oral gestagens. *Endocrinology* **69**: 638–647.

FEKETE, G. and SZEBERÉNYI, S. (1965a) Data on the mechanism of adrenal suppression by medroxyprogesterone. *Steroids* **6**: 159–166.

FEKETE, G. and SZEBERÉNYI, S. (1965b) The effect of 6α-methyl-17α-acetoxy-progesterone (MAP) on adrenal steroidogenesis. *Acta Physiol. Hung.* **26**, Suppl. 56.

FEUER, G. and GRANDA, V. (1970) Steroid hormones as possible regulators of the development of the hepatic microsomal drug metabolizing system in the fetus and the newborn. In: *Third International Congress on Hormonal Steroids*, p. 169, James, V. H. T. (Ed.). Internat. Congress Series 210, Excerpta Medica, Amsterdam–New York.

FOLCH-PI, A., ORIOL, A., HERRERA LASSO, L., MAQUEO, M., DORFMAN, R. I. and KINCL, F. A. (1965) Inhibition of fertility in mice by steroid implants. *Acta Endocr. (Kbh.)* **48**: 602–608.

FOLMAN, Y. and POPE, G. S. (1964) The inter-action of strong and weak uterotrophic-vaginotrophic agents in the immature mouse. *J. Endocrinol.* **30**: x–xi.

FOOTE, W. D., FOOTE, W. C. and FOOTE, L. H. (1968) Influence of certain natural and synthetic steroids on genital development in guinea pigs. *Fertil. Steril.* **19**: 606–615.

FRANCE, E. S. and PINCUS, G. (1964) Biologically active substances affecting gonadotrophin-induced ovulation in immature rats. *Endocrinology* **75**: 359–364.

FRITH, D. A. (misspelt as FIRTH) and HOOPER, K. C. (1968) The effect of 17α-ethynyl-estradiol-17β on the metabolism of polypeptides in the hypothalamus. *Biochem. J.* **108**: 510–511.

FRITH, D. A. and HOOPER, K. C. (1971) The action of some ovulation inhibitors on the rabbit hypothalamus. *Acta Endocr. (Kbh.)* **66**: 221–228.

FUCHS, A.-R. (1964) Effect of intra-amniotic administration of progesterone and

6-methyl-17-acetoxy-progesterone on oxytocin-induced labour in rabbits. *Acta Endocr. (Kbh.)* **46**: 235–244.

FUCHS, F. and KOCH, F. (1963) Inhibition of oxytocin-induced labour in rabbits with various gestagens. *Acta Endocr. (Kbh.)* **42**: 403–411.

FUSSGÄNGER, R. (1934) Ein Beitrag zum Wirkungsmechanismus des männlichen Sexualhormons. *Med. u. Chem.* **2**: 194–212.

GALLO, R. V. and ZARROW, M. X. (1970) Effect of progesterone and other steroids on PMS-induced ovulation in the immature rat. *Endocrinology* **86**: 296–304.

GARCIA, C.-R. (1968) Oral Contraception. *Clinical Obstetrics and Gynecology*, Vol. 11, no. 3. Hoeber Medical Division, Harper & Row, New York.

GAZZANIGA, P. P., SONNINO, F. F., ZICHELLA, L. and HECHT-LUCARI, G. (1962) The effect *in vitro* of a series of hormonal steroids on the motility of the isolated guinea-pig uterus (with a contribution concerning the mechanism of action). In: *International Congress on Hormonal Steroids*. Internat. Congress Series No. 51, Abstr. 383. Excerpta Medica, Amsterdam–New York.

GERARD, G., VIGNOLO, W. H., RODRIGUEZ, R. and CORDOSO, T. (1963) Accion del acetato de nor-etisterona sobre la hipofisis de la rata macho. *Anales de la Facultad de Medicina de Montevideo* **48**: 367–371.

GIANNINA, T., STEINETZ, B. G., RASSAERT, C. L., MCDOUGALL, E. A. and MELI, A. (1969) Biological profile of quingestanol acetate. *Proc. Soc. Exp. Biol. Med.* **131**: 781–789.

GLENN, E. M., RICHARDSON, S. L. and BOWMAN, B. J. (1959) Biologic activity of 6-alpha-methyl compounds corresponding to progesterone, 17-alpha-hydroxy-progesterone acetate and compound S. *Metabolism* **8**: 265–285.

GOISIS, M. (1964) Effects of progestational steroids on the morphology and function of anterior pituitary and ovaries in the baboon. *Int. J. Fertil.* **9**: 175–176.

GOLDMAN, A. S. and BONGIOVANNI, A. M. (1967) Induced genital anomalies. *Ann. N.Y. Acad. Sci.* **142**: 755–767.

GORSKI, R. (1966) Localization and sexual differentiation of the nervous structures which regulate ovulation. *J. Reprod. Fertil. Suppl.* **1**: 67.88.

GREENE, R. R., BURRILL, M. W. and IVY, A. C. (1939a) Experimental intersexuality: the effect of antenatal androgens on sexual development of female rats. *Amer. J. Anat.* **65**: 415.

GREENE, R. R., BURRILL, M. W. and IVY, A. C. (1939b) Experimental intersexuality: the paradoxical effects of estrogens on the sexual development of the female rat. *Anat. Rec.* **74**: 429–438.

GREENE, R. R., BURRILL, M. W. and IVY, A. C. (1939c) Progesterone is androgenic. *Endocrinology* **24**: 351–357.

GREENWALD, G. S. (1964) Mechanisms by which norethynodrel and ethynyl-oestradiol inhibit ovulation in the hamster. *Acta Endocr. (Kbh.)* **47**: 10–14.

GREENWALD, G. S. (1965) Antiovulatory potency of various steroids, determined by single injection into female hamsters. *J. Endocrin.* **33**: 25–32.

GRIFFITH, D. R., WILLIAMS, R. and TURNER, C. W. (1963) Effects of orally administered progesterone-like compounds on mammary gland growth in rats. *Proc. Soc. Exp. Biol. Med.* **113**: 401–403.

GRISWOLD, D. P., SKIPPER, H. E., LASTER, W. R., WILCOX, W. S. and SCHABEL, JR., F. M. (1966) Induced mammary carcinoma in the female rat as a drug evaluation system. *Cancer Res.* **26**: 2169–2180.

GRUMBACH, M. M., DUCHARME, J. R. and MOLOSHOK, R. E. (1959) On the fetal masculinizing action of certain oral progestins. *J. Clin. Endocr.* **19**: 1369–1380.

HALLER, J. (1964) Reversibility of norethisterone-acetate induced inhibition of gonadotropic function in the splenic ovarian graft planimetric test. In: *Excerpta Med. Intern. Congr. Ser. no.* **72,** 455–462.

HALLER, J. (1968) *Ovulationshemmung durch Hormone.* Georg Thieme Verlag, Stuttgart.
HALLER, J. (1969) *Hormonal Contraception.* Geron-X Inc., Los Altos (Calif.).
HALLER, J. (1970) Direct effect of medroxyprogesterone acetate (MPA) on the intrasplenic ovarian graft in guinea pigs. In: *Third Internat. Congress on Hormonal Steroids*, p. 215, James, V. H. T. (Ed.). Internat. Congress Series 210, Excerpta Medica, Amsterdam–New York.
HALMI, N. S. (1950) Two types of basophils in the anterior pituitary of the rat and their respective cytophysiological significance. *Endocrinology* **47**: 289–299.
HAMADA, H., NEUMANN, F. and JUNKMANN, K. (1963) Intrauterine antimaskuline Beeinflussung von Rattenfeten durch ein stark gestagen wirksames Steroid. *Acta Endocr. (Kbh.)* **44**: 380–388.
HARPEL, P. C., HOMBURGER, F., and TREGER A. (1968) Mouse uterine plasminogen activator, acid phosphatase, and contraceptive hormones. *Amer. J. Physiol.* **215**: 928–931.
HARPER, M. J. K. (1964) The effect of chlormadinone on the response of the ovaries and uterus of the immature rat to gonadotrophic stimulation. *J. Endocr.* **30**: 235–245.
HARPER, M. J. K. (1965) Augmentation by chlormadinone of the uterine weight response to human chorionic gonadotrophin in intact immature rats. *J. Endocr.* **33**: 443–454.
HARRIS, G. W. and SHERRATT, R. M. (1969) Reaction of chlormadinone acetate (6-chloro-Δ^6-dehydro-17α-acetoxyprogesterone) upon experimentally induced ovulation in the rabbit. *J. Physiol.* **203**: 59–66.
HAYLES, A. B. and NOLAN, R. B. (1958) Masculinization of female fetus, possibly related to administration of progesterone during pregnancy. *Proc. Staff Meet. Mayo Clin.* **33**: 200–203.
HECHT-LUCARI, G. (1966) Antioestrogene und antiandrogene Effekte gewisser oral wirksamer Gestagene. *Geburtsh. Frauenheilk.* **26**: 620–623.
HECHT-LUCARI, G., KRAFT, H. G. and KIESER, H. (1966) Estrogenic, antiestrogenic and antifertility activity of chlormadinone acetate and other steroidal and nonsteroidal compounds. In: *Research on Steroids*, vol. 2, pp. 357–370. Cassano, C. (Ed.). Il Pensiero Scientifico, Rome.
HEIKEL, T. A. J. and LATHE, G. H. (1970) The effect of 17α-ethynyl-substituted steroids on adenosine triphosphatases of rat liver membrane. *Biochem. J.* **118**: 187–189.
HERTZ, R., TULLNER, W. and RAFFELT, E. (1954) Progestational activity of orally administered 17α-ethynyl-19-nortestosterone. *Endocrinology* **54**: 228–230.
HERVEY, E., HERVEY, G. R. and JEFFERY, J. D. A. (1967) The effects of some synthetic progestational agents on body weight and composition in the female rat. *J. Endocr.* **38**: iv.
HERVEY, E., HERVEY, G. R. and JEFFERY, J. D. A. (1968) Dissociation of progesterone-like effects of certain compounds upon body weight and body composition in the female rat from other progestational activity. *J. Endocr.* **41**: vi.
HILL, R., AVERKIN, E., BROWN, W., GAGNE, W. E. and SEGRE, E. (1970) Progestational potency of chlormadinone acetate in the immature beagle bitch: preliminary report. *Contraception* **2**: 381–390.
HILLIARD, J., HAYWARD, J. N., CROXATTO, H. B. and SAWYER, C. H. (1966a) Norethindrone blockade of pituitary gonadotropin release, counteraction by estrogen. *Endocrinology* **78**: 151–157.
HILLIARD, J., CROXATTO, H. B., HAYWARD, J. N. and SAWYER, C. H. (1966b) Norethindrone blockade of LH release to intrapituitary infusion of hypothalamic extract. *Endocrinology* **79**: 411–419.
HOLMES, R. L. and MANDL, A. M. (1962) The effect of norethynodrel on the ovaries and pituitary gland of adult female rats. *J. Endocr.* **24**: 497–515.
HOLUB, D. A., KATZ, F. H. and JAILER, J. W. (1961) Inhibition by 6-methyl-17-acetoxyprogesterone of ACTH synthesis and release in the rat. *Endocrinology* **68**: 173–177.

HOOPER, K. C. (1968) The effects of ovariectomy and injected oestradiol monobenzoate on polypeptide metabolism in the hypothalamus. *Biochem. J.* **110**: 151–153.

HUGGINS, C., BRIZIARELLI, G. and SUTTON, JR., H. (1959) Rapid induction of mammary carcinoma in the rat and the influence of hormones on the tumors. *J. Exp. Med.* **109**: 25–41.

HUGGINS, C., GRAND, L. C. and BRILLANTES, F. P. (1961) Mammary cancer induced by a single feeding of polynuclear hydrocarbons and its suppression. *Nature* **189**: 204–207.

HUGGINS, C., TORRALRA, Y. and MAINZER, K. (1956) Hormonal influences on mammary tumors of the rat. 1. Acceleration of growth of transplanted fibroadenoma in ovariectomized and hypophysectomized rats. *J. Exp. Med.* **104**: 525–539.

HULKA, J. F., MOHR, K. and LIEBERMAN, M. W. (1965) Effect of synthetic progestational agents on allograft rejection and circulating antibody production. *Endocrinology* **77**: 897–901.

HUMPHREY, K. W. (1970) Mechanisms concerned in ovum transport. In: *Advances in the Biosciences*, vol. 4, pp. 133–163. Schering Symposium on Mechanisms Involved in Conception. Pergamon, Vieweg, Oxford, Braunschweig.

JADRIJEVIĆ, D., MARDONES, E. and LIPSCHÜTZ, A. (1956) Antifibromatogenic activity of 19-nor-α-ethynyl-testosterone in the guinea pig. *Proc. Soc. Exp. Biol. Med.* **91**: 38–39.

JAKOBOVITS, A., GECSE, A., PIUKOVICH, I., SZONTAGH, F. and KARADY, M. (1970) Effect of 19-nor steroids on the mobility of human Fallopian tubes. *Int. J. Fertil.* **15**: 36–39.

JONES, R. C., EDGREN, R. A. and TAYLOR, R. J. (1966) An assay for progestagens by the intravenous route. *Steroids* **7**: 551–556.

JONGH, S. E. DE (1968) Recollections of the heyday of experimental endocrinology under Laqueur at the Amsterdam Polderweg. *Acta Endocr. (Kbh.)* **57**: 1–15.

JOST, A. (1963a) Hormones et tératogénèse. In: *Effects of Drugs on the Foetus. Proceedings of the European Society for the Study of Drug Toxicity*, Vol, 1, pp. 35–47. Internat. Congress Series no. 64. Excerpta Medica, Amsterdam, New York.

JOST, A. (1963b) Maintien de la gestation chez la lapine par un stéréo-isomère voisin de la progestérone (6-dehydro-rétro-progestérone). Action sur les foetus. *Acta Endocr. (Kbh.)* **43**: 539–544.

JOST, A. and MOREAU, M. G. (1963) Action sur l'appareil génital des foetus de rat d'une substance progestative de synthèse, l'allylestrénol; importance des conditions d'administration. *C.R. Acad. Sci.* **256**: 502–503.

JOST, A. and MOREAU-STINNAKRE, M. G. (1970) Action d'une substance progestative synthetique (17α-allyl-4 oestrène-17β-ol) sur la differenciation sexuelle des foetus de rat. Remarques méthodologiques. *Acta Endocr. (Kbh.)* **65**: 29–49.

JUNKMANN, K. (1963) Experimentelle Gesichtspunkte bei der Prüfung synthetischer Gestagene. *Dt. Med. Wschr.* **88**: 629–638.

JUNKMANN, K. (1964) Die Tierexperimentelle Prüfung antikonzeptioneller Steroide. *Der Internist* **5**: 237–242.

JUNKMANN, K. (1968) *Die Gestagene*, Teil 1. Handbook of Experimental Pharmacology, Vol. XXII/1. Springer-Verlag, Berlin, New York.

JUNKMANN, K. and NEUMANN, F. (1964) Zum Wirkungsmechanismus von an Feten antimaskulin wirksamen Gestagenen. *Acta Endocr. (Kbh.)* Suppl. **90**, 139–154.

KAHN, R. H. (1966) Effect of long term treatment of mice with norethynodrel. *Anat. Rec.* **154**: 364.

treatment with norethynodrel. *Acta Endocr. (Kbh.)* **51**: 411–414.

KAHN, R. H. and BAKER, B. L. (1964) Effect of norethynodrel alone or combined with mestranol on the mammary glands of the adult female rat. *Endocrinology* **75**: 818–821.

KAHN, R. H. and BAKER, B. L. (1966) Prolactin content of the rat hypophysis following

KAHN, R. H. and BAKER, B. L. (1969) Effect of long-term treatment with norethynodrel on A/J and C_3H/HeJ mice. *Endocrinology* **84**: 661–668.

KAHN, R. H., BAKER, B. L. and ZANOTTI, D. B. (1965) Factors modifying the stimulatory action of norethynodrel on the mammary gland. *Endocrinology* **77**: 162–168.

KAISER, R. and MOHR, U. (1961) Zur Frage der Wirkung von Äthinylnortestosteronacetat auf das Wachstum bestimmter Sarkome. *Z. Krebsforsch.* **64**: 122–124.

KANEMATSU, S. and SAWYER, C. H. (1965) Blockade of ovulation in rabbits by hypothalamic implants of norethindrone. *Endocrinology* **76**: 691–699.

KAR, A. B. and CHANDRA, H. (1965) Effect of some progestational steroids on the response of the ovary of prepuberal rhesus monkeys to exogenous gonadotrophin. *Steroids* **6**: 463–472.

KAR, A. B., SETTY, B. S. and KAMBOJ, V. P. (1968) Postcoital contraception by topical application of some steroidal and nonsteroidal agents. *Amer. J. Obstet. Gynecol.* **102**: 306–307.

KARADY, S. and HOOTON FRAYN, A. (1967) Gonadotrophins and tumour growth. *Med. Pharmacol. Exp.* **17**: 1–5.

KAWAKAMI, M. and SAWYER, C. H. (1967) Effects of sex hormones and antifertility steroids on brain thresholds in the rabbit. *Endocrinology* **80**: 857–871.

KENDLE, K. E. and TELFORD, J. M. (1970) Investigations into the mechanism of the antifertility action of minimal doses of megestrol acetate in the rabbit. *Brit. J. Pharmacol.* **40**: 759–774.

KINCL, F. A. (1961) Steroide CLV: Progestative Wirksamkeit von 6-substituierten 17α-Acetoxyprogesteron-Derivaten. *Endokrinologie* **40**: 257–266.

KINCL, F. A. (1963) Notiz über den Mechanismus der Anti-Ovulation mit 6-chloro-Δ^6-17α-Acetoxy-progesteron in Kaninchen. *Endokrinologie* **44**: 67–71.

KINCL, F. A. (1964a) Copulatory reflex response to steroids. In: *Methods in Hormone Research*, vol. 3, pp. 477–483. R. Dorfman (Ed.). Academic Press Inc., New York.

KINCL, F. A. (1964b) Induction of ovulation in rats by steroids. In: *5. Congresso internazionale per la riproduzione animale e la fecondazione artificiale. Trento 6–13 Settembre 1964.* Estratto dalle communicazioni libere, vol. III.

KINCL, F. A. (1965) Failure of various steroids to block ovulation at the ovarian level. In: *Research on Steroids*, vol. 2, pp. 353–356. Cassanole C. (Ed.) Il pensiero scientifico, Rome.

KINCL, F. A., ANGEE, I., CHANG, C. C. and RUDEL, H. W. (1970) Sustained release hormonal preparations. 9. *Acta Endocr. (Kbh.)* **64**: 508–518.

KINCL, F. A. and DORFMAN, R. I. (1961) Copulatory reflex in guinea pigs induced by, progesterone and related steroids. *Acta Endocr. (Kbh.)* **38**: 257–261.

KINCL, F. A. and DORFMAN, R. I. (1962) Influence of progestational agents on the genetic female foetus of orally treated pregnant rats. *Acta Endocr. (Kbh.)* **41**: 274–279.

KINCL, F. A. and DORFMAN, R. I. (1963a) Anti-ovulatory activity of subcutaneously injected steroids in the adult oestrous rabbit. *Acta Endocr. (Kbh.)*, Suppl. **73**: 3–15.

KINCL, F. A. and DORFMAN, R. I. (1963b) Anti-ovulatory activity of steroids administered by gavage in the adult oestrous rabbit. *Acta Endocr. (Kbh.)*, Suppl. **73**: 17–30.

KINCL, F. A. and DORFMAN, R. I. (1963c) Orally active steroidal ovulation inhibitors in the adult oestrus rabbit. *Steroids* **2**: 521–525.

KINCL, F. A. and DORFMAN, R. I. (1965a) Antifertility activity of various steroids in the female rat. *J. Reprod. Fertil.* **10**: 105–113.

KINCL, F. A. and DORFMAN, R. I. (1965b) The biological activity of estrogen-free norethindrone. *Proc. Soc. Exp. Biol. Med.* **119**: 340–344.

KINCL, F. A. and DORFMAN, R. I. (1966) Inhibition of ovulation in the adult estrus rabbit by vaginal deposition. *Steroids* **8**: 5–11.

KINCL, F. A. and FOLCH-PI, A. (1962) Actividad progestacional de derivados del pregnano. *Ciencia (Mex.)* **22**: 31–34.

KINCL, F. A., MAQUEO, M. and DORFMAN, R. J. (1965a) Influence of various steroids on testes and accessory sex organs in the rat. *Acta Endocr. (Kbh.)* **49**: 145–154.

KINCL, F. A., FOLCH-PI, A., MAQUEO, M., HERRERA LASSO, L., ORIOL, A., and DORFMAN, R. I. (1965b) Inhibition of sexual development in male and female rats treated with various steroids at the age of five days. *Acta Endocr. (Kbh.)* **49**: 193–206.

KINCL, F. A. and RUDEL, H. W. (1970). Sustained release hormonal preparations. *Acta Endocr. (Kbh.)* Suppl. 150.

KINCL, F. A. and SICKLES, J. S. (1969) The influence of progestational agents on ovulation in the Japanese quail (*Coturnix Coturnix Japonica*). *Acta Endocr. (Kbh.)* **60**: 512–516.

KING, T. O. and LUBANSKY, J. (1963) A two-year toxicity study of a norethindrone-mestranol combination in rats. *Federation Proceedings* **22**: 481.

KING, T. O. and LUBANSKY, J. (1965) Chronic toxicity study of anapregnone in rats. *Toxicol. Appl. Pharmacol.* **7**: 488.

KISTNER, R. W. (1969) *The Use of Progestins in Obstetrics and Gynecology.* Year Book Medical Publishers Inc., Chicago.

KOBAYASHI, T. (1963) The fundamental and clinical studies on 6-dehydro-retro-progesterone. Report I. *The World of Obstetrics and Gynecology* **15**: 57 (1097)–63 (1103).

KOBAYASHI, T., FURUHATA, T. and TSUYUGUCHI, M. (1962) Biological and clinical effects of allylestrenol (Gestanon). *Sanka to Fujinka (Obstet. and Gynec.)* **29**: 142.

KÖNIG, ANNEMARIE and HALLER, J. (1965) Über die Wirkung synthetischer Gestagene auf den Uterusmuskel der Ratte *in vitro*. *Arch. Gynäk.* **202**: 53–55.

KRAAY, R. J. and BLACK, L. J. (1970) Influence of progestins on the uptake of radioactive estradiol. In: *Third Internat. Congress on Hormonal Steroids*, p. 150. James, V.H.T.(Ed.). Internat. Congress Series 210, Excerpta Medica, Amsterdam, New York.

KRAAY, R. J. and BRENNAN, D. M. (1936) Evaluation of chlormadinone acetate and other progestagens for foetal masculinization in rats. *Acta Endocr. (Kbh.)* **43**: 412–418.

KRAEHAHN, G. and VON BERSWORDT-WALLRABE, R. (1969) Effects of 17α-ethynyl-19-nortestosterone acetate on pituitary and serum levels of ICSH and FSH in female rats. *Europ. J. Pharmac.* **6**: 303–311.

KRAFT, H. G. and HARTING, J. (1968) Antiandrogenic activities of some pregnane derivatives. In: *Testosterone. Proceedings of the Workshop Conference held from April* 20*th to* 22*nd* 1967 *at Tremsbüttel*, pp. 144–150. Tamm, J. (Ed.), Georg Thieme Verlag, Stuttgart.

KRAUSE, R. (1966) Comparative deciduoma-inducing activities of various steroids of the normal and 9β,10α-series. In: *Second Internat. Congress on Hormonal Steroids.* Internat. Congress Series no. 111, p. 343, abstr. 671. Romanoff, E. B. and Martini, L. (Eds.) Excerpta Medica Foundation, Amsterdam.

LABHSETWAR, A. P. (1966a) Mechanism of action of medroxyprogesterone (17α-acetoxy-6α-methylprogesterone) in the rat. *J. Reprod. Fertil.* **12**: 445–451.

LABHSETWAR, A. (1966b) Induction of pseudopregnancy in the rat with norethynodrel. Program of 48th meeting of the Endocrine Society held in Chicago, June 1966. Abstract no. 200.

LABHSETWAR, A. P. (1968) Studies on the mode of action of oral contraceptives: effect of chlormadinone on pituitary FSH and LH contents of the female rat. *J. Reprod. Fertil.* **17**: 101–110.

LACROIX, E., EECHAUTE, W. and LEUSEN, I. (1968) Influence of lynestrenol on estrogen production by rat ovaries. *Arch. Int. Pharmacodyn.* **172**: 240–243.

LECOCQ, F. R., BRADLEY, E. M., and GOLDZIEHER, J. W. (1967) Metabolic balance studies with norethynodrel and chlormadinone acetate. *Amer. J. Obstet. & Gynec.* **99**: 374–381.

LEE, A. E. and WILLIAMS, P. C. (1964) Oestrogen antagonists: assay by inhibition of vaginal cornification. *J. Endocrin.* **28**, 199–203.

LENNON, H. D. (1966) Effects of various 17α-alkyl substitutions and structural modifications of steroids on sulfobromophthalein (BSP) retention in rabbits. *Steroids* **7**: 157–170.

LEONORA, J. and CRANE, M. G. (1970) Effect of long term administration of medroxyprogesterone acetate (MPA) and estrogens in the rat. *Clin. Res.* **18**: 169.

LERNER, L. J. (1964) Hormone antagonists, inhibitors of specific activities of estrogen and androgen. In: *Rec. Progr. Horm. Res.* Vol. 20, pp. 435–490. Pincus, G. (Ed.) Academic Press, New York and London.

LERNER, L. J., DE PHILLIPO, M., YIACAS, E., BRENNAN, D. and BORMAN, A. (1962) Comparison of the acetophenone derivative of 16α,17α-dihydroxyprogesterone with other progestational steroids for masculinization of the rat fetus. *Endocrinology* **71**: 448–451.

LINDSAY, D. R. and SCARAMUZZI, R. J. (1969) Oestrogenic and antioestrogenic activities of a number of steroids in behavioural oestrus and vaginal smear assays in the ewe. *J. Endocr.* **45**: 549–555.

LIPSCHÜTZ, A. (1950) *Steroid Hormones and Tumors.* Williams & Wilkins, Baltimore.

LIPSCHÜTZ, A., IGLESIAS, R., PANASEVICH, V. I. and SALINAS, S. (1967) Pathological changes induced in the uterus of mice with the prolonged administration of progesterone and 19-nor-contraceptives. *Brit. J. Cancer* **21**: 160–165.

LITTLE, K. (1970) The production of platelet thrombi. *Curr. Ther. Res.* **12**: 677–694.

LIU, F. T. Y. and LIN, H. S. (1970) Effect of some contraceptive steroids on pituitary growth hormone content in female rats. *Proc. Soc. Exp. Biol. Med.* **133**: 1354–1357.

LOGOTHETOPOULOS, J., SHARMA, B. B. and KRAICER, J. (1961) Effects produced in rats by the administration of 6α-methyl-17α-hydroxyprogesterone acetate from birth to maturity. *Endocrinology* **68**: 417–430.

LUBANSKY, J. and KING, T. O. (1965) Chronic toxicity study of anapregnone (6α-Me-4 pregnene-17α-ol-20-one acetate) in dogs. *Toxicol. Appl. Pharmacol.* **7**: 489.

LUPO, C. and POGGI, G. (1964) Effetti del Vinilestrenolone sulla dinamica uterina *in vitro* (The effects of vinyl-estrenolone on the uterine dynamic *in vitro*). *Riv. Biol.* (*Perugia*) Suppl. to Vol. **67**: 79–88.

LURASCHI, C. (1958) Effetti dei progestazionali di sintesi sulla dinamica uterina. *Ann. Ostet. Ginec.* **80**: 443–448.

MADJEREK, Z. (1960) Deciduoma formation in mice as a criterion of progestational activity. *Acta Endocr.* (*Kbh.*), Suppl. **51**: 901.

MADJEREK, Z. (1961) Influence of some new oral pre-gestagens and gestagens on the symphysis pubis of the guinea pig. *Arch. Int. Pharmacodyn.* **130**: 473–476.

MADJEREK, Z., DE VISSER, J., VAN DER VIES, J. and OVERBEEK, G. A. (1960) Allylestrenol, a pregnancy maintaining oral gestagen. *Acta Endocr.* (*Kbh.*) **35**: 8–19.

MAEKAWA, K. (1960) Difference in response between uterus and vagina to estrogen given concurrently with progestogen. *Endocrinol. Japon.* **7**: 91–95.

MANALO-ESTRELLA, P., DANFORTH, D. N. and BUCKINGHAM, J. C. (1965) Regression rate of vascular effects induced by pregnancy and by norethynodrel-mestranol. *Fertil. Steril.* **16**: 81–84.

MANNING, J. P., SCHWARTZ, E., TORNABEN, J. A., BOXILLE, G. C., and RUSSEL, T. J. (1969) Influence of an oral contraceptive progestin-estrogen combination on simian uterine phosphatases. *Fertil. Steril.* **20**: 745–756.

MAQUEO, M. and KINCL, F. A. (1965) Macro- and microscopic evaluation of the feminization or masculinization of rats treated with various steroids. In: Internat. Congress. Series no. 99, Abstr. 712, p. 89. Excerpta Medica, Amsterdam and New York.

MAROIS, G. (1968) Actions de sept stéroides progestatifs de synthèse sur la distance ano-génitale et sur la différenciation sexuelle somatique du rat. *Biologie Médicale* **56**: 103–198.

MAROIS, M. (1962a) Action d'un progestatif actif par voie buccale, la dydrogestérone, sur la corne utérine de la lapine. *Bull. Acad. Nat. Méd.* **146**: 324–328.

MAROIS, M. (1962b) Maintien de la gestation chez la ratte sous l'action d'un progestatif actif par voie buccale: la dydrogestérone. *Bull. Acad. Nat. Méd.* **146**: 329–334.

MAROIS, M. (1962c) Action d'un progestatif actif par voie buccale, la dydrogestérone sur la symphyse pubienne du cobaye. *Bull. Acad. Nat. Méd.* **146**: 349–353.

MAROIS, M. (1962d) Absence de propriétés masculinisantes ou féminisantes d'un progestatif actif per os, la dydrogestérone, chez le rat male ou femelle adulte et chez le foetus de rat. *Bull. Acad. Nat. Méd.* **146**: 354–364.

MATSCHER, R. (1958) Action of some synthetic steroids on the adrenocortical atrophy from prednisone in the rat. *Boll. Soc. Ital. Biol. Sper.* **34**: 437–440 (*Chem. Abstr.* **55**, 11, 669c (1961)).

MATSCHER, R. and LUPO, C. (1959) Attivitá del 6α-metil-17α-idrossiprogesterone acetato (MAP) sulla motilità uterina del ratto in paragone al 17αidrossiprogesterone acetato (AP). *Boll. Soc. Ital. Biol. Sper.* **35**: 20–22.

MATSCHER, R. and LUPO, C. (1960) L'azione antigonadotropa di alcuni nuovi ormoni sintetici ad azione progestativa studiata sul ratto maschio adulto. *Arch. Sci. Biol.* (*Bologna*) **44**: 350–358.

MCCARTHY, J. D. (1965) Influence of two contraceptives on induction of mammary cancer in rats. *Amer. J. Surg.* **110**: 720–723.

MCCORMACK, C. E. and MEYER, R. K. (1965) Facilitative action of progestational compounds on ovulation in PMS-treated immature rats. *Fertil. Steril.* **16**: 384–392.

MCDONALD, P. G. (1968) The effect of a single injection of norethindrone with or without estrogen, on ovulation in the rat. *J. Endocr.* **41**: v.

MCDONALD, P. G. and GILMORE, D. P. (1969) Effects of ovarian steroids on the norethisterone blockade of ovulation in the rat. *J. Endocr.* **45**: 51–56.

MCGINTY, D. (1959) Discussion of paper presented by V. A. Drill. *Fed. Proc.* **18**: 1048–1050.

MCGINTY, D. A. and DJERASSI, C. (1958) Some chemical and biological properties of 19-nor-17α-ethynyltestosterone. *Ann. N.Y. Acad. Sci.* **71**: 500–515.

MCKINNEY, G. R. and BRASELTON, J. P. (1970) Antiandrogens and antiuterotropic activities of three synthetic progestagens. *Steroids* **15**: 405–411.

MCKINNEY, G. R. and WEIKEL, J. H. (1965) The adrenal response to stress of rats treated with certain progestagens. *Toxicol. Appl. Pharmacol.* **7**: 491.

MCKINNEY, G. R., WEIKEL, J. H., WEBB, W. K. and DICK, R. G. (1968) Use of the life-table technique to estimate effects of certain steroids on probability of tumor formation on a long-term study in rats. *Toxicol. Appl. Pharmacol.* **12**: 68–79.

MEY, R. (1963a) Zur Frage einer maskulinisierenden Wirkung von Allylestrenol. *Acta Endocr.* (*Kbh.*) **44**: 27–35.

MEY, R. (1963b) Untersuchungen zur Frage einer intrauterinen Maskulinisierung durch 6-chlor-6-dehydro-17α-acetoxyprogesteron. *Arzneimittelforsch.* **13**: 906–908.

MEYERSON, B. J. (1966) The effect of imipramine and related anti-depressive drugs on estrus behaviour in ovariectomised rats activated by progesterone, reserpine or tetrabenazine in combination with estrogen. *Acta physiol. scand.* **67**: 411–422.

MEYERSON, B. J. (1967) Relation between the anesthetic and gestagenic action and estrous behavior-inducing activity of different progestins. *Endocrinology* **81**: 369–374.

MICHAEL, R. P. (1968) Gonadal hormones and the control of primate behaviour. In: *Endocrinology and Human Behaviour*, pp. 69–93. Michael, R. P. (Ed.). Oxford University Press, London.

MICHAEL, R. P. (1969) Behavioral effects of gonadal hormones and contraceptive steroids in primates. In: *Metabolic Effects of Gonadal Hormones and Contraceptive Steroids*, pp. 706–721. Salhanick, H. A., Kipnis, D. M. and van de Wiele, R. L. (Eds.). Plenum Press, New York, London.

MISCHLER, T., GAWLAK, D., GIANNINA, T. and MELI, A. (1969) The biological profile of three 19-nortestosterone-3-cyclopentyl enol ethers (34207). *Proc. Soc. Exp. Biol. Med.* **132**: 323–327.

MIYAKE, T. (1961) Inhibitory effect of various steroids on gonadotrophin hypersecretion in parabiotic mice. *Endocrinology* **69**: 534–546.

MIYAKE, T., KAKUSHI, H. and HARA, K. (1963a) Bioassay of progestational steroids based on the deciduoma formation in spayed mice. *Steroids* **2**: 739–748.

MIYAKE, T., KAKUSHI, H. and HARA, K. (1963b) Deciduomatogenic and anti-deciduomatogenic activity of steroids. *Steroids* **2**: 749–763.

MIYAKE, T. and KOBAYASHI, F. (1960) Effects of norethisterone (17α-ethynyl-19-nortestosterone) and certain other steroids on the female gonads of hypophysectomized immature rats. *Endocrinol. Japon.* **7**: 215–224.

MIYAKE, T. and PINCUS, G. (1958) Progestational activity of certain 19-nor steroids and progesterone derivatives. *Endocrinology* **63**: 816–824.

MOGGIAN, G. (1959) Progestational activity of 17α-methyl-19-nortestosterone. *Endocrinology* **64**: 363–366.

MONTUORI, E., BUR, G. E. and KOROMPAY, A. (1960) Acción de algunos gestagenos sinteticos sobre la evolución de la preñez de la rata. *Rev. Soc. Argent. Biol.* **36**: 45–53.

MUNSHI, S. R. (1964) The effect of norethynodrel in mice and rats. In: *Proc. Seventh Conference Internat. Planned Parenthood Federation, Singapore*, 1963. Internat. Congress Series 72, Excerpta Medica, Amsterdam, New York.

MURPHY, E. D. (1961) Carcinogenesis of the uterine cervix in mice: effect of diethylstilbestrol after limited application of 3-methylcholanthrene. *J. Nat. Cancer Inst.* **27**: 611–653.

NEILL, J. D., JOHANSSON, E. D. B. and KNOBIL, E. (1968). Patterns of circulating progesterone concentrations during the fertile menstrual cycle and the remainder of gestation in the Rhesus monkey. In. *Proc. 3rd Int. Congress of Endocrinology*, pp. 157–158. So quoted by Beck (1969).

NERI, R. (1970) Anti-androgenic properties of chlormadinone acetate and its 16-methylene analogue Sch 12600. In: *Third International Congress on Hormonal Steroids*, p. 69. James, V. H. T. (Ed.). International Congress Series no. 210, Excerpta Medica, Amsterdam, New York.

NETTER, A. (1970) *L'Inhibition de l'ovulation*. Masson and Cie, Paris.

NEUMANN, F. (1968) Chemische Konstitution und pharmakologische Wirkung. In: *Handbook of Experimental Pharmacology*, Vol. XXII, 1, Die Gestagene, Teil 1, pp. 680–1025. Junkmann, K. (Ed.). Springer Verlag, Berlin, New York.

NEUMANN, F., BERSWORDT-WALLRABE, R. VON, ELGER, W. and STEINBECK, H. (1968a) Activities of antiandrogens. Experiments in prepuberal and puberal animals and in foetuses. In: *Testosterone. Proceedings of the Workshop Conference held from April 20th to 22nd 1967 at Tremsbüttel*, Tamm, J. (Ed.). Georg Thieme Verlag, Stuttgart.

NEUMANN, F., BERSWORDT-WALLRABE, R. VON, ELGER, W., STEINBECK, H. and HAHN, J. D. (1968b). Effects of antiandrogens. In: *Progress in Endocrinology*. International Congress Series 184, pp. 823–836. Excerpta Medica, Amsterdam, New York.

NEUMANN, F., BERSWORDT-WALLRABE, R. VON, ELGER, W., STEINBECK, H., HAHN, J. D. and KRAMER, M. (1970) Aspects of androgen-dependent events as studied by antiandrogens. *Recent Progr. Hormone Res.* **26**: 337–410.

NEUMANN, F. and DOMENICO, A. (1964) Untersuchungen zur Ovulationshemmung an der Ratte mit Kombinationen von Steroiden verschiedener Stoffklassen. In: *11. Symposion der Deutschen Gesellschaft für Endokrinologie*, pp. 274–278. Springer-Verlag, Berlin, Heidelberg, New York.

NEUMANN, F., ELGER, W. and STEINBECK, H. (1969) Drug-induced intersexuality in mammals. *J. Reprod. Fertil. Suppl.* **7**: 9–24.

NEUMANN, F., ELGER, W., STEINBECK, H. and BERSWORDT-WALLRABE, R. VON (1967) Antiandrogene. In: *13. Symposion der Deutschen Gesselschaft für Endokrinologie*, pp. 78–81. Springer-Verlag, Berlin, Heidelberg, New York.

NEUMANN, F. and HEMPEL, R. (1965) Hemmung der Uteruswirkung von Oxytocin durch Gestagene. *Acta Endocr. (Kbh.)* **48**: 645–655.

NEUMANN, F. and JUNKMANN, K. (1963) A new method for determination of virilizing properties of steroids on the fetus. *Endocrinology* **73**: 33–37.

NEUMANN, F. and KRAMER, M. (1964) Antagonism of androgenic and anti-androgenic agents in their action on the rat fetus. *Endocrinology* **75**: 428–433.

NEUMANN, F., KRAMER, M. and JUNKMANN, K. (1964) Experimental studies of 17α-ethynyl-19-nortestosterone acetate in animals. Supplement of *Medicina Experimentalis*, vol. 11.

NEVINNY-STICKEL, J. (1960) Verzögerung der Ei-Implantation durch hormonale Beeinflussung bei der Ratte. *Geburtsh. Frauenheilk.* **20**: 1082.

NISHINO, Y. and NEUMANN, F. (1971) Untersuchungen zur oestrogenen und antioestrogenen Wirkung von Gestagenen gemessen am Sialinsäuregehalt der Mäusevagina. In: *17 Symposion der Deutschen Gesellschaft für Endokrinologie*, Springer-Verlag, Berlin, Heidelberg, New York.

NOMINÉ, G., BUCOURT, R., TESSIER, J., PIERDET, A., COSTEROUSSE, G. and MATHIEU, J. J. (1965) Agencements stéroides triéniques et activité progestative. *C.R. Acad. Sci. (Paris)* **260**: 4545–4548.

NUTTING, E. F. and MARES, S. E. (1970) Inhibition of fertilization in rabbits during treatment with progesterone. *Biol. Reprod.* **2**: 230–238.

NUTTING, E. F. and MEYER, R. K. (1964) Effects of various steroids on nidation and fetal survival in ovariectomized rats. *Endocrinology* **74**: 573–578.

NUTTING, E. F. and SOLLMAN, P. B. (1967) Delay of implantation in intact rats treated with progestins. *Acta Endocr. (Kbh.)* **54**: 8–18.

OVERBEEK, G. A. (1962) Progestogens and the foetus. *Brit. Med. J.* **1962**: 1339–1340.

OVERBEEK, G. A., MADJEREK, Z. and DE VISSER, J. (1962) The effect of lynestrenol on animal reproduction. *Acta Endocr. (Kbh.)* **41**: 351–370.

OVERBEEK, G. A., MADJEREK, Z. and DE VISSER, J. (1963) Animal studies on steroids useful in the field of human fertility. *Bull. Soc. Roy. Belge Gynec. Obstet.* **33**: 345–348.

OVERBEEK, G. A. and DE VISSER, J. (1956) A new substance with progestational activity. *Acta Endocr. (Kbh.)* **22**: 318–329.

OVERBEEK, G. A. and DE VISSER, J. (1964a) Difficulties in determining the site of action of ovulation inhibitors. *Int. J. Fertil.* **9**: 177–179.

OVERBEEK, G. A. and DE VISSER, J. (1964b) Different modes of action of two antiovulatory compounds. *Acta Endocr. (Kbh.)* Suppl. **90**: 179–190.

PAESI, F. J. A., DE JONGH, S. E., and ENGELBREGT, A. (1957) Some notable differences between the results of FSH-estimations in rat hypophyses by the extraction and implantation methods respectively. *Acta Endocr.* **25**: 412–418.

PAESI, F. J. A. and VAN REES, G. P. (1960) Differences between the results of FSH-measurements in hypophyses of rats with extraction and implantation techniques respectively. *Acta Endocr. (Kbh.)* **34**: 366–374.

PALMER, R. H., GALLAGHER, JR., T. F., MUELLER, M. N. and KAPPAS, A. (1969) The effect of natural and synthetic estrogens on the excretion of BSP by the liver. In: *Metabolic Effects of Gonadal Hormones and Contraceptive Steroids*, pp. 19–29. Salhanick, H. A., Kipnis, D. M. and van de Wiele, R. L. (Eds.). Plenum Press, New York and London.
PASTEELS, J. L. and ECTORS, F. (1967) Mode d'action de la médroxyprogestérone (Provera) sur le système hypothalamohypophysaire de la ratte. *C.R. Acad. Sci. (Paris)*, Série D, **264**: 106–109.
PEÑA REGIDOR, P. (1967) La acción del linestrenol y etinil estradiol asociados, frente a la reacción de Friedman. *Rev. Ibér. Endocr.* **14**: 39–49.
PETERSON, D. L. and EDGREN, R. A. (1965) The effect of various steroids on mating behaviour, fertility and fecundity of rats. *Int. J. Fertil.* **10**: 327–332.
PETERSON CLANCY, D. and EDGREN, R. A. (1968) The effects of norgestrel, ethynyl estradiol and their combination, Ovral, on lactation and the offspring of rats treated during lactation. *Int. J. Fertil.* **13**: 133–141.
PETERSON, D. L., EDGREN, R. A. and JONES, R. C. (1964) Steroid-induced block of ovarian compensatory hypertrophy in hemicastrated female rats. *J. Endocr.* **29**: 255–262.
PETROW, V. (1960) Claudogens—a new term for antifertility steroids. *J. Pharm. Pharmacol.* **12**, 704.
PINCUS, G. (1956) Some effects of progesterone and related compounds upon reproduction and early development in mammals. *Acta Endocr. (Kbh.) Suppl.* **28**: 18–36.
PINCUS, G. (1965) *The Control of Fertility*. Academic Press, New York.
PINCUS, G., CHANG, M. C., ZARROW, M. X., HAFEZ, E. S. E. and MERRILL, A. (1956) Studies of the biological activity of certain 19-nor steroids in female animals. *Endocrinology* **59**: 695–707.
POEL, W. E. (1966) Pituitary tumors in mice after prolonged feeding of synthetic progestins. *Science* **154**: 402–403.
POSSANZA, G. J., OLIVER, J. T., SAWYER, M. J. and TROOP, R. C. (1964) Effects of 6-methyl-17-acetoxyprogesterone on pituitary-adrenal function. *Biochem. Pharmacol.* **13**: 361–364.
PRIEDKALNS, J. (1969) Effect of melengestrol acetate on ovarian follicles, interstitial gland and corpora lutea in the rat: a quantitative morphological study. *Z. Zellforsch.* 56–73.
PURSHOTTAM, N., MASON, M. M. and PINCUS, G. (1961) Induced ovulation in the mouse and the measurement of its inhibition. *Fertil. Steril.* **12**: 346–352.
PURVES, H. D. and GRIESBACH, W. E. (1951) The site of thyrotrophin and gonadotrophin production in the rat pituitary studied by McManus–Hotchkiss staining for glycoprotein. *Endocrinology* **49**: 244–264.
PURVES, H. D. (1961) Morphology of the hypophysis related to its function. In: *Sex and Internal Secretions*, Vol. 1, pp. 161–239. Young, W. C. (Ed.). Williams & Wilkins (Baltimore).
RAMIREZ, V. D. and SAWYER, C. H. (1965) Suppression of the initiation of natural puberty and of pubertas praecox induced by estrogen in rats treated with norethindrone. *VI. Pan. Am. Congress of Endocrinology*, page E 175, Abstract 384. Internat. Congress Series, no. 99, Excerpta Medica, Amsterdam.
REVESZ, C. and CHAPPEL, C. I. (1966) Biological activity of medrogestone: A new orally active progestin. *J. Reprod. Fertil.* **12**: 473–487.
REVESZ, C., CHAPPEL, C. I. and GAUDRY, R. (1960) Masculinization of female fetuses in the rat by progestational compounds. *Endocrinology* **66**: 140–144.
RICHARDS, M. P. M. (1966) Progesterone and pseudopregnancy in the golden hamster. *J. Reprod. Fertil.* **11**: 463–464.
RICHTER, R. H. H. (1963) Über die Wirkung einiger Steroide auf die embryonale und foetale Entwicklung der Ratte. *Gynaecologia* **156**: 41–46.

RINGLER, I. (1966) Efficacy of topically applied progestational agents. *Steroids* **7**: 341–349.
ROGERS, A. W. and JOHN, P. N. (1970) The distribution of 3H-progesterone and 3H-megestrol acetate in the uterus of the ovariectomized rat. In: *Third Internat.Congress on Hormonal Steroids*. Internat. Congress Series 210, p. 153. Excerpta Medica, Amsterdam, New York.
ROUSSEL, (1966) *Documentation Medicale* no. 1077. Laboratoires Roussel, Paris.
RUDEL, H. W. and KINCL, F. A. (1966) The biology of anti-fertility steroids. *Acta Endocr. (Kbh.)* Suppl. 105.
RUGGIERI, P. DE and MATSCHER, R. (1959) Sintesi e attivita biologica di un nuovo 19-nor-steroide il "17α-vinyl-estr-5(10)-en-17β-ol-3 one". *Boll. Soc. Ital. Biol. Sper.* **35**: 24–27.
RUGGIERI, P. DE, MATSCHER, R., LUPO, C. and SPAZZOLI, G. (1965) Biological properties of 17α-vinyl-5(10)-estrene-17β-ol-3 one (norvinodrel) as a progestational and claudogenic compound. *Steroids* **5**: 73–91.
RUIZ-GIJÓN, J. (1962) Accion progesterinica de la 6-dehidro-retroprogesterona (Duphaston). *Acta Ginec. Madrid* **13**: 213–220.
SAGER, D. B., SCHUETZ, A. W. and MEYER, R. K. (1966) Effect of estrone and progestational steroids on human chorionic gonadotrophin (HCG)-induced ovarian augmentation in parabiotic rats. *Endocrinology* **78**: 445–452.
SALA, G., BALDRATTI, G. and ARCARI, G. (1960) Influence of 6 alpha-methyl-17 alpha-acetoxyprogesterone on female sexual functions. In: *Moderne Entwicklungen auf dem Gestagengebiet*, pp. 58–63. Nowakowski, H. (Ed.). Springer Verlag, Berlin, Göttingen, Heidelberg.
SALA, G., CAMERINO, B. and CAVALLERO, C. (1958) Progestational activity of 6α-methyl-17α-hydroxyprogesterone acetate. *Acta Endocr. (Kbh.)* **29**: 508–512.
SALHANICK, H. A. and SWANSON, J. (1960) Structure activity relationship of progestational steroids. *Acta Endocr. (Kbh.)* Suppl. **51**, 903.
SALLOCH, R. R., NEUMANN, F., and BÖHNISCH, G. (1971) Einfluss verschiedener Gestagene auf den Eitransport bei Ratten. In: *17. Symposium der Deutschen Gesellschaft für Endokrinologie*. Springer-Verlag, Berlin, Heidelberg–New York.
SANWAL, P. C., PANDE, J. K., DASGUPTA, P. R., KAR, A. B. and SETTY, B. S. (1970) Long-term effect of a continuous low dose of megestrol acetate on the genital organs and fertility of female rats. *Steroids* **15**, 711–722.
SAS, M., KOVÁCS, L. and RESCH, B. (1965) Die Ergebnisse der während der Lynestrenol-Belastung durchgeführten Schwangerschaftsreaktionen. *Endokrinologie* **48**: 289–292.
SAS, M., RAPCSÁK, V. and OROJÁN, I. (1966) Die Wirkung der Gestagenbehandlung auf die Hoden. *Endokrinologie* **49**: 133–137.
SAS, M., RESCH, B., KOVÁCS, L. and SZONTÁGH (1967) Die Wirkung ovulationshemmender Steroide auf die einzelnen Phasen des Fortpflanzungsprozesses bei Kaninchen. (Postovulatorische Hemmwirkung). *Endokrinologie* **51**: 170–174.
SAUNDERS, F. J. (1958a) The effects of several steroids on fecundity in female rats. *Endocrinology* **63**: 561–565.
SAUNDERS, F. J. (1958b) The effects of several steroids on mating behavior, ovulation and pregnancy in female rats. *Endocrinology* **63**: 566–569.
SAUNDERS, F. J. (1964) Some notes on the mode of action of norethynodrel in preventing fertility in rats. *Acta Endocr.* **46**: 157–160.
SAUNDERS, F. J. (1965) Effects on the course of pregnancy of norethynodrel with mestranol (Enovid) administered to rats during early pregnancy. *Endocrinology* **77**: 873–878.
SAUNDERS, F. J. (1967) Effects of norethynodrel combined with mestranol on the offspring when administered during pregnancy and lactation in rats. *Endocrinology* **80**: 447–452.

SAUNDERS, F. J. and DRILL, V. A. (1958) Some biological activities of 17-ethynyl and 17-alkyl derivatives of 17-hydroxyestrenones. *Ann. N.Y. Acad. Sci.* **71**: 516–530.
SAUNDERS, F. J., EDGREN, R. A. and DRILL, V. A. (1957) On the progestational activity of 17α-ethynyl-17-hydroxy-5(10)-estren-3-one (norethynodrel). *Endocrinology* **60**: 804–805.
SAUNDERS, F. J. and ELTON, R. L. (1959) Progestational action of some newer steroids with special reference to maintenance of pregnancy. In: *Recent Progress in the Endocrinology of Reproduction*, pp. 227–253. Lloyd, C. W. (Ed.). Academic Press, New York.
SAWYER, C. H. (1965) Blockade of the release of gonadotrophic hormones by pharmacological agents. In: *Proceedings 2nd Internat. Congr. Endocrinology*, Int. Congr. Ser. 83, Vol. I, pp. 629–634. Taylor, S. (Ed.). Excerpta Medica, Amsterdam.
SCHALLY, A. V., ARIMURA, A., KASTIN, A. J., MATSUO, H., BABA, Y., REDDING, T. W., NAIR, R. M. G. and DEBELJUK, L. (1971) Gonadotropin-releasing hormone: One polypeptide regulates secretion of luteinizing and follicle-stimulating hormones. *Science* **173**: 1036–1038.
SCHALLY, A. V. and BOWERS, C. Y. (1964) *In vitro* and *in vivo* stimulation of the release of luteinizing hormone. *Endocrinology* **75**: 312–320.
SCHALLY, A. V., CARTER, W. M., SAITO, M., ARIMURA, A. and BOWERS, C. Y. (1968) Studies on the site of action of oral contraceptive steroids. I. Effect of antifertility steroids on plasma LH levels and on the response to luteinizing hormone-releasing factor in rats. *J. Clin. Endocr.* **28**: 1747–1755.
SCHALLY, A. V., PARLOW, A. F., CARTER, W. H., SAITO, M., BOWERS, C. Y. and ARIMURA, A. (1970) Studies on the site of action of oral contraceptive steroids. II. Plasma LH and FSH levels after administration of antifertility steroids and LH-releasing hormone (LH-RH). *Endocrinology* **86**: 530–541.
SCHARDEIN, J. L., KAUMP, D. H., WOOSLEY, E. T. and JELLEMA, M. M. (1969) Long-term toxicologic and tumorigenesis studies on an oral contraceptive agent in albino rats. *Toxicol. Appl. Pharmacol.* **14**: 649.
SCHERMUND, H. J. and NAPP, J. H. (1962) Über die Wirkung von Äthinyl-Nortestosteron-Azetat auf verschiedene Impftumoren. *Zbl. Gynäk.* **84**: 761–762.
SCHNEIDER, W. and RAUSCHER, H. (1959) Tierexperimentelle Untersuchungen über die biologische Wirksamkeit von 19-Nortestosteron-Verbindungen. *Arch. Int. pharmacodyn.* **119**: 345–351.
SCHOFIELD, BRENDA, M. (1964) Myometrial activity in the pregnant guinea-pig. *J. Endocr.* **30**: 347–354.
SCHÖLER, H. F. L. (1960) Biological properties of 9,10-isomeric steroids. I. Progestational activity of 9β,10α-steroids. *Acta Endocr. (Kbh.)* **35**: 188–196.
SCHÖLER, H. F. L. (1964) The actions of "retro" progestagens. In: *Hormonal Steroids. Proceedings of the First International Congress on Hormonal Steroids*, Vol. 1, pp. 53–63. Martini, L. and Pecile, A. (Eds.). Academic Press, New York and London.
SCHÖLER, H. F. L. and WACHTER, A. M. DE (1961) Evaluation of androgenic properties of progestational compounds in the rat by the female foetal masculinization test. *Acta Endocr.* **38**: 128–136.
SEGALOFF, A. (1963) The enhanced local androgenic activity of 19-nor steroids and stabilization of their structure by 7α- and 17α-methyl substitutes to highly potent androgens by any route of administration. *Steroids* **1**: 299–315.
SEGALOFF, A. and GABBARD, R. B. (1962) Steroid structure and androgenicity. *Endocrinology* **71**: 949–959.
SELF, L. W. (1965) Pituitary cytology of rats receiving ethynodiol diacetate and mestranol for 2 years. *Metabolism* **14**: 311–312.
SHIMIZU, H. and OKAZAKI, Y. (1967) Effect of chlormadinone acetate on the body weight of female rats. *J. Endocr.* **39**: 305–306.

SHIPLEY, E. G. (1965) Effectiveness of topical application of a number of progestins. *Steroids* **5**: 699–717.
SHIPLEY, E. G. and MEYER, R. K. (1965) Effects of corticoids and progestins on pituitary gonadotropic functions in immature rats. In: *Hormonal Steroids*, Vol. 2, pp. 293–300. Martini, L. and Pecile, A. (Eds.). Academic Press, New York.
SICHUK, G., FORTNER, J. G. and DER, B. K. (1967) Evaluation of the influence of norethynodrel with mestranol (Enovid) in middle-aged male Syrian (golden) hamsters, with particular reference to spontaneous tumours. *Acta Endocr. (Kbh.)* **55**: 97–107.
SMITH, B. D. and BRADBURY, J. T. (1966) Influence of progestins on ovarian responses to estrogens and gonadotrophins in immature rats. *Endocrinology* **78**: 297–301.
SMITH, R. E. and HENZL, M. R. (1969) Role of mucopolysaccharides and lysosomal hydrolases in endometrial regression following withdrawal of estradiol and chlormadinone acetate. I. Epithelium and stroma. *Endocrinology*, **85**: 50–66.
SODERWALL, A. L., CONNOR, F. J. and SAKINEN, F. M. (1966) Some observations of Enovid effects on female hamster reproductive processes. *Anat. Res.* **154**: 489.
SPIEGEL, E. and WYCIS, H. (1945). Anticonvulsant effects of steroids. *J. Lab. Clin. Med.* **30**: 947–953.
STEGNER, H.-E. and BELTERMANN (1969) Die Elektronenmikroskopie des Cervixdrüsenepithels und der sog. Reservezellen. *Arch. Gynäk.* **207**: 480–504.
STEINBECK, H., CUPCEANCU, B., MEHRING, M. and NEUMANN, F. (1971) Influence of neonatal gestagen injection on the differentiation of psychosexuality in female rats. *Acta Endocr. (Kbh.)* **67**: 544–550.
STEINETZ, B. G., BEACH, V. L., DIPASQUALE, G. and BATTISTA, JR., J. V. (1965) Effects of different gestagenic steroid types on plasma-free corticosteroid levels in ACTH-treated rats. *Steroids* **5**: 93–108.
STITT, S. L. and KINNARD, J. (1968) The effect of certain progestins and estrogens on the threshold of electrically induced seizure patterns. *Neurology* **18**: 213–216.
STUCKI, J. (1958) Maintenance of pregnancy in ovariectomized rats with some newer progestins. *Proc. Soc. Exp. Biol.* **99**: 500–504.
SUCHOWSKY, G. K. (1960) Remark in discussion. In: *Moderne Entwicklungen auf dem Gestagengebiet.* 6. *Symposium der Deutschen Gesellschaft für Endokrinologie*, p. 68. Nowakowski, H. (Ed.). Springer-Verlag, Berlin, Heidelberg.
SUCHOWSKY, G. K. (1963) Pregnancy maintaining effect of synthetic progestagens in the rat. *Acta Endocr. (Kbh.)* **42**: 533–536.
SUCHOWSKY, G. K. (1964) Oestrogens, androgens and progestagens. In: *Evaluation of Drug Activities: Pharmacometrics* Vol. 2, pp. 703–727. Laurence, D. R. and Bacharach, A. L. (Eds.). Academic Press, London and New York.
SUCHOWSKY, G. K. and BALDRATTI, G. (1964) Relationship between progestational activity and chemical structure of synthetic steroids. *J. Endocrin.* **30**: 159–170.
SUCHOWSKY, G. K., BALDRATTI, G., ARCARI, G. and SCRASCIA, E. (1965). Die Beeinflussung von zentralen Regulations-mechanismen durch Steroide. *Arzneimittelforsch.* **15**: 437–439.
SUCHOWSKY, G. K., BALDRATTI, G., SCRASCIA, E. and ARCARI, G. (1966) Biological activities of a combination of medroxyprogesterone acetate and ethynyloestradiol. *Acta Endocr. (Kbh.)* **51**: 439–446.
SUCHOWSKY, G. and JUNKMANN, K. (1960) Zur Frage der Virilisierung des Foetus durch Behandlung der Mutter mit Gestagenen. *Geburtsh. Frauenheilk.* **20**: 1019–1023.
SUCHOWSKY, G. K. and JUNKMANN, K. (1961) A study of the virilizing effect of progestagens on the female rat fetus. *Endocrinology* **68**: 341–349.
SUCHOWSKY, G. K., PEGRASSI, L. and BONSIGNORI, A. (1969) The effects of steroids on aggressive behaviour in isolated male mice. In: *Aggressive Behaviour*, pp. 164–171. Garattini, S. and Ligg, E. B. (Eds.). Excerpta Medica, Amsterdam.

SUCHOWSKY, G. K., TUROLLA, E. and ARCARI, G. (1967) Studies of the so-called virilizing effects of steroids in female rat fetuses. *Endocrinology* **80**: 255–262.

SULMAN, F. G., EVIATAR, A. and DANON, A. (1959) Duration of progestational effect in rabbit endometrium after prolonged administration of progestogens. *Proc. Soc. Exp. Biol.* **102**: 641–644.

SZONTÁGH, F. E., VARGA, L., BARDOCZY, A. and FÖLDI, M. (1964) The effect of orally administered gestagen on the anaphylactic reactions in rats. *J. Endocr.* **28**: 159–161.

TAUBERT, H. D. (1967) Maintenance of delayed nidation in the rat by single dose injection of depot 6α-methyl-17-acetoxyprogesterone. *Endocrinology* **80**: 218–220.

TAUSK, M. (1967) Synthetic progestational substances. In: *Endocrine Functions of the Ovary*. International symposium under the direction of M. F. Jayle. *Europ. Rev. Endocrin.* Suppl. 2: Vol. 2, pp. 419–435. Soulairac, A. and Marois, M. (Eds.). Pergamon Press, Oxford.

TERRAGNO, N., TERRAGNO, A. and CAVANAGH, D. (1968) Effects of anovulatory agents on isolated human Fallopian tube. *J. Amer. med. Ass.* **204**: 534.

THOMAS, J. A. (1963) Modification of glucagon-induced hyperglycemia by various steroidal agents. *Metabolism* **12**: 207–212.

THOMAS, J. A. and STRAUSS, A. J. (1965) The effect of steroids on mouse sex accessory fructose levels. *Acta Endocr. (Kbh.)* **48**: 619–629.

THOMSEN, K. and NAPP, J. H. (1960) Nebenwirkungen bei hochdosierter Nortestosteronmedikation in der Gravidität. *Geburtsh. Frauenheilk.* **20**: 508–513.

TOKUDA, G., AOKI, Y. and HIGASHIYAMA, S. (1963) The effect of 6α-methyl-17α-acetoxyprogesterone and 6α-methyl-Δ6-17α-acetoxyprogesterone on the central nervous system, especially the adrenal-hypophysis (Jap.). *Horumon To Rinshō (Clin. Endocr.)* **11**: 68–74. Abstr.: *Cancer Chem. Abstr.* **5**: 133–134 (1964).

TÓTH, F. (1964) Die Wirkungen von Progesteron und Progesteroiden auf Leber und Nieren. *Z. Geburtsh. Gynäk.* **162**: 152–159.

TÓTH, F. (1966) Hepatic and renal changes induced by synthetic progestagens and natural progesterones. *Acta Morphol. Acad. Scient. Hung.* **14**: 1–6.

TÓTH, F. and SZÓNYI, I. (1966) The inhibiting effect of a norsteroid on tumor formation and on the metabolism of tumor cells. *Amer. J. Obstet. Gynecol.* **94**: 518–523.

TUCKER, M. J. (1971) Some effects of prolonged administration of a progestagen to dogs. In: The correlation of adverse effects in man with observations in animals; *Proceedings of the European Society for the Study, of Drug Toxicity*, Vol. 12, pp. 228–238. Baker, S. B. De C. (Ed). Excerpta Medica, Amsterdam, New York.

TULLNER, W. and HERTZ, R. (1957) Progestational activity of 19-norprogesterone and 19-norethisterone in the Rhesus monkey. *Proc. Soc. Exp. Biol. Med.* **94**: 298–300.

TUROLLA, E. (1960) Modificazioni morfologiche ed istochimiche del surrene e dell' apparato genitale della ratta con 6 alfa-metil-17 alfa-acetossiprogesterone. *Ann. Ost. Ginec.* **6**: 751–762.

TUROLLA, E., SUCHOWSKY, G. K. and ARCARI, G. (1963) Valutazione degli effetti cosiddetti virilizzanti del testosterone propionato ed etinilestradiolo. *Boll. Atti. Soc. Ital. Endocr.* **11**: 301–308.

UHLARIK, S., KOVÁCS, L., VISKI, S. and SZONTÁGH, F. E. (1964) ICSH-Gehalt der Hypophyse und die Veränderungen des genitalen Zyklus von Rattenweibchen bei Gestagenbelastung. *Endokrinologie* **47**: 82–90.

USHER, D. R. (1968) The influence of norethindrone and mestranol on pituitary-adrenal function. *Can. J. Physiol. Pharmac.* **46**: 694–697.

VAN DER VIES, J., BAKKER, F. M. and DE WIED, D. (1960) Correlated studies on plasma free corticosterone and on adrenal steroid formation rate *in vitro*. *Acta Endocr. (Kbh.)* **34**: 513–523.

VAN DER VIES, J. (1960) The effects of steroids on adrenocortical function. *Acta Physiol. Pharmacol. Neerl.* **9**: 122–123.

VAN DER VIES, J. (1965) On the mechanism of action of nandrolone phenylpropionate and nandrolone decanoate in rats. *Acta Endocr. (Kbh.)* **49**: 271–282.

VAN DER VIES, J. and FEENSTRA, H. (1967) The effects of ovarian hormones on the placenta of rats. *Acta Endocr. (Kbh.)* Suppl. **119**: 235.

VELARDO, J. T. and FEDDEN, G. A. (1964) Influence of braxorone, prodox and provera on vaginal estrous cycles of rats. *Amer. Zool.* **4**: 329.

VICKERY, B. H. and BENNETT, J. P. (1969) Mechanisms of antifertility action of chlormadinone acetate in the rabbit. *Biol. of Reprod.* **1**: 372–377.

WAKELING, A. (1965) Effect of norethynodrel on spontaneous ovulation and fertilization in adult female rats. *J. Reprod. Fertil.* **10**: 1–7.

WARD, C. J. and DE PROSPO, N. D. (1968) Effects of norethynodrel in hypo- and hyperthyroid rats. *J. Endocr.* **40**: 263–264.

WATNICK, A. S., GIBSON, J., VINEGRA, M. and TOLKSDORF, S. (1965) The comparative contraceptive activities of 10β-hydroperoxy-17α-ethynyl-4-estren-17β-ol-3-one (Sch 10015) and norethynodrel. *J. Endocrin.* **33**: 241–248.

WATNICK, A. S., TOLKSDORF, S., KOSIEROWSKI, J. and TABACHNICK, I. A. (1966) Postovulatory contraceptive actions of 10β-hydroperoxy-17α-ethynyl-4 estren-17β-ol-3-one (Sch 10015) and norethynodrel. In: International Congress Series 111, p. 83. Excerpta Medica, Amsterdam–New York.

WEIFENBACH, H. (1965) Der Einfluss von FSH, HCG und Gestagenen auf die kompensatorische Superovulation der Ratte. *Acta Endocr. (Kbh.)* **50**: 7–14.

WEIKEL, JR., J. H. and WHEELER, A. G. (1965) Toxicology of progestagens with special reference to dimethisterone and megestrol acetate. *Toxicol. Appl. Pharmacol.* **2**: 502.

WEISBURGER, J. H., WEISBURGER, E. K., GRISWOLD, JR., D. P., and CASEY, A. E. (1968) Reduction of carcinogen-induced breast cancer in rats by an anti-fertility drug. *Life Sciences* **7**: 259–266.

WEISSMANN, G. (1964) Labilization and stabilization of lysosomes. *Fed. Proc.* **23**: 1038–1044.

WHARTON, L. R. and SCOTT, R. B. (1964) Experimental production of genital lesions with norethindrone. *Amer. J. Obstet. Gynec.* **89**: 701–715.

WILKINS, L., JONES, JR., H. W., HOLMAN, G. H. and STEMPFEL, JR., R. S. (1958) Masculinization of the femal fetus associated with administration of oral and intramuscular progestins during gestation: non-adrenal female pseudohermaphrodism. *J. Clin. Endocr.* **18**, 559–585.

WILLEMS, J. L. and DE SCHAEPDRIJVER, A. F. (1966) Adrenergic receptors in the oestradiol and allyl-oestrenol dominated rabbit uterus. *Arch. Int. Pharmacodyn.* **161**: 269–274.

WISLOCKI, G. B. and SNIJDER, F. F. (1933) The experimental acceleration of the rate of transport of ova through the Fallopian tube. *Bull. Johns Hopkins Hosp.* **52**: 379–400.

WOOLLEY, D. E. and TIMIRAS, P. S. (1962) The gonad–brain relationship: effects of female sex hormones on electroshock convulsions in the rat. *Endocrinology* **70**: 196–209.

WU, D. H. (1962) Gestational effect of allylestrenol. *Endocr. Jap.* **9**: 187–192.

ZANDER, J. (1953) Die Ausscheidung der freien Corticoide bei verschiedenen Funktionszuständen der Frau; die Ausscheidung im mensuellen Zyklus. *Klin. Wschr.* **13**: 504–507.

ZARROW, M. X., ANDERSON, JR., N. C. and CALLANTINE, M. R. (1963) Failure of progestogens to prolong pregnancy in the guinea pig. *Nature (Lond.)* **198**: 690–692.

ZARROW, M. X. and GALLO, R. V. (1969) Action of progesterone on PMS-induced ovulation in the rat. *Endocrinology* **84**: 1274–1276.

CHAPTER 29

THE METABOLISM OF ORALLY ACTIVE SYNTHETIC PROGESTATIONAL COMPOUNDS

J. H. H. Thijssen

Department of Medicine, University Hospital, The Netherlands

INTRODUCTION

During recent years, many steroids have been synthesized which are not naturally occurring, some of which are particularly important therapeutic agents. The metabolism of these steroids *in vivo* and *in vitro* has been documented by Langecker (1968). Our knowledge of the metabolism of synthetic steroid hormones will become of great value, as it contributes to studies on the mechanism of steroid hormone action and on the relationship between structure and biological activity (Dorfman and Ungar, 1965).

Of the large number of synthetic steroids having progestational activity (by definition an activity in the Clauberg-assay) only a relatively small number have therapeutic value and have found practical application. Although some compounds are widely used, the metabolism of these steroids is in general little understood. In those instances where the metabolism of therapeutic agents has been investigated, only low yields of metabolites have been isolated.

METHODS

Usually the metabolism is studied after administration of the radioactive progestational compound labeled with either ^{3}H or ^{14}C, by monitoring the excretion of radioactivity of excreta, estimation of the yields being generally based on the recovery of radioactivity excreted in the urine and sometimes in the feces. Only rarely has the amount of radioactivity in the blood been measured.

When tritiated steroids are studied, a significant loss of tritium can be recorded, due to exchange with protons in the organism after administration, or to metabolism at the point where the tritium is attached (Besch *et al.*, 1965). Losses of radioactivity can also occur with ^{14}C-labeled compounds when ^{14}C is present in one of the substituents of the steroid ring system. However, the use of radioactivity is very helpful during initial studies for detecting unknown metabolites of a drug.

In several studies an attempt has been made to identify the radioactive metabolites excreted in the urine. The methods used in these studies were almost invariably the same:

1. Urine is extracted with non-polar solvents, e.g. diethylether, chloroform or ethylacetate, in order to extract unconjugated steroids (called *free steroids*).
2. Following this preliminary treatment, the urine is subjected to hydrolysis, either with enzymes (a specific β-glucuronidase or a mixture of various hydrolytic enzymes such as are present in the digestive juice of *Helix pomatia*, the Roman snail) or with mineral acids. The radioactivity released is extracted from the water phase with a non-polar solvent.
3. Radioactive metabolites obtained in this way are isolated via several chromatographic purifications and identified by comparison with authentic reference compounds or characterized by other techniques such as infrared analysis, formation of a derivative, etc.

METABOLISM OF ORALLY ACTIVE SYNTHETIC PROGESTATIONAL COMPOUNDS

The results obtained in studies of the metabolism of synthetic progestational compounds is discussed for each substance separately, in Section I compounds derived from progesterone (having a pregnane ring system), and in Section II those estrane derivatives, the metabolism of which has been studied.

The available data on excretion of radioactivity after administration of labeled synthetic progestational compounds to human subjects are given in Table 1.

SECTION I

I-1. A substance closely related to progesterone is its *cyclopentyl-3-enol ether*. Unlike progesterone itself, this derivative is active after oral administration in man. It is likely that it is hydrolyzed in the human organism since the excretion of pregnanediol in the urine increases after oral administration of the cyclopentyl-3-enol-ether of progesterone (Caie and Klopper,

TABLE 1. EXCRETION OF RADIOACTIVITY AFTER ADMINISTRATION OF RADIOACTIVE PROGESTATIONAL COMPOUNDS TO HUMAN SUBJECTS
The range found is given in parentheses.

Compound	Administration	Excretion (% of dose/days) in			Reference
		Urine	Feces	Milk	
Dydrogesterone	p.o.	20/6			Houki (1966)
Medroxyprogesterone acetate	i.v.	33/4 (20–42)	8/4 (5–13)		Slaunwhite and Sandberg (1961)
	i.v.	37/3–6 (31–45)			Fotherby et al. (1965)
	p.o.	4/1	85/5		Besch et al. (1966)
Megestrol acetate	p.o.	66/7 (57–78)	20/7 (8–30)		Cooper and Kellie (1968)
Melengestrol acetate	p.o.	74/10 (44–87)			Cooper et al. (1967)
Norethisterone	i.v.	70/5			Layne et al. (1963)
	p.o.	50/5			
	i.v.	54/5 (37–81)			Kamyab et al. (1968a)
	p.o.	33/5			Murata (1967)
	p.o.	43/10 (38–48)	39/10 (35–43)		Gerhards et al. (1971)
Norethynodrel	p.o.	38/5 (28–40)	32/5 (27–37)		Layne et al. (1963)
	p.o.			0.1/4	Pincus et al. (1966)
	p.o.			1.0/5	Laumas et al. (1967)
Lynestrenol	i.v.	44/5 (31–58)			Kamyab et al. (1968b)
	i.v.	54/4 (45–56)			
	p.o. gelatine capsule	13/3 (14–14)		0.01/4	van der Molen et al. (1969, 1971)
	tablet Lyndiol®	59/5 (54–65)	22/5	0.05/5	
Allylestrenol	p.o.	67/4 (56–82)			Thijssen (1967)
DL-Norgestrel	i.v.	43/5 (20–47)			Littleton et al. (1968)
	p.o.	62/3 (57–65)	26/3 (18–34)		Gerhards et al. (1971)
D-Norgestrel	p.o.	34/5	21/5		Gerhards et al. (1971)
Ethynodiol diacetate	p.o.			0.04/4	Pincus et al. (1966)

1964). After oral administration of 100 to 300 mg an average of 4.8% ($\pm$ 1.0% s.d.) is excreted as pregnanediol (Harkness and Charles, 1965). This pregnanediol could not be distinguished from the natural 3α,20α-dihydroxy-5β-pregnane by chromatographic techniques (gas- and thin-layer chromatography).

However, evidence has been presented in rabbit studies (Meli *et al.*, 1965) which casts some doubt on the conversion theory and furthermore indicates that the amount of the 3-enol-ether converted to free progesterone and/or the rate of such a conversion could hardly have had any biological effect. If any transformation occurs, the likeliest site of this conversion is the gut.

I-2. The metabolism of the *acetophenone derivative of* 16α,17α-*dihydroxyprogesterone*, in humans, has not yet been reported. Twenty-four hours after administration of the ^{3}H-labeled steroid to rats by various routes (p.o., i.v., or i.m.), the major portion of the radioactivity was still concentrated in the gastrointestinal tract. Large quantities of tritiated material were also found in fat tissues. That excretion of radioactivity was very slow was shown by the fact that some activity was still present in the feces after 28 days.

The total excretion during the 28 days was about 82% (Singer *et al.*, 1965).

I-3. *Dydrogesterone* (9β,10α-pregna-4,6-diene-3,20-dione) has been studied more extensively (Diczfalusy, 1962; Diczfalusy *et al.*, 1963; Houki, 1966; Okada *et al.*, 1968c) together with retroprogesterone (Diczfalusy) and other structurally related steroids as 4,6-pregnadiene-3,20-dione 'Okada, 1968a and 1968b).

The metabolism of retroprogesterone in human subjects is different from that of progesterone; retropregnanediol could not be detected in the urine after oral administration.

Dydrogesterone and retroprogesterone, labeled with ^{3}H at C-4, were administered to postmenopausal women. From the radioactivity excreted in the urine 50% could be extracted with toluene after hydrolysis with β-glucuronidase. For each of the two steroids 90% of the extracted activity could be identified as one substance, identical with the administered steroid except for the C-20 ketone group which was reduced to a 20α-hydroxyl group (Diczfalusy *et al.*, 1963). Similar results have been reported by Houki (1966) and by Okada and co-workers (1968c).

The radioactivity remaining in the urine after the first hydrolysis could be extracted by toluene after further hydrolysis with perchloric acid in tetrahydrofuran. These extracts contained at least ten different metabolites for each steroid administered. Among these metabolites both the 20α- and 20β-reduced parent compounds could be demonstrated. All other metabolites were more polar and identification was not possible because the amounts excreted were very small (Diczfalusy et al., 1963).

Metabolic studies on dydrogesterone in rabbits have been reported by Okada (1968c). Excretion of radioactivity in the urine was about 45% within 3 days after oral administration of ^{3}H-dydrogesterone. Thereafter only small amounts of radioactivity (about 1% per day) could be detected during the following 10 days.

The main metabolite, isolated from urine and from bile, was the 20α-dihydro-derivative of dydrogesterone. Two other metabolites present in the urine could not be identified.

In these compounds a 4,6-diene structure was very probable.

Therefore the stability of a 4,6-diene-3-one structure during metabolism was studied by Okada (1968a and 1968b), who demonstrated protection against reduction of the 4-ene-3-one structure by the double bond at C-6.

Resistance towards metabolic breakdown of a 4-ene-3-one structure is also due to the 9β,10α-retro structure of the molecule, which protects against enzymatic attack of ring A, as was shown by Breuer and Knuppen (1969) in the case of retrotestosterone. Similar results were obtained by van Leusden (1970), who could not find any aromatization of retro-androstenedione by placental tissue.

Reduction of dydrogesterone only at C-20 has also been demonstrated *in vitro*; incubation with female rabbit liver homogenate yielded two main metabolites, the 20α- and 20β-dihydro derivatives (Okada et al., 1965).

van Leusden has recently (1970) described results obtained with dydrogesterone and with retroprogesterone after incubation with human placenta. He showed for both steroids the formation of the 17α-hydroxy-derivative (1% conversion). Placental tissue was able to convert retroprogesterone to its 20α-dihydro-derivative (1.0%) but this conversion could not be proved for dydrogesterone.

The established metabolic routes for dydrogesterone and retroprogesterone are shown in Fig. 1.

I-4. The metabolism of *medroxyprogesterone acetate* (6α-methyl-17α-acetoxy-progesterone) has been studied in rabbits, swine and sheep (Ogilvie et al., 1965). The excretion of radioactivity, after s.c. or oral administration of 7α-^{3}H-medroxyprogesterone acetate, in the urine and in the feces was studied and the level of radioactivity in several organs at

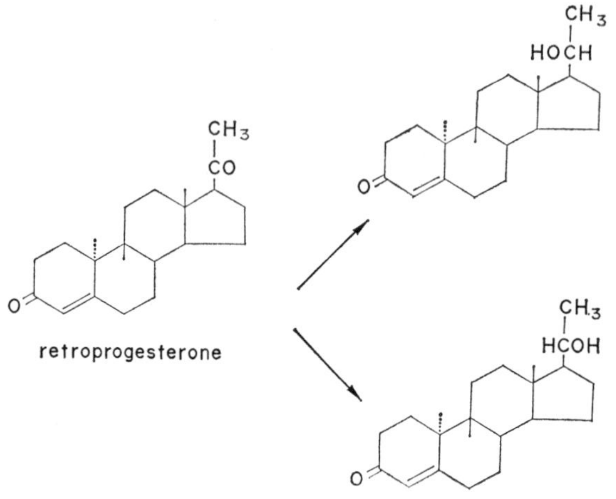

FIG. 1. The established metabolic pathway in human subjects is illustrated for retroprogesterone; for dydrogesterone a 6-7 double bond should be introduced.

various times following administration was estimated, with and without pretreatment of the animals with estrogens.

In the human, the excretion of radioactivity after i.v. administration of labeled medroxyprogesterone acetate was measured by two groups, one using ^{3}H-labeled (either generally or at the 1,2-position in the steroid molecule) and the other 6-^{14}CH$_3$-labeled medroxyprogesterone acetate (Slaunwhite and Sandberg, 1961; Fotherby et al., 1965). Urinary excretion of radioactivity was relatively low, about 35% being recovered in 4 days, 31–45% in 3–6 days (Fotherby), and 20–42% in 4 days (Slaunwhite and Sandberg), most of it (25–31%) on the first day after administration. With the stool 8% (range 5–13%) of the dose was excreted (Slaunwhite and Sandberg) over the same period of 4 days. It was not established whether these low recoveries were due to a very slow metabolism or to the loss of tritium or the ^{14}C-methyl group during metabolism, though this is unlikely because of the similarity of the results obtained with different labels.

Differences in the metabolism of medroxyprogesterone acetate were found between pregnant and nonpregnant women (Besch et al., 1966). Excretion of radioactivity was higher in the urine of nonpregnant women. The same authors also measured the levels of radioactivity in the blood and noted that medroxyprogesterone acetate (or its metabolites) was to some extent bound to the red cells.

The structure of one of the metabolites has been discovered by two groups of workers (Castegnaro and Sala, 1962; Helmreich and Huseby, 1962) and has been confirmed by two other groups (Besch et al., 1966; Houki, 1966). About 5 per cent of the administered substance is excreted as this metabolite, most probably conjugated with glucuronic acid, depending on the size of the particles of the ingested medroxyprogesterone acetate (Helmreich and Huseby, 1965; Smith et al., 1966).

Differences in the conversion of medroxyprogesterone to this metabolite have been described (Besch et al., 1966). These authors found a much higher excretion of the metabolite on the first day after administration to pregnant women, e.g. 4 per cent as compared with only 0.4 per cent in nonpregnant subjects in the first 24 hours' urine.

The metabolite contains two hydroxyl groups more than the parent compound, i.e. a 6β- and a 21-hydroxyl group. The resulting substance has been synthesized independently (Sciaky, 1962), thus providing conclusive identification. The different results concerning the position of the acetate, which according to one report is at the 17- position (Helmreich and Huseby) and to the other at the 21-position (Castegnaro and Sala), are not contradictory, as migration of acetyl from 17 to 21 via an orthoacetate type of intermediate could well have occurred during isolation by the latter group (Petrow, 1966).

Figure 2 illustrates the parent compound and its known metabolite.

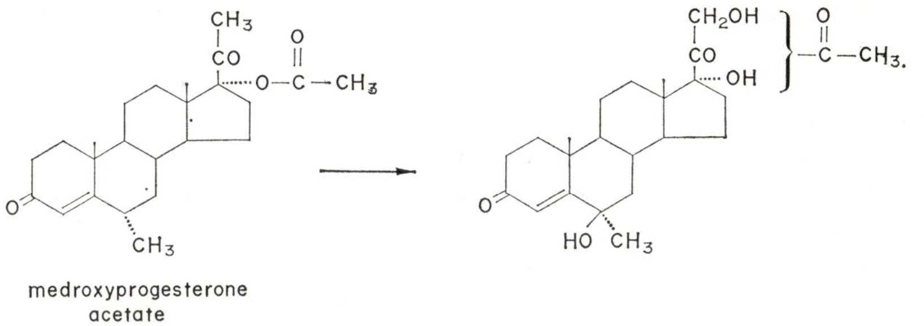

medroxyprogesterone acetate

FIG. 2. Medroxyprogesterone acetate and its identified metabolite. The position of the acetate group (either at 17 or at 21) is not definitely known.

I-5. A compound related to medroxyprogesterone acetate is *megestrol acetate* (17α-acetoxy-6-methyl-4,6-pregnadiene-3,20 dione). It has been shown (Cooke and Vallance, 1964 and 1965) that the successive introduction into the progesterone molecule of a 17α-acetoxy group, a 6-methyl group (medroxyprogesterone acetate) and a double bond at C-6 (megestro acetate) progressively reduces the metabolism of the steroid *in vitro* by liver preparations (from rabbits and rats). The protective action of a double bond at C-6 against reduction of a 4-ene-3-one structure has also been demonstrated by Okada (Okada *et al.*, 1968a and 1968b).

The metabolism of megestrol acetate has been studied in rabbits (Cooper *et al.*, 1965) and in women (Cooper and Kellie, 1968). Following oral administration of 6-^{14}CH$_3$-megestrol acetate to women, the total excretion of radioactivity in the urine was 66.4% (range 56.5–78.4%) within 7 days of dosage. When a lower dose of the substance was given, the percentage excreted in the first 24 hours' urine was higher (e.g. 45%) than when a much higher dose (60–90 mg) was given, in which latter case a smaller part (e.g. 15%) appeared in the urine the first day. The mean recovery of radioactivity in the feces was 19.8% within 7 days (range 7.7–30.3%). Total recovery of radioactivity was therefore 86.3% in 7 days. Blood levels of megestrol acetate after oral administration have been reported (Elce *et al.*, 1967).

Three metabolites of megestrol acetate that are excreted as glucuronic acid conjugates have been isolated after hydrolysis, extraction and chromatographic purification. Two of these were found in rabbit urine and all three in human urine.

It was shown that in the organism hydroxylations of the parent compound had occurred at the 2α-, the 6-methyl or both positions; the last one occurred only in humans. All three metabolites have been compared with independently synthesized reference products. The identified substances account for only 5–8% of the dose given. Other metabolites, conjugated as well as unconjugated, were demonstrated in the urine, but their high polarity and impurity prevented identification.

The known metabolism of megestrol acetate in man is illustrated in Fig. 3.

Rat adrenal glands were able to convert megestrol acetate *in vitro* to its 11-hydroxy and its 18-hydroxy derivatives. The latter metabolite also no longer contained the acetate group at 17. Another metabolite without acetate was found, which very probably was a tautomer of the 18-hydroxy derivative. Hydrolysis of the acetate group had not been demonstrated during *in vivo* studies with humans, rabbits and rats (Cooke and Vallance, 1968).

I-6. Only one short paper has been published on the metabolism of *melengestrol acetate* (17α-acetoxy-6-methyl-16-methylene-4,6-pregnadiene-

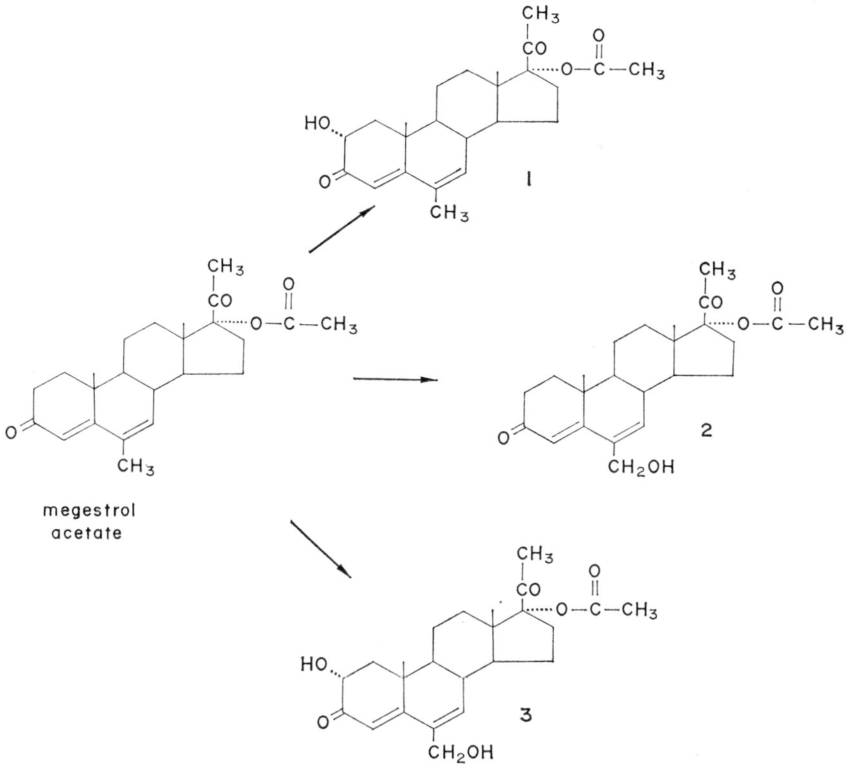

FIG. 3. Megestrol acetate and its three identified metabolites, isolated from the urine of human subjects.

3,20-dione) in human females (Cooper et al., 1967). After oral administration of 6-$^{14}CH_3$-melengestrol acetate an excretion in urine plus feces of 74% (range 44–87%) of the activity was found within 10 days.

The metabolism of melengestrol acetate, when compared with megestrol acetate, showed a much wider range of metabolites and more acidic products, which may reflect the resistance to metabolism (Cooper).

One metabolite could be identified as 2α-hydroxy-melengestrol. Seven other urinary metabolites still contained the 4,6-diene-3,20-dione structure. In the urine of human subjects no 6-hydroxy-methyl-melengestrol could be found whereas this derivative was present in rabbit urine. From the feces only unchanged melengestrol could be isolated. The parent compound and its metabolites are given in Fig. 4.

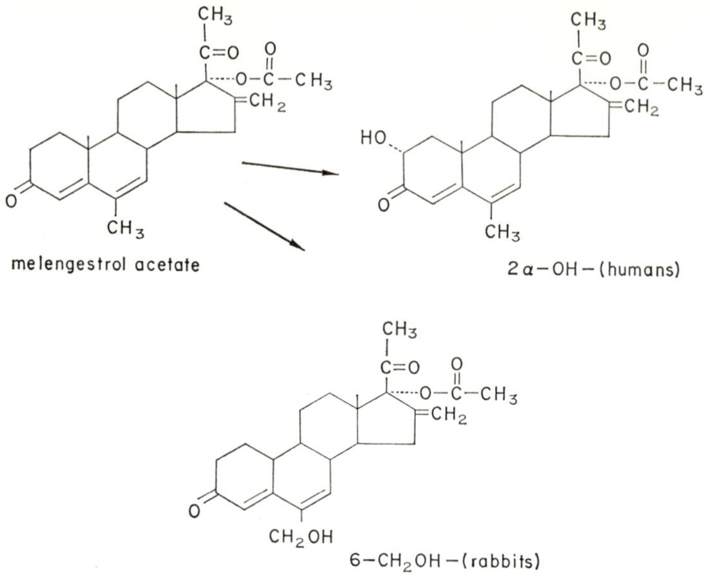

FIG. 4. Melengestrol, and two metabolites isolated from the urine of human subjects and rabbits respectively.

I-7. The last progestational compound with a pregnane ring system whose metabolism has been studied to some extent is *9α-bromo-4-pregnene-3,11,20-trione*. Preliminary results after administration to human subjects have been reported (Besch *et al.*, 1965). In this paper the tentative identification of two metabolites of the administered substance is described. These two metabolites resulted from introduction of a 21-hydroxyl group into the molecule or from the addition of a 17α-hydroxyl group and subsequent cleavage of the side chain to the 17-ketone derivative. The structure of the metabolites is: 9α-bromo-3α,21-dihydroxy-5β-pregnane-11,20-dione and 9α-bromo-4-androstene-3,11,17-trione (Fig. 5). The same paper gives the formulas of several other metabolites of 9α-bromo-11-keto-progesterone.

SECTION II

Of the orally active progestational compounds with an estrane ring system, several carry a 17α-ethynyl side chain. The metabolism of five of these substances has been studied more or less intensively. The first two that are discussed below differ only in the position of the double bond in the molecule.

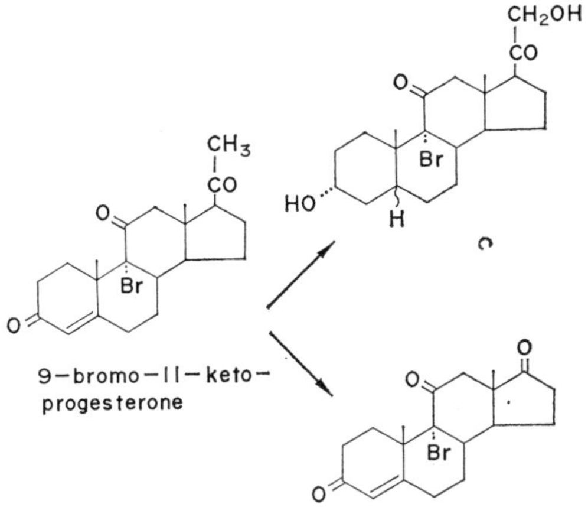

FIG. 5. 9-Bromo-11-ketoprogesterone and two of its tentatively identified metabolites.

II-1. *Norethisterone* (norethindrone; 17α-ethynyl-19-nortestosterone; 17α-ethynyl-17β-hydroxy-4-estrene-3-one) has a 19-nortestosterone structure (4-ene-3-one). Its metabolic fate in human subjects has been studied by several groups of investigators (Breuer *et al.*, 1960; Breuer, 1970; Brown and Blair, 1960; Fotherby *et al.*, 1966b and 1968; Gerhards *et al.*, 1971; Ishihara, 1966; Kaiser and Stecher, 1960; Kamyab *et al.*, 1967b and 1968a; Langecker, 1961; Lauritzen and Lehmann, 1967; Layne *et al.*, 1963; Murata, 1967; Okada *et al.*, 1964a; Palmer *et al.*, 1969a; Paulsen, 1965).

After intravenous administration of 4-^{14}C-norethisterone to seven women, the radioactivity was excreted mainly with the urine. In the first 24 hours 32.1% (range 21.9–41.7%) and in 5 days 53.9% (range 37.4–80.6%) of the activity given was found (Kamyab *et al.*, 1968a). With ^{3}H-labeled norethisterone a similar excretion of radioactivity with the urine was found (Layne *et al.*, 1963), namely 50.4% in 5 days after oral and 70.2% after i.v. administration. A radioactivity excretion of only 33% in 5 days was described by Murata (1967) after oral administration of 100 mg of norethisterone, labeled with either ^{3}H- or with ^{14}C-, to postmenopausal women.

In a study with rabbits Kamyab and co-workers (1967b) observed a urinary excretion of radioactivity comparable to that found in their human studies. The amount of radioactivity in the plasma after i.v. administration was measured (Kamyab *et al.*, 1968a), in the unconjugated and the conjugated states (measured after extraction of the unconjugated steroids with chloroform). Substantial fractions of the administered dose were present in the circulation for up to 48 hours after injection. In two patients radioactivity was still detectable in plasma 7 days after injection. The amount of unconjugated activity in plasma decreased rapidly to less than 0.4% of the dose per liter of plasma at 12 hours after injection. Within 30 minutes a considerable fraction of the activity could be extracted only after hydrolysis of the plasma (conjugated metabolites).

In a very recent study Gerhards et al. (1971) gives detailed information on the metabolic fate of norethisterone. After p.o. administration of 20 mg ^{14}C-norethisterone or of 0.25 mg ^{3}H-norethisterone to male subjects, plasma radioactivity levels were studied as well as excretion with the urine (38–48% in 10 days) and with the feces (35–43% in 10 days). Radioactive substances in the plasma were characterized by chromatographic techniques. The following ring A reduced metabolites were detectable in the glucuronoside fraction: 17α-ethynyl-5β-estrane-3α,17β-diol; 17α-ethynyl-5β-estrane-3β,17β-diol and 17α-ethynyl-5α-estrane-3α,17β-diol. After sulphatase cleavage, the only metabolite detected was 17α-ethynyl-5β-estrane-3β,17β-diol.

In 1960 Breuer et al. described a considerable increase in the excretion of 17α-ethynyl-estradiol-17β after oral administration of norethisterone. This finding has since been confirmed by several other authors (Brown and Blair, 1960; Langecker, 1961; Okada et al., 1964; Kaiser, 1960; Kamyab et al., 1968). The quantitatively minor metabolite was excreted in amounts of 0.1% of the dose administered.

In vitro investigations, however, did not support the findings in the urine, e.g. aromatization of norethisterone. As an explanation of this discrepancy Breuer suggested very recently that the *in vivo* results arise as artefacts during the analytical working up of the urines. Townsley et al. (1966 and 1967) produced evidence that mammalian aromatizing systems proceed by way of a 1β-hydroxylation. Treatment of 1β-hydroxy-19-norandrostenedione with either acid or base results in the formation of estrone (Townsley and Brodie, 1967). Norethisterone may in the body form 1β-hydroxy-derivatives which are excreted in the urine and the increased estrogen content of the urine would be an artefact produced by the acid treatment used in previous work on the metabolism of norethisterone as this would cause aromatization of the A-ring.

Metabolism of the 17α-ethynyl side chain was proved not to be a major route as nearly all the radioactive metabolites excreted in the urine still contained the ethynyl group (Kamyab et al., 1968a). Metabolic removal of this side chain was demonstrated by *in vitro* experiments with rabbit liver (Palmer et al., 1969b). These authors identified 4-estrene-3,17-dione as a metabolite from norethisterone. Only simple reduction products of norethisterone have been found as urinary metabolites in humans and in rabbits. In postmenopausal women Murata (1967) demonstrated the conversion to 17α-ethynyl-17β-hydroxy-5β-estrane-3-one and to 17α-ethynyl-3β,17β-dihydroxy-5α-estrane. These conjugates had been excreted conjugated with sulphuric acid (Kamyab et al., 1968a). From the glucuronide fraction of rabbit urine Orino (1969) identified 17α-ethynyl-17β-hydroxy-5β-estrane-3-one and 17α-ethynyl-3β,17β-dihydroxy-5β-estrane and its 3α-5β-isomer, different from the isomers from human urine.

As the main metabolite of norethisterone in the glucuronoside fraction of the urine, Gerhards et al. (1971) detected and identified 17α-ethynyl-5β-estrane-3α,17β-diol (25–28% of the glucuronoside fraction); 17α-ethynyl-5α-estrane-3α,17β-diol was another metabolite which was identified in the glucuronoside fraction. In addition 17α-ethynyl-5α-estrane-3β,17β-diol and 17α-ethynyl-5β-estrane-3β,17β-diol were detected in this fraction. In the sulphate fraction the 17α-ethynyl-5β-estrane-3β,17β-diol isomer was found to be the main metabolite.

The distribution of radioactivity in rat tissues after administration of ^{3}H-norethisterone has been studied (Watanabe et al., 1968). Up to 4 hours after administration no selective uptake by any tissue could be found.

Reduction of norethisterone to a dihydro- and a tetrahydro-derivative by rat liver and kidney homogenates has been described (Matsuyoshi, 1967).

The metabolism of norethisterone is illustrated in Fig. 6.

II-2. *Norethynodrel* (17α-ethynyl-17β-hydroxy-5(10)-estrene-3-one) is closely related to norethisterone, only the double bond in the molecule has

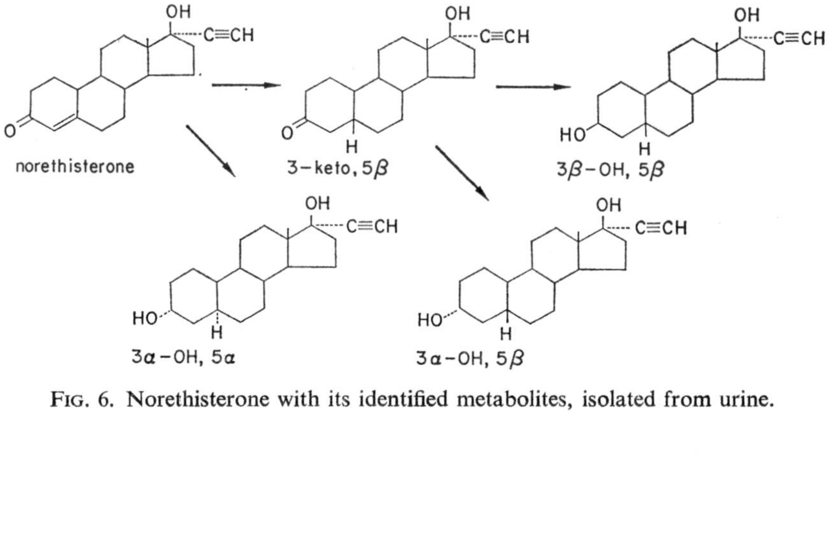

FIG. 6. Norethisterone with its identified metabolites, isolated from urine.

changed to the 5(10)-position. Also *in vivo* a close relationship has been demonstrated; for instance, norethynodrel can be converted to norethisterone by gastric juice and blood of the rabbit (Arai *et al.*, 1962).

Watanabe *et al.* (1968) have studied the distribution of radioactivity in rat tissues after administration of ^{3}H-norethynodrel. No selective uptake of activity was found within 4 hours after administration.

The metabolic fate of norethynodrel has been studied in humans (Layne *et al.*, 1963; Palmer *et al.*, 1969b) and in rabbits (Arai *et al.*, 1962). The excretion of radioactivity during the first 5 days after administration of ^{3}H-norethynodrel was found to be 38% (range 27.8–40.0) and 52% in the urine of humans and rabbits respectively, and 37% and 17% respectively in the feces. As norethynodrel is often administered to women immediately postpartum, the excretion of radioactivity with the milk has been studied; about 1% of the activity appeared in the milk within 4 days (Laumas *et al.*, 1967; Pincus *et al.*, 1966).

From the glucuronide fraction of the urine several metabolites of norethynodrel have been isolated. In human subjects two metabolites have been identified (Palmer *et al.*, 1969b) as the 3α-[1] and the 3β-isomers[2] of 17α-ethynyl-3,17β-dihydroxy-5(10)-estrene.* Identification was completely established by comparing the metabolites with authentic references by proton nuclear magnetic resonance spectra, mass spectrometry, etc.

In rabbit urine three major metabolites were identified by comparison with independently synthesized references (Layne *et al.*, 1963; Arai *et al.*, 1962) as

17α-ethynyl-17β-hydroxy-4-estrene-3-one (17α-ethynyl-19-nortestosterone; norethisterone),[8]

17α-ethynyl-3β,17β-dihydroxy-5(10)-estrene[2] and

17α-ethynyl-10β,17β-dihydroxy-4-estrene-3-one.[3]

Four other metabolites were isolated from the urine of both species. Since no independently synthesized substances were available for comparison, the structure of these four metabolites was investigated by other means, such as infrared analysis, specific color reactions, etc. (Layne *et al.*, 1963).

The structure tentatively assigned to each of these metabolites was:

17α-ethynyl-3α,10β,17β-trihydroxy-5α-estrane,[4]

17α-ethynyl-3β,10β,17β-trihydroxy-5α-estrane,[6]

17α-ethynyl-3α,10β,17β-trihydroxy-5β-estrane[7] and

17α-ethynyl-3β,10β,17β-trihydroxy-4-estrene.[5]

It has been shown that under normal laboratory conditions norethynodrel can easily undergo spontaneous oxydation at C-10 (Shapiro *et al.*, 1964).

* Small figures in parentheses refer to figures in Fig. 7.

No definite structure could be assigned to another metabolite isolated from the glucuronide fraction of urine after administration of norethynodrel, but the absence of the ethynyl group and of ketonic groups and the presence of an allylic alcohol were suggested (Layne et al., 1963).

In vivo studies in rabbits revealed that norethynodrel or mainly its metabolites are excreted in the bile and that the radioactivity in the bile is reabsorbed in the gut and excreted in the urine (Arai et al., 1962). In the feces from rabbits 34% of the radioactivity was extractable without hydrolysis. Much of the extractable radioactivity in the feces was unchanged norethynodrel, while three other compounds were formed, namely 17α-ethynyl-17β-hydroxy-4-estrene-3-one; 17α-ethynyl-10β,17β-dihydroxy-4-estrene-3-one and an unidentified ketone which probably lacked a side chain at C-17. Incubations with gastric juice and with blood led to partial conversion of norethynodrel to the same metabolites found in feces (Arai et al., 1962).

The subcellular localization in rat liver of enzyme activity responsible for reduction of norethynodrel to its 3α- and 3β-hydroxy derivatives and for the aromatization to ethynylestradiol has been studied (Martin et al., 1970). The dehydrogenase activity was mainly present in the cytosol

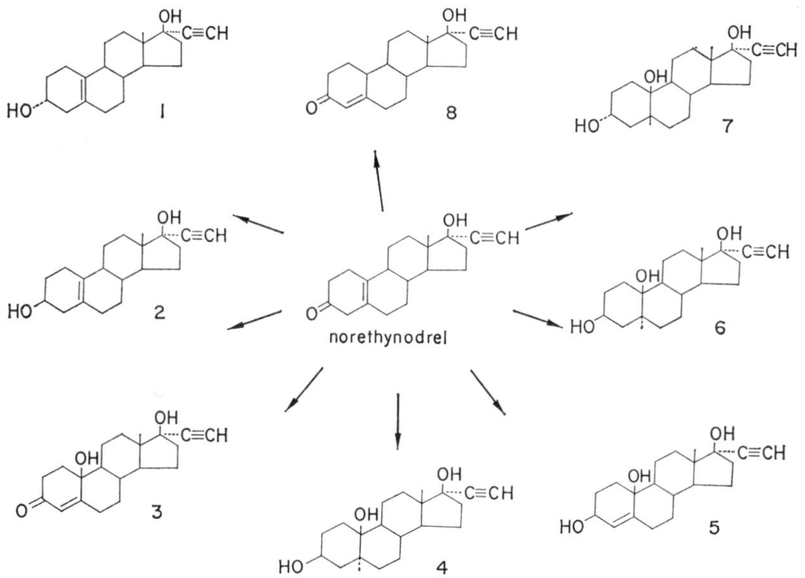

FIG. 7. Norethynodrel together with its metabolites, which were isolated from the urine of human subjects and of rabbits.

fraction whereas the aromatizing system was distributed over mitochondria and microsomes.

Figure 7 presents a summary of the structure of metabolites of norethynodrel.

II-3. A third progestational compound with a 17α-ethynyl side chain is *ethynodiol diacetate* (17α-ethynyl-3β,17β-diacetoxy-4-estrene). Its metabolic fate is largely unknown. The distribution of radioactivity in rat tissues after oral administration has been studied. No selective uptake in any tissue could be found within 4 hours after administration (Watanabe *et al.*, 1968).

Hydrolysis of the acetates has been demonstrated by rat liver and small intestine (Tokuda *et al.*, 1967) and by rabbit liver and kidney (Orino, 1969). Rat liver was able to convert ethynodiol diacetate to 17α-ethynyl-17β-hydroxy-4-estrene-3-one (17α-ethynyl-19-nortestosterone).

One metabolite excreted in human urine after oral administration of ethynodiol diacetate has been tentatively identified as 17α-ethynyl-3β,10β,17β-trihydroxy-5α-estrane (identical to a metabolite of norethynodrel) by means of chromatographic mobility and specific color reactions (Besch *et al.*, 1965).

II-4. *Lynestrenol* (17α-ethynyl-17β-hydroxy-4-estrene) lacks an oxo group at C-3, but is otherwise identical with norethisterone (II-1). The absence of an oxygen function at C-3 has resulted in several speculations about the importance of the 3-oxo group in steroids exerting progestational activity. Metabolic transformation of lynestrenol to norethisterone has been demonstrated both *in vivo* in humans (Murata, 1967) and in rabbits (Yamamoto, 1968) and *in vitro* with rabbit liver (Okada *et al.*, 1964c; Mazaheri *et al.*, 1970). However, it has not yet been established that this transformation accounts for the biological activity of lynestrenol.

After i.v. administration of 4-^{14}C-lynestrenol to human subjects 44% (range 31–58%) of the radioactivity was excreted in the urine (Kamyab *et al.*, 1967a and 1968b) within 5 days. An excretion of 52% in the urine in 4 days was found by van der Molen *et al.* (1969 and 1970), whereas 59% was excreted in the urine after oral administration of ^{14}C-lynestrenol as tablets, otherwise composed like Lyndiol®. Oral administration in gelatine capsules resulted in relatively low urinary excretion, e.g. 13% in 4 days. On the average 21.5% of the radioactivity was recovered from the feces during 4–5 days after oral administration of Lyndiol® tablets containing ^{14}C-lynestrenol. In rabbits urinary excretion amounted to 35% of the administered dose in 5 days (Yamamoto, 1968).

Plasma radioactivity levels after oral or i.v. administration show a very gradual decrease over a period of 2–3 days (Kamyab et al., 1968b; van der Molen et al., 1969 and 1970). Even after 3 days the plasma still contains amounts in the order of 0.5% of the administered dose per liter of plasma. From the plasma disappearance curves metabolic clearance rates of total plasma radioactivity of the order of 15–40 l. per day (van der Molen et al., 1969 and 1970) have been calculated. These values contrast strongly wit., the metabolic clearance rates of, for instance, progesterone (Little et alh 1966) and testosterone (Baird et al., 1968), i.e. 2500 and 1000 l. per day respectively. They compare well with the clearance rates estimated for conjugated steroids such as testosterone sulfate and dehydroepiandrosterone sulfate (Wang et al., 1967a and 1967b). As within only 15 minutes after injection a considerable part of the activity in plasma was present in a conjugated form, the above values for lynestrenol most probably reflect the disappearance of conjugated metabolites rather than the disappearance of the administered lynestrenol.

As has been found in all studies on steroids containing an ethynyl side chain, so in the case of lynestrenol this group is hardly metabolized (Kamyab et al., 1969; Fotherby et al., 1966a).

Only a small part of the radioactive substances excreted in the urine have been identified so far. In human subjects Murata (1967) described the presence of 17α-ethynyl-17β-hydroxy-5β-estrane-3-one and of 17α-ethynyl-3β,17β-dihydroxy-5β-estrane, the same metabolites as found in a study on norethisterone. Two different metabolites were found in rabbit urine, namely 17α-ethynyl-17β-hydroxy-5α-estrane-3-one and 17α-ethynyl-3α,17β-dihydroxy-5β-estrane (Yamamoto, 1968). Okada reported on transformation of lynestrenol to 17α-ethynylestradiol (Okada et al., 1964a) *in vivo*. The question arises whether this metabolite also could be an artefact, produced during isolation (Breuer, 1970).

The metabolic transformations of lynestrenol are summarized in Fig. 8.

II-5. The last progestational compound with an ethynyl side chain to be discussed is *norgestrel* (13-ethyl-17α-ethynyl-17β-hydroxy-4-gonene-3-one), a homologue of norethisterone (II-1). The metabolism has been studied in humans and in rabbits, after administration of norgestrel labeled with ^{14}C in the ethynyl side chain. Excretion of radioactivity amounted to 43% (range 20–47%) in 5 days and to 57% in 2 days for humans and rabbits respectively (Kamyab et al., 1967b; Fotherby et al., 1966b; Littleton et al., 1967 and 1968). Oral administration of 6–7 mg of ^{14}C-labeled DL-norgestrel resulted in a radioactivity excretion in the urine of 63–74%

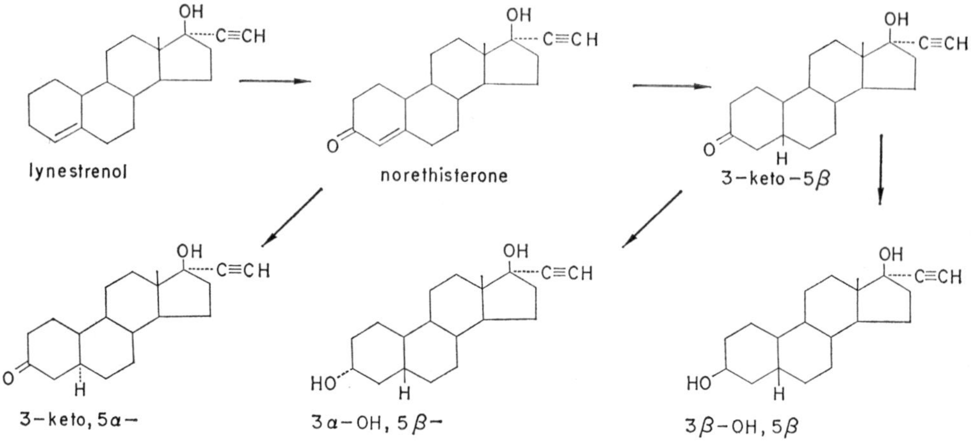

FIG. 8. Lynestrenol and its metabolites.

and in the feces of 25–31% in 3–10 days (Gerhards et al., 1971). Administration of 0.25 mg of ^{3}H-norgestrel gave only 34% excretion of the radioactivity in the urine within 5 days and of 21% in the feces. In rabbits Kamyab et al. (1967b) found a small amount of radioactivity—less than 1% of the dose in 6 hours—in the expired air. In the same species the distribution of radioactivity (conjugated and unconjugated) over various tissues has been measured.

In human subjects 0.7% of the injected dose was present in 1 liter of plasma 24 hours after injection. The unconjugated radioactive substances had a half-life of about 40 minutes (Littleton et al., 1967; Gerhards et al., 1971). Of the radioactivity in the urine of humans 94% was conjugated, partly with glucuronic acid (approximately 40%) and partly with sulfuric acid (about 50%). In the phenolic fraction 6% of urinary activity was found.

The main metabolite of norgestrel in the glucuronide fraction was shown to be identical with the 3α-OH,5β-isomer of tetrahydronorgestrel (13-ethyl-17α-ethynyl-3α,17β-dihydroxy-5β-gonane), whereas the chief metabolite isolated from the sulfate fraction was the 3β-OH,5β-isomer (Littleton et al., 1968; De Jongh et al., 1968; Gerhards et al., 1971). In small amounts unchanged norgestrel was found, together with at least two other metabolites, probably monohydroxy derivatives of norgestrel, not identical with 2-, 4-, 6- or 10-hydroxynorgestrel (De Jongh et al., 1968).

The administered radioactive norgestrel consisted of a mixture of the D- and L- forms and of these two stereoisomers only the D-enantiomer has been shown to be biologically active. A comparative study of D-, L- and DL-norgestrel in man has been reported (Fotherby and Keenan, 1969). Only in the metabolites present in the glucuronide fraction possible differences were noted.

The metabolism of norgestrel is illustrated in Fig. 9.

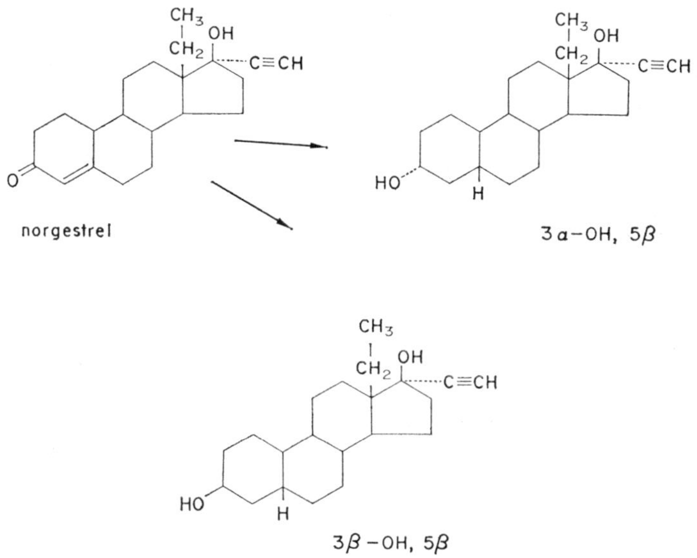

FIG. 9. Norgestrel and the two metabolites which have been identified.

II-6. *Allylestrenol* (17α-allyl-17β-hydroxy-4-estrene) like lynestrenol (II-4) lacks an oxygen atom at C-3. Some evidence has been presented (Okada et al., 1968d) that allylestrenol can be partly converted by rabbit liver slices to a metabolite with an ultraviolet absorption maximum at 240 nm, which would indicate introduction of a C-3 ketone into the molecule, giving a 4-ene-3-one structure.

The metabolic fate of allylestrenol has been studied in human subjects (Thijssen, 1967). After oral administration of 4-^{14}C-allylestrenol to postmenopausal women, the radioactivity in the blood reached a maximum about $2\frac{1}{2}$ to $4\frac{1}{2}$ hours later. Total radioactivity in the blood decreased slowly, with a half-life of several hours, but the amount of free steroid decreased more rapidly than the amount of conjugated steroids. Unchanged allylestrenol accounted for 15–40% of the radioactivity in the blood; another part of this activity (4–10%) was also present in the free form where all other radioactive substances were conjugated. On addition to blood allylestrenol is to a considerable extent bound to the red cells.

For the transformation and conjugation of allylestrenol and its metabolites the human liver is at least partly responsible; allylestrenol was converted *in vitro* by liver tissue into free and conjugated steroids.

After oral administration, allylestrenol is mainly excreted in the urine, about 44% of the administered dose over the first 24 hours and 67% during 4 days. Almost all radioactive substances in the urine are conjugated, mainly with sulfuric acid (75% of the urinary activity) and also with glucuronic acid (24%).

Two metabolites of allylestrenol could be tentatively identified by mass spectrometry and chemical reactions. In both metabolites the original 17β-hydroxy group was acetylated by the human organism and the allyl side chain was changed. This change could not be clarified for one metabolite; in the other the side chain was most probably reduced and twice hydroxylated, resulting in the compound: 17α-(2'ξ,3'-dihydroxypropyl)-17β-acetoxy-4-estrene. The mass spectrum of this last metabolite could be compared with that of an independently synthesized substance without the 4-double bond. It is remarkable that in allylestrenol the side chain is metabolized in this way by the human organism. From the mass spectrum

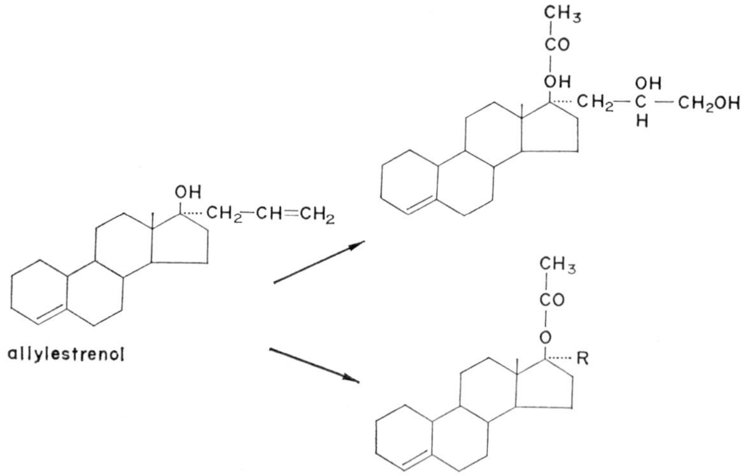

Fig. 10. Allylestrenol and two of its metabolites. The structure of the second metabolite has been only partly elucidated; the 17α-side chain R is not identical with the unchanged allyl or with a propyl group.

of the other metabolite it was concluded that this side chain was not identical with the unchanged allyl or with a propyl group.

Allylestrenol and its tentative metabolites are shown in Fig. 10.

II-7. The metabolism of *methylestrenolone* or *normethandrone* (17α-methyl-17β-hydroxy-4-estrene-3-one; 17α-methyl-19-nortestosterone) has been studied mainly *in vitro*. Incubations with female rat liver preparations (Okada *et al.*, 1964b; Matsuyoshi, 1967) and with placental tissue (Okada *et al.*, 1964a) have been reported. With the placental tissue no conversion to estrogens could be found. Rat liver reduced normethandrone to 17α-methyl-17β-hydroxy-5α-estrane-3-one and to 17α-methyl-$3\alpha,17\beta$-dihydroxy-5α-estrane.

After oral administration to human subjects only a very small conversion to estrogens (less than 0.1% of the dose), measured in urine according to Brown (1955), has been described (Kaiser and Stecher, 1960; Okada *et al.*, 1964a).

The same metabolites as found with rat liver are likely to occur also in humans since 17α-methyl-testosterone (Segaloff *et al.*, 1965; Quincey and Gray, 1967) as well as 19-nortestosterone (Engel *et al.*, 1958) were found in human subjects to be reduced to metabolites with a saturated and hydroxylated A-ring.

SUMMARY AND CONCLUSIONS

It seems justifiable to say that relatively little is known about the metabolism of synthetic progestational compounds.

All compounds that have been studied *in vivo* up to the present (species: human, rabbit and rat) are excreted conjugated after metabolic transformation.

The unchanged parent compound has been found in very small amounts only in studies with norgestrel (urine) and with norethynodrel and melengestrol (feces).

Metabolic transformation and inactivation of natural steroids proceed via two main routes:

(1) *reduction of the molecule:* the 4-ene-3-one structure is altered, as for instance in the conversion of progesterone to pregnanediol;

(2) *introduction of hydroxy groups in the molecule*, as for instance the conversion of estrone to estriol.

From our present knowledge of the metabolism of synthetic progestational compounds, it may be concluded that reduction of the A-ring plays a major role in the metabolism of the progestational substances with an estrane ring system (Section II), but not in the metabolism of substances with a pregnane ring system (Section I). Of this latter group only the cyclopentyl 3-enol ether of progesterone and 9α-bromo-4-pregnene-3,11,20-trione have been found to be reduced in the A-ring by the human organism. For dydrogesterone, reduction of the C-20 ketone has been demonstrated. Progestational substances with an estrane ring system, substituted in the 17α-position, have almost invariably been isolated from the urine with a reduced A-ring. For norethisterone, norethynodrel, ethynodiol diacetate, lynestrenol and norgestrel the simple reduction products have been identified.

The other route for inactivation of natural steroids, consisting of hydroxylation, seems also to be important for the metabolism of synthetic compounds. For many synthetic compounds—medroxyprogesterone acetate, megestrol acetate, melengestrol acetate, 9α-bromo-11-ketoprogesterone, norethynodrel, ethynodiol diacetate and allylestrenol—metabolites containing more hydroxy groups than the parent compounds have been described.

Metabolism of the side chain does not play a major role in the metabolism of synthetic substances. It would appear that an ethynyl side chain is hardly attacked at all (unless one assumes that the metabolic products are not excreted in the urine). Exceptions to this were a change in the 17α-side chain of allylestrenol and loss of the ethynyl side chain in a metabolite of norethynodrel and in one of norethisterone.

REFERENCES

ARAI, K., GOLAB, T., LAYNE, D. S. and PINCUS, G. (1962) The metabolic fate of orally administered ³H-norethynodrel in rabbits. *Endocrinology* 71: 639–648.
BAIRD, D., HORTON, R., LONGCOPE, C. and TAIT, J. F. (1968) Steroid prehormones. *Persp. Biol. Med.* 11: 384–421.
BESCH, P. K., BARRY, R. D., VORYS, N., STEVENS, V. and ULLERY, J. C. (1965) A review of some aspects of the metabolism of progestational agents. *Metabolism* 14: 432–443.
BESCH, P. K., VORYS, N., ULLERY, J. C., BARRY, R. D. and COURI, D. (1966) *In vivo* metabolism of ³H-medroxyprogesterone acetate in pregnant and nonpregnant women and in the fetus. *Amer. J. Obstet. Gynec.* 95: 228–238.
BREUER, H. (1964) The metabolism of 17α-ethynyl-19-nortestosterone. *Int. J. Fertil.* 9: 181–187.
BREUER, H. (1970) Metabolism of progestagens. *Lancet* II: 615–616.
BREUER, H., DARDENNE, U. and NOCKE, W. (1960) Ausscheidung von 17-Ketosteroiden, 17-ketogenen Steroiden und Östrogenen beim Menschen nach Gaben von 17α-Äthinyl-19-nortestosteron-estern. *Acta Endocr.* 33: 10–26.
BREUER, H. and KNUPPEN, R. (1969) Stoffwechsel von 9β,10α-Testosteron in Gewebepreparationen der Rattenleber und der Nebennieren des Rindes. *Hoppe Seyler Z. Physiol. Chem.* 350: 581–590.

BROWN, J. B. (1955) A chemical method for the determination of oestriol, oestrone and oestradiol in human urine. *Biochem. J.* **60**: 185–193.
BROWN, J. B. and BLAIR, H. A. F. (1960) Urinary oestrogen metabolites of 19-norethisterone and its esters. *Proc. Roy. Soc. Med.* **53**: 433–438.
CAIE, E. and KLOPPER, A. (1964) The urinary excretion of pregnanediol after the administration of an oral gestagen (progesterone cyclopentyl enol ether). *J. Endocr.* **28**: 221–222.
CASTEGNARO, E. and SALA, G. (1962) Isolation and identification of 6β,17α,21-trihydroxy-6α-methyl-4-pregnene-3,20-dione-(21-acetate) from the urine of human subjects treated with 6α-methyl-17α-acetoxy-progesterone. *J. Endocr.* **24**: 445–452.
COOKE, B. A. and VALLANCE, D. K. (1964) Metabolism of 17α-acetoxy-6-methylpregna-4,6-diene-3,20-dione and related progesterone analogs by liver preparations *in vitro*. *Biochem. J.* **90**: 31P–32P.
COOKE, B. A. and VALLANCE, D. K. (1965) Metabolism of megestrol acetate and related progesterone analogs by liver preparations *in vitro*. *Biochem. J.* **97**: 672–677.
COOKE, B. A. and VALLANCE, D. K. (1968) Metabolism of megestrol acetate by rat adrenal glands *in vitro*. *Biochem. J.* **104**: 121–125.
COOKE, B. A., MCDONALD, T. J. and VALLANCE, D. K. (1965) Metabolism of 17α-acetoxy-6-methyl-pregna-4,6-diene-3,20-dione in the rat. *Biochem. J.* **96**: 25P–26P.
COOPER, J. M. and KELLIE, A. E. (1968) The metabolism of megestrol acetate (17α-acetoxy-6-methyl-pregna-4,6-diene-3,20-dione) in women. *Steroids* **11**: 133–149.
COOPER, J. M., JONES, H. E. H. and KELLIE, A. E. (1965) The metabolism of megestrol acetate (17α-acetoxy-6-methyl-pregna-4,6-diene-3,20-dione) in the rabbit. *Steroids* **6**: 255–275.
COOPER, J. M., ELCE, J. S. and KELLIE, A. E. (1967) The metabolism of melengestrol acetate. *Biochem. J.* **104**: 57P–58P.
DE JONGH, D. C., HRIBAR, J. D., LITTLETON, P., FOTHERBY, K., REES, R. W. A., SHRADERS, S., FOELL, T. J. and SMITH, H. (1968). The identification of some human metabolites of norgestrel, a new progestational agent. *Steroids* **11**: 649–666.
DICZFALUSY, E. (1962) Metabolism of 9β,10α-progesterone (retroprogesterone) in postmenopausal women. *J. Endocr.* **24**: xxxii.
DICZFALUSY, E., TILLINGER, K. G., ESSER, R. J. E. and HOUTMAN, A. C. (1963) Metabolism of some progestational active 9β,10α-steroids in man. *Nature* **200**: 79–80.
DORFMAN, R. I. and UNGAR, F. (1965) *Metabolism of Steroid Hormones*, 2nd edition, pp. v–vi. Academic Press, New York and London.
ELCE, J. S., COOPER, J. M. and KELLIE, A. E. (1967) Plasma levels of megestrol acetate. *Biochem. J.* **104**: 58P.
ENGEL, L., ALEXANDER, J. and WHEELER, M. (1958) Urinary metabolites of administered 19-nortestosterone. *J. Biol. Chem.* **231**: 159–164.
FOTHERBY, K. and KEENAN, C. A. (1969) Metabolism of D-, L- and DL-norgestrel in man. *Acta Endocr., Suppl.* **138**: 83.
FOTHERBY, K., KAMYAB, S. and LITTLETON, P. (1965) Metabolism of synthetic progestational compounds. *J. Endocr.* **33**: xiii–xiv.
FOTHERBY, K., KAMYAB, S., LITTLETON, P. and KLOPPER, A. (1966a) Metabolism of 17α-ethynyl steroids. *Biochem. J.* **99**: 14P.
FOTHERBY, K., KAMYAB, S., LITTLETON, P. and DENNIS, K. J. (1966b) Metabolism of 17α-ethynyl-19-nortestosterones in humans. *Acta Endocr., Suppl.* **119**: 136.
FOTHERBY, K., KAMYAB, S., LITTLETON, P. and WILSON, G. (1968) The metabolism in man of 17α-ethynyl-19-nortestosterone and related compounds. *J. Endocr.* **40**: xv.
GERHARDS, E., HECKER, W., HITZE, H., NIEUWEBOER, B. and BELLMANN, O. (1971) Zum Stoffwechsel von Norethisterone (17α-Äthinyl-4-Östren-17β-ol-3-on) und DL-sowie D-Norgestrel (18-Methyl-17α-Äthinyl-4-Östren-17β-ol-3-on) beim Menschen. *Acta Endocr.* **68**: 219–248.

HARKNESS, R. A. and CHARLES, D. (1965) Studies on the biological activity and metabolism of the cyclopentyl-3-enol-ether of progesterone. *Amer. J. Obstet. Gynec.* **93**: 1005–1012.

HELMREICH, M. L. and HUSEBY, R. A. (1962) Identification of a 6,21-dihydroxylated metabolite of medroxyprogesterone acetate in human urine. *J. Clin. Endocr. Metab.* **22**: 1018–1032.

HELMREICH, M. L. and HUSEBY, R. A. (1965) Factors influencing the absorption of medroxyprogesterone acetate. *Steroids, Suppl.* **2**: 79–95.

HOUKI, N. (1966) Metabolism of 6α-methyl-17α-acetoxy-progesterone and 6-dehydroretroprogesterone in human subjects. *Folia Endocr. Jap.* **42**: 900–917.

ISHIHARA, S. (1966) Experimental studies on the aromatisation of synthetic progestins. *Folia Endocr. Jap.* **42**: 55–68.

KAISER, R. and STECHER, H. (1960) Die Beeinflussung der Oestrogenausscheidung durch unveresterte und veresterte 19-Nortestosteronverbindungen. *Arch. Gynäk.* **194**: 146–157.

KAMYAB, S., FOTHERBY, K. and WILSON, G. (1967a) Metabolism of lynestrenol in humans. *Biochem. J.* **103**: 14P.

KAMYAB, S., LITTLETON, P. and FOTHERBY, K. (1967b) Metabolism and tissue distribution of norethisterone and norgestrel in rabbits. *J. Endocr.* **39**: 423–435.

KAMYAB, S., FOTHERBY, K. and KLOPPER, A. (1968a) Metabolism of 4-^{14}C-norethisterone in women. *J. Endocr.* **41**: 263–272.

KAMYAB, S., FOTHERBY, K. and KLOPPER, A. (1968b) Metabolism of 4-^{14}C-lynestrenol in man. *J. Endocr.* **42**: 337–343.

LANGECKER, H. (1961) Die Metabolite im menschlichen Harn nach Verabreichung von 17α-Aethinyl-19-nortestosteron (Noraethisteron). *Acta Endocr.* **37**: 14–18.

LANGECKER, H. (1968) Resorption, Verteilung und Ausscheidung der Gestagene. In: *Handbook of Experimental Pharmacology*, Vol. XXII, Die Gestagene, Part I, pp. 264–351. Springer Verlag, Berlin, Heidelberg, New York.

LAUMAS, K. R., MALKANI, P. K., BHATNAGAR, S. and LAUMAS, V. (1967) Radioactivity in the breast milk of lactating women after oral administration of ^{3}H-norethynodrel. *Amer. J. Obstet. Gynec.* **98**: 411–413.

LAURITZEN, C. and LEHMANN, W. D. (1967) Untersuchungen zur Ausscheidung von Hormonen mit der Muttermilch. *Arch. Gynäk.* **204**: 212–213.

LAYNE, D. S., GOLAB, T., ARAI, K. and PINCUS, G. (1963) The metabolic fate of orally administered ^{3}H-norethynodrel and ^{3}H-norethisterone in humans. *Biochem. Pharmac.* **12**: 905–911.

LEUSDEN, H. A. I. M. VAN (1970) Wat is er aan de hand met progestativa in de placenta? Een experimenteel onderzoek naar het lot van 9β,10α-steroiden (retrosteroiden) in de menselijke placenta. *Ned. T. Verlosk.* **70**: 349–358.

LITTLE, B., TAIT, J. F., TAIT, S. A. S. and ERLENMEYER, F. (1966) The metabolic clearance rate of progesterone in males and ovariectomized females. *J. Clin. Invest.* **45**: 901–912.

LITTLETON, P. and FOTHERBY, K. (1967) Metabolites of norgestrel (Wyeth 3707) in humans. *Acta Endocr., Suppl.* **119**: 162.

LITTLETON, P., FOTHERBY, K. and WILSON, G. (1967) Metabolism of norgestrel in humans. *Biochem. J.* **103**: 14P–15P.

LITTLETON, P., FOTHERBY, K. and DENNIS, K. J. (1968) Metabolism of ^{14}C-norgestrel in man. *J. Endocr.* **42**: 591–598.

MARTIN, A. P., HALTERMAN, D. R., VORBECK, M. L., KUO, M. C. and LUCAS, F. V. (1970) Metabolism of norethynodrel, a 19-nor-progestin. Subcellular localization of enzyme activity. *Steroids* **16**: 487–493.

MATSUYOSHI, K. (1967) Studies on metabolism of some progestational 19-norsteroids. *Folia Endocr. Jap.* **43**: 91–105.

MAZAHERI, A., FOTHERBY, K. and CHAPMAN, J. R. (1970) Metabolism of lynestrenol to norethisterone by liver homogenate. *J. Endocr.* **47**: 251–252.

MELI, A., WOLFF, A., LUCKER, W. E. and STEINETZ, B. G. (1965) The biological profile of progesterone 3-cyclopentyl enol ether as compared with that of progesterone. *Proc. Soc. Exp. Biol. Med.* **118**: 714–717.

MURATA, S. (1967) Metabolism of 17α-ethynyl-19-nortestosterone and 17α-ethynylestrenol *in vivo*. *Folia Endocr. Jap.* **43**: 1083–1096.

OGILVIE, M. L., CASIDA, L. E. and FIRST, N. L. (1965) Tissue incorporation and excretion of tritium-labelled progestins in rabbits, sheep and swine. *J. Animal Sci.* **24**: 1051–1060.

OKADA, H., AMATSU, M., ISHIHARA, S. and TOKUDA, G. (1964a) Conversion of some synthetic progestins to oestrogens. *Acta Endocr.* **46**: 31–36.

OKADA, H. MATSUYOSHI, K. and TOKUDA, G. (1964b) *In vitro* metabolism of 17α-methyl-19-nortestosterone by female rat liver homogenate. *Acta Endocr.* **46**: 40–46.

OKADA, H., OTA, S., TAKE, K. and YAMAMOTO, H. (1964c) Conversion of 17α-ethynyl-4-estrene-17β-ol to 17α-ethynyl-19-nortestosterone in rabbit liver. *Folia Endocr. Jap.* **40**: 1095–1098.

OKADA, H., IWASAKI, S., TAKE, H., MATSUYOSHI, K. and HOUKI, N. (1965) *In vitro* metabolism of 6-dehydro-retroprogesterone. I. Reduction of C-20 ketone. *Folia Endocr. Jap.* **41**: 856–859.

OKADA, H., HIGASHI, Y., NISHIMURA, T. and AHARA, M. (1968a) Metabolism of 6-dehydro-6-chloro-17α-acetoxyprogesterone in rabbit. *Folia Endocr. Jap.* **44**: 1103–1106.

OKADA, H., HIGASHI, Y., YAMAMOTO, H., SUMI, M. and AHARA, M. (1968b) Metabolism of 6-dehydro-progesterone in rabbit. *Folia Endocr. Jap.* **44**: 885–888.

OKADA, H., HAYASHI, H., YAMAMOTO, H., SUMI, M. and ISHIHARA, M. (1968c) Metabolism of 6-dehydro-retroprogesterone in rabbit. *Folia Endocr. Jap.* **44**: 15–18.

OKADA, H., SUMI, M., AHARA, M. and ISHIHARA, M. (1968d) Metabolism of 3-deoxo steroids in rabbit liver. II. Experiments with liver slices. *Folia Endocr. Jap.* **44**: 1274–1276.

ORINO, K. (1969) Hydrolysis of steroid esters *in vivo* and *in vitro*. *Folia Endocr. Jap.* **45**: 851–865.

PALMER, K. H., FEIERABEND, J. F., BAGGETT, B. and WALL, M. E. (1969a) Metabolic removal of a 17α-ethynyl group from the antifertility steroid, norethisterone. *J. Pharmac. Exp. Ther.* **167**: 217–222.

PALMER, K. H., ROSS, F. T., RHODES, L. S., BAGGETT, B. and WALL, M. E. (1969b Metabolism of antifertility steroids. I. Norethynodrel. *J. Pharmac. Exp. Ther.* **167**: 207–216.

PAULSEN, C. A. (1965) Progestin metabolism: special reference to oestrogenic pathways. *Metabolism* **14**: 313–319.

PAULSEN, C. A., LEACH, R. B., LANMAN, J., GOLDSTON, N., MADDOCK, W. O. and HELLER, C. G. (1962) Inherent estrogenicity of norethindrone and norethynodrel: comparison with other synthetic progestins and progesterone. *J. Clin. Endocr. Metab.* **22**: 1033–1039.

PETROW, V. (1966) Steroidal oral contraceptive agents. In: *Essays in Biochemistry*, Vol. II, pp. 117–145. Campbell, P. N. and Greville, G. D. (Eds.).

PINCUS, G., BIALY, G., LAYNE, D. S., PANIAGUA, M. and WILLIAMS, K. I. H. (1966) Radioactivity in the milk of subjects receiving radioactive 19-norsteroids. *Nature* **212**: 924–925.

QUINCEY, R. V. and GRAY, C. H. (1967) The metabolism of (1,2-^{3}H)-17α-methyltestosterone in human subjects. *J Endocr.* **37**: 37–55.

SCIAKY, R. (1962) 6-Hydroxy-6-methylsteroids. Note I: Synthesis of 6α-methyl-4-pregnene-6β,17α,21-triol-3,20-dione-21-acetate, a metabolite of 6α-methyl-17α-acetoxy-progesterone. *Gazz. chim. ital.* **92**: 539–548.

SEGALOFF, A., GABBARD, R. B., CARRIERE, B. T. and RONGONE, E. L. (1965) The metabolism of 4-^{14}C-methyltestosterone. *Steroids, Suppl.* **1**: 149–158.

SHAPIRO, E. L., LEGATT, T. and OLIVETO, E. P. (1964) 10-Hydroxy peroxy-19-norsteroids. *Tetrahedron Letters*: 663–667.

SINGER, F. M., JANUSCHKA, J. P., TAFT, A., YIACAS, E., LERNER, L. J. and BORMAN, A. (1965) Radioactive distribution of tritium-labelled acetophenone derivative of 16α,17α-dihydroxyprogesterone. *Proc. Soc. Exp. Biol. Med.* **118**: 1051–1054.

SLAUNWHITE, W. R. and SANDBERG, A. A. (1961) Disposition of radioactive 17α-hydroxyprogesterone, 6α-methyl-17α-acetoxyprogesterone and 6α-methyl-prednisolone in human subjects. *J. Clin. Endocr. Metab.* **21**: 753–764.

SMITH, D. L., PULLIAM, A. L. and FOREST, A. A. (1966) Comparative absorption of micronized and nonmicronized medroxyprogesterone acetate in man. *J. Pharmac. Sci.* **55**: 398–403.

THIJSSEN, J. H. H. (1967) The metabolism of progestational compounds. Ph.D. Thesis, Utrecht.

TOKUDA, G., MURAKAMI, A, HIGASHIYAMA, S., MIZOGUCHI, S., IWASAKI, S., KOBAYASHI, H. and ORINO, K. (1967) Biological effects of 17α-ethynyl-4-estrene-3β,17β-diol diacetate. *Folia Endocr. Jap.* **43**: 905–914.

TOWNSLEY, J. D., POSSANZA, G. and BRODIE, H. J. (1966) A new placental metabolite of oestr-4-ene-3,17-dione: a possible source of error in oestrogen estimation. *Biochem. J.* **101**: 25c–27c.

TOWNSLEY, J. D. and BRODIE, H. J. (1967) Studies on the mechanism of estrogen biosynthesis. IV. Ovarian metabolism of estr-4-ene-3,17-dione. *Biochim. Biophys. Acta* **144**: 440–445.

VAN DER MOLEN, H. J., HART, P. G. and WIJMENGA, H. G. (1969) Studies with 4-^{14}C-lynestrenol in normal and lactating women. *Acta Endocr.* **61**: 255–274.

VAN DER MOLEN, H. J., WIEDHAUP, K. and WIJMENGA, H. G. (1971) Clearance and metabolism of some contraceptive steroids in normal and lactating women. *Proceedings of the Third International Congress on Hormonal Steroids*. Excerpta Medica Foundation Internat. Congress Series no. 219, pp. 898–906.

WANG, D. Y., BULBROOK, R. D., SNEDDON, A. and HAMILTON, T. (1967a) The metabolic clearance rates of dehydroepiandrosterone, testosterone and their sulphate esters in man, rat and rabbits. *J. Endocr.* **38**: 307–318.

WANG, D. Y., BULBROOK, R. D., ELLIS, F. and COOMBS, M. M. (1967b) Metabolic clearance rates of pregnenolone, 17α-acetoxypregnenolone and their sulphate esters in man and rabbit. *J. Endocr.* **39**: 395–403.

WATANABE, H., SAHA, N. N. and LAYNE, D. S. (1968) Distribution of radioactivity in rat tissues after administration of tritiated 17α-ethynyl-19-norsteroids. *Steroids* **11**: 97–101.

YAMAMOTO, H. (1968) Metabolism of 17α-ethynyl-estrenol in rabbit. *Folia Endocr. Jap.* **44**: 1309–1319.

SECTION EDITOR'S NOTE

THE reader is reminded that Chapters 23 and 24 of Volume I also contain data on the effects of orally active synthetic substitutes for progesterone in the human.

CHAPTER 30

ORALLY ACTIVE PROGESTATIONAL COMPOUNDS. HUMAN STUDIES: EFFECTS ON THE UTERO-VAGINAL TRACT

J. Ferin

Department of Obstetrics and Gynecology,
University Hospital, Belgium

A. PROGESTATIONAL POTENCY

I. EFFECTS ON THE ENDOMETRIUM

As has been pointed out before (see Chapters 22 and 26), the complete secretory transformation of the estrogen-primed endometrium is, according to the present state of our knowledge, the only truly specific effect of progesterone. Any compound which can bring about this transformation in a woman without endogenous progesterone production will therefore be called progestational. Table 1 lists the compounds we have so defined. Our bibliography is representative, but by no means exhaustive. We have selected references concerning particularly well-documented observations.

TABLE 1. COMPOUNDS HAVING PROGESTATIONAL ACTIVITY ON ORAL ADMINISTRATION IN THE HUMAN

Trivial name
(Generic name)
[Systematic name]

A. Progesterone derivatives

    Progesterone cyclopentyl enol ether
    (Quingesterone)
        (Hecht-Lucari and Scarpellini, 1961)
        (Klopper, 1961)
    9-α-Bromo-11-ketoprogesterone
        (Wied and Davis, 1957)

(continued overleaf)

TABLE 1—cont.

6,17α-Dimethyl-6-dehydro-progesterone
(Medrogestone)
[6,17α-Dimethyl-4,6-pregnadiene-3,20-dione]
   (Carter et al., 1964)

B. 17-alpha-Hydroxyprogesterone derivatives

17α-Hydroxy-progesterone caproate
   (Boschann and Drews, 1961)
17α-Acetoxyprogesterone
[17α-Hydroxy-4-pregnene-3,20-dione acetate]
   (Goldzieher et al., 1958)
   (Davis and Wied, 1957)
17α-Acetoxyprogesterone 3-cyclopentyl-enol ether
   (Loskant, 1966)
6α-Methyl-17α-acetoxyprogesterone
(Medroxyprogesterone acetate)
[17α-Hydroxy-6α-methyl-4-pregnene-3,20-dione acetate]
   (Boschann and Drews, 1961)
   (Wied and Davis, 1963)
6-Chloro-17α-acetoxy-6-dehydro-progesterone
(Chlormadinone acetate)
[6-Chloro-17α-hydroxy-pregna-4,6-diene-3,20-dione acetate]
   (Martinez-Manautou et al., 1962)
[17α-Hydroxy-1,2α-methylene-6α-chloro-pregna-4,6-diene-3,20-dione acetate]
   (Vokaer and Kridelka, 1963)
[17α-Hydroxy-9α-fluoro-11-hydroxy-16-methylene-4-pregnene-3,20-dione acetate]
   (Nevinny-Stickel, 1963)
[17α-Hydroxy-6α-methyl-pregna-1,4-diene-3,20-dione]
   (Martinez-Manautou et al., 1962)
[17α-Hydroxy-6α-chloro-pregna-1,4-diene-3,20-dione]
   (Martinez-Manautou et al., 1962)
[17α-Hydroxy-6α-methyl-pregna-4,6-diene-3,20-dione]
   (Martinez-Manautou et al., 1962)
6-Dehydro-6-methyl-17-acetoxyprogesterone
(Megestrol acetate)
[17α-Hydroxy-6α-methyl-4,6-pregna-diene-3,20-dione acetate]
   (Greenblatt et al., 1963)
   (Østergaard, 1965)

C. Nor-progesterone derivatives

17α-Hydroxy-nor-progesterone acetate
   (Nevinny-Stickel, 1962)

D. Retro-progesterone derivatives

6-Dehydroretroprogesterone
(Dydrogesterone)
[9α,10α-Pregna-4,6-diene-3,20-dione]
   (Tillinger and Diczfalusy, 1960)
   (Vokaer and Ferin, 1961)

TABLE 1—*cont.*

[6-Chloro-9β,10α-pregna-1,4,6-triene-3,20-dione]
(Ferin, unpublished results)

E. Testosterone derivatives

17-ethynyltestosterone
(Ethisterone)
[17α-ethynyl-17β-4-androsten-3-one]
(Ferin, 1954)
(Davis and Wied, 1957)
6α:21-Dimethyl-ethynyltestosterone
(Dimethisterone)
[17β-Hydroxy-6α-methyl-17-propinyl-4-androsten-3-one]
(Douglas, 1959)

F. Retro-testosterone derivatives

[17α-(2'-Methallyl)-9β,10α-4,6-androsta-diene-17-ol-3-one]
(Ferin, unpublished results)

G. 19-Nortestosterone derivatives

1. *Derivatives of $\triangle^4$-estrenolone*
   19-Nor-17α-ethynyltestosterone
   (Norethindrone)
   [17α-Ethynyl-17β-hydroxy-4-estren-3-one]
   (Hertz *et al.*, 1956)
   (Pots, 1957)
   19-Nor-17-ethynyltestosterone acetate
   (Nor-ethindrone acetate)
   (Pots, 1958)
   19-Nor-17-methyltestosterone or 17-methyl-estrenolone
   (Nor-methandrolone)
   [17α-Methyl-17β-hydroxy-4-estren-3-one]
   (Ferin, 1957b)
   (Netter *et al.*, 1957)
   19-Nor-17-ethyltestosterone
   (Nor-ethandrolone)
   [17α-Ethyl-17β-hydroxy-4-estren-3-one]
   (Kaiser, 1957)
   (Epstein *et al.*, 1958)
   19-Nor-17-propynyltestosterone
   17α-Propynyl-17β-hydroxy-4-estrene-3-one]
   (Ferin and Schlikker, unpublished results)
   19-Nor-17-ethynyltestosterone diacetate
   (Ethynodiol diacetate)
   [17α-Ethynyl-4-estren-3β,17β-diol diacetate]
   (Ferin, unpublished results)
   (Ferin and Schlikker, unpublished results)
   (Norgestrienone)
   [17α-ethynyl-17β-hydroxy-4,9,11-estratriene-3-one]
   (Netter *et al.*, 1967)
   (Ferin and Mingeot, unpublished results)   (*continued overleaf*)

1. *Derivatives of* $\triangle^4$-*estrenolone*—*cont.*
18-Homonorethisterone
(Norgestrel, dl)
[d-13β-Ethyl-17α-ethynyl-17β-hydroxy-gon-4-ene-3-one]
    (Ferin, unpublished results)
 	
2. *Derivatives* of $\triangle^{5(10)}$-*estrenolone*
(Norethynodrel)
[17α-Ethynyl-17β-hydroxy-5(10)-estren-3-one]
    (Epstein *et al.*, 1958)
17-Vinylestrenolone
(Norvinodrel)
[17α-Vinyl-17β-hydroxy-estr-5(10)-en-3-one]
    (D'Incerti Bonini and Pagani, 1962)
    (Ferin and Schlikker, unpublished results)
 	
3. *Derivatives of estrenol*
17-Ethynyl-estrenol or 17-ethynyl-3-desoxy-nortestosterone
(Lynestrenol)
[17α-Ethynl-17β-hydroxy-4-estrene]
    (Nevinny-Stickel, 1963)
    (Ferin, unpublished results)
    (Ferin and Schlikker, unpublished results)
 	
    17-Ethynyl-estrenol acetate
        (Ferin and Schlikker, unpublished results)
    17-Allyl-estrenol
        (Nevinny-Stickel, 1963)
    17-Ethyl-estrenol
        (Nevinny-Stickel, 1963)
        (Ferin and Schlikker, unpublished results)
    17-Propargyl-estrenol
        (Ferin and Schlikker, unpublished results)

Quantitative comparison of the endometrial progestational activity of the various compounds is difficult. Endogenous estrogen should be very low and progesterone production should be virtually nil. The ovariectomized woman is therefore undoubtedly the ideal subject for these studies. The following conditions must be strictly adhered to in order to obtain valid results.

1. The genital tract should be in a state of maximum sensitivity. The effects of prolonged estrogen deprivation should be eliminated by artificial cycles induced before the test treatments.

2. Estrogen priming must be adequate. When this priming has been strongly reduced or suppressed, as by the use of the combined type of oral contraception—in this case because of the antiestrogenic effect of the

progestational substance—secretory transformation is very incomplete; after stunted proliferative and early secretory phases the glands undergo rapid involution. The spiral arteries are undeveloped or underdeveloped. Venous lakes appear in the stroma, which becomes edematous and finally undergoes decidual transformation, mostly localized and not accompanied by the development of the dense reticulin network that characterizes the normal premenstrual endometrium (Waidl et al., 1968). This has been shown by many workers in this field (Rock et al., 1957; Pincus et al., 1958; Maqueo et al., 1963; Rice-Wray et al., 1963; Roland et al., 1964; Goldzieher and Rice-Wray, 1966).

Estrogen priming should be uniform, by the administration of identical doses of the same estrogen during a fixed period of time.

3. The same strict conditions should apply to estrogen treatment *during* the administration of the progestational compound; the same dosage of the same estrogen should always be given.

Estrogen loading before and during progestational treatment is probably an important factor in determining the endometrial response and for each dose of estrogen there is an optimum dose of the gestagen. It is certain that an excess of estrogen during the estrogen–progestational phase of the artificial cycle causes pronounced morphological disturbances of the endometrium (Ferin and Schlikker, 1960; Ferin, 1963; Ferin, 1966) (Table 2). Similar phenomena are seen in women with normal cycles who receive large doses of estrogens after ovulation (Morris and Van Wagenen, 1966).

On the other hand, too little estrogen during the estrogen–progestational phase of the artificial cycle can easily provoke break-through bleeding (Ferin, 1954a).

In castrated monkeys (*Macaca mulatta*) an equilibrated action of estradiol and progesterone is needed to produce a normal secretory differentiation of the endometrium (Good and Mayer, 1968).

In view of possible individual variations in sensitivity to progestational substances, particularly those due to differences in body weight (Good and Mayer, 1968) (volume of fat tissue?), any compounds which are to be compared should be given to the same woman in succession, if possible in different doses.

The practical execution of such a program may be extremely difficult and valid studies are therefore rare. The number of patients studied is always too small to permit a statistical evaluation. To some extent this deficiency may be compensated by a greater number of cycles induced in the same woman.

Responsiveness to estrogens and gestagens appears not to change with

TABLE 2. EXPERIMENTAL ESTROGENIC EXCESS IN OVARIECTOMIZED WOMEN

Estrogenic priming: 1st–14th days: 0.05 mg ethynyl-estradiol (E.E.).
Progestational treatment: constant dose, from day 15 to day 28.
(Ferin and Schlikker, 1960; Ferin, 1963; Ferin, 1966; Ferin and Mingeot, unpublished results.)

	Progestational treatment, daily dosage	Daily dosage of estrogen (E.E.), from day 15 to day 28	Endometrium
Patient no. 4	Ethisterone 500 mg	0.1 mg	Late secretory
	Ethisterone 500 mg	0.25 mg	Slightly atypical*
	Ethisterone 500 mg	0.5 mg	Pattern of 18th–19th days
Patient no. 1	Norethisterone 5 mg	0.05 mg	Late secretory
	Norethisterone 5 mg	0.1 mg	Late secretory
	Norethisterone 5 mg	0.25 mg	Atypical*
Patient no. 2	Norethisterone 5 mg	0.05 mg	Late secretory
	Norethisterone 5 mg	0.1 mg	Late secretory
	Norethisterone 5 mg	0.25 mg	Atypical*
Patient no. 1	Chlormadinone 5 mg	0.025 mg	Late secretory
	Chlormadinone 5 mg	0.05 mg	Late secretory
	Chlormadinone 5 mg	0.1 mg	Late secretory
	Chlormadinone 5 mg	0.25 mg	Late secretory
Patient no. 6	Dydrogesterone 17.5 mg	0.05 mg	Late secretory
	Dydrogesterone 17.5 mg	0.25 mg (from day 1)	Pattern of 18th–19th days

* The atypical endometrial pattern has been described in Chapter 22.: reduction or disappearance of the excretory phenomena; elliptic form of the glandular nuclei; superficial spiral arterioles and sometimes predecidual and granular stromal cells. Similar patterns have been observed by Wied and Davis (1961) after excessive estrogenic priming.
Delay in the secretory transformations has been observed in cyclic women receiving large doses of stilbestrol after ovulation (Morris and Van Wagenen, 1966).

age. This is at least the present author's personal experience, covering a period of 30 years.

In none of the studies published so far has sufficient attention been paid to size and shape of crystals of active substances, administered orally, yet these factors might greatly influence intestinal absorption. It has been shown that micronization increases urinary excretion of the metabolite of medroxyprogesterone acetate during the first 8 hours following its administration (Smith et al., 1966).

The influence of the distribution of doses throughout the day has not been studied, nor has enough distinction been made between perlingual and gastro-intestinal routes of absorption. The existence of a significant difference between the effectiveness of these ways of absorption cannot be excluded *a priori*.

Comparative studies of the endometrial effects of progestational substances have been done mainly by two different methods. *The first* consists in producing the endometrial characteristics of the estrogen–progesterone phase in ovariectomized women. Two tests (called short test and long test) have been used to study this phenomenon. In the short test one tries to establish the dose needed to induce a massive glycogen deposition in the endometrial glands (Ferin, 1954) (Table 3). The result is easy to interpret. The final, semi-quantitative, criterion is the volume and the number of vacuoles at the base of the glandular cells, taking the place of glycogen deposits which have been removed by the fixation fluid. Although this reaction is not fully specific for progestational substances (see Chapter 22) it is nevertheless produced by all of them.

The aim in the long test is to determine the dose of a compound that will induce complete secretory transformation of the endometrium (Tables 4, 5, 6). The final interpretation of the result is not simple. Attention should be paid to the intensity of the process of secretion, the shape of the glands and in particular the occurrence of connective tissue projections into the glands ("tufts" or "thorns" of connective tissue), shape and position of nuclei of the epithelial cells, development of the spiral arteries, degree of interstitial edema and differentiation of the fibroblasts into predecidual cells or endometrial granulocytes.

According to some authors (Nevinny-Stickel, 1963) different progestational substances act differently on the various endometrial structures, glands, arteries and stroma. Medroxyprogesterone acetate, for example, is reported to influence glandular transformation more than decidualization of the stroma, in contrast with alkyl derivatives of 3-desoxy-nor-testosterone, described as acting predominantly on the stroma. These

TABLE 3. PROGESTATIONAL ACTIVITY OF VARIOUS STEROIDS AT THE ENDOMETRIAL LEVEL COMPARATIVE ASSAYS IN OVARIECTOMIZED WOMEN

End point: endometrial glandular subnuclear vacuolization ("short test").
Graded response 1+ to 4+:
  1+ a small vacuole in several cells of a few glandular sections.
  2+ a vacuole in several cells of the majority of glandular sections.
  3+ a vacuole in all the glandular cells.
  4+ a large vacuole in all the glandular cells.

Estrogenic priming: 0.05 mg ethynyl-estradiol daily, day 1 to day 20.
Progestational treatment: x mg daily, day 16 to day 20.
Endometrial biopsy: on day 20 or 21.
Interval of 8 to 10 days between each course.
Three selected ovariectomized women: V.d.H.; V.A.; D. (Body weights, respectively: 75–90 kg; 60–70 kg.; 48–50 kg.) D is patient 4 in Tables 2 and 6 and V.d.H. is patient 5 in Table 6.

Asterisk(*) denotes compounds whose progestational activity in the human species is uncertain. (Ferin, 1957; Ferin, 1960; Ferin, 1962a; Ferin, unpublished results.)

		V.d.H.	V.A.	D.
A. Progesterone and progesterone derivatives				
Progesterone intramuscularly	5mg			3+
	2			0
Sublingually	150		1+	
	100	0	0	1+
	50		0	
	25	0		
Progesterone cyclopentylenolether orally	75		2+	
	50		1+	
	25			1+
6,17α-Dimethyl-6-dehydro-progesterone orally	5		4+	4+
B. 17α-Hydroxyprogesterone derivatives				
17α-Hydroxyprogesterone* orally	500	0		
	300			0
17α-Acetoxyprogesterone orally	50		0	
	25		0	
6α-Methyl-17α-acetoxyprogesterone orally (Medroxyprogesterone acetate)	5		2+	
	2.5	3+	2+	1+
	1.25	2+	0	0
6-Chloro-17α-acetoxy-6-dehydro-progesterone (chlormadinone acetate) orally	3		3+	
	2	3+	1+	
	1	2+	0	3+
	0.5	2+	0, 0	2+,2+,0
	0.1	0		0

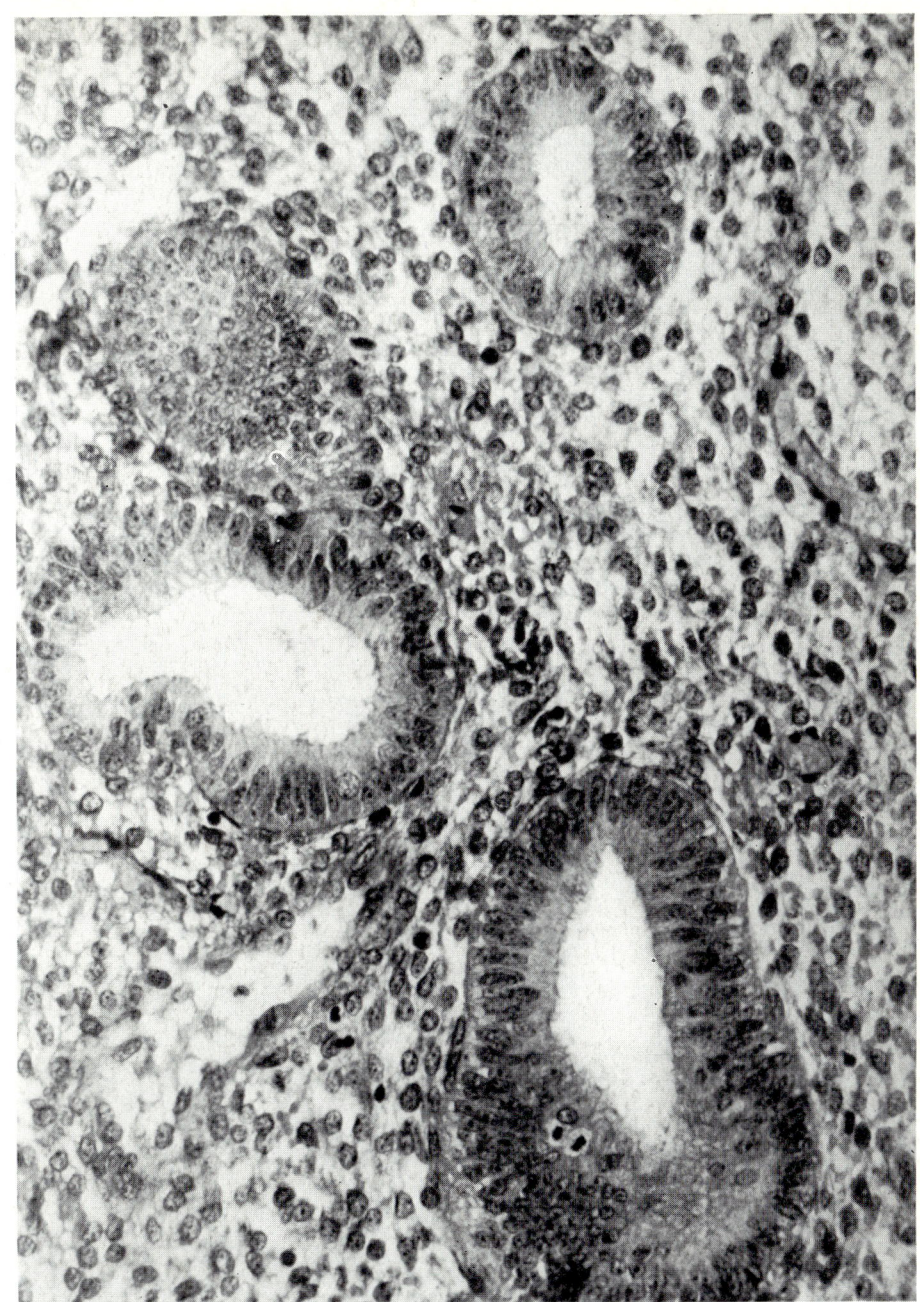

FIG. 1. Patient V.A. (V.A.; Table 3). Day 1 to day 20: 0.05 mg ethynyl-estradiol. Day 16 to day 20: 50 mg quingesterone. No. 98.527: proliferative endometrial glands. Small basal vacuoles in several glandular cells (Type 1+ of response in the so-called "short test"). High-power view (magnification 620×). Fixation in Bouin's fluid.

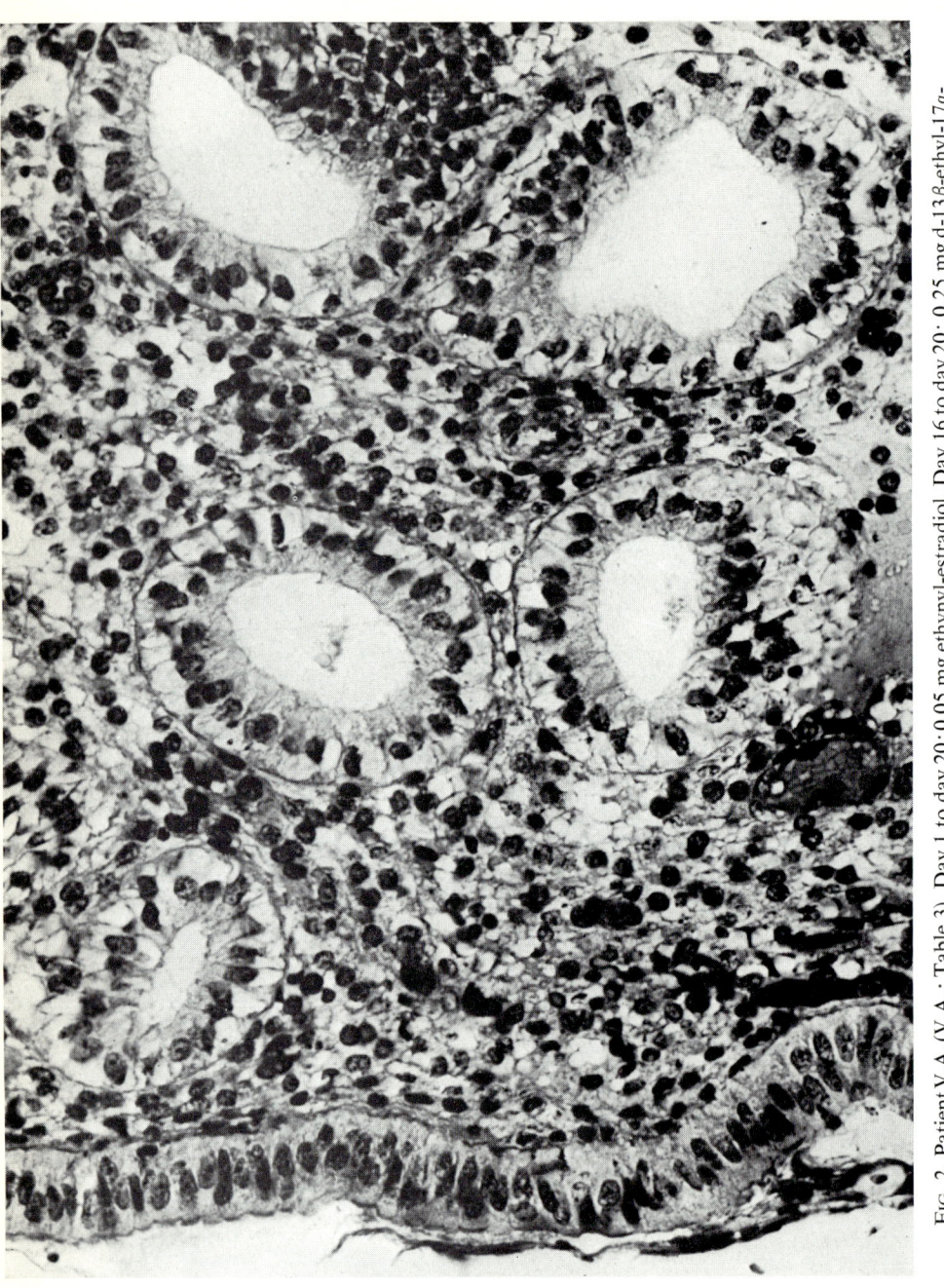

FIG. 2. Patient V.A. (V.A.; Table 3). Day 1 to day 20: 0.05 mg ethynyl-estradiol. Day 16 to day 20: 0.25 mg d-13β-ethyl-17α-ethynyl-17-hydroxy-gon-4-ene-3-one (d-Norgestrel). No. 99,801: large basal vacuole in each glandular cell (Type 4+ of response in the so-called "short test"). High-power view (magnification 620×). Fixation in Bouin's fluid.

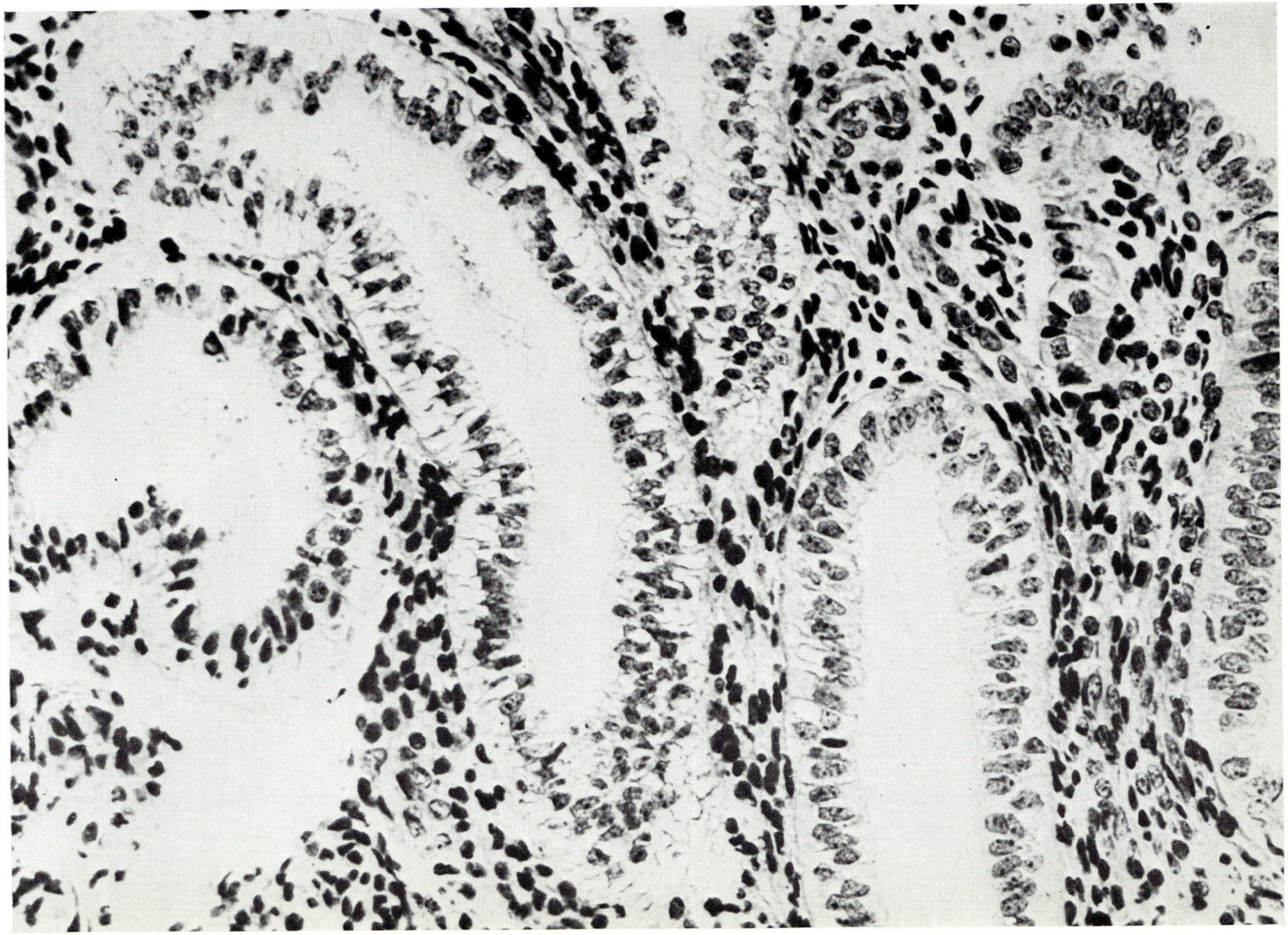

FIG. 3. Patient V.A. Idem.

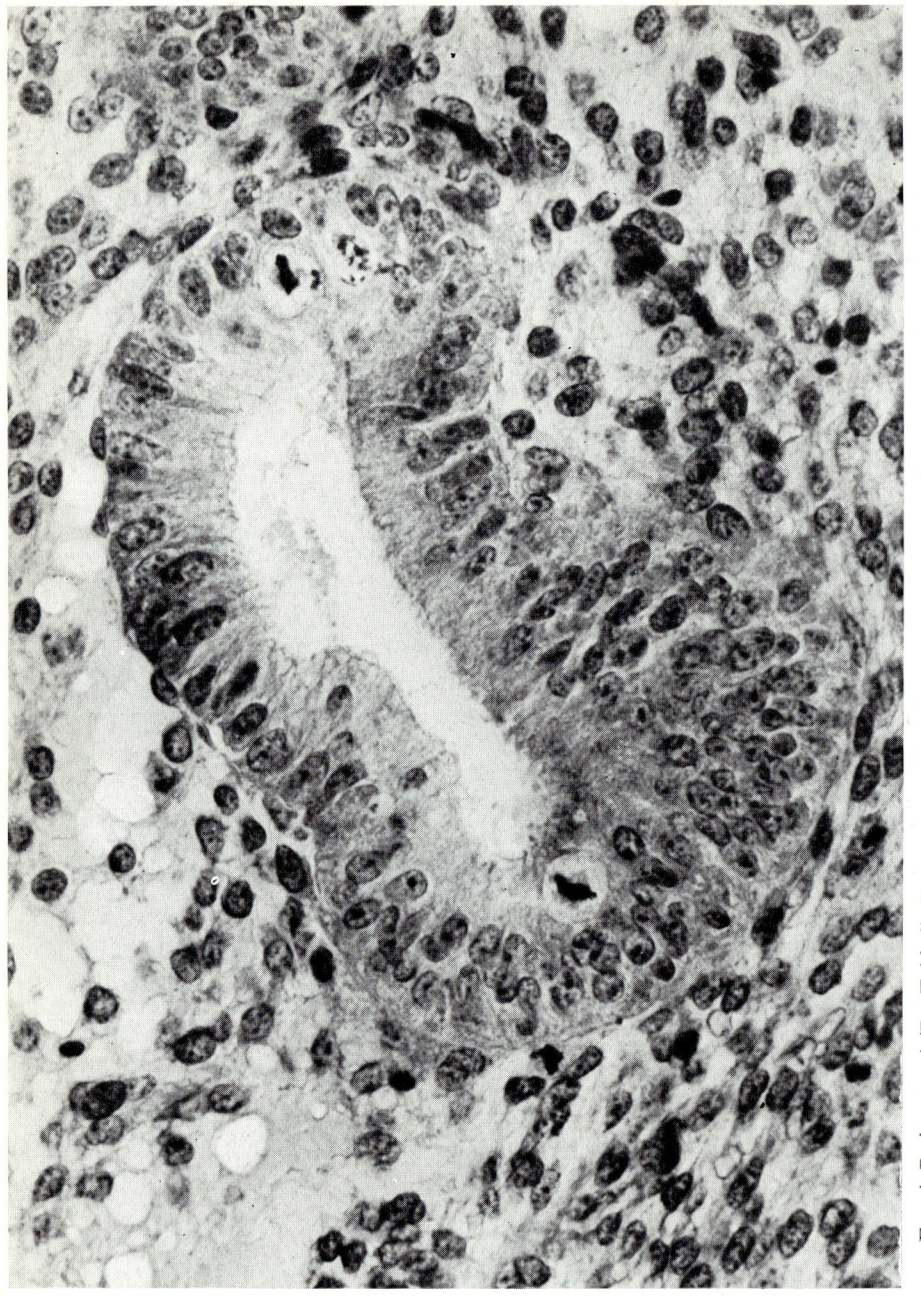

FIG. 4. Patient no. 4 (D.; Table 3). Day 1 to day 20: 0.05 mg ethynyl-estradiol. Day 16 to day 20: 1 mg 17α-(2'-methallyl)-17-hydroxy-9β,10α-androsta-4,6-diene-3-one. No. 86.554: proliferative gland. Absence of basal vacuolization (Type O of response in the so-called "short test"). High-power view (magnification 1000×). Fixation in Bouin's fluid.

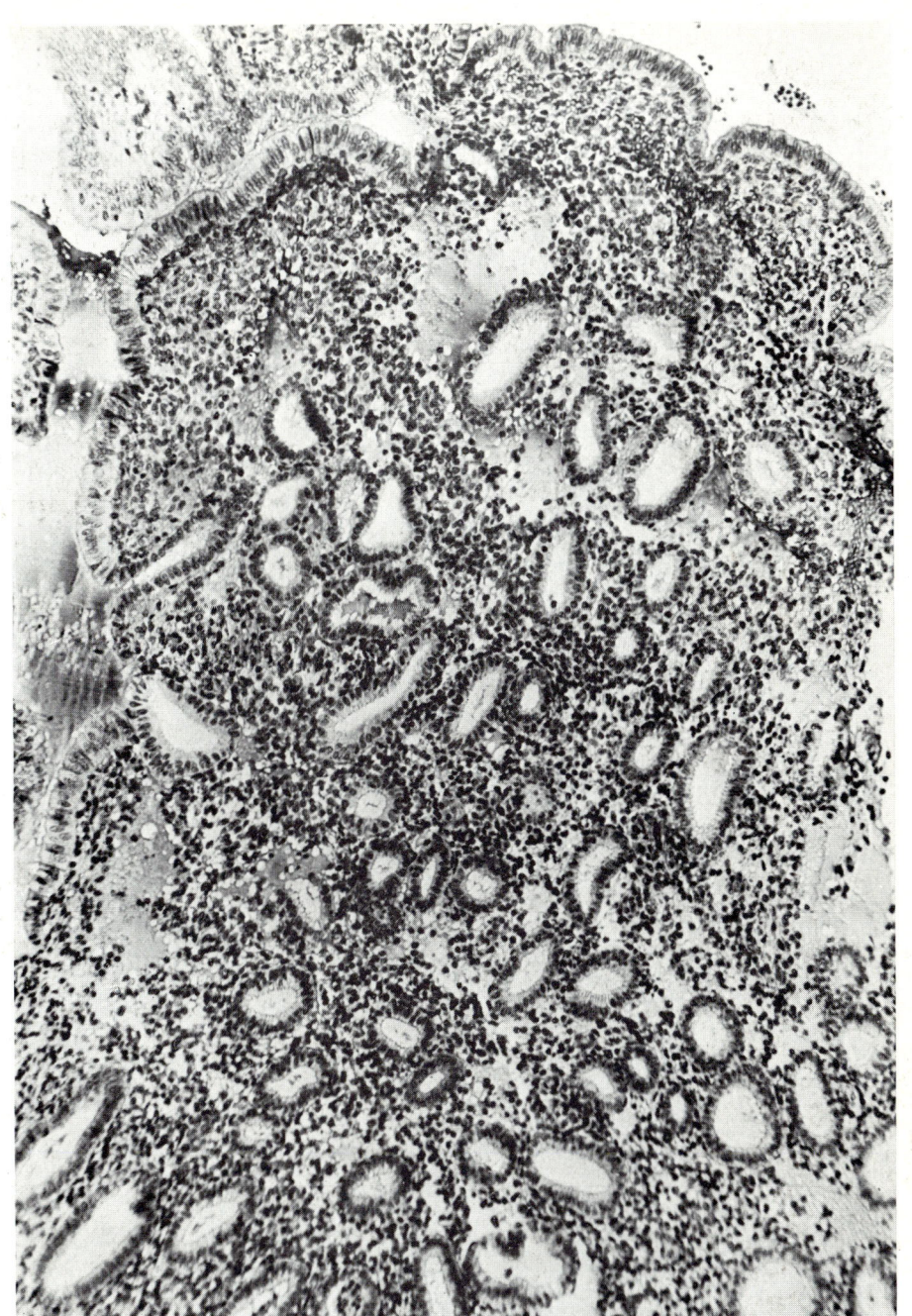

Fig 5. Patient no. 6 (Table 6). Day 1 to day 28: 0.05 mg ethynyl-estradiol. Day 15 to day 28: 0.25 mg norgestrienone. No. 12.240: inadequate secretory changes. Small glandular sections with elliptic nuclei. No arteriolar fields. Low-power view (magnification 250×). Fixation in Bouin's fluid.

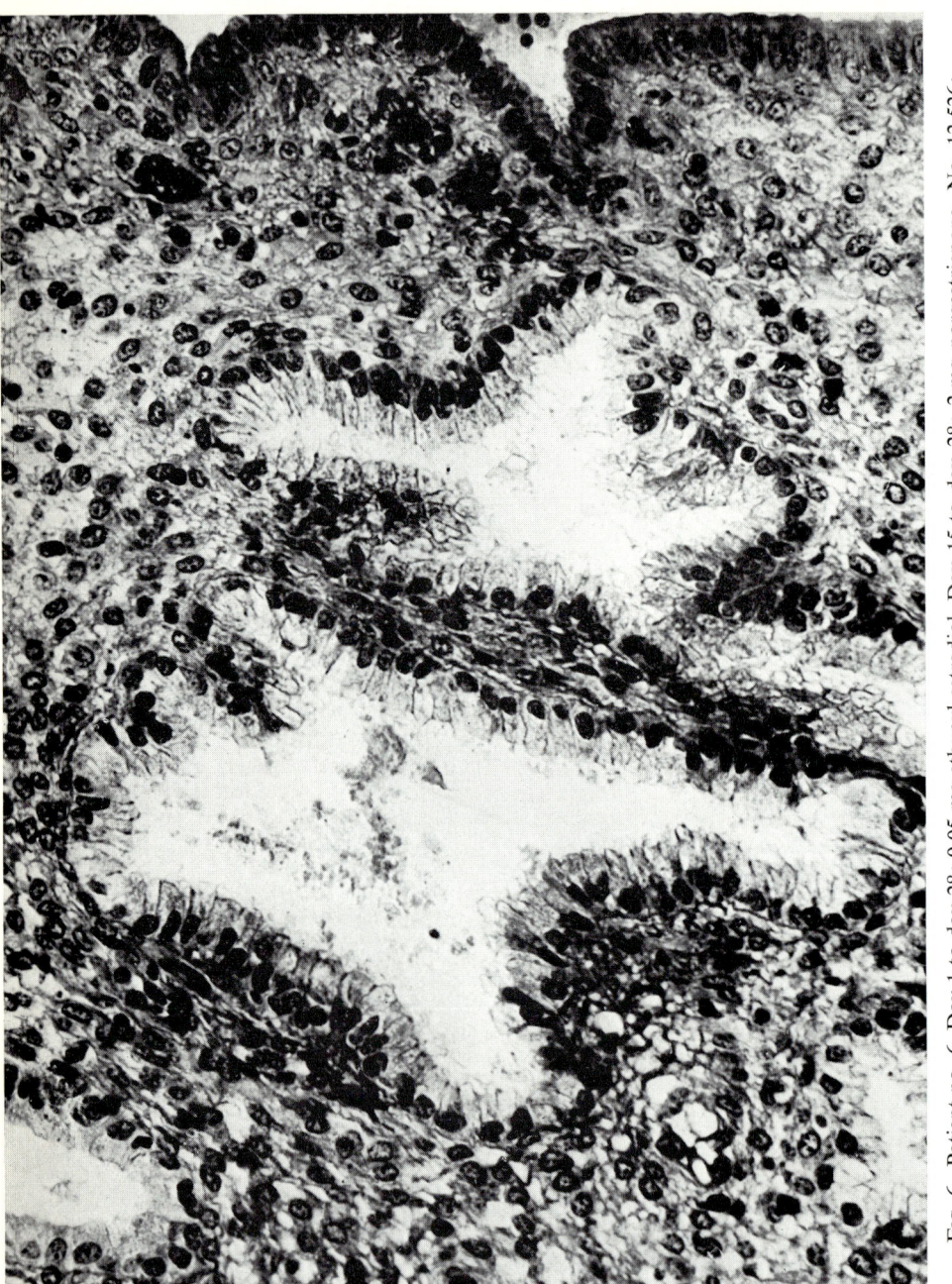

Fig 6. Patient no. 6. Day 1 to day 28: 0.05 mg ethynyl-estradiol. Day 15 to day 28: 2 mg norgestrienone. No. 12.526: adequate secretory changes. Large glandular sections with round basal nuclei. Secretory material in glandular lumina. Some small tuft-like invaginations distorting the glandular walls. High-power view (magnification 620×). Fixation in Bouin's fluid.

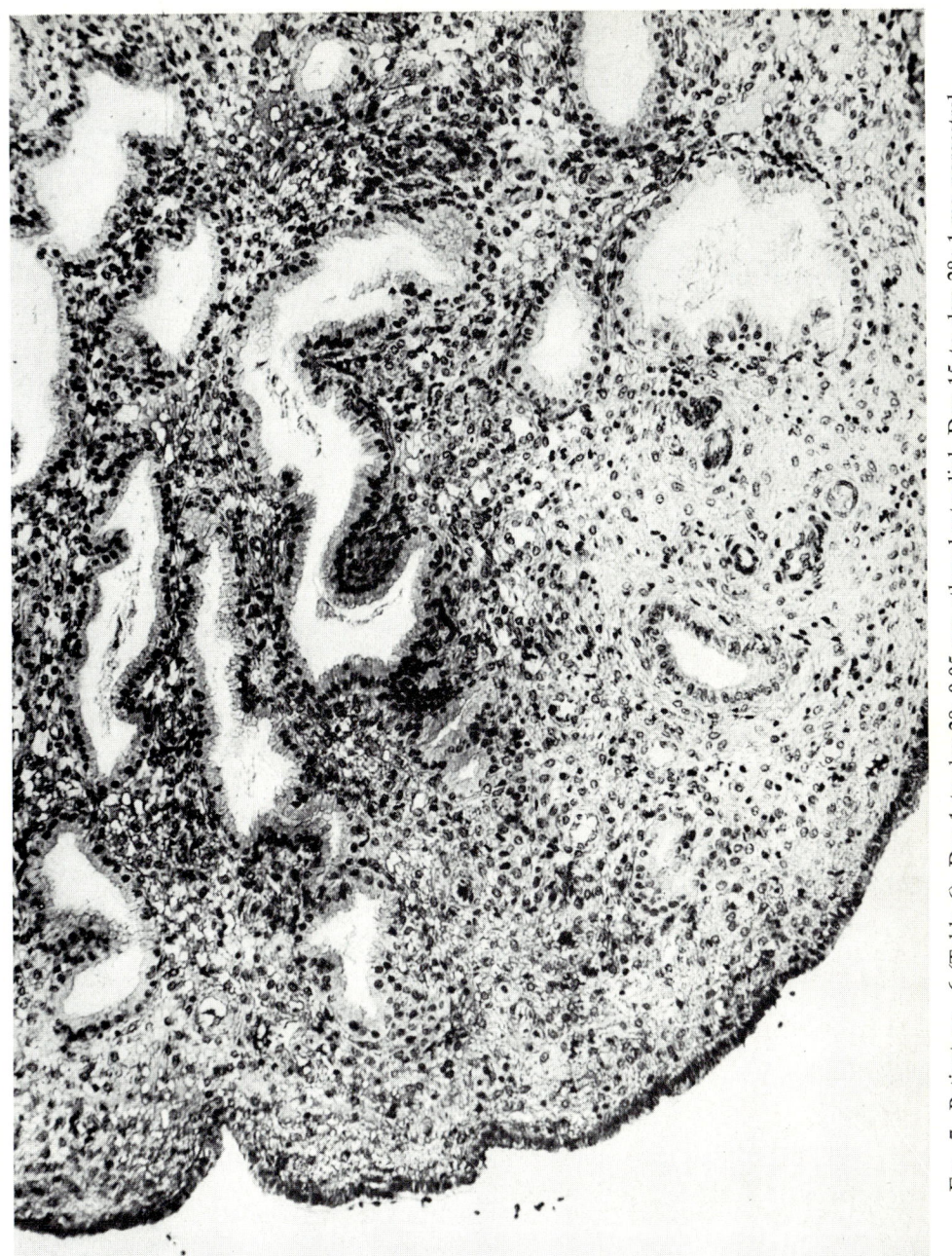

FIG. 7. Patient no. 6 (Table 6). Day 1 to day 28: 0.05 mg ethynyl-estradiol. Day 15 to day 28: 1 mg norgestrel. No. 12.929: adequate secretory changes. Large glandular sections with round basal nuclei. Superficial arteriolar field. Low-power view (magnification 250×). Fixation in Bouin's fluid.

Orally Active Progestational Compounds: Human Studies

TABLE 3—cont.

		V.d.H.	V.A.	D.
B. 17α-Hydroxyprogesterone derivatives—cont.				
6-Methyl-17α-acetoxy-6-dehydro-progesterone (Megestrol acetate)				
orally	2		2+	
	1		0	
	0.5		0	1+
6,16α-Dimethyl-6-dehydro-17α-acetoxy-progesterone*				
orally	1	0	0	
9α-Fluoro-17α-acetoxy-4-pregnene-3,11,20-trione*				
orally	1	0	0	0
3,17α-Dihydroxy-16-methylene-2,4,6-pregnatriene-20-one-diacetate*				
orally	10		0	0
	6	0		0
	1.5	0	0	0
	0.75			0
C. Nor-progesterone derivatives	25			
19-Nor-progesterone	2			4+
intramuscularly	0.5			4+
	0.1			3+
				0
17α-Acetoxy-4,6-19-nor-pregnadiene-3,20-dione*				
orally	25		0	
	15		0	
D. Retro-progesterone derivatives				
6-Dehydroretroprogesterone (Dydrogesterone)				
orally	10		1+	
	5		0	
	2.5	1+	0	2+
	2	1+,2+,2+		
	1	1+		1+
	0.5	0		
6-Chloro-9β,10α-1,4,6-pregnatriene-3,20-dione				
orally	2	3+	2+	2+
	1	2+	0	0
6-Chloro-9β,10α-4,6-pregnadiene-3,20-dione*				
orally	4	4+		
	2		0	0
	1	1		0

(continued overleaf)

TABLE 3—cont.

		V.d.H.	V.A.	D.
D. Retro-progesterone derivatives—*cont.*				
16α,17α-isopropylidenedihydroxy-9β,10α-4,6-pregnadiene-3,20-dione*				
orally	1	0	0	0
16α-Ethoxy-9β,10α-4,6-pregnadiene-3,20-dione*				
orally	10	0		0
	5		0	
E. Testosterone derivatives				
17α-Methyl-testosterone				
sublingually	50		0	
	30			2+,2+
Ethisterone				
sublingually	100		3+	
	50	1+	1+	3+
	25	0	0	0
6α-21-Dimethyl-ethisterone				
sublingually	10		0	1+
	5	0	0	0
orally	25	1+	1+	
F. Retrotestosterone derivatives				
17α-(2'-Methallyl)-9β,10α-androst-4-en-17-ol-3-one*	25	3+		
	5		0	0
orally	1	0	0	
17α-(2'-Methallyl)-9β,10α-4,6-androstadiene-17-ol-3-one				
orally	5		2+	
	2.5	4+		
	1	2+		0
G. 19-Nor-testosterone derivatives				
1. *Derivatives of △⁴-estrenolone*				
17α-Methyl				
(Normethandrone)				
sublingually	75			
	25	4+	4+	4+
	12.5	4+	4+	4+
	5		4+	4+
	2	4+		
	1		2+	4+
	0.5	3+	2+	4+
	0.3	1+		3+
	0.2	0	0	
	0.1	0	0	0
orally	10	4+		
	1	4+	2+	4+
	0.5		0	
intramuscularly	0.5			4+

TABLE 3—cont.

		V.d.H.	V.A.	D.
G. 19-Nor-testosterone derivatives—cont.				
1. Derivatives of $\triangle^4$-estrenolone—cont.				
17α-Ethyl (Norethandrolon)	25		4+	
sublingually	2	4+	3+	3+
	1	4+	1+	
	0.5	1+	0	0
17α-Ethynyl (Norethisterone)	10	4+	4+	
sublingually	1	4+	4+	
	0.2	3+	1+	4+
	0.1	2+	0	0
	0.05	0	0	
17α-Ethynyl-17-acetate (Norethisterone acetate)	1		3+	
sublingually	0.5		1+	4+
	0.1	2+	0	3+
	0.05	0		0
17α-(2 Methallyl)*				
sublingually	1	2+	0	0
orally	2		0	0
17α-Propynyl				
sublingually	1	3+		3+
	0.3	2+	0	2+
	0.1	0		0
orally	1		2+	
16β-Hydroxy-16α-n-propyl-19-nor-testosterone acetate*				
sublingually	2.5		2+	2+
	1	3+	2+	2+
17α-Ethynyl diacetate (Ethynodiol diacetate)				
orally	0.3		2+	
	0.1	3+	0	2+
	0.05	0	0	0
17α-ethynyl-17β-hydroxy-estra-4,9,11-trien-3-one (Nor-gestrienone)	0.25			0
orally	0.05		0	
2. Derivatives of $\triangle^{5(10)}$-estrenolone				
17α-ethyl (Norethynodrel), so-called "pure" norethynodrel, with an undetermined amount of ethynyl-estradiol-3-methyl ether (EEME)				
orally	20	4+	4+	
	2	4+	1+	4+
	1	0	0	0
17α-Vinyl (Norvinodrel)				
sublingually	1	3+, 4+	2+	3+

(continued overleaf)

TABLE 3—cont.

		V.d.H.	V.A.	D.
G. 19-Nor-testosterone derivatives—*cont.*				
3. *Derivatives of estrenol*				
17α-Methyl				
sublingually		2		3+	4+
		1	3+	1+	4+
orally		2		3+	
		0.3	2+	0	1+
		0.1	0		
17α-Ethyl				
sublingually		2.5		2+, 3+	
		1	4+	0	2+
		0.5	1+		0
		0.25	0		
17α-Propyl*				
sublingually		10	3+		3+
		5	2+		
		2	0		
		1			0
orally		10		0	
		1		0	
17α-Allyl (Allylestrenol)				
sublingually		15		1+	
		10		0	2+
		5	4+,3+,4+	0	0
		3			0
		2		0	0
		1	0		
orally		10	4+		
17α-Ethynyl (Lynestrenol)				
sublingually		5	4+	4+	4+
		2.5		4+	
		1	4+	2+	3+
		0.3	3+	1+	2+
		0.125			0
		0.1	1+	0	1+
		0.05	0		0
orally		0.25		2+	4+
17α-Ethynyl acetate				
orally		0.5	4+	2+	2+
		0.1	0	0	0
17α-Ethynyl-6α-methyl*				
sublingually		1	2+		
		0.5	1+	1+	2+
		0.25	1+	0	
17α-Propargyl				
sublingually		2.5		0	
		1.25	2+		
orally		0.5		0	0

TABLE 3—cont.

		V.d.H.	V.A.	D.
H. d-13β-Ethyl-17α-ethynyl-17-hydroxy-gon-4-ene-3-one (d-Norgestrel) orally	0.25 0.05 0.025		4+ 1+ 0, 1+	0, 0

differences in the effects of various progestational compounds might depend on their intrinsic estrogenic or antiestrogenic properties. The great importance of the preceding and concomitant estrogen loading for the progestational differentiation of the endometrium has already been emphasized. In any event, for every progestational substance a formulation can be found that will assure the development of a secretory endometrium, comparable in every respect to a normal mucosa.

The second method consists in the postponement of menstruation in women who have normal cycles by producing a state of pseudopregnancy. This test has been proposed by Greenblatt *et al.* (1958b) and standardized by Swyer *et al.* (1960). Varying doses of progestational substances are administered together with a standard dose of mestranol during 20 successive days, starting on the 20th day of the cycle. The dose is determined which in half of the cases causes a delay of menstruation (Tables 7, 8). It might be asked whether this is entirely due to the progestational activity of the drug administered. Some observations (Østergaard *et al.*, 1966) do in fact indicate that a central inhibiting action seems to be involved: menstruation is not delayed unless the level of urinary gonadotrophins is decreased during treatment. It is difficult to visualize how the lack of such a central inhibition could interfere with the delay of menstruation, since the administered steroids act directly on the uterus and take the place of the endogenous hormones there.

A third method has been proposed: the determination of the threshold dose of a progestational substance capable of producing a withdrawal bleeding in an estrogenized woman. However, uncontrollable factors, such as emotions, may intervene in the mechanism of hemostasis and consequently the results are too erratic (Swyer *et al.*, 1960).

TABLE 4. COMPARATIVE PROGESTATIONAL ACTIVITY OF VARIOUS STEROIDS IN OVARIECTOMIZED WOMEN

End point: endometrial late secretory changes.
Fern abolition (cervix); late luteal vaginal smear.
Estrogenic priming: 1 mg diethylstilbestrol daily, 1st to 28/30th days.
Progestational compound: orally, from the 14th or 16th day to 28th or 30th day.
Exploration of the genital tract: at the end of the treatment.
Effective dose (ineffective dose in brackets).

	Endometrium	Cervix	Vaginal smear
Progesterone (intramuscularly), daily	20 mg (10 mg)	10 mg (5 mg)	20 mg (10 mg), Wied and Davis (1958)
Ethisterone, daily	250 mg (150–200 mg)	250–300 mg (150–200 mg)	250–300 mg (150–200 mg), Davis and Wied (1957)
17-α-Acetoxyprogesterone, daily	100–125 mg (50–75 mg)	50–75 mg (25–50 mg)	100–125 mg (50–125 mg), Davis and Wied (1957)
9-α-Bromo-11-keto-progesterone, daily	120–160 mg (80–100 mg)	80–100 (60–80 mg)	100–160 mg (60–80 mg), Wied and Davis (1957)
	100–140 mg (60–80 mg)	80 (60 mg)	100–140 mg (60–80 mg), Wied and Davis (1958)

TABLE 5. PROGESTATIONAL ACTIVITY OF VARIOUS STEROIDS AT THE ENDOMETRIAL LEVEL.
COMPARATIVE ASSAYS IN OVARIECTOMIZED WOMEN; EFFECTIVE DOSES

End point: endometrial late secretory changes.
Estrogenic priming: 7 × 5 mg estradiobenzoate in oily solution, intramuscularly from day 1 to day 22.
Progestational treatment: orally, from day 15 to day 24 or 28.
Endometrial biopsy: at the end of the treatment.
(Boschann and Drews, 1961)

Progesterone	daily intramuscularly	20 mg
	orally	200 mg
17α-Acetoxy-progesterone	daily	70 mg
17α-Hydroxy-progesterone caproate	daily	70 mg
6α-Methyl-17α-acetoxy progesterone	daily	2.5 mg
Ethisterone	daily	50 mg
17α-Methyl-19-nortestosterone	daily	10 mg
17α-Ethyl-19-nortestosterone	daily	10 mg
17α-Ethynyl-19-nortestosterone	daily	10 mg
17α-Ethynyl-19-nortestosterone acetate	daily	2.5 mg

(*Table 6 appears on pages* 260–264.)

TABLE 7. POSTPONEMENT OF MENSTRUATION

Twenty-day course of progestogen *without estrogen*, orally, from the 20th day of the cycle in normal cyclic women. A positive response is a cycle length of at least 40 days. (Swyer *et al.*, 1960; Swyer and Little, 1961, 1962, 1968; *Handbook on Oral Contraception*, 1965.)

	No. of observations	Approx. ED_{50} (mg)
Norethindrone	89	4.25
Norethindrone acetate	51	10.5
Norethynodrel	16	20
Vinylestrenolone	12	>10
Ethynodiol diacetate	9	>4
Megestrol acetate	30	>10
Melengestrol acetate	17	>10
17α-Acetoxyprogesterone cyclopentyl-3-enolether	7	>20
Dimethisterone	21	>80
Dydrogesterone	9	>20
Norgestrel	28	4

N.B. The effectiveness of certain compounds could be ascribed to an intrinsic estrogenic property, or more likely to estrogenic metabolites. (Brown and Blair, 1960; Breuer *et al.*, 1960; Langecker, 1961; Okada *et al.*, 1964.)

TABLE 6. COMPARATIVE PROGESTATIONAL ACTIVITY OF VARIOUS STEROIDS, ORALLY ADMINISTERED, IN OVARIECTOMIZED WOMEN

End point: late secretory endometrial changes.
Fern abolition (cervix) and disappearance of the highly proliferated cell type (<5%) (vaginal smear).
Estrogenic priming: 0.05 mg ethynyl-estradiol, daily, 1st to 26th, 27th or 28th day.
Progestational compound: from the 15th day to the 26th, 27th or 28th day.
Break-through-bleeding (BTB): duration, in days, before endometrial biopsy.
(Ferin, Ferin and Schlikker; Ferin and Mingeot, unpublished results.)

S: typical secretory changes   IS: inadequate secretory changes   BTB: breakthrough bleeding

	Daily dose (mg)	Endometrium	Cervix	Vaginal smear	BTB
Medroxyprogesterone acetate					
Patient no. 1	5	IS	abolition	no disappearance	—
Patient no. 2	10	S	partial abolition		—
	5	IS			—
Patient no. 3	5	IS	abolition	no disappearance	—
	10	S			—
Chlormadinone acetate					
Patient no. 1	1	desquamation			+1 d
	5	S			—
Patient no. 2	1	desquamation			+1 d
	5	S	no abolition		—
Patient no. 3	1	IS	partial abolition		—
	5	S	no abolition		—
Patient no. 4	2	IS	partial abolition	no disappearance	—
	5	S	abolition		—
Patient no. 5	4	S			+2 d
	2	S			—
Patient no. 6	5	S			—

Orally Active Progestational Compounds: Human Studies

Compound / Patient	Dose		Effect 1	Effect 2	Days
17α-Acetoxy-4,6-19-norpregnadiene-3,20-dione					
Patient no. 1	50				+6 d
Patient no. 3	50	IS			—
Dydrogesterone					
Patient no. 1	5	S	partial abolition	no disappearance	+1 d
Patient no. 2	10	S	abolition	no disappearance	—
	5	IS		no disappearance	+2 d
	10	S		no disappearance	—
Patient no. 3	5	S	partial abolition		—
Patient no. 6	10	S			—
	5	IS			—
	10	S			—
6-Chloro-9β,10α-pregna-1,4,6-triene-3,20-dione					
Patient no. 3	5	S	abolition	disappearance	—
Patient no. 4	5	S	abolition	no disappearance	—
Patient no. 5	5	S			—
Patient no. 6	5	S			—
17α-(2′-Methallyl)17-Hydroxy-9β,10α-androsta-4,6-diene-3-one					
Patient no. 1	5	S			+6 d
	10	S			—
Patient no. 3	5	S	abolition	disappearance	—
	10	IS			—
Patient no. 5	40				—
Patient no. 6	5	IS			—

(continued overleaf)

TABLE 6—*cont.*

	Daily dose (mg)	Endometrium	Cervix	Vaginal smear	BTB
Normethandrolone					
Patient no. 1	5	IS	abolition	disappearance	—
Patient no. 2	5	S	abolition	disappearance, but numerous parabasal cells	+1 d
Patient no. 3	5	S			—
Norethindrone					
Patient no. 1	5	S	abolition	no disappearance	—
Patient no. 2	5	S	abolition		—
Patient no. 3	5	S	partial abolition		—
17α-Ethynyl-19-nortestosterone acetate					
Patient no. 1	5	S	abolition	no disappearance	—
Patient no. 2	5	S	abolition	no disappearance	—
Patient no. 3	5	S	no abolition		—
17α-Propynyl-19-nortestosterone					
Patient no. 1	5	IS		no disappearance	—
Ethynodiol diacetate					
Patient no. 1	1	desquamation			+1 d
	2	S			—
Patient no. 3	1	IS			—
Patient no. 4	2	S	partial abolition	no disappearance	—
	2	S	abolition		—
Patient no. 6	3	S		disappearance	—
	2	S			—

Compound / Patient	Dose				
Norgestrienone					
Patient no. 3	2.5	S			—
	5	S			—
	0.25	IS			+2 d
Patient no. 6	1	IS/S			—
	2	S			—
	2.5	S			—
	5	S			—
	10	S			—
Norgestrel (dl)					
Patient no. 6	1	S	abolition	no disappearance	—
d-13β-Ethyl-17α-ethynyl-17β-ol-gon-4-en-3-one (d-Norgestrel)					
Patient no. 4	0.25	S	partial abolition	no disappearance	—
Patient no. 6	0.25	S	partial abolition	no disappearance	—
16β-Hydroxy-16α-n-propyl-19-nortestosterone acetate					
Patient no. 1	5	IS	partial abolition		—
Patient no. 2	5	IS	partial abolition		—
Patient no. 3	5	IS		no disappearance	+10 d
*17α-Ethynyl-Δ$^{5(10)}$ estrenolone**					
Patient no. 1	5	S	partial abolition	no disappearance	—
Patient no. 2	5	S	partial abolition	no disappearance	—
17α-Vinyl-Δ$^{5(10)}$ estrenolene					
Patient no. 1	5	IS	abolition	no disappearance	+1 d
Patient no. 2	5	S	abolition	disappearance	—
Patient no. 3	5	IS			—

* Contains 0.94% of so-called impurities; not all of these, are of course, estrogenic.

(*continued overleaf*)

TABLE 6—cont.

	Daily dose (mg)	Endometrium	Cervix	Vaginal smear	BTB
Lynestrenol					
Patient no. 1	5	S	abolition		+ 1 d
Patient no. 2	5	IS	abolition		—
Patient no. 3	5	S			—
	10	S			—
	15	S			—
Patient no. 4	5	IS	abolition		—
Lynestrenol acetate					
Patient no. 1	5	S			—
	10	S			—
Patient no. 2	5	S	abolition		—
	10	IS			—
Patient no. 3	5	S			—
17α-Propargyl-estrenol					
Patient no. 1	5	S			—
	10	S			—
Patient no. 2	5	S			—
	5	IS			+ 2 d
Patient no. 3	10	S			—
17α-Allyl-estrenol					
Patient no. 1	15	desquamation			+ 2 d
Patient no. 2	15	desquamation			+ 5 d
Patient no. 3	15	desquamation	no abolition	no disappearance	+ 2 d
17α-Ethyl-estrenol					
Patient no. 1	5	IS	abolition		+ 1 d
Patient no. 2	5	S			—

TABLE 8. POSTPONEMENT OF MENSTRUATION

Twenty-day course of progestogen *with estrogen*, orally, from the 20th day of the cycle in normal cyclic women. A positive response is a cycle length of at least 40 days. (Swyer et al., 1960; Swyer and Little, 1961, 1962, 1968; *Handbook on Oral Contraception*, 1965.)

	Daily dose P/E (mg)	No. of observations	No. of + responses	Approx. ED_{50} (mg)
Norethynodrel + mestranol	0.15–0.075	28		5.3
Vinylestrenolone + mestranol	/0.1	13		7
Ethynodiol diacetate + mestranol	/0.1	32		1.5
Medroxyprogesterone acetate + mestranol	/0.1	21		22.5
Megestrol acetate + mestranol	/0.1 5/0.1[a] 10/0.2[a]	51 23 8	19 8	1.8
Melengestrol acetate + mestranol	/0.1	16		2.5
Progesterone cyclopentyl-enolether + mestranol	/0.1 100/0.18[b]	4 4		>25
17α-acetoxyprogesterone cyclopentyl-3-enolether + mestranol	/0.1	22		>10
Norgestrel + mestranol	/0.1	70		0.125
Dydrogesterone + mestranol	/0.1	4		>10

[a] Østergaard (1965); Østergaard et al. (1966). [b] Harkness and Charles (1965).

II. EFFECTS ON THE ENDOCERVICAL MUCOSA

In the ovariectomized woman, administration of most artificial progestogens easily reproduces the effect of progesterone on an estrogen-type endocervical secretion (see Tables 4 and 6).

In the cyclic woman daily doses of 0.25 mg of chlormadinone acetate and megestrol acetate or 0.05 mg of norgestrel appear to be able to change the mucus quality and to reduce sperm invasion and sperm activity within the mucus. However, although a dose of 0.025 mg of norgestrel changes the mucus quality and sperm *activity*, sperm *penetration* does not seem to be affected (Swyer and Little, 1968).

Roland (1968), using a daily dose of 0.075 or 0.05 mg of the same compound, observed a reduction of the mid-cycle spinnbarkeit and a lower degree of ferning. The post coital sampling demonstrated actively motile spermatozoa in the endocervical mucus, but not in the uterine fundus.

Mason et al. (1967) gave small daily doses (0.5 mg) of megestrol acetate for 3 weeks per cycle to normally menstruating women and found no sperm penetration in the cervical mucus although this was of normal appearance and consistency. Under continuous medication with the same dose of megestrol acetate van Leusden (1969) found the cervical mucus to become opaque, with absence of spinnbarkeit, and similar to that occurring during the second half of the menstrual cycle before the administration of the drug.

III. EFFECTS ON THE SQUAMOUS VAGINAL EPITHELIUM

The squamous epithelium of the vagina in its estrogen-dominated phase undergoes the transformation which characterizes the action of progesterone when exposed to the action of artificial progestational compounds. A few comparative studies have been made to establish the doses needed in order to make the estrogenic appearance of the smears disappear (see Tables 4 and 6).

B. ANTI-ESTROGENIC POTENCY

The anti-estrogenic activity of a drug is shown by the suppression of estrogen effects in various parts of the genital tract. The ideal method of demonstrating this activity consists in the administration of a standard dose of an estrogen together with varying doses of the substance to be tested to subjects whose endogenous estrogen production is very low such as ovariectomized women.

1. *The endometrium*

When the anti-estrogenic activity is high one can obtain complete inhibition of endometrial growth in an ovariectomized woman. In this respect testosterone and its derivatives are typical anti-estrogens (Ferin, 1943, 1946, 1950, 1951, 1954b, 1955). There is no progestational compound with which one can obtain the same result. When the anti-estrogenic activity is low, thinning of the endometrial mucosa as a consequence of reduced proliferation is seen. This is difficult to measure in the material obtained by biopsies. The absence of mitoses from the glandular epithelium is also noticeable. As an example we may state that at least 0.25 mg of ethynodiol-diacetate is needed daily to suppress the glandular mitoses provoked by 0.1 mg of mestranol (Ferin, 1966).

To some extent massive deposition of glycogen in the endometrial glands might be considered as an expression of anti-estrogenicity. This phenomenon is observed in cultures of proliferating endometrium entirely deprived of the stimulation by sex hormones (Ehrmann et al., 1961). So it looks as if progestational substances, while inhibiting the proliferative stimulus of the estrogens on the endometrium, bring out its secretory potential. In this connection it should be noted that under certain conditions testosterone and methyltestosterone can also induce massive glycogen loading in the endometrium, as do progestational substances (see Chapter 22). However, these androgens do not bring about the complete secretory transformation of the human endometrium. This shows the fundamental difference between the effects of androgens and those of gestogens in the female genital tract.

Rudel et al. (1967) studied the effects of progestational substances on the endometrial glands of cyclic women, by administration beginning on the 5th day of the cycle.

In this glandular suppression test, estrogen-free norethindrone is three times as potent as chlormadinone acetate. It should be noted that this technique disregards the possibility of an inhibition of endogenous estrogen production through an effect of the drug on the hypothalamo-pituitary system or on the ovary. This could create an exaggerated impression of the magnitude of the anti-estrogenic potency of the compound tested.

2. *The endocervical mucosa*

An anti-estrogenic effect of progestogens on the endocervical mucus can easily be demonstrated. The secretion of the estrogen-type mucus is inhibited. Here the effects of androgens can apparently not be distinguished from those of the progestogens (Ferin, 1950, 1951, 1954b, 1955).

3. *The vagina*

The anti-estrogenic effect is characterized by the disappearance of "estrogen cells" (eosinophilic, karyopycnotic superficial type of cell) from the vaginal smears. This effect can be elicited by androgens (Shorr et al., 1938; Rothermich, 1939; Ferin, 1950, 1954b; Boschann, 1958a) and by all the progestational substances, provided they are administered for a sufficiently long period in relation to the *dose* of estrogen (Boschann, 1958b). See Tables 4, 6 and 9.

TABLE 9. DISAPPEARANCE OF EOSINOPHILIC KARYOPYCNOTIC SUPERFICIAL CELL TYPE IN ESTROGENIZED OVARIECTOMIZED WOMEN

Estrogenic priming	Progestational compound 10 to 14 days	Effective daily dose (mg)	Ineffective daily dose (mg)	Author(s)
Estradiol benzoate 5 mg × 7 intramuscularly (twice weekly)	norethindrone	10	5	Boschann (1958b)
Diethylstilbestrol 1 mg daily	norethindrone acetate methandrolone norethindrone	4 10 10	3	Boschann (1958b) Del Sol and Rohrbach (1962b) Del Sol and Rohrbach (1962b)

C. SUMMARY

The results of the comparative study of the progestational activity of a number of compounds are shown in Table 10.

It cannot be denied that these data are open to statistical criticism. They are, nevertheless, the best we could obtain, considering the extreme difficulties of human studies of this kind.

TABLE 10

	Endometrial test in ovariectomized women (Ferin)		Postponement of menstruation test Approx. ED_{50} (Swyer and Little, 1968)
	Short test	Long test	
Medroxyprogesterone acetate	1.25–2.5 mg	> 5 mg (2.5 mg[a]) ⩽ 10 mg	22.5 mg (+ 0.1 mestranol)
Chlormadinone acetate	0.5–2 mg	> 2 mg ⩽ 4 mg	
Dydrogesterone	1–10 mg	> 5 mg ⩽ 10 mg	> 10 mg (+ 0.1 mestranol)
Norethindrone	0.1–0.2 mg	⩽ 5 mg (10 mg[a])	4.25 mg
Norethindrone acetate	0.1–0.5 mg	⩽ 5 mg (2.5 mg[a])	10.5 mg
Ethynodiol diacetate	0.1–0.3 mg	2 mg	1.5 mg (+ 0.1 mestranol)
Lynestrenol	0.1–0.3 mg	⩾ 5 mg	
Norgestrel		⩽ 1 mg	0.125 mg (+ 0.1 mestranol)

[a] Boschann and Drews (1961).

The great differences between individual figures only show that progestational substances are really different, both qualitatively and quantitatively, not only from progesterone but also amongst each other.

REFERENCES

ALLEN, W. M. and WU, D. H. (1959) Effects of 17-α-ethinyl-19-nortestosterone on pregnancy in rabbits. *Fertil. Steril.* **10**: 424–438.

AYDAR, C. K. and GREENBLATT, R. B. (1964) 6 dehydro-retroprogesterone (Duphaston), an interesting progesterone-like compound. *Int. J. of Fertil.* **9**: 585–595.

BOLTON, C. H., HAMPTON, J. R. and MITCHELL, J. R. A. (1968) Effect of oral contraceptive agents on platelets and plasma-phospholipids. *Lancet*, **i**: 1336–1341.

BOSCHANN, H. W. (1955) Cytologische Untersuchungen über die Wirkung von Androgenen am atrophischen Vaginalepithel in Abhängigkeit von Dosierung und Applikationsart. *Arch. f. Gynäk.* **187**: 39–64.

BOSCHANN, H. W. (1957) Effect of administered androgens on the vaginal epithelium of women exhibiting the atrophic menopausal cell type (and discussion thereafter). *Acta Cytol.* **1**: 87–89.

BOSCHANN, H. W. (1958a) What are the relative dosages of androgens plus estrogens which suppress the occurrence of the highly proliferated cell type? *Acta Cytol.* **2**: 414–416.

BOSCHANN, H. W. (1958b) Discussion after Ferin, J. *Acta Cytol.* **2**: 421–423.

BOSCHANN, H. W. (1962) Discussion after Del Sol and Rohrbach. *Acta Cytol.* **6**: 232.

BOSCHANN, H. W. and DREWS, R. (1961) The effect of 6α-methyl-17α-acetoxyprogesterone on the endometrium. In: *Progesterone, Brook Lodge Symposium*, pp. 133–145. Brook Lodge Press, Augusta, Michigan.

BREUER, H., DARDENNE, U. and NOCKE, W. (1960) Ausscheidung von 17-Ketosteroiden, 17-Ketogenensteroiden und Östrogenen beim Menschen nach Gaben von 17α-Athynyl-nor-Testosterone-Estern. *Acta Endocr. (Kbh.)* **33**: 10–26.

BROWN, J. B. and BLAIR, H. A. F. (1960) Urinary oestrogen metabolites of 19-norethisterone and its esters. *Proc. Roy. Soc. Med. (London)* **53**: 433.

CARTER, W. F., FAUCHER, G. L. and GREENBLATT, R. B. (1964) Evaluation of a new progestational agent, 6,17α-dimethyl 6-dehydroprogesterone. *Amer. J. Obst. and Gynec.* **89**: 635–641.

DAVIS, M. E. and WIED, G. L. (1957) 17α-Hydroxyprogesterone acetate; effective oral progestational substance. *J. Clin. Endocr. Met.* **17**: 1237–1244.

DEL SOL, J. R. and ROHRBACH, C. (1962a) The effect of progestogens on the atrophic epithelium. *Acta Cytol.* **6**: 231–232.

DEL SOL, J. R. and ROHRBACH, C. (1962b) Effects of progestogens on the highly proliferated vaginal epithelium. *Acta Cytol.* **6**: 278–279.

D'INCERTI BONINI, L. and PAGANI, C. (1962) Indagine clinica sull'attivita progestativa del vinilestrenolone. *Ann. Ost. Ginec.* **84**: 279–285.

DOUGLAS, M. G. (1959) Observations on the use of 6α:21-dimethyl-ethisterone in secondary amenorrhoea. *J. Obst. Gyn. Brit. Emp.* **66**: 914–916.

DUNCAN, G. W., LYSTER, S. C., HENDRIX, J. W., CLARK, J. J. and WEBSTER, H. D. (1964) Biologic effects of melengestrol acetate. *Fertil. Steril.* **15**: 419–432.

EHRMANN, R. L., MCKELVEY, H. A. and HERTIG, A. T. (1961) Secretory behavior of endometrium in tissue culture. *Obst. Gynec.* **17**: 416–433.

EPSTEIN, J. A., KUPPERMAN, H. S. and CUTLER, A. (1958) Comparative pharmacological and clinical activity of 19-nortestosterone and 17-hydroxyprogesterone derivatives in man. *Ann. N.Y. Acad. Sci.* **71**: 560–571.

FERIN, J. (1943) Sur l'antagonisme entre les substances oestrogènes et androgènes chez la femme. *Ann. Endocr.* **4**: 195–197.

FERIN, J. (1946) L'inhibition par le propionate de testostérone de l'action oestrogène du diéthylstilboestrol chez les femmes ovariectomisées. *C.R. Soc. Biol.* **140**: 594–596.

FERIN, J. (1947) L'hémorragie utérine de privation androgène chez la femme oestrogénisée. *Ann. Endocr.* **8**: 171–176.

FERIN, J. (1950) Inhibition des effets oestrogènes par la méthyl-testostérone chez la femme ovariectomisée. *Ann. Endocr.* **11**: 676–678.

FERIN, J. (1951) Stéroides antioestrogènes non virilisants chez la femme ovariectomisée. *Ann. Endocr.* **12**: 1082–1086.

FERIN, J. (1954a) Doses d'hormones nécessaires pour provoquer les modifications morphologiques utérines et vaginales de la phase lutéale chez la femme ovariectomisée. In *La Fonction lutéale*, pp. 207–234. Masson, Paris.

FERIN, J. (1954b) Exposition scientifique. Documents de recherches cliniques et expérimentales. *Congrès International de Gynécologie et d'Obstétrique, Génève*, p. 51.

FERIN, J. (1955) Les effets chez la femme de la 19-nortesterone et du cyclopentylpropionate de 19-nortestosterone. *Ann. Endocr.* **16**: 895–899.

FERIN, J. (1957a) Progestational activity of certain 19-nor-steroids. Comparative assays in oophorectomized women. *J. Clin. Endocr. Metab.* **17**: 1252–1255.
FERIN, J. (1957b) La méthyloestrénolone (norméthandrolone), nouvelle substance progestogène, active par la voie perlinguale. *Geburtsh. Frauenheilk.* **17**: 10–24.
FERIN, J. (1962a) Activité progestative comparée chez la femme ovariectomisée des 17-alkyls correspondants de l'oestrénolone et de l'oestrénol. *Ann. Endocr.* **23**: 103–104.
FERIN, J. (1962b) Effects of 19-nor-steroidal progestogens on the vaginal smears of normally menstruating women. *Acta Cytol.* **6**: 305–306.
FERIN, J. (1963) Critères endométriaux de l'activité du corps jaune non gravidique. In: *L'Insuffisance lutéale*, pp. 235–243. Masson, Paris.
FERIN, J. (1966) Antagonism of sex steroids as determined on the genital tract. *Europ. Rev. Endocrin.*, suppl. 2, part **1**: 135–144.
FERIN, J. and SCHLIKKER, E. (1960) Artificial cycles in oophorectomized women. *Int. J. Fert.* **5**: 19–25.
GOLDZIEHER, J. W., PETERSON, W. F. and GILBERT, R. A. (1958) Comparison of the endometrial activities in man of anhydrohydroxyprogesterone and 17-acetoxy-progesterone, a new oral progestational compound. *Ann. New York Acad. Sci.* **71**: 722–726.
GOLDZIEHER, J. W. and RICE-WRAY, E. (1966) *Oral Contraception.* Ch. Thomas, Springfield, Illinois.
GOOD, R. G. and MAYER, D. L. (1968) Estrogen–progesterone relationships in the development of secretory endometrium. *Fertil. Steril.* **19**: 37–49.
GREENBLATT, R. B. and JUNGCK, E. C. (1958a) Delay of menstruation with norethindrone, an orally given progestational compound. *J.A.M.A.* **166**: 1461–1463.
GREENBLATT, R. B., JUNGCK, E. C. and BARFIELD, W. E. (1958b) A new test for efficacy of progestational compounds. *Ann. New York Acad. Sci.* **71**: 717–720.
GREENBLATT, R. B. and BARFIELD, W. E. (1959) The progestational activity of 6-methyl-17-acetoxyprogesterone. *South. Med. J.* **52**: 345–351.
GREENBLATT, R. B., JUNGCK, E. C., BIGGER, J. T. and GREER, M. V. (1963) Progestational activity of a new acetoxyprogesterone derivative (6α-methyl-6-dehydro-17α-acetoxyprogesterone). *Fertil. Steril.* **14**: 393–401.
Handbook on Oral Contraception (1965) Edit. by E. MEARS, pp. 17–18. J. and A. Churchill Ltd., London.
HARKNESS, R. A. and CHARLES, D. (1965) Studies on the biological activity and metabolism of the cyclopentyl-3-enol ether of progesterone. *Amer. J. Obstet. Gynec.* **93**: 1005–1012.
HECHT-LUCARI, G. and SCARPELLINI, L. (1961) Esperienze cliniche con l'etere ciclopentilenolico del progesterone in ginecologia. *Folia Endocrinol.*, Suppl. **14**: 359–373.
HERTZ, R., WAITE, J. H. and THOMAS, L. B. (1956) Progestational effectiveness of 19-nor-ethynyl testosterone by oral route in women. *Proc. Soc. Exper. Biol. Med.* **91**: 418–420.
KAISER, R. (1957) Über die progestative Wirkung von 19-Nortestosteronverbindungen bei oraler Verabreichung. *Geburtsh. Frauenheilk.* **17**: 24–37.
KLOPPER, A. (1961) A comparison of the clinical effects of various progestational compounds. *Folia Endocrinol.*, Suppl. **14**: 286–293.
LANGECKER, H. (1961) Die Metabolite im menschlichen Harn nach Verabreichung von 17α-Aethinyl-19-Nortestosteron. *Acta Endocr.* **37**: 14–18.
LOSKANT, G. (1966) Klinische Untersuchung einer oral wirksamen Progesteronverbindung. *Zbl. f. Gynäk.* **88**: 930–933.
MAQUEO, M., PEREZ-VEGA, E., GOLDZIEHER, J. W., MARTINEZ-MANAUTOU, J. and RUDEL, H. (1963) Comparison of the endometrial activity of 3 synthetic progestins used in fertility control. *Amer. J. Obstet. Gynec.* **85**, 427–432.

MARTINEZ-MANAUTOU, J. (1967) Hormonal fertility control without ovulation suppression. *Fertility and Sterility. Proc. Fifth World Congress 1966*. Excerpta Medica Foundation, Internat. Congress Series no. 133, pp. 999–1003.
MARTINEZ-MANAUTOU, J. M., MAQUEO, M., GILBERT, R. A. and GOLDZIEHER, J. W. (1962) Human endometrial activity of several new derivatives of 17-acetoxy progesterone. *Fertil. Steril.* **13**: 169–183.
MASON, B. A., COX, M. J. E., MASON, D. W. and GRANT, V. (1967) Chemical and experimental studies with low doses of megestrol acetate. *Postgraduate Medical J.*, September Supplement.
MORRIS, J. MCL. and VAN WAGENEN, G. (1966) Compounds interfering with ovum implantation and development. The role of estrogens. *Amer. J. Obstet. Gynec.* **96**: 804–815.
NETTER, A., LAMBERT, A. and LUMBROSO, P. (1957) Effets progestatifs de la méthyl-oestrénolone. *C.R. Soc. Fr. Gyn.* **27**: 397–400.
NETTER, A., LAMBERT, A., YANEVA, H. and PELISSIER, C. (1967) Etude d'un nouveau progestatif de synthèse, la norgestrienone. *Rev. Franc. Endocr. Clin.* **8**: 231–240.
NEVINNY-STICKEL, J. (1962) Die gestagene Wirkung von Hydroxy-nor-Progesteron-estern bei der Frau. 8. *Symposion der Deutschen Gesellschaft für Endokrinologie*, pp. 248–255. Springer, Berlin.
NEVINNY-STICKEL, J. (1963) Die unterschiedliche morphologische Wirkung verschiedener synthetischen Gestagene auf das Endometrium. 9. *Symposion der Deutschen Gesellschaft für Endokrinologie*, pp. 177–180. Springer, Berlin.
OKADA, H., AMATSU, M., ISHIKARA, S. and TOKUDA, G. (1964) Conversion of some synthetic progestins to oestrogen. *Acta Endocr.* **46**: 31–36.
ØSTERGAARD, E. (1965) The oral progestational and antiovulatory properties of megestrol acetate and its therapeutic use in gynaecological disorders. *J. Obstet. Gynec. Brit. Commonwealth* **72**: 45–58.
ØSTERGAARD, E., ARENDS, J., HAMBURGER, CHR. and JOHNSON, S. G. (1966) Postponement of menses, suppression of urinary gonadotrophins, 17-KGS and 17-KS in normal women treated with a megestrol acetate/mestranol combination (delpregnin) from day 20 of the cycle. *Acta Endocr.* **53**: 13–23.
PINCUS, G., ROCK, J. and GARCIA, C. R. (1958) Effects of certain 19-nor-steroids upon reproductive processes. *Ann. N.Y. Acad. Sci.* **71**: 677–690.
POTS, P. (1957) Die perorale Wirksamkeit synthetischer Gestagne. *Zbl. f. Gynäk.* **79**: 529–539.
POTS, P. (1958) Testierung der peroralen Gestagenwirkung von Aethinyl-nor-testo-steronacetät. *Klin. Wschr.* **36**: 824–825.
PUNDEL, J. P. (1957) *Acquisitions récentes en cytologie vaginale hormonale*. Masson, Paris.
RICE-WRAY, E., ARANDA-ROSELL, A., MAQUEO, M. and GOLDZIEHER, J. W. (1963) Comparison of the long-term endometrial effects of synthetic progestins used in fertility control. *Amer. J. Obstet. Gynec.* **87**: 429–433.
ROCK, J., GARCIA, C. R. and PINCUS, G. (1957) Synthetic progestins in the normal human menstrual cycle. *Recent Progr. in Hormone Research* **13**: 323–339.
ROLAND, M. (1968) Norgestrel-induced cervical barrier to sperm migration. *J. Reprod. Fertil.*, suppl. **5**: 173–177.
ROLAND, M., CLYMAN, M. J., DECKER, A. and OBER, W. B. (1964) Classification of endometrial response to synthetic progestogen–estrogen compounds. *Fertil. Steril.* **15**: 143–163.
ROTHERMICH, N. O. (1939) Comparative study of effects of male and female sex hormones on human vaginal smear. *Endocrinology* **25**: 520–524.

RUDEL, H. W., LEBHERZ, T., MAQUEO-TOPETE, M., MARTINEZ-MANAUTOU, J. and BESSLER, S. (1967) Assay of the anti-oestrogenic effects of progestogens in women. *J. Reprod. Fertil.* **13**: 199–203.

SHORR, E., PAPANICOLAOU, G. N. and STIMMEL, B. F. (1938) Neutralization of ovarian follicular hormone in women by simultaneous administration of male sex hormones. *Proc. Soc. Exper. Biol. Med.* **38**: 759–762.

SMITH, D. L., PULLIAM, A. L. and FORIST, A. A. (1966) Comparative absorption of micronized and nonmicronized medroxyprogesterone acetate in man. *J. Pharmac. Sci.* **55**: 398–403.

STOKES, P. E., HORWITH, M., PENNINGTON, T. G. and CLARKSON, B. (1959) 17α-ethyl 19-nortestosterone as an anabolic agent and its effect on creatine metabolism and vaginal cytology in humans. *Metabolism* **8**: 709–721.

SWYER, G. I. M., SEBOK, L. and BARNS, D. F. (1960) The determination of the relative potency of some progestogens in the human. *Proc. R. Soc. Med. (London)* **53**: 435–436.

SWYER, G. I. M. and LITTLE, V. (1961) Some clinical studies with 17α-acetoxyprogesteron cyclopentyl enol ether. *Folia Endocr.*, Suppl. **14**: 312–318.

SWYER, G. J. and LITTLE, V. (1962) Action and uses of orally active progestational steroids. *Proc. Roy. Soc. Med.* **55**: 861–868.

SWYER, G. I. M. and LITTLE, V. (1968) Clinical assessment of relative potency of progestogens. *J. Reprod. Fert.*, Suppl. **5**: 63–68.

TILLINGER, K. G. and DICZFALUSY, E. (1960) Progestational activity of stereoisomeric progesterone-analogues following oral administration in amenorrhea. *Acta Endocr.* **35**: 197–203.

TYLER, E. T. (1968) in "Medical News". *J.A.M.A.* **204**: 35–36.

VAN LEUSDEN, H. A. (1969) Continuous oral administration of megestrol acetate to women. *J. Reprod. Fert.* **19**: 537–539.

VOKAER, R. and FERIN, J. (1961) La 6-déhydro-rétro-progestérone. Nouvelle hormone progestative. *Bull. Soc. Roy. Belge Gyn. Obst.* **31**: 431–444.

VOKAER, R. and KRIDELKA, J. C. (1963) Etude clinique de l'activité chez la femme d'un nouveau stéroide progestatif: le 17-acétate de 1,2-α-méthylène-6-chlore, Δ4,6-pregnadiène 17-α-ol-3,20-dione. *Ann. Endocr.* **24**, 49–57.

WAIDL, E., FIKENTSCHER, H. and BRUCKNER, W. (1968) Die interzellulären Strukturen des Endometriums bei der oralen Kontrazeption. *Geburtsh. Frauenheilk.* **28**: 159–166.

WASCHKE, G. (1957) Beitrag zum Aethylnortestosteron und Aethinyl-nortestosteron-Effekt bei verschiedenen Zyklusstörungenen. *Zbl. f. Gynäk.* **79**: 1199.

WIED, G. L. and DAVIS, E. (1957) 9α-bromo-11-ketoprogesterone. Another new orally effective substance with progestational activity. *Obstet. Gynec.* **10**: 411–417.

WIED, G. L. and DAVIS, E. (1958) Comparative activity of progestational agents on the human endometrium and vaginal epithelium of surgical castrates. *Ann. N.Y. Acad. Sci.* **71**: 599–616.

WIED, G. L. and DAVIS, E. (1959) A new orally progestational agent: increased effectiveness in the human of a progestational agent by attaching a methyl group at carbon position six of the steroid ring. *Obstet. Gynec.* **14**: 305–308.

WIED, G. L. and DAVIS, E. (1961) The parenteral effectiveness of 6-methyl-17-α-OH-progesterone acetate under varying dosages of estrogenic priming of the endometrium of surgical castrates. *Brook Lodge Symposium: Progesterone*, pp. 147–150 Brook Lodge Press, Augusta, Mich.

WIED, G. L. and DAVIS, E. (1963) Provest and provera: a comparative study. *Int. J. Fertil.* **8**: 601–603.

CHAPTER 31

OTHER EFFECTS OF SYNTHETIC PROGESTATIONAL COMPOUNDS IN THE HUMAN

M. Tausk
Utrecht, The Netherlands

and

J. de Visser
Oss, The Netherlands

IN THIS chapter a number of observations will be discussed, concerning effects of synthetic substitutes for progesterone, which did not seem to fit more adequately into other chapters, such as: effects on the utero-vaginal tract (Chapter 30), therapeutic effects (Chapter 32), contraceptive effects and side effects (Chapter 34). For terminology and spelling of non-proprietary names see Chapter 28 (introduction and Table 1), though the present chapter is not strictly limited to the compounds discussed in Chapter 28.

1. INDUCTION (FACILITATION) OF OVULATION

During the last 3 years a number of papers have appeared, describing an ovulation-inducing effect of a "retrosteroid", Ro 4-8347, to which recently a trademark, Retroid®, and a non-proprietary name (Trengestone) have been assigned. The structure is shown in Fig. 1. Stamm *et al.* (1968) gave it to fifty-five women with amenorrhea or anovulatory cycles (in daily doses varying between 4 and 12 mg for 3 to 20 days per treatment cycle, and sometimes for as long as 12 months). They saw signs of ovulation in fifty-one of these women, including seven pregnancies. In the authors' opinion the results are comparable with those of clomiphene treatment.

The drug apparently acts by stimulating the secretion of gonadotrophins (and thereby the secretion of estrogens); it produces a secretory endometrium in total doses of 40–60 mg divided over 10 days. It does not increase body temperature. In this respect it is comparable to another progestational restrosteroid, dydrogesterone (see Chapter 28, Table 1). Other reports on essentially similar findings include those of Dapunt (1969), Dapunt and Windbichler (1969) and Taubert and Jürgensen (1970a). These authors found that twenty-seven out of sixty patients showed biphasic temperature curves after treatment. "A presumptive rate of ovulation of 45% is certainly much lower than the ovulation rate with

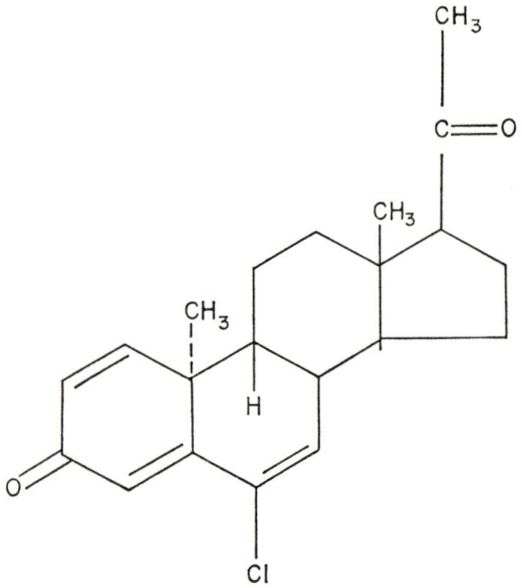

Fig. 1.

clomiphene, but it is also noticeably higher than a placebo effect" (Taubert and Jürgensen, 1970b).

Odell and Swerdloff (1968) found that medroxyprogesterone acetate, given orally for 3 days to estrogen-treated postmenopausal women, alone or in combination with progesterone (10 mg i.m. as a single injection), would induce a FSH and LH peak in the plasma, which would fit in with the authors' hypothesis that in the normal cycle "small preovulatory rises in a blood *progestogen* represent the ovarian signal that induces the LH–FSH ovulatory peak in women". The tenability of this hypothesis will not be discussed here but we shall revert to the whole problem in Chapter 35 (general summary).

2. INHIBITION OF OVULATION, INFLUENCES ON THE SECRETION OF GONADOTROPHINS AND POSSIBLE DIRECT EFFECTS ON THE OVARY

There is a striking scarcity of data regarding the antiovulatory potency of the various progestational drugs, assessed in women (in contrast to the abundance of data on this potency of oral contraceptives which contain estrogens in addition).

A number of results are presented in Chapter 34 (Table 3, p. 392), which show remarkably small differences between five progestational steroids, whose activities differ much more in animal tests, as discussed in Chapter 28. Similar conclusions can be derived from comparative figures, presented by Haller (1968). The minimum effective human (oral) dose is stated to be approximately 5 mg for norethisterone acetate and norethynodrel, 5–10 mg for lynestrenol and medroxyprogesterone acetate, 3–6 mg for chlormadinone acetate and 10–20 mg for norethisterone. Obviously the assessment of such potencies in the human is infinitely more difficult than in animals and Haller stresses the point that these are rough approximations.

Comparative studies in which the occurrence of ovulation was judged by pregnanediol determinations were published by Nevinny-Stickel (1963 a and b, 1964). Some data from the last mentioned paper are presented in our Table 1.

TABLE 1. ANTIOVULATORY ACTIVITY OF VARIOUS STEROIDS ADMINISTERED ORALLY FROM THE 5TH TO THE 24TH CYCLE DAY. Adapted from Nevinny-Stickel (1964).

Compound	Daily dose (mg)	No. of cycles	Ovulation inhibited	Ovulation not inhibited	Success %
Chlormadinone acetate	1–2	13	11	2	85
Chlormadinone acetate	3–4	4	4	—	100
Allylestrenol	20	6	3	3	50
Allylestrenol	25	3	3	—	100

McCormick et al. (1968) found that Anovlar® (4 mg norethisterone acetate and 50 mcg ethynyl estradiol) inhibited ovulation (as judged from gonadotrophin peaks in the urine, pregnanediol and body temperature) in at least four of six women during one treatment cycle. Norethisterone acetate alone (in a dose of only 1 mg per day) was compatible with rises in pregnanediol excretion in three out of six women (of which one occurred on the 33rd day of treatment. Random ovulation?)

Diczfalusy *et al.* (1969) gave (estrogen-free) norethisterone cyclically to two normal women and found that 0.1 mg/day abolished the "ovulatory" pregnanediol excretion pattern in only one of them. In the other it was not affected at this dose but disappeared on a dose of 2.5 mg, while the LH excretion pattern ("diminished and broadened") was the same on either dose.

A progestational drug which has repeatedly been shown *not* to inhibit ovulation in women is dydrogesterone, even in doses as high as 400 mg daily (Bishop *et al.*, 1962; Loraine *et al.*, 1966).

Nevertheless Jaffe *et al.* (1969) showed that its administration during two consecutive cycles to five women, who according to all parameters ovulated normally before and after the treatment period, caused the disappearance of both the midcycle FSH and LH peak from the serum and prevented the rise in body temperature and in pregnanediol excretion during the second half of the treatment cycles. Intriguing is the observation by Stolte *et al.* (1969) that the urinary LH peak was suppressed by daily administration of 20 mg dydrogesterone (Duphaston®) for 20 days in cycles during which ovulations occurred as demonstrated by biphasic temperature curves, rise of pregnanediol and in one case by inspection of the ovaries.

Superlutin (16-methylene-6-dehydro-17α-acetoxy-progesterone, MDAP) did not consistently inhibit ovulation in doses up to 6 mg daily unless combined with at least 75 mcg ethynyl estradiol (Štěrba *et al.* 1965).

Lynestrenol in daily doses of 5 mg (orally, from day 5 to 25 of the cycle) suppressed the mid-cycle peak in urinary excretion of LH only, as reported by Schmidt-Elmendorff and Kopera (1966). At the 15-mg/day level the FSH peak was equally eliminated, as would be the case with 2.5 or 5 mg supplemented by mestranol (75 or 150 mcg respectively). Lynestrenol has been shown to have intrinsic estrogenic activity (see Chapter 28, subsection 13.2, p. 103).

It is not only—and probably not even mainly—the difficulty of choosing reliable criteria for the occurrence of ovulation in steroid-treated women, which stands in the way of a more accurate determination of activities, but also the impossibility of doing enough frequent measurements in sufficiently large numbers of women. The problem is, of course, quite different from what one encounters in an investigation of the reliability of an oral contraceptive, taken routinely at the same dose level by great numbers of women, whereby the occurrence or absence of ovulation is determined by one relatively simple parameter (such as pregnanediol excretion). It is therefore still questionable whether more sophisticated methods, such as plasma LH determinations by means of radio-immunoassays, will produce more reliable pharmacological data, permitting a quantitative assessment of antiovulatory potency in the human, though they appear to yield very interesting qualitative results, as will be illustrated now.

Franchimont et al. (1970) found that one single injection of 150 mg medroxyprogesterone acetate on the 5th day of the cycle suppressed the mid-cycle FSH peak or the LH peak (each in one case) and did not interfere with either in two other cases. On the other hand, small oral doses of norethisterone acetate suppressed both the FSH and the LH peak in the plasma without changing the basal plasma levels of these hormones. In postmenopausal women this compound in daily oral doses of 0.3 mg was found to decrease plasma LH levels preferentially, while FSH remained unchanged in three out of four cases. Single doses of 200 mg i.m. depressed FSH and more strongly LH plasma levels for periods of 1 to 2 months.

Schally et al. (1970) found that the administration of the oral contraceptive Lyndiol could not prevent the rise of FSH or LH in the serum of postmenopausal women when these were injected with a porcine LH releasing preparation, which indicates that contraceptive steroids act by suppressing the secretion of releasing hormones, not their effect on the pituitary.

Larsson-Cohn et al. (1970a) reported that norethisterone administered continuously in daily doses of 0.5 mg to four normally menstruating women caused the disappearance of the urinary mid-cycle LH peak in all cases, while the basal LH excretion showed considerable day-to-day variations. In two cases all signs of luteal activity (as judged from plasma progesterone and urinary pregnanediol) disappeared immediately when this treatment was instituted. On a continuous regimen of 0.3 mg/day (Larsson-Cohn et al., 1970c) seven normal women showed signs of cyclical luteal activity, though in most cases plasma progesterone and urinary pregnanediol values were lower than during corresponding control cycles. It seems that 0.3 mg has a weaker effect on the hormone levels than 0.5 mg but a stronger effect than 0.5 mg chlormadinone acetate. Chlormadinone acetate, according to the same group of authors (Larsson-Cohn et al., 1970b) given continuously to six normal young women in daily doses of 0.5 mg, permitted the persistence of a normal LH excretion pattern during all three treatment cycles in two women whereas the others also had periodical variations in the LH excretion but no distinct mid-cycle peaks. The plasma concentration of progesterone showed regular periodic increases, but was lower than normal in many cycles, though seldom below the lowest normal value. The authors consider it as possible that a defective corpus luteum function would account for the low plasma progesterone values, as suggested by Østergaard and Starup (1968) who saw corpora lutea in a few women on cyclical megestrol acetate plus mestranol treatment, and on megestrol alone, in spite of low pregnanediol excretion values.

While none of these authors specifically ascribe the defective hormone production to a direct drug effect on the corpora lutea, such an effect should, we believe, be considered as possible (see also Chapter 28, subsection 23.1, p. 177). In the studies of Larsson-Cohn et al. there were also changes in the patterns of gonadotrophins, which might have been instrumental in bringing about changes in progesterone production.

Collins et al. (1971) in a similar study found that 0.5 mg of chlormadinone acetate given daily markedly depressed the mid-cycle urinary LH peak in all of six women treated, but only in three of these were the production rates of progesterone (mg/24 h) markedly suppressed and did pregnanediol excretion fail to rise. In the others, where progesterone production remained relatively high (according to phase of cycle) there was, however a significant change in progesterone metabolism (from pregnanediol to pregnanolone). The occurrence of "ovulatory" progesterone secretion without preceding LH rises (in the urine) makes the authors wonder, whether minimal increases in LH secretion could have caused ovulation or whether follicles may have become luteinized, without having ovulated. It stands to reason that further studies including those of plasma levels of FSH and LH will throw light upon these important problems.

Effects of the administration of norgestrel in daily small doses of only 50 mcg from the 1st day of the cycle in which patients (fifteen women) were to undergo an operation for tubal ligature, continued until and including the day of operation, were studied by Wright et al. (1970). In eleven of these cases histologically normal corpora lutea were found and the endometrium appeared to be more or less in phase. Nevertheless pregnanediol excretion values were lower than on the corresponding days of normal cycles. A direct effect on progesterone secretion of the corpus luteum is considered by the authors as a possibility.

With comparable doses of 0.03 mg of d-norgestrel Larsson-Cohn et al. (1971) found a tendency to a decrease of the estrogen excretion and low progesterone levels in some cycles. The authors conclude that the effect of this drug on the corpus luteum activity seemed to be "about equal to that of chlormadinone acetate 0.5 mg daily, while 0.3 and 0.5 mg of norethindrone depressed the function more markedly".

The peripheral plasma levels of progesterone (believed to reflect secretion of the corpus luteum) were found to be lowered by the administration of norethisterone, chlormadinone acetate or norgestrel in the post-ovulatory period of normal women (Johansson, 1970).

A direct influence of a progestational drug, medroxyprogesterone acetate (MAP), has also been suggested by Lunenfeld *et al.* (1963) who studied this in two young women with (long-standing) amenorrhoea. They were shown to respond to gonadotrophin therapy (HMG followed by HCG) by increased excretion of estrogens, ovulation (pregnanediol) and menstruation. When during a second course of treatment these subjects received daily doses of 5 mg medroxyprogesterone acetate (MAP) with 50 mcg ethynyl estradiol (EE), ovulation was suppressed (but not with MAP or EE alone). The authors' cautious conclusion was that "the anti-ovulatory capacity of MAP–EE may be due, in particular, to a direct action on the ovary, resulting in a decrease of its sensitivity to stimulation by pituitary gonadotrophins".

Leaving aside the many problems that need further studies, in the context of the present chapter it would still appear justified to quote Swyer (1970) saying: we are still missing reliable data on the relative potency to inhibit ovulation in women of the numerous progestatives now used in oral contraceptives.

3. RELATED ASPECTS OF HYPOTHALAMIC (PITUITARY) INHIBITION

The possibilities now available of modifying hypothalamic (gonadotrophic) activity in the human are beginning to shed a new light on some old problems. In particular we are referring to the mechanism of climacteric vasomotor symptoms. There have been discussions in the early days of gynecological endocrinology, about the mechanism of the so-called hot flushes, whether they were due to estrogen deficiency or to the increased levels of gonadotrophins in the body. The latter are now interpreted as being due to increased activity (de-inhibition) of hypothalamic centres. The fact that hot flushes have repeatedly been described as side effects of clomiphene therapy seems to indicate that increased hypothalamic activity—caused either by estrogenic deficiency or by pharmacological stimulation—causes the vasomotor reactions. This is corroborated by the interesting finding, reported by Reiffenstuhl and Hohlweg (1968), that these symptoms can be suppressed, not only by estrogens but also by a progestational compound, known to have an inhibitory influence on the

TABLE 2. EFFECT ON BODY TEMPERATURE IN THE HUMAN

Compound	Conditions and dosages (p.o. unless otherwise indicated) under which thermogenicity		Reference
	has been shown	has not been shown	
Allylestrenol	Castrated women and gonadal dysgenesis, 20–25 mg/day		Nevinny-Stickel (1963)
Chlormadinone acetate		0.5 mg continuous daily administration (not suppressing ovulation)	Larsson-Cohn et al. (1970b)
Dydrogesterone		Dysmenorrhea 10 mg/day for 15 days	Kobayashi (1963)
		Amenorrhea, 10 to 20 mg/day	Bishop et al. (1962)
Ethisterone	Castrated women 60 to 80 mg/day		Israel and Schneller (1950)
17α-Hydroxyprogesterone caproate	Primary or secondary amenorrhea or ovulatory failure, 125 mg i.m.		Epstein et al. (1958)
Lynestrenol	Normal women, ovulation inhibited by drug (2.5 mg + 75 mcg mestranol, cyclically)		Knutsson et al. (1964)
Megestrol acetate	Amenorrhea, 2.5 mg/day		Knutsson et al. (1965) Greenblatt et al. (1963)

Norethisterone	Amenorrhea, "patients with uniphasic records" 20 mg/day	Greenblatt (1956)
	Primary or secondary amenorrhea or ovulatory failure 10 mg/day	Epstein et al. (1958)
	Normal women with inhibited ovulation; continuous daily administration of 0.5 mg	Larsson-Cohn et al. (1970a)
	Normal women, contin. daily administration of 0.3 mg	Larsson-Cohn et al. (1970c)
Norethisterone enanthate	Normal women long-acting injections of 300 mg	Gilfrich et al. (1969)
Norethynodrel	Primary or secondary amenorrhea or ovulation failure, 10 mg/day	Epstein et al. (1958)
Norgesterone	Ovariectomy with estrogen priming 10 mg/day	d'Incerti Bonini and Pagani (1962)
Norgestriénone	Amenorrhea 1 mg/day	Netter et al. (1967)
Normethandrone	Primary or secondary amenorrhea or ovulatory failure 10 mg/day	Epstein et al. (1958)
Superlutin	Oligo-amenorrhea, temperature rise dose-dependent (4–6 mg/day)	Štěrba et al. (1962)
Trengestone (Retroid®)	Amenorrhea and anovulatory cycles 4 to 12 mg daily	Stamm et al. (1968)

hypothalamus, chlormadinone acetate. It was used in doses of 20–30 mg (or less) daily p.o. or 100 mg of a crystal suspension i.m. every 3 to 6 weeks.

A hypothalamic-pituitary effect was assumed to be involved in a phenomenon described by Rauscher et al. (1969). These authors gave several progestational drugs in single doses to women with various types of amenorrhea or otherwise disturbed cycles, either i.m. (17α-hydroxyprogesterone caproate, 100 mg or 500 mg of the 19-nor analogue) or p.o. (20 mg of norethisterone, 10 mg of its acetate, 20 mg of normethandrone, or 10 mg of cyproterone acetate) and found that each of these compounds in a number of cases produced not only one uterine ("withdrawal") bleeding but that, without further medication this was often followed by several "subsequent bleedings" with regular intervals of about 14 days. These observations may well deserve further studies.

The remarkable observation by Lawrence and Kirsteins (1970) that medroxyprogesterone acetate (in oral doses of 4 to 5 times 10 mg per day) drastically reduced plasma-growth hormone in acromegalic patients (both under basal conditions and after arginine stimulation) was tentatively put down to a hypothalamic inhibitory effect on growth hormone secretion.

4. INFLUENCES ON BODY TEMPERATURE

The well-known thermogenic effect of progesterone (see Chapter 14) which causes the biphasic curve of body temperature in the normal cycle is probably also due to a hypothalamic effect. It is mimicked by most but not all synthetic progestational compounds. In studying this property of a new drug one must obviously exclude any possibility of an effect of endogenous progesterone being involved. This can best be done by administration of the substance to women who have no functioning ovaries. Dydrogesterone is notable as a steroid which does not inhibit ovulation nor increase body temperature in doses exceeding those needed for progestational transformation of the endometrium.

A great number of references on the thermogenicity of progestational compounds are to be found in the review by Gibian and Unger (1968). A selection of data is presented in Table 2.

5. INFLUENCES ON CONTRACTILITY OF THE NON-PREGNANT UTERUS

Some observations concerning effects of synthetic progestational compounds were already mentioned in Chapters 5 and 24.

Eskes and his group in Amsterdam devoted a study to the influence of a few progestational compounds on the spontaneous contractility of the human non-pregnant uterus (see Eskes *et al.*, 1970 a and b; Braaksma, 1970). They chose the "open-tip catheter" for pressure recording, having convinced themselves by very careful measurements that this yields very accurate tracings without the deformation of the pressure curves obtained with "all types of closed fluid systems", which introduce "a non-linear factor" due to the resistance of the rubber balloon (Braaksma, 1970, p. 21). They studied spontaneous pressure waves throughout the cycle and found a characteristic pattern during the "ovulatory phase" (days 11–14), consisting in high-frequency–low-amplitude waves, with high basal pressure (more than 20 mm Hg) between contractions (Eskes *et al.*, 1970a) which disappeared under cyclic treatment with Lyndiol or Lyndiol 2.5 (lynestrenol 5 mg + 150 mcg mestranol or half these doses respectively). The persistent activity during these anovulatory cycles (low-frequency, high-amplitude, low basal pressure) resembled that seen during labor or menstruation "or at the best the premenstrual phase". It is evident—and was to be expected—that a combination of these steroids, which does not produce normal cyclic endometrial changes, does not reproduce a physiological contractility pattern either. The progestational compound lynestrenol alone (Orgametril®) "gave these pictures".

The authors conclude that the addition of 75 or 150 mcg of mestranol to the progestational compound cannot be detected in the response of the myometrium.

It seemed therefore of particular interest to study a progestational compound which is by many authors considered *not* to inhibit ovulation in the human and as such they chose dydrogesterone (Eskes *et al.*, 1970b). The drug (Duphaston®) was given in large doses (20–40 mg per day orally from days 5–25 of the cycle or 100 mg by injection on the 1st, 2nd or 3rd day of the cycle). Each patient served as her own control. Dydrogesterone did not interfere with the development of an ovulatory pattern of spontaneous uterine contractions, though there were some minor differences when compared with normal control cycles (a slight increase in amplitude and a slight decrease in frequency with somewhat stronger arterial pulsations). These might well be due to a direct drug effect on the myometrium in the absence of inhibition of ovulation.

6. INFLUENCE ON THE FALLOPIAN TUBE

A number of observations concerning effects of progestational compounds on the human oviduct were included in the corresponding section in Chapter 28 (Section 18, p. 154).

7. INFLUENCES ON THE BIOLOGY OF THE HUMAN CERVIX

In view of the importance of the cervix as a target of contraceptive drugs, any pharmacological effects on this structure deserve attention.

As briefly mentioned in Chapter 30 (p. 266) "Roland (1968) using a daily dose of 0.075 or 0.05 mg of norgestrel observed a reduction of the midcycle spinnbarkeit and a lower degree of ferning. The postcoital sampling demonstrated actively motile spermatozoa in the endocervical mucus, but not in the uterine fundus." In another paper Roland (1968) comments on this interesting observation by saying: "the progestagen appears rather to exert a profound effect upon the cervical mucus in some way other than by producing a hostile barrier."

Chlormadinone acetate, in daily doses of 0.4 mg, given p.o. for contraception, according to a study by Gregoire and Ustay (1969), without inhibiting ovulation, reduced the amount of cervical mucus drastically, with complete elimination of the midcycle peak, but without affecting the glycogen content of the mucus (The glycogen content of the human cervical secretions, unlike that of the hamster, appears not to be steroid dependent.)

In a study on mucus formation in the mouse vagina Carlborg (1966) made the interesting discovery that the content of sialic acid in the vagina, which served as a good parameter of mucification, was lowered in spayed animals by exceedingly small doses of estradiol (0.005 to 0.05 mcg daily per animal), lower than those which produced estrous smears. Progesterone, on the other hand, when given alone did not change the sialic acid content (in doses ranging from 1.0 to 5 mg). Only with combinations of both hormones in an optimal ratio (1.5 mg progesterone plus 0.015 mcg estradiol) were sialic acid levels reached, corresponding to those in midpregnancy. Some time later the author (Carlborg et al., 1968) went on to study the sialic acid in the human cervix under the influence of norethisterone acetate with or without ethynyl estradiol.

The subjects were five healthy young women studied for nine cycles and five other ones (also studied by McCormick et al. for suppression of gonadotrophin excretion, see p. 277), who were given either Anovlar® or 1 mg of norethisterone acetate alone, from the 5th to the 25th day of the cycle. In all the untreated cycles there was a very distinct minimum of sialic acid concentration in the cervical mucus on or about the 16th day (see Fig. 2). In the cycles with Anovlar treatment the determination of sialic acid concentration indicated a constant value of 40 mcg/mg dry cervical mucus. In two out of five cycles with norethisterone acetate alone an increase in pregnanediol excretion was recorded and in one of these there was a mid-cycle nadir of sialic acid. In the other cycles of this group it decreased continuously. Although the reader gets the impression that the occurrence or absence of ovulation is of predominant influence on the behavior of cervical sialic acid concentration, the one case of a woman who, while on norethisterone acetate, apparently ovulated (pregnanediol increase) but had a low sialic acid value would seem to lend support to the authors' suggestion that the dose of norethisterone had a direct and demonstrable effect on the sialic acid content of the mucus. ("It is suggested that more effort should be directed in obtaining agents which produce

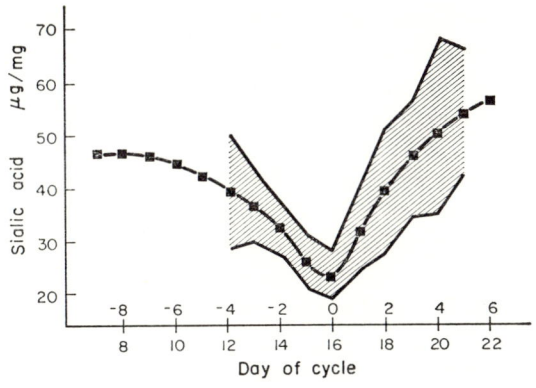

Fig. 2.

peripheral obstacles to sperm migration rather than inhibition of ovulation".) Sperm receptivity was negative in all cycles under treatment with either Anovlar or norethisterone acetate.

In this context the following observation will be of interest.

The distribution of tritium labeled chlormadinone acetate (CA) and progesterone (P) in women who had to undergo hysterectomy were studied after intravenous injection of 250 mcg by Gallegos et al. (1970). the highest concentration (dpm per g wet tissue) of CA was found in the subcutaneous abdominal fat. In the genital tract, the greatest amount of radioactivity was found in the Fallopian tube, the endocervix or the cervical mucus itself (six out of seven cases). By contrast P was concentrated in the subcutaneous fat only in three patients in the the proliferative phase. Those who were in the secretory phase had the highest activity in the skin, the uterus and uterine fibroids but none in the "mucus producing tissues of the genital tract".

8. INFLUENCES ON ADRENAL FUNCTION

It has been shown in animal studies (Chapter 28, subsections 20.1 and 20.2, p. 160) that medroxyprogesterone acetate (MAP) and other chemically related progestational compounds depress adrenal size and function, which in several instances could be explained by a corticosteroid-like activity of the compound.

This has been investigated in the human. Cammanni *et al.* studied the effects of MAP in four adrenalectomized patients and one woman, whose pituitary had been destroyed by ^{90}Y implantation, using the diuretic response to a waterload, glucose tolerance and insulin resistance tests as criteria. In all these respects 100 mg MAP injected daily s.c. proved to be equal or superior to 50 mg of cortisone given p.o. One patient who 3 days after discontinuation of cortisone maintenance developed a critical state of adrenal insufficiency recovered under i.v. cortisol treatment and was put back on her maintenance dose of 50 mg. When this was replaced by 100 mg MAP s.c., no symptoms of insufficiency were seen within 16 days.

MAP was much less active on oral administration.

Most studies which could reveal an influence of progestational compounds on adrenal function were undertaken with a view to testing the safety of oral contraceptives and therefore an estrogen was almost always administered concomitantly (see Chapter 34). Since estrogens are known to increase the level of the cortisol-binding globulin transcortin and of (protein-bound) cortisol in the plasma, and to increase the size of the adrenals in animals, it is difficult to draw conclusions from such studies regarding the influence of the progestational component of the drug. There are, however, a few cases where the latter was given separately, such as in the report by Layne *et al.* (1962) who found that Enovid in a dose of 10 mg per day (containing 9.85 norethynodrel and 0.150 mg mestranol*) increased cortisol levels in plasma and binding of cortisol to plasma proteins about as much as the two components separately. This was accompanied by a significant reduction in cortisol secretion rate since norethynodrel is notably estrogenic; it was concluded, that "the effects of Enovid and of Norethynodrel on cortisol metabolism are due to their estrogenic potency."

* Ethynyl estradiol 3-methyl ether, also abbreviated as EE3ME.

Dodek et al. (1965), who studied the same phenomena in the same population of (psychiatric) patients as Layne et al., by a slightly different technique (continuous infusion instead of single dose injections of radioactive, labeled cortisol), found the same increase in plasma levels and a great reduction in metabolic clearance of cortisol, but failed to demonstrate a decrease in cortisol production rate, due to (long-term and short-term) administration of Enovid. Though they did not give the two components separately, they also ascribe the overall effect of the drug to its estrogenicity.

Normethandrone without added estrogen was studied by Vermeulen and Ferin (1962, 1963), who gave the drug p.o. in daily doses of 5 or 2.5 mg, continuously or cyclically, to women with menstrual disturbances for periods of at least 2 months and found depressed urinary excretion of cortisol metabolites, increased levels of transcortin, and a decreased cortisol production. All the observations, including a prolonged half-life of 4-^{14}C-cortisol, were interpreted as at least partly due to a reduced cortisol inactivation rate, which for several reasons was supposed to be caused by interference with the cortisol-inactivating enzymes in the liver. Normethandrone is not estrogenic. Its effect on certain liver functions in women had been described earlier by Feldman and Carter (1960), who gave it in very high doses (30 mg daily for long periods of time). Dodek et al. considered an effect on liver enzymes as a possible mechanism to reduce metabolic clearance rates of Enovid but rejected it.

A long-acting ester of norethisterone, the enanthate, injected in single doses of 300 mg to healthy female volunteers, did not change plasma corticoid levels, nor their response to the injection of ACTH and had no influence on 17-ketosteroid excretion (Gilfrich et al., 1969).

De Moor et al. (1966) reported that normethandrone in daily doses of 5 mg did not change the cortisol binding capacity of the plasma during the first week of treatment, but lynestrenol (a weakly estrogenic substance) increased it greatly in four out of six patients, treated for at least 3 months.

In summary, the impression is gained that only those progestational compounds which by themselves have some estrogenic activity increase the level of (protein-bound) cortisol in the blood and lower its metabolic clearance, mainly by increasing the concentration of the cortisol binding globulin. So far no indications have been found that the adrenal-inhibiting effect of certain progestational compounds, demonstrated in the rat, manifests itself in the human at dose levels practically employed, e.g. in oral contraception. Even in doses of 100 mg daily for 10 days Castegnaro and Sala (1962) found medroxyprogesterone acetate (MAP) without effect on adrenal function as judged from the excretion of cortisol metabolites and the response to metyrapone and ACTH. Earlier Mazza and Hecht-Lucari (1960) had found a transient decrease in 17-ketosteroid excretion but only a doubtful depression of 17-OH-corticosteroids in ten normal women (including three pregnant ones) after one or two i.m. injections of 100 mg of MAP.

Chlormadinone acetate in daily doses of 0.5 mg was found to be without consistent influence on corticoid excretion, cortisol plasma levels or adrenal response to ACTH and hypoglycemia (Daly et al., 1969). In some tests megestrol acetate was also examined and its behavior was similar.

In doses of 20 mg daily for 3 weeks medroxyprogesterone acetate (MAP) according to Crane and Harris (1969) caused a significant decrease in aldosterone excretion rates in the third week of treatment on unrestricted sodium intake but the response to sodium restriction was unchanged. When combined with ethynyl estradiol, MAP (as Provest®) was found to increase aldosterone excretion, but this was entirely accounted for by the effect of the estrogen.

9. OTHER EFFECTS OF PROGESTATIONAL COMPOUNDS ON THE PRODUCTION AND METABOLISM OF STEROIDS

Mauvais-Jarvis (1966) found that lynestrenol influenced the metabolism of dehydro-*epi*-androsterone-sulfate (DHAS) in normal men and hirsute women suffering from the Stein–Leventhal syndrome. The effects were similar to those of ethynyl estradiol or the combination of lynestrenol and mestranol (Lyndiol®) and are attributed to the estrogenicity of these substances. Lyndiol enhanced sulfate conjugation of steroids (17-ketones and testosterone) and the production of DHA. It is assumed that Lyndiol specifically stimulates sulfurylation of certain steroids in the liver or outside it. It inhibits 5α-$\Delta 4$-reductase and activates 17β-hydroxysteroid dehydrogenase. Attention is called to the importance of the peripheral hydrogenation of testosterone in the target organs (inhibited by Lyndiol?) which would lead to compounds biologically more active than testosterone.

The effect of medroxyprogesterone acetate (MAP) on the metabolism of testosterone was studied by Gordon et al. (1970) who gave it p.o. in high doses (40 mg daily) for periods of 4 to 12 weeks to four men and three women. The effects were far more pronounced in the males, where it increased metabolic clearance and decreased plasma concentrations and production rates. (The subjects complained of diminished libido.) Influence on plasma protein binding was variable. There was no significant decrease in production rate in women. Plasma LH values decreased significantly in all but one subject, but FSH only in one (a postmenopausal woman).

Supplementary to this were some animal experiments. MAP did not interfere with the effect of testosterone proprionate, given simultaneously, on the seminal vesicles or prostates of rats, but pretreatment of the animals (2.5 mg every other day, 4 times) significantly inhibited the growth promoting effect of testosterone. The administration of the drug to male rats (5 mg, 3 times weekly, seven doses s.c.) resulted in a highly *significant increase* in hepatic testosterone A-ring reductase activity.

The authors speculate that MAP may have such an effect in the human which could account for the increased metabolic clearance rate. The decreased production rate would be due to decreased LH secretion.

As a matter of fact, the same group (Gordon *et al.*, 1971) showed that treatment with MAP (40 mg daily p.o. for about 3 weeks) caused an increase in A-ring reductase activity of 200–500 per cent in human liver biopsies and of 30 to 60 per cent in the metabolic clearance of testosterone.

For influences on the progesterone secretion of an established corpus luteum see above, Section 2, p. 280.

10. GENERAL METABOLIC EFFECTS OF PROGESTATIONAL COMPOUNDS

10.1. BODY-MASS

In view of the known effects of progesterone on bodyweight and the composition of body-mass (see Chapter 15), the results of some animal studies (see Chapter 28, subsection 21.1, p. 168), and numerous reports on weight changes in women taking oral contraceptives, studies concerning the effects of synthetic progestational compounds on these parameters in women would seem to be important.

Lecocq *et al.* (1967) examined the effects of such drugs, norethynodrel and chlormadinone acetate, on lean body-mass and nitrogen balance in six healthy young women on an individually established caloric intake and a regimen of 80 mcg mestranol daily, beginning 3 weeks before the administration of the progestational compounds, viz. 5 mg norethynodrel or 2 mg chlormadinone acetate daily for another 3 weeks. Body density was measured twice weekly in a specially designed volumeter.

Because of the fixed caloric diet there were little changes in bodyweight (and changes in appetite could not have become very effective). Main results: "Every subject manifested an increase in lean body-mass and, because weight was stable, a decrease in body fat. The average increase was 2.14 kg for 3 studies on norethynodrel and 1.43 kilograms for 4 studies on chlormadinone acetate. Except for a single instance . . . the rise in lean body-mass on norethynodrel was significantly higher than that in the chlormadinone acetate studies, which were remarkably consistent. . . . With chlormadinone acetate, the calculated accumulation of lean tissue, as derived from nitrogen balance, compared favorably with that from body densimetric techniques. However, this was not true of the norethynodrel studies. . . . With norethynodrel in addition to the accumulation of protein, body water retention was probable in one subject, and loss of body water in the other 2. . . . The nitrogen retention with both progestins was substantial, averaging over 1 gm per day more than during the control mestranol week."

There was a rather surprising negative phosphorus balance with either compound that remained unexplained.

10.2. BLOOD CHEMISTRY

Small changes in blood chemistry were observed by Tronconi and Ferrero (1960) in women taking large oral doses of medroxyprogesterone acetate (60 mg daily for 4 days: slight decrease of total plasma proteins and of clearing factor activity, very slight increase in α-lipoproteins and decrease in β); no changes in blood electrolytes, but slight increase in diuresis (Tronconi and Santi, 1960).

In view of the well-known effects of oral contraceptive tablets on copper and iron levels in the serum Briggs and Briggs (1970) studied the effects of two progestational compounds and of ethynyl estradiol separately. Norethisterone acetate in daily doses of 0.3 to 1.0 mg or norgestrel (1.0 mg) given orally for 3 to 4 weeks caused rises in serum iron and total iron-binding capacity but not in serum copper levels. Ethynyl estradiol caused a rise in copper only. It is assumed that these changes are secondary to effects on the liver. Medroxyprogesterone acetate (MAP) as a single long-action injection of 300 mg (Depo Provera®) had no effect on the serum levels of iron, total iron-binding capacity, transferrin, and protein-bound iodine in women, in whom estrogen-containing oral contraceptives had previously raised these levels (Powell *et al.*, 1970).

The same compound and 5 other synthetic progestational agents were studied by Barbosa *et al.* (1971) for their effects on plasma protein levels in healthy volunteers in high oral doses (15 to 40 mg daily for 4 weeks).

The main results are summarized by us in Table 3. It can be seen that the (weakly estrogenic) estrane derivatives increase the carrier proteins for cortisol (as is known of estrogens) and that dydrogesterone is remarkably free of any effect on plasma proteins.

Chlormadinone acetate in daily oral contraceptive doses of 0.5 mg for 6 to 9 months was without effect on the homeostasis of 17 plasma proteins (Laurell et al., 1969). *The general impression is thus gained that most of the biochemical changes in the plasma of women taking oral contraceptives are mainly caused by the estrogenic components of these drugs.*

10.3. SALT AND WATER EXCRETION

The effect of norethisterone on sodium and potassium excretion was studied by Jenkins (1961) and compared with that of progesterone. The subjects were four women suffering from cyclical edema and one man

TABLE 3. INFLUENCES OF SYNTHETIC PROGESTATIONAL COMPOUNDS ON PLASMA PROTEINS IN MAN. (Data from Barbosa et al. 1971.)
Symbols used: + significantly increased; − no significant change.
Abbreviations for names of compounds (followed by dose in mg/day): DY: dydrogesterone; ET: ethisterone; MAP: medroxyprogesterone acetate; NE: norethisterone; NAC: norethisterone acetate; FC: free (non-protein bound) cortisol.
Abbreviations for plasma proteins: CBG: cortisol binding globulin; Fib.: fibrinogen; Glu.: β-glucuronidase; HAP: haptoglobin; PL: plasminogen; TBG: thyroxin binding globulin; TBPA: thyroxin binding prealbumin; TP: total proteins.

	ET 30	MAP 40	NE 30	NAC 15	DY 40
CBG	−	−	+	+	−
FC			−	−	
Fib.	−	−	−	−	−
Glu.	−	−	+	+	−
HAP	+	+	+	+	−
PL	−	+	+	+	−
TBG	−	−	−	−	−
TBPA	−	−	+	−	−
TP	−	−	−	−	−

with cirrhosis of the liver and marked ascites. Whereas large doses of progesterone (100–200 mg daily i.m.) produced some increase in sodium excretion (though much less than 2 g of chlorothiazide) norethisterone (in daily oral doses of 30 mg) had no such effect. It has been assumed (see Chapter 15) that progesterone behaves as an aldosterone antagonist and in fact in the cirrhotic patient 200 mg of progesterone had an effect comparable to that of 400 mg of spironolactone. No such effects were seen with norethisterone. It even caused some sodium retention. The doses of norethisterone were, of course, much smaller than those of progesterone, even taking into account the ratio of biological activities (e.g. in the Clauberg test, see Chapter 28, Table 3).

By contrast medroxyprogesterone acetate as reported by D'Alessandro *et al.* (1961) in daily doses of 40 to 80 mg caused a distinct increase in volume of urine in four patients, suffering from liver cirrhosis and ascites, with heart and renal failure or congestive heart failure and hepatic congestion. The effect was increased by hydrochlorothiazide. Secondary hyperaldosteronism was suspected to have been antagonized by the treatment.

10.4. GLUCOSE METABOLISM

Low doses of chlormadinone acetate (0.5 mg daily) were studied by Taft *et al.* (1969) with respect to their influence on glucose utilization and insulin secretion. Though the number of subjects treated was small, the data suggest that the exaggerated insulin response to glucose seen with norethisterone plus mestranol is not observed with chlormadinone acetate (see also Chapter 28, subsection 21.2, p. 172). Dittmar and Waidle (1969) equally found chlormadinone acetate (0.5 mg daily) without influence on blood glucose and insulin levels during glucose tolerance tests in twenty normal women.

Beck (1970) arrived at the same conclusion after a study of sixteen women with subclinical diabetes and eight normal subjects during treatment with either conventional contraceptive steroids or chlormadinone acetate 0.5 mg p.o. per day. After 6 months treatment with the latter compound glucose tolerance became abnormal in only two subclinical diabetic subjects and deteriorated in one other (as against two and three respectively after 2.5 months of conventional contraceptive treatment).

Medroxyprogesterone acetate, though lowering growth hormone levels in acromegalics according to Lawrence and Kirsteins (1970), was without significant influence on glucose tolerance in most of these patients and "unlike progesterone ... was not associated with evidence of increased insulin resistance noted in the studies reported by Beck (1969)".

Deterioration of glucose tolerance in diabetic subjects treated with 17α-hydroxyprogesterone caproate was reported by Schreibman (1968).

11. EFFECTS ON THE LIVER

There are good reasons to assume that the occasional occurrence of jaundice and increased BSP-retention in women taking oral contraceptive drugs is primarily or solely due to their estrogenic component. In this context studies on the progestational components are, of course, relevant. One such report is by Boake (1967), who studied a woman that had previously developed intrahepatic cholestatic jaundice during each of three pregnancies. It is now well known that these patients are particularly prone to jaundice on oral contraception. The author found that she showed hepatic dysfunction with pruritus and nausea on estrogens (Premarin, estradiol or stilbestrol) but had no alterations of liver functions when treated with medroxyprogesterone acetate (10 mg/day for 1 week) or lynestrenol (10 mg/day for 5 days). (See also subsection 9, p. 290, Gordon et al. (1971).)

Routier et al. (1967) described a case of jaundice and edema of the legs in a woman who for half a year had taken 10 mg of norethisterone daily during the last 8 days of each cycle. Complete normalization after cessation of treatment. Three other cases quoted from literature, in two of which still higher doses had been given. Routier's case was complicated by an eruption of acne which could point to an androgenic steroid effect.

No impairment of liver function was observed during depot treatment with norethisterone enanthate, 200 mg i.m. every 12 weeks for 9 months (Petry et al., 1970), nor after single injections of 300 mg (Gilfrich et al., 1970).

Clinch and Tindall (1969) could show that megestrol acetate in daily oral doses of 20 to 30 mg, given to puerperal women with the purpose of suppressing lactation, did not influence BSP-retention in comparison with normally lactating women and in contrast with the same dose of stilbestrol, which significantly reduced the excretion of the dye by the liver into the bile.

12. EFFECTS ON BLOOD-COAGULATION FACTORS

Numerous studies on blood-coagulation factors and behavior of platelets, undertaken to elucidate the causes of thromboembolic episodes as a rare side effect of oral contraception, have in general implicated the estrogenic component of the drugs. In one of these (Bolton et al., 1968) it was shown that various combination-type contraceptive drugs increase the sensitivity of blood-platelets to adenosine diphosphate (ADP), which manifests itself by a change in electrophoretic mobility of the platelets and is presumably caused by an abnormality in the low-density lipoproteins. These platelets then resemble those found in arterial disease. The estrogens in these drugs, ethynyl estradiol or mestranol, were indicted. Chlormadinone acetate in daily doses of 0.5 mg or 1.0 was found not to affect platelet ADP sensitivity (see also Hampton, 1970).

Chlormadinone acetate (referred to as progesterone), given continuously in 0.5-mg daily doses, was reported to be without effect on coagulability or increased platelet aggregation by Poller et al. (1969; Poller, 1970). Menon et al. (1970) found a slight decrease in fibrinolytic activity in the blood of women who had been on the same regimen for 6 to 24 months, as compared with normal women (no drugs) and a group on a "combined pill". The scatter amongst these groups was very high. Pregnant women had very much lower fibrinolytic activities than any of these groups.

Norethisterone enanthate in single long-acting injections of 300 mg did cause significant changes in thromboplastin time, recalcification time and fibrinogen, suggesting an increased coagulability (Gilfrich et al., 1969).

13. VARIOUS OBSERVATIONS, INCLUDING EFFECTS ON THYROID FUNCTION, RELEASE FROM DEPOT CAPSULES, PREGNANCY TESTS, AND INFLUENCE ON LACTATION

The absence of any abnormalities in babies born to mothers who had been treated with medroxyprogesterone acetate, in some cases up to 50 or 60 mg per day and sometimes for the entire duration of pregnancy, was reported by Tronconi (1962). The babies were observed during the whole first year of life.

The same compound was found to have no effect on the thyroid (^{131}I-uptake) in "normal or medium doses" whereas "large doses" yielded thyroid tests temporarily "similar to those in severe hypothyroidism" (Maneschi et al., 1962).

Whereas estrogens—usually contained in oral contraceptives—increase thyroxin-binding globulin (TBG) and thereby PBI in the plasma, no such effect was found with the daily administration of low dosage (0.5 mg) of chlormadinone acetate, without added estrogen in normal women as judged by PBI, T_3-resin uptake and electrophoretic index (Taft et al., 1969).

The release of three progestational compounds from implanted silicone rubber (Silastic) capsules was studied by Coutinho et al. (1970). Megestrol acetate, norgestrel and norgestrienone were effective in preventing conception and release rates were stable after the first 2 weeks of treatment. Megestrol acetate under similar conditions according to Benagiano et al. (1970) showed declining diffusion rates.

The use of medroxyprogesterone acetate as an oral pregnancy test was recommended by Walther and Platt (1964). Combinations of estrogens with progesterone or orally active progestational compounds have been used for quite some time (particularly in Europe) for the diagnosis of pregnancy in women with short-lasting amenorrhea since these drugs (parenterally or orally, respectively) would cause a withdrawal bleeding, when the patient is not pregnant. Walther and Platt found that single oral doses of 50 mg medroxyprogesterone acetate (5 tablets of 10 mg Provera®) gave accurate results in most of the tests. Babies born to the women so treated were normal. Results are shown on thirty patients of whom twenty were pregnant, with a total of one false negative (incipient abortion) and two false positives.

The effect of lynestrenol on lactation was studied by Kamal *et al.* (1969) in an Arab population in Cairo. The drug was given continuously in doses of 0.5 mg daily and compared with three combination-type oral contraceptives as well as with a placebo. All these "medications" were ranked on the basis of points given for five parameters of lactation and growth of the baby. As a non-inhibitor lynestrenol came out on top of placebo. (Twenty-four women in each group, studied until the baby was 24 weeks old. Those on lynestrenol performed even better than those on placebo.) On the other hand, as reported for the same group by Abdel Kader *et al.* (1969), lynestrenol like the other drugs reduced the protein and fat content of the milk as well as that of Na, K, Ca and Mg, though growth curves of babies stayed within the normal range.

REFERENCES

ABDEL KADER, M. M., ABDEL HAY, A., EL-SAFOURI, S., ABDEL AZIZ, M. T., SAAD EL-DIN, J., KAMAL, I., HEFNAWI, F., GHONEIM, M., TALAAT, M., YOUNIS, N., TAGUI, A. and ABDALLA, M. (1969) Clinical, biochemical, and experimental studies on lactation. III. Biochemical changes induced in human milk by gestagens. *Amer. J. Obstet. Gynec.* **105**: 978–985.

BARBOSA, J., SEAL, U. S. and DOE, R. (1971) Effects of steroids on plasma proteins—progestational agents. *J. Clin. Endocr.* **32**: 547–554.

BECK, P. (1969) Progestin enhancement of the plasma insulin response to glucose in Rhesus monkeys. *Diabetes* **18**: 146–152.

BECK, P. (1970) Comparison of the metabolic effects of chlormadinone acetate and conventional contraceptive steroids in man. *J. Clin. Endocr.* **30**: 785–791.

BENAGIANO, G., ERMINI, M., DONINI, S. and OLIVIERI, V. (1970) Sustained release hormonal preparations as long acting contraceptive agents. In: *Third International Congress on Hormonal Steroids.* Internat. Congress Series, no. 210, Abstr. 465, p. 217. Excerpta Medica, Amsterdam, New York.

BISHOP, P. M. F., BORELL, U., DICZFALUSY, E. and TILLINGER, K. G. (1962) Effect of dydrogesterone on human endometrium and ovarian activity. *Acta Endocr. (Kbh.)* **40**: 203–216.

BOAKE, W. C. (1967) Effects of natural and synthetic oestrogens and progestogens on hepatic function. *Acta Endocr. (Kbh.)* Suppl. **119**: 169.

BOLTON, C. H., HAMPTON, J. R. and MITCHELL, J. R. A. (1968) Effect of oral contraceptive agents on platelets and plasma-phospholipids. *Lancet* **1**: 1336–1341.

BRAAKSMA, J. T. (1970) Drukregistratie in de niet zwangere uterus *in vivo*—onderzoek van een methode. (Pressure recording in the non pregnant uterus *in vivo.*) Dutch with English Summary. Thesis, The Free University, Amsterdam.

BRIGGS, M. H. and BRIGGS, M. (1970) Contraceptives and serum proteins. *Brit. Med. J.* **2**: 521.

CAMMANNI, F., MASSARA, F. and MOLINATTI, G. M. (1963) The cortisone-like effect of 6α-methyl-17-acetoxy-progesterone in the adrenalectomized man. *Acta Endocr. (Kbh.)* **43**: 477–483.

CARLBORG, L. G. (1966) Quantitative determination of sialic acids in the mouse vagina. *Endocrinology* **78**: 1093–1099.

CARLBORG, L., MCCORMICK, W. and GEMZELL, C. (1968) Effect of norethisterone acetate with or without ethynyl oestradiol on sialic acid concentration and sperm receptivity of the cervical mucus. *Acta Endocr. (Kbh.)* **59**: 636–643.

CASTEGNARO, E. and SALA, G. (1962) The influence of MAP in man. II. A determination of the adrenal function. In: *Internat. Congress on Hormonal Steroids*. Internat. Congress Series no. 51, Abstr. 261, p. 196. Excerpta Medica, Amsterdam, New York.

CLINCH, J. and TINDALL, V. R. (1969) Effect of oestrogens and progestogens on liver function in the puerperium. *Brit. Med. J.* **1**: 602–605.

COLLINS, W. P., KOULLAPIS, E. N. and SOMMERVILLE, I. F. (1971) The effect of chlormadinone acetate on progesterone secretion and metabolism. *Acta Endocr.* **68**: 271–284.

COUTINHO, E. M., FERREIRA, D. A. M., PRATES, H., TATUM, H., SANTANO, A. R. and MATTOS, C. E. R. (1970) Long term steroid administration in humans by subcutaneous Silastic capsules. In: *Third International Congress on Hormonal Steroids*. International Congress Series no. 210, Abstr. 464, p. 217. Excerpta Medica, Amsterdam, New York.

CRANE, M. G. and HARRIS, J. J. (1969a) Plasma renin activity and aldosterone excretion rate in normal subjects. I. Effect of ethynyl estradiol and medroxyprogesterone acetate. *J. Clin. Endocr.* **29**: 550–557.

CRANE, M. G. and HARRIS, J. (1969b) Plasma renin activity and aldosterone excretion rate in normal subjects. II. Effect of oral contraceptive agents. *J. Clin. Endocr.* **29**: 558–562.

D'ALESSANDRO, B., BRANCACCIO, A. and JACONO, G. (1961) Sull'effetto diuretico del 6α-metil-17α-idrossiprogesterone acetato (MAP). Possibilitá di una azione competitiva dell'aldosterone. *Boll. Soc. Ital. di Biologia Sper.* **37**: 724–727.

DALY, J. R., ELSTEIN, M. and MURRAY, J. (1969) Adrenocortical function studies during oral contraception with chlormadinone acetate. In: *Chlormadinone Acetate. A New Departure in Oral Contraception*, pp. 73–77. Christie, G. A. and Moore-Robinson, M. (Eds.). Syntex Pharmaceuticals Ltd., Maidenhead.

DAPUNT, O. (1969) Unsere Ergebnisse der Amenorrhoe- und Sterilitätsbehandlung mit dem Retrosteroid Ro 4-8347. In: *Second European Congress on Sterility*, Abstr. 278. Drobnjak, P. (Ed.). Tiskara izdavačkog Zavoda Jugoslavenske Akademije, Zagreb.

DAPUNT, O. and WINDBICHLER, H. (1969) Behandlungsergebnisse mit dem Retrosteroid Ro 4-8347. *Wien. Klin. Wschr.* **81**: 785–861.

DE MOOR, P., STEENO, O., BROSENS, I. and HENDRIKX, A. (1966) Data on transcortin activity in human plasma as studied by gel filtration. *J. Clin. Endocr.* **26**: 71–78.

DICZFALUSY, E., GOEBELSMANN, U., JOHANNISSON, E., TILLINGER, K. G. and WIDE, L. (1969) Pituitary and ovarian function in women on continuous low dose progestogens; effect of chlormadinone acetate and norethisterone. *Acta Endocr. (Kbh.)* **62**: 679–693.

D'INCERTI BONINI, L. and PAGANI, C. (1962) Indagine clinica sull'attivitá progestativa del vinilestrenolone (Clinical investigation of the progestational activity of vinylestrenolone). (Italian.) *Ann. Ost. Ginec.* **84**: 279–285.

DITTMAR, F. W. and WAIDL, E. (1969) Die Wirkungen von kleinsten Gestagen-Dosen auf den Kohlenhydratstoffwechsel. *Geburtsh. Frauenheilk.* **29**: 1026–1031.

DODEK, O. I., SEGRE, E. J. and KLAIBER, E. L. (1965) Effects of Enovid on cortisol metabolism. *Amer. J. Obstet. Gynec.* **93**: 173–177.

EPSTEIN, J. A., KUPPERMAN, H. S. and CUTLER, A. (1958) Comparative pharmacological and clinical activity of 19-nortestosterone and 17-hydroxyprogesterone derivatives in man. *Ann. N.Y. Acad. Sci.* **71**: 560–571.

ESKES, T. K. A. B., CRONE, A., HEIN, P. R., KARS-VILLANUEVA, E. B., BRAAKSMA, J. T. and JANSSENS, J. (1970a) The influence of oral contraceptive and progestational drugs upon the mechanical activity of the non-pregnant human uterus *in vivo*. *Nederl. T. Verlosk.* **70**: 47–56.

ESKES, T. K. A. B., HEIN, P. R., STOLTE, L. A. M., KARS-VILLANUEVA, E. B., CRONE, A., BRAAKSMA, J. T. and JANSSENS, J. (1970b) Influence of dydrogesterone on the activity of the non-pregnant human uterus. *Amer. J. Obstet. Gynec.* **106**: 1235–1241.

FELDMAN, E. B. and CARTER, A. C. (1960) Endocrinologic and metabolic effects of 17α-methyl-19-nortestosterone in women. *J. Clin. Endocr.* **20**: 842–857.

FRANCHIMONT, P., CESSION, G., GASPARD, U., LEGROS, J. J. and AYALON, D. (1970) Action des progestatifs anticonceptionnels sur les gonadotrophines sériques. In: *Inhibition de l'ovulation*, pp. 189–197. Netter, A. (Ed.). Masson & Cie, Paris.

GALLEGOS, A. J., GONZÁLEZ DIDDI, M. and MARTINEZ MANAUTOU, J. (1970) Tissue deposit of progestogens and possible correlation to contraceptive activity. In: *Third Internat. Congress on Hormonal Steroids*. Internat. Congress Series no. 210, Abstr. 128, p. 67. Excerpta Medica, Amsterdam, New York.

GIBIAN, H. and UNGER, R. (1968) Wirkungen der Gestagene auf den Stoffwechsel. In: *Die Gestagene*, Teil 1, pp. 352–449. Junkmann, K. (Ed.), being Vol. XXII/1 of *Handbook of Experimental Pharmacology*. Springer-Verlag, Berlin, Heidelberg, New York.

GILFRICH, H. J., NIESCHLAG, E., DUDECK, J. and OVERZIER, C. (1969) Norethisteronönanthat. Untersuchungen während der Anwendung eines langwirkenden Kontrazeptivum. *Deutsch. Med. Wschr.* **94**: 2473–2477.

GORDON, G. G., ALTMAN, K., SOUTHREN, A. L. and OLIVO, J. (1971) Human hepatic testosterone. A-ring reductase activity: effect of medroxyprogesterone acetate. *J. Clin. Endocr.* **32**: 457–461.

GORDON, G. G., SOUTHREN, A. L., TOCHIMOTO, S., OLIVO, J., ALTMAN, K., RAND, J. and LEMBERGER, L. (1970) Effect of medroxyprogesterone acetate (Provera) on the metabolism and biological activity of testosterone. *J. Clin. Endocr.* **30**: 449–456.

GREENBLATT, R. (1956) The progestational activity of 17α-ethynyl-19-nortestosterone. *J. Clin. Endocr.* **16**: 869–875.

GREENBLATT, R. B., JUNGCK, E. C., BIGGER, JR., J. T. and GREER, M. V. (1963) Progestational activity of a new acetoxy-progesterone derivative (6α-methyl-6-dehydro-17α-acetoxyprogesterone). *Fertil. Steril.* **14**: 393–401.

GREGOIRE, A. T. and USTAY, K. (1969). Effect of chlormadinone on amount of human cervical mucus and its glycogen content. *Fertil. and Steril.* **20**: 938–943.

HALLER, J. (1968) *Ovulationshemmung durch Hormone*, p. 19. Georg Thieme Verlag, Stuttgart. English translation: *Hormonal Contraception*. Geron-X Inc., Los Altos, Calif. (1969).

HAMPTON, J. R. (1970) Platelet abnormalities induced by the administration of oestrogens. *J. Clin. Path.* **23**: Suppl. 3: 75–80.

ISRAEL, S. L. and SCHNELLER, O. (1950) The thermogenic property of progesterone. *Fertil. Steril.* **1**: 53–64.

JAFFE, R. B., MIDGLEY, JR., A. R. and GOEBELSMAN, U. (1969) Regulation of human gonadotropins. V. Effect of dydrogesterone on serum levels of follicle-stimulating and luteinizing hormones in women. *Amer. J. Obstet. Gynec.* **104**: 1031–1037.

JENKINS, J. S. (1961) Progesterone and norethisterone in cyclical oedema and ascites. *Brit. Med. J.* **2**: 861–863.

JOHANSSON, E. D. B. (1970) Luteolytic effects of gestagens. In: *Third Internat. Congress on Hormonal Steroids*, p. 215. James, V. H. T. (Ed.). Internat. Congress Series 210, Excerpta Medica, Amsterdam, New York.

KAMAL, I., HEFNAWI, F., GHONEIM, M., TALAAT, M., YOUNIS, N., TAGUI, A., and ABDALLA, M. (1969) Clinical, biochemical and experimental studies on lactation. *Amer. J. Obstet. Gynec.* **105**: 324–334.

KNUTSSON, F., RYBO, G. and ÅNBERG, Å. (1964) The inhibitory effect on ovulation of lynestrenol combined with mestranol. *Acta Obstet. Gynec. Scand.* **43**: Suppl. 7: 38–39.

KNUTTSSON, F., RYBO, G. and ÅNBERG, Å. (1965) Anovulatory effect of lynestrenol in combination with mestranol. *Acta Obst. Gynec. Scand.* **44**: 325.

KOBAYASHI, T. (1963) The fundamental and clinical studies on 6-dehydro-retro-progesterone. Report I. *The World of Obstetrics and Gynecology* **15**: 57 (1097)–63 (1103). (Jap.).

LARSSON-COHN, U., JOHANSSON, E. D. B. and GEMZELL, C. (1971) Effects of continuous daily administration of 0.03 mg of d-norgestrel on the plasma levels of progesterone and the urinary excretion of oestrogens. *Acta Endocr. (Kbh.)* **66**: 702–710.

LARSSON-COHN, U., JOHANSSON, E. D. B., WIDE, L. and GEMZELL, C. (1970a) Effects of continuous administration of 0.5 mg of norethindrone on the plasma levels of progesterone and on the urinary excretion of luteinizing hormone, pregnanediol and total oestrogens. *Acta Endocr. (Kbh.)* **63**: 216–224.

LARSSON-COHN, U., JOHANSSON, E. D. B., WIDE, L. and GEMZELL, C. (1970b) Effects of continuous daily administration of 0.5 mg of chlormadinone acetate on the plasma levels of progesterone and on the urinary excretion of luteinizing hormone and total oestrogens. *Acta Endocr. (Kbh.)* **63**: 705–716.

LARSSON-COHN, U., JOHANSSON, E. D. B. and GEMZELL, C. (1970c) Effects of continuous daily administration of 0.3 mg of norethindrone on the plasma levels of progesterone and on the urinary excretion of pregnanediol and total oestrogens. *Acta Endocr. (Kbh.)* **64**: 38–46.

LAURELL, C.-B., KULLANDER, S. and THORELL, J. (1969). Plasma proteins after continuous, oral use of a progestogen-chlormadionone (*Sic*) acetate as a contraceptive. *Scand. J. Clin. Lab. Invest.* **24**: 387–389.

LAWRENCE, A. M. and KIRSTEINS, L. (1970) Progestins in the medical management of active acromegaly. *J. Clin. Endocr.* **30**: 646–652.

LAYNE, D. S., MEYER, C. J., VAISHWANAR, P. S. and PINCUS, G. (1962) The secretion and metabolism of cortisol and aldosterone in normal and in steroid-treated women. *J. Clin. Endocr.* **22**: 107–118.

LECOCQ, F. R., BRADLEY, E. M. and GOLDZIEHER, J. W. (1967) Metabolic balance studies with norethynodrel and chlormadinone acetate. *Amer. J. Obstet. Gynec.* **99**: 374–381.

LORAINE, J. A., BELL, E. T. and HARKNESS, R. A. (1966) The effect of various compounds on ovulation in human subjects as judged by hormone assays. In: *Ovulation*, pp. 271–282. Greenblatt, R. B. (Ed.). J. B. Lippincott, Philadelphia & Toronto.

LUNENFELD, B., SULIMOVICI, S. and RABAU, E. (1963) Mechanism of action of antiovulatory compounds. *J. Clin. Endocr.* **23**: 391–395.

MANESCHI, M., CITTADINI, E. and QUARTARARO, P. (1962) The effects of administration of certain synthetic progestative substances on the function of the thyroid. In: *International Congress on Hormonal Steroids*. International Congress Series no. 51, Abstr. 278, p. 206. Excerpta Medica, Amsterdam, New York.

MAUVAIS-JARVIS, P. (1966) Etudes *in vivo* sur le métabolisme des androgènes après administration de stéroides inhibiteurs de l'ovulation. II: Métabolisme de la testostérone et du sulfate de déhydroépiandrostérone radioactifs, chez les sujets traités par le lynoestrénol, des oestrogènes de synthèses et leur association. *Acta Endocr. (Kbh.)* **53**: 37–52.

Mazza, A. and Hecht-Lucari, G. (1960) Effetto del 6α-metil-17α-acetossiprogesterone (MAP) sulla eliminazione urinaria dei 17-chetosteroidi e dei 17-idrossicorticosteroidi nella donna. *Monitore Ostet. Ginecol. di Endocrin. e del Metabolismo* **2** (nuova serie), 1–8.

McCormick, W. G., Carlborg, L. and Gemzell, C. (1968) Urinary FSH and LH excretion following combined treatment with norethisterone acetate and ethynyl oestradiol and norethisterone acetate only. *Acta Endocr. (Kbh.)* **57**: 536–548.

Menon, S., Rannie, G. H., Weightman, D. and Dewar, H. A. (1970) A comparative study of blood fibrinolytic activity in normal women, pregnant women and women on oral contraceptives. *J. Obst. Gynaec. Brit. Commonwealth* **77**: 752–756.

Netter, A., Lambert, A., Yaneva, H. and Pelissier, C. (1967) Etude d'un nouveau progestatif de synthèse, la norgestriénone. *Rev. Franc. Endocr. Clin.* **8**: 231–240.

Nevinny-Stickel, J. (1963a) Die gestagene Wirkung von zwei halogenierten Derivaten des 17α-Hydroxyprogesteron-acetats bei der Frau. *Z. Geburtsh. Gynäk.* **161**: 168–187.

Nevinny-Stickel, J. (1963b) Untersuchungen über die gestagene Wirksamkeit von 17αAllyl-3 Desoxy-19-Nortestosteron (Allyl-Oestrenol) bei der Frau. *Zbl. Gynäk.* **85**: 865–870.

Nevinny-Stickel, J. (1964) Inhibition of ovulation determined by estimation of pregnanediol excretion. *Int. J. Fertil.* **9**: 57–67.

Odell, W. D. and Swerdloff, R. S. (1968) Progestogen-induced luteinizing and follicle-stimulating hormone surge in postmenopausal women: a simulated ovulatory peak. *Proc. Nat. Acad. Sci.* **61**: 529–536.

Østergaard, E. and Starup, J. (1968) Occurrence and function of corpora lutea during different forms of oral contraception. *Acta Endocr. (Kbh.)* **57**: 386–394.

Petry, R., Tenhaeff, D., Senge, Th. and Rausch-Stroomann, J.-G. (1970) Clinical and biochemical observations under treatment with the depot-contraceptive agent norethisterone enanthate. In: *Third Internat. Congress on Hormonal Steroids.* International Congress Series no. 210, Abstr. 462, p. 216. Excerpta Medica, Amsterdam, New York.

Poller, L. (1970) Relation between oral contraceptive hormones and blood clotting. *J. Clin. Path.* **23**: suppl. 3: 67–74.

Poller, L., Thomson, J. M., Tabiowo, A. and Priest, C. M. (1969) Progesterone, oral contraception and blood coagulation. *Brit. Med. J.* **1**: 554–556.

Powell, L. W., Jacobi, J. M., Gaffney, T. J. and Adam, R. (1970) Failure of a pure progestogen contraceptive to affect serum levels of iron, transferrin, protein-bound iodine, and transaminase. *Brit. Med. J.* **3**: 194–195.

Rauscher, H., Schneider, W. and Voigt, K. (1969) Neue Beobachtungen über den Effekt von Gestagenen. I. *Arch. Gynäk.* **208**: 103–112.

Reiffenstuhl, G. and Hohlweg, W. (1968) Die Behandlung klimakterischer Beschwerden mit einem antigonadotrop wirkenden Gestagen. *Med. Klin.* **63**: 1194–1196.

Roland, M. (1968) Effects of a progestagen on cervical physiology and sperm capacitation. *Ob./gyn. Digest.* **10**: 41–48.

Routier, G., Corette, L. and Darras, P. (1967) Hepatite severe et progestatifs de synthèse. *J. Sc. Medicales de Lille* **85**: 229–234.

Schally, A. V., Arimura, A., Kastin, A. J., Reeves, J. J., Bowers, C. Y., Baba, Y. and White, W. F. (1970) Hypothalamic LH-releasing hormone: chemistry, physiology and effect in humans, pp. 45–83. In *Mammalian Reproduction*, 21. Colloquium der Gesellschaft für biologische Chemie, Mosbach. Gibian, H. and Plotz. E. J. (Eds.), Springer-Verlag, Berlin, New York.

SCHMIDT-ELMENDORFF, H. and KOPERA, H. (1966) The effect of oral contraceptives on gonadotrophin excretion. In: *Social and Medical Aspects of Oral Contraception. A Round Table Conference*, pp. 89–94. Scheveningen, The Netherlands. Dukes, M. N. G. (Ed.). Internat. Congress Series no. 130, Excerpta Medica, Amsterdam, New York.

SCHREIBMAN, P. H. (1968) Alterations in carbohydrate and lipid metabolism by a progestin. *Diabetes* 17 (suppl. 1), 341–342.

STAMM, O., CAVENG, B., GERARD, J. and KELLER, M. (1968) Ovulationsauslösung mittels Retrosteroid Ro 4-8347. *Z. Geburtsh. Gynäk.* 169: 225–241.

ŠTĚRBA, R., KRÁLOVÁ, A., ULRYCH, J. and VALOVÁ, B. (1965) Die ersten klinischen Erfahrungen mit 16-Methylen-6-dehydro-17α-acetoxyprogesteron (MDAP). *Zbl. Gynäk.* 87: 540–548.

STOLTE, L. A. M., WESSELIUS-DE CASPARIS, A., GEUENS, I., VAN KESSEL, H. and BROSENS, (1969) Dydrogesterone (6-dehydroretroprogesterone, Duphaston®) and ovulation. I. Investigations in the human. *Acta Endocr. (Kbh.)*, Suppl. 138: 205.

SWYER, G. L. M. (1970) L'inhibition de l'ovulation par les oestrogènes et les progestatifs. In: *L'Inhibition de l'ovulation*, pp. 49–56. Netter, A. (Ed.). Masson & Cie, Paris.

TAFT, P., WINIKOFF, D., TAYLOR, K., PAGE, D. and BRITTINGHAM, L. C. (1969) The influence of oral contraceptives with and without an ovulation suppressant action on thyroid function tests. Preliminary observations on differences in insulin response to glucose. In: *Chlormadinone Acetate. A New Departure in Oral Contraception*, pp. 60–72. Christie, G. A. and Moore-Robinson, M. (Eds.). Syntex Pharmaceuticals Ltd., Maidenhead.

TAUBERT, H. D. and JÜRGENSEN, O. (1970a) The treatment of monophasic cycles with a new retroprogesterone (Ro 4-8347). In: *Proceedings 6th World Congress of Gynaecology and Obstetrics*, Abstr. 105. Jones, H. W. and Baramki, Th.A. (Eds.). Williams & Wilkins Co., Baltimore.

TAUBERT, H. D. and JÜRGENSEN, O. (1970b) The treatment of monophasic cycles with the retroprogesterone Ro 4-8347. *Bull. Schweiz. Akad. Wiss.* 503–511.

TRONCONI, G. (1962) Long term observations of the offspring of patients given synthetic progestative substances in the course of their pregnancy. In: *Internat. Congress on Hormonal Steroids*. Internat. Congress Series no. 51, Abstr. 266, p. 199. Excerpta Medica, Amsterdam, New York.

TRONCONI, G. and FERRERO, A. (1960) Quadro elettroforetico proteico, lipoproteico e attivitá chiarificante plasmatica in corso di trattamento con 6 alfa-metil-17 alfa-acetossiprogesterone. *Ann. Ostet. Ginec.* 82: 735–741.

TRONCONI, G. and SANTI, F. (1960). Alcuni aspetti dell'equilibrio elettrolitico in corso di trattamento con 6 alfa-metil-17 alfa-idrossiprogesterone acetate. *Ann. Ostet. Ginec.* 82: 742–750.

VERMEULEN, A. and FERIN, J. (1962) The influence of 17α-methyl-19-nortestosterone (MNT) on the metabolism of Cortisol. *Acta Endocr. (Kbh.)* 39: 22–31.

VERMEULEN, A. and FERIN, J. (1963) Invloed van synthetische progestogenen op de bijniercortex. (Dutch.) *Bull. Soc. Roy. Belge Gynec. Obstet.* 33: 337–344.

WALTHER, R. A. and PLATT, W. R. (1964) Medroxyprogesterone test for the diagnosis of first trimester pregnancy. A five tablet oral (single dose). *Missouri Med.* 61: 678–681.

WRIGHT, S. W., FOTHERBY, K. and FAIRWEATHER, F. (1970) Effect of daily small doses of norgestrel on ovarian function. *J. Obstet. Gyn. Brit. Cwlth.* 77: 65–68.

CHAPTER 32

THERAPEUTIC APPLICATION OF PROGESTATIONAL DRUGS

K. Semm
*Department of Obstetrics and Gynecology,
Universitäts-Frauenklinik, Kiel*

A. APPLICATIONS IN THE NON-PREGNANT WOMAN

Our knowledge of the possibility of producing a secretory endometrium in ovariectomized women by the administration of estradiol benzoate and the corpus luteum hormone is closely associated with the name of C. Kaufmann (1933). It has become customary to speak of a transformation dose, meaning the total dose of progesterone or of one of its derivatives needed to convert an estrogen-primed endometrium into a secretory one. This should be fully developed, as distinguished from a "rigid secretory phase" (Winter and Pots, 1956).

Progesterone therapy was decisively advanced by the introduction of 17α-hydroxyprogesterone caproate (Junkmann, 1954). The free alcohol has been isolated and has been considered as a weak androgen having no progestational activity. The prolonged effect of the ester stimulated interest in other long-acting substitutes for progesterone. In this connection the acetate of 17α-hydroxyprogesterone and 17α-ethynyl-19-nortestosterone enanthate should be mentioned. According to Davis and Wied (1957) the transformation dose of the latter compound amounts to 100 mg, whereas 350 mg of 17α-hydroxyprogesterone caproate or acetate were needed to obtain the same endometrial picture. A rise in body temperature was obtained with 150 mg of norethisterone enanthate or 350 mg of 17α-hydroxyprogesterone caproate or acetate. The same doses rendered the ferning test negative. According to these studies norethisterone enanthate is the most active of the three compounds, but its action lasts too long for appropriate use in the menstrual cycle. In the prevention or treatment of abortion, where this prolonged effect would be desirable, it cannot be used because of a strong virilizing activity, which the compound shares with several nortestosterone derivatives (Pots, 1958).

17α-Hydroxyprogesterone caproate in oily solution was found to be far less active in inducing (and maintaining) decidual changes in the endometrium than 17α-hydroxy-6α-methyl-progesterone acetate in aqueous suspension. When these two drugs were combined with an estrogen, 100–150 mg of the latter substance were found equal in activity to 250–375 mg of the former.

On the basis of laboratory and clinical studies regarding the progesterone requirements throughout the cycle, Ober *et al.* (1954) developed a simple and economical method of progesterone treatment, suited for all the known disturbances of the cycle and for the postponement of menstruation. By the use of suspensions of progesterone crystals they laid the foundation for the therapeutic use of long-acting progestational compounds.

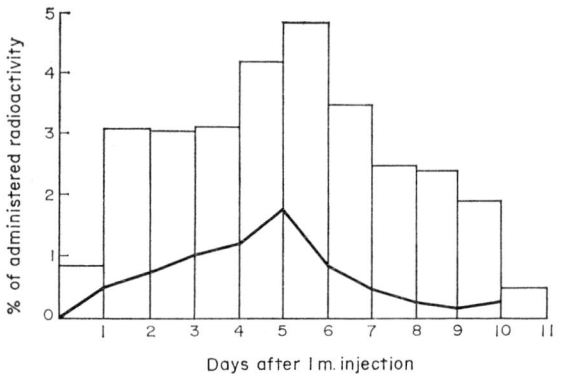

FIG. 1. Radioactivity in plasma (curve) and in urine (columns) after a single injection of 4-^{14}C-labeled 17α-hydroxyprogesterone caproate. From Plotz (1959).

By injecting 4-^{14}C-labeled 17α-hydroxyprogesterone caproate and by measuring the radioactivity in plasma and urine Plotz (1959) could demonstrate the prolonged availability of the compound in the human organism (Fig 1). This may be helpful in determining the dosage of the drug and the frequency of administration. The prolonged effect is due to delayed resorption from the injection site rather than to storage within fat tissue.

Progestational therapy aims essentially at the production of a few phenomena in a great variety of abnormal conditions. One of these aims is the establishment of a (sometimes prolonged) secretory phase, often referred to in clinical terminology as pseudopregnancy. Examples of the conditions where the induction of this state may be desirable are the following: uterine hypoplasia, general hypogenitalism, sterility, disturbances of the cycle (including poly-hypermenorrhea), juvenile uterine hemorrhages and certain severe extra-genital disturbances of a cyclical character.

We now discuss the therapeutic uses of progestational drugs. For the sake of convenience some classic pictures are listed alphabetically and discussed in that order with reference to progestational therapy.

1. Carcinoma of the endometrium.
2. Endometriosis.
3. Fibromyoma.
4. Mammary carcinoma.
5. Mastopathia cystica.
6. Menstrual disorders
    (a) amenorrhea,
    (b) anovulatory cycles,
    (c) dysfunctional bleeding,
    (d) dysmenorrhea,
    (e) polymenorrhea (shortened luteal phase) and the postponement of menstruation,
    (f) premenstrual tension.
7. Pruritus vulvae.
8. Skin diseases.
9. Sterility.
10. Surgical removal of corpora lutea.
11. Uterine hypoplasia.

1. CARCINOMA OF THE ENDOMETRIUM

Some authors have found indications associating the occurrence of carcinoma of the endometrium with prolonged and increased secretion of estrogens and a deficiency of progesterone. The literature was reviewed by de Waard (1958). Together with Bruinsma (Bruinsma and de Waard, 1959) this author was able to show that the association of endometrial carcinoma with diabetes, obesity or hypertension, reportedly established in earlier literature, may be equally due to increased or prolonged estrogen secretion, witness the fact that, at least as far as diabetic women are concerned, a significantly higher percentage was found to have estrogenic vaginal smears after the menopause than amongst a carefully chosen control group. These estrogens were assumed to be of adrenal origin and it was further shown (Baanders-van Halewijn, 1962; Baanders-van Halewijn et al., 1963) that this postmenopausal adrenal estrogen secretion was associated with both obesity and endometrial carcinoma, over-nutrition probably playing a key role in this mechanism, as is borne out by epidemiological studies (de Waard and Oettlé, 1965; de Waard and Schwarz, 1964.)

Kistner was the first to try progestational drugs for the treatment of carcinoma of the corpus uteri and even recommended them for its prevention (Kistner and Baginski, 1961).

D'Incerti Bonini (1964) treated thirty-four cases with either medroxyprogesterone acetate (MAP) or vinylestrenolone* in daily oral doses of 80 mg or less, combined with more or less extended surgery. Histological improvement was significant in nineteen patients,† appreciable in twelve, and poor or nil in three cases.

Favorable results in advanced recurrent and/or metastatic endometrial carcinoma were obtained by Bergsjö (1965) by intramuscular injections of progesterone in oil, 17α-hydroxy-19-norprogesterone caproate or 17α-hydroxyprogesterone p-butoxyphenyl propionate. Anderson (1965) used medroxyprogesterone acetate with good results. Schmidt-Matthiesen and Wellers (1968) have critically reviewed the subject, covering almost 500 cases and emphasizing the need for high doses. Results include permanent cures as well as temporary remissions for periods of 20 to 30 months. Objective improvement is reported in 20–40% of cases, subjective improvement in about 70%. Side effects are infrequent and slight. Other papers: Behrens (1957); Frick (1965); Heckmann (1965); Skov Jensen and Lass (1965); Kottmeier (1962); Curchod, 1970).

2. ENDOMETRIOSIS

The often very painful condition of endometriosis is encountered in two forms: (1) Endometriosis interna: the mucosa of the corpus penetrates into the myometrium. (2) Endometriosis externa: endometrial tissues settle outside the uterus, especially retrocervically in the region of the sacrouterine ligament and in the posterior segment of the excavatio rectouterina. Complaints due to endometriosis tend to diminish or to disappear during or after pregnancy. It is assumed that under the increased influence of estrogens and progesterone the ectopical endometrium also undergoes decidual changes and becomes partly necrotic.

Kistner (1958 a, b) was the first to treat endometriosis with progestational drugs in combination with estrogens. It was suggested that the changes

* Ormonoterapia Richter; Vestalin®.
† The paper gives a figure of twenty-nine, which is clearly due to an error.

brought about are a combination of (1) anovulation and amenorrhea, (2) decidual transformation of functioning endometriotic tissue, and (3) decidual necrosis and absorption. Kistner (1960) reported on comparative studies with three progestational compounds in various combinations with estrogens, viz. (1) 17α-hydroxyprogesterone caproate, (2) norethynodrel, (3) medroxyprogesterone acetate.

The first compound (Delalutin®) was injected in weekly doses of 62.5 mg for 2 weeks and these were gradually increased every 2 weeks so that at the end of 12 weeks the patient was receiving 500 mg. At the same time an estrogen was given—diethylstilbestrol (0.5 mg) or ethynyl estradiol 0.05 mg daily—and these doses were increased at weekly intervals up to a level of 60.0 mg of diethylstilbestrol or 0.6 mg of ethynyl estradiol. As a later variation of the regimen estradiol valerate (Delestrogen®) was injected (10 mg weekly) instead of the oral estrogens previously given, but it caused severe uterine cramps and bleeding in several patients. On the other hand, a mixture of 250 mg of 17α-hydroxyprogesterone caproate and 5 mg of estradiol valerate per ml used by Thomas (quoted by Kistner, 1960) gave satisfactory results in 85% of cases, comparable to the improvement rate obtained by others with "oral progestins". This mixture is given every 2 weeks and the dose is kept constant until "break-through" bleeding occurs. It produces less nausea in the early phase.

Norethynodrel was given as Enovid® (containing 1.5% of ethynyl estradiol 3-methyl ether) in a dose of 10 mg daily for 2 weeks, with an increase of 10 mg every 2 weeks up to a maintenance dose of 30 or 40 mg. Improvement rate was 80–85% in over 200 cases. One of the major side-effects, nausea, could be diminished by beginning with a 5-mg rather than 10-mg tablet. It seemed related to the estrogen. Other side-effects included fluid retention, irritability and, occasionally, severe headache. Break-through bleeding was infrequent but sometimes made it necessary to increase the dosage considerably. This state of pseudopregnancy should be continued for at least 6, sometimes 9 or 12 months. It did not cause virilization. According to later reports (Kistner, 1962), this dosage was reduced to 2.5 mg Enovid® daily for 1 week, 5 mg daily for 1 week, 10 mg daily for 2 weeks, 15 mg daily for 2 weeks and 20 mg daily indefinitely. Norlutin® is recommended with a similar schedule and the advice: "add estrogen for break-through bleeding."

Medroxyprogesterone acetate. This was given parenterally, 100 mg every 2 weeks in conjunction with ethynyl estradiol (0.05 mg daily p.o.). Excellent results in eight cases.

Andrews et al. (1959) gave 17α-hydroxyprogesterone caproate in doses of 250 mg every 7th or 10th day and 2 mg of stilbestrol daily for 3 months. Because of relatively frequent break-through bleeding they then changed to an oral combination product.

Since orally active progestational drugs have become available the therapy of endometriosis has become their domain, as illustrated by Helpap (1963) who described his results with norethisterone acetate. Through their inhibiting effect on pituitary gonadotrophin secretion and the suppression of endometrial proliferation these substances, particularly those derived from 19-nortestosterone, when given for long periods, can maintain endometrial tissue in an almost non-functional state. Norethisterone or lynestrenol are given in increasing doses (5 to 20 mg per day). On the other hand, *continuous* progestational treatment without the addition of an estrogen has been recommended by Ferin (1964), who gave lynestrenol (Orgametril®) 5 mg per day for 6 to 9 months. Haller (1968) finds this schedule very satisfactory. He doubles the doses for short periods in case of break-through bleeding. Instead of 5 mg of lynestrenol 10 mg of norethisterone acetate (Primolut-nor®) or 4 mg of chlormadinone acetate (Gestafortin®) may be given. See also Cohen (1964).

Some authors prefer cyclic administration of oral contraceptives of the combined estrogen–progestagen type (no sequentials!) mainly because of the simplicity of the treatment and the favorable psychological effect of the maintenance of periodic bleeding. Treatment should be continued for at least 1 year.

If hormonal treatment of endometriosis remains unsuccessful, the possibility of stroma endometriosis should be considered. It occurs in 20% of all cases (differential diagnosis: endometrial sarcoma!). According to Stoll and Rummel (1964) treatment should be surgical only.

Bayer, from his experience with 255 cases, recommends surgical treatment to be followed by progestational therapy for up to 8 months (or androgen–gestagen therapy only).

Numerous papers deal with the treatment of endometriosis by parenteral or oral medication. Their number reflects the importance of the disease. The following is a list of such papers; they do not contain suggestions for treatment essentially different from those discussed above. Antoine (1963), Balina (1962), Borglin et al. (1965), Carol and Müller (1964), Carter (1962), Chalmers (1962), Chartier et al. (1966), Cromer (1965), Dujovich (1960), Durham (1961), Finke (1963), Grant (1961), Gray (1965), Gregoire et al. (1963), Guiot et al. (1965), Hofmann (1966), Hvidt (1962), Joosse (1961), Käser (1962), Kolstad (1964), Korte (1963), Lax (1961), Lebherz and Fobes (1961), Mach (1965), Mills (1962), Murray and Ramella (1961), Nevinny-Stickel (1962), Novak and Hoge (1958), Palmer (1964), Pschyrembel (1964), Puck and Polenz (1963), Richter (1964, 1965), Riva *et al.* (1961, 1962), Scott and Wharton (1962), Snaith (1962), Soiva and Castrén (1963, 1964), Thomas (1960), Upton (1962), Williams (1962), Wright (1962).

3. FIBROMYOMA

Fibromyomatosis of the uterus may or may not be accompanied by disturbances of the menstrual blood flow (usually initially menorrhagias). In both cases therapy with progestational compounds also would appear to be justified in view of the experimental work of Lipschütz and Iglesias (1938) and Lipschütz (1950). After their basic studies on the growth of fibromyomas (in rats) under the influence of estrogens, a conservative therapy of fibromyomatosis by progesterone was attempted. With 10-mg doses of progesterone in solution 3 to 6 times a week, Goodman (1946) observed arrested growth or even involution of tumors. Oral preparations are now used practically exclusively for this purpose (Mixon and Hammond, 1961).

Data on the results of conservative (hormone) therapy of fibromyomatosis of the uterus are given by Bolck (1960), Krater (1960), Ufer (1966).

4. MAMMARY CARCINOMA

A discussion of the many facets of the etiology of carcinoma of the breast and its possible hormone dependence would be outside the scope of this chapter.

Crowley and MacDonald (1965) reported on twenty-two cases of mammary carcinoma, resistant to estrogen therapy alone which were treated with additional weekly doses of 1000 mg 17α-hydroxyprogesterone caproate. Remissions involving the primary tumor and metastases occurred in six patients and lasted for 2 to 24 months. For further observations see Geller *et al.* (1961), Jelle (1962), Curwen (1963), Huggins (1958), Kleibel and Becker (1960), Landau *et al.* (1962).

5. MASTOPATHIA CYSTICA

Mastopathia cystica as distinguished from simple premenstrual engorgement of the breasts is characterized by benign proliferation and cyst formation of the mammary ducts (sharply delineated nodules, painful on pressure), mainly arising from estrogenic stimulation. In our experience if hormonal treatment is indicated (malignancy having been excluded) androgens are to be preferred. Combination with progesterone preparations sometimes gives favorable results. Clark and Greenblatt (1957) gave 17α-hydroxyprogesterone caproate in a case of juvenile mammary hypertrophy, which reduced the size of the breasts and led to the disappearance of nodules. Further therapeutic schedules have been proposed by Bacigalupo (1961), Cunningham and Lang (1962), Riisfeldt (1942).

6. MENSTRUAL DISORDERS

(a) Amenorrhea

Amenorrhea may be physiological, uterine or dysfunctional. In the treatment of uterine or dysfunctional, primary or secondary amenorrhea mixtures of estrogens and gestagens are now almost exclusively used, usually in a ratio of 1:10 to 1:20 and for producing withdrawal bleeding. However, Lacny (1962) reported excellent results in primary or secondary amenorrhea by the injection of 250 mg of 17α-hydroxyprogesterone caproate every 28 days, either alone or in combination with estradiol valerate (2 × 5 mg i.m.), for periods up to 3 to 4 months.

Matsumoto and Watanabe (1958), gave a complete transformation dose (125 mg) of 17α-hydroxyprogesterone caproate together with 5 to 10 mg of an estrogen depot preparation to 20 women, and invariably produced withdrawal bleeding 10 to 14 days later. Further treatment schedules have been proposed by Alvarez and Seahle (1954), Buschbeck (1962), Dauria (1960), Gitsch (1964), Greenblatt (1963), Igarashi (1957), Käser (1958), Monzo (1960), Pujohl (1960), Staemmler (1963, 1964), Zander *et al.* (1962).

(b) Anovulatory cycles

Anovulatory cycles are normal soon after the menarche, postpartum and preceding the menopause. They occur frequently during reproductive life in cases of inflammation of the adnexa and of physical or psychological stress, in other words, under exogenous influences which may also bring about amenorrhea. These cycles—characterized by a monophasic temperature curve—are usually neither regular nor of 4 weeks' duration. Though progesterone has been shown to induce ovulations (Rust, 1956; Haskins, 1959) other and far more effective ways of treatment are, of course, now available for that purpose. On the other hand, when the induction of ovulation is not essential, progesterone therapy may be used (mainly in the

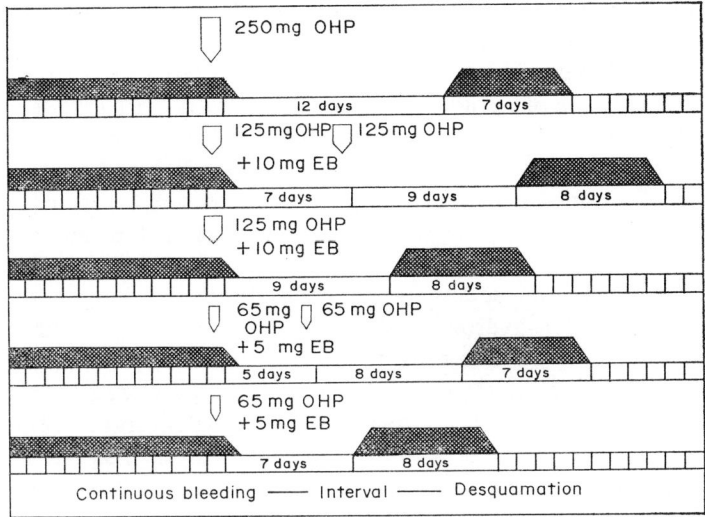

Fig. 2. Treatment of dysfunctional bleeding. From Pots (1955). OHP, 17α-hydroxyprogesterone caproate; EB, estradiol benzoate.

climacteric and pre-climacteric) with the object of rendering the endometrial changes more normal. The recommended dose is 125–250 mg of 17α-hydroxyprogesterone caproate on day 18 of the cycle. The same regimen is used in the treatment of irregular anovulatory cycles, which are caused by precocious involution of the follicles. For literature see Bickenbach and Doering (1959), Kaufmann (1953), Schwartz and Sefgar (1957).

(c) *Dysfunctional bleeding*

This term is used by us to designate excessive and persistent uterine hemorrhage as part of the classic picture of glandular cystic hyperplasia of the endometrium, caused by persistent follicles and the absence of corpora lutea. For effective treatment some authors recommend administration not only of a gestagen but also of an estrogen, since the sudden creation of a relative estrogen deficiency would cause desquamation of the endometrium and thereby further bleeding.

The dose-dependence of this effect was shown (Fig. 2) by Pots (1955) who also pointed out that the moderate depot-effect of estradiol benzoate is to be preferred to that of a crystal suspension and does not cause "second bleeding" as described by Ober *et al.* (1954) and attributed to the different duration of action of the two components in depot-mixtures.

Thomas (1958) found dysfunctional bleeding to stop on an average about 19 hours after the administration of 125 mg of 17α-hydroxyprogesterone caproate and 10 mg of ethynyl estradiol.

Using combinations of 125-375 mg of 17α-hydroxyprogesterone caproate and 10 mg of estradiol benzoate or valerate, Zorn (1958) was able to stop dysfunctional bleeding within 2 to 3 days in over 90% of his cases. Any atypical reponse to the injection of such a mixture should raise the suspicion of an organic disease and warrant further exploration.

Ober (1957b) considers a crystal suspension of esters of estradiol and 17α-hydroxyprogesterone in a ratio of 1:20 as particularly suitable. Rauscher and Kofler (1958) induced a therapeutic withdrawal bleeding by the injection of 125 mg of 17α-hydroxyprogesterone caproate in 110 out of 116 such treatments given to 76 women with disturbed cycles. Fiducial limits for expected success were 85% to 99%. The interval between treatment and withdrawal bleeding varied between 8 and 16 days (average 11½) and the duration of the bleeding between 3⅓ and 8 days (average 5½).

Orally active progestational compounds have been successfully used for the treatment of dysfunctional bleeding, either alone or in combination with estrogens, in the form of the usual contraceptive tablets.

Haller (1968) points out that dysfunctional uterine bleeding in adolescence is particularly amenable to this form of therapy; while not actually curing the condition it controls bleeding and thus permits the patient to await the spontaneous maturation of the organism. It also prevents the development of a sometimes severe anemia.

Relatively high doses of Envoid® or Norlutin® (20 to 30 mg, in exceptional cases even 60 mg, a day) were used. Quoting from the European literature Haller states that the usual contraceptive preparations (containing chlormadinone, lynestrenol or norethisterone acetate) have all been used in doses of two to three tablets per day for 4 to 10 days and that the rate of success varies between 86% and 100%. Dydrogesterone (not a contraceptive drug) is included in the list. Following cessation of this treatment, a withdrawal bleeding is to be expected, the first day of which should be considered day 1 of a new cycle, during which the usual "contraceptive" regimen should be applied from day 5 to day 24.

Other treatment schedules for the control of dysfunctional bleeding are proposed by Arrighi (1964), Boschann (1955), Beyl (1959), Fries (1962), Froewis and Leeb (1960), Geipel and v. Loehr (1963), Hamada (1965), Henzl et al. (1962), Hauser et al., (1960), Jann (1956), Leinzinger (1959), Markle (1950), Napp (1962), Ober (1953, 1957), Prill (1957), Rauscher and Romberg (1956), Robey (1958), Schlösser (1958), Schmidt-Mathiessen (1963).

(d) *Dysmenorrhea*

Two types of dysmenorrhea or algomenorrhea are distinguished, viz. primary and secondary. Primary dysmenorrhea is usually associated with a biphasic cycle and with disturbances of the autonomous nervous system along with some psychasthenia (anxiety neurosis). It is amenable to gestagen therapy, like the secondary type which is usually seen in association with organic abnormalities such as endometriosis, faulty position of the uterus, fibromyomas, inflammation, etc.

Primary dysmenorrhea is often thought to be caused by hypoplasia of the uterus (Döring, 1959). It can best be treated by repeated prolongation of the cycle (induction of so-called pseudopregnancy). Injections of 125 mg of 17α-hydroxyprogesterone caproate are given on days 20, 25, 30 and 38, combined with 10 mg of estradiol valerate on day 20. This treatment is aimed at an enlargement of the uterus which, in turn, causes the painful menstruations to disappear. These recommendations are in agreement with those of Aydar and Greenblatt (1964). It is generally assumed that in anovulatory cycles menstruation is not painful; ovulation inhibitors have therefore been widely recommended for the treatment of dysmenorrhea. This is reported to be successful in 50% to 100% of cases (Haller, 1968). On the other hand, dydrogesterone (Duphaston®) is generally considered to be effective in this condition although it does not normally inhibit ovulation (Bishop, 1961; Backer 1962). The percentage of successful results is comparable with that obtained with ovulation inhibitors.

(e) *Polymenorrhea (shortened luteal phase) and postponement of menstruation*

The term polymenorrhea designates menstrual bleeding with intervals of less than 25 days duration. Such cycles may be ovulatory (with biphasic temperature curve) but with an inadequate corpus luteum or they may be anovulatory. Therapy aims at substituting for endogenous progesterone secretion (see Rauscher, 1958) but stimulation of such secretion by means of gonadotrophic preparations (human chorionic gonadotrophin, HCG) has also been reported (Staemmler, 1965) (Fig. 3).

When postponement of a menstruation is desirable for medical or other reasons, inhibition of ovulation by estrogens or oral contraceptive drugs may be the preferred treatment. However, a progesterone derivative may be needed if treatment is begun late in the cycle. Husslein and Hofhansl (1959) could consistently delay menstruation for 2 to 7 days by one intramuscular injection of 250 mg of 17α-hydroxyprogesterone acetate plus

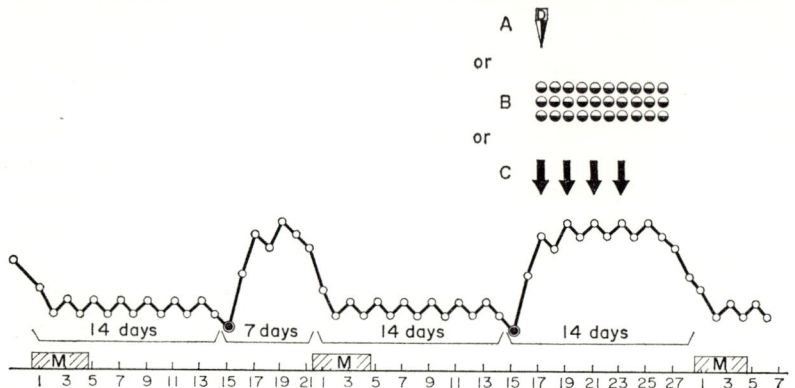

FIG. 3. Treatment of insufficient luteal function. From Staemmler (1965). Depot injection (estrogen + gestagen). ◓ tablet (estrogen + gestagen). ↓ injection of HCG.

10 mg of estradiol benzoate, provided this was given not later than 2 days before the expected end of the cycle (Fig. 4). When two injections were given, viz. on the 26 and 32nd day of the cycle, the delay amounted to 8 to 12 days.

However, in the opinion of the authors this parenteral treatment is not to be preferred to oral medication, such as norethisterone acetate, 2 mg, plus 10 mcg of ethynyl estradiol daily. These results agree with those of Matsumoto and Watanabe (1958).

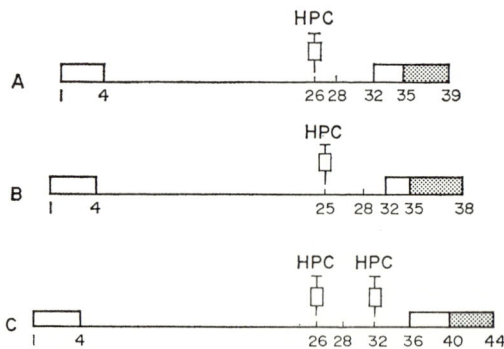

FIG. 4. Postponement of menstruation. From Husslein and Hofhansl (1959.)HPC, 250 mg of 17α-hydroxyprogesterone caproate plus 1mg of estradiol benzoate. Figures: days of cycle.

By giving the conventional ovulation inhibiting contraceptive drugs from day 5 to day 28 (24 days) a brief delay of menstruation is observed but in the ensuing (usually ovulatory) cycle without treatment menstrual bleeding will again be 1 week later than the normal date in the particular regular cycle, if the patient had not been treated. Such postponement by about 1 week can be obtained immediately by giving the tablets for 28 days (day 5 to day 32) (Haller, 1968).

Delay of menstruation by postovulatory administration of progestational compounds has been recommended by Greenblatt and Rose (1962) as a test for the activity of a drug.

(f) *Premenstrual tension*

The syndrome of premenstrual tension is characterized by a very labile mood, depression, irritability, insomnia, nausea and other disturbances such as headache, back pain, cramps in the lower abdomen irradiating into the thighs, etc. All this looks like a strong exaggeration of symptoms normally occurring in the late premenstrual phase. The syndrome is supposed to be caused by an excess of estrogens in relation to progesterone —though this has never been proven—or to a special sensitivity towards estrogens. In her well-known classification of side effects of oral contraception, Mears (1967) lists premenstrual tension as the first amongst estrogenic effects. Psychogenic factors are undoubtedly involved. Next to psychotherapy, progesterone—e.g. 250 mg of 17α-hydroxyprogesterone caproate —in the second half of the cycle should be tried (Davis, 1958).

In the opinion of Parker (1960) premenstrual retention of water is the main factor, though he also considers vitamin-B-deficiency, autonomic nervous disturbances, menotoxins and hormonal dysfunctions. He also emphasizes treatment with 17α-hydroxyprogesterone (apart from psychotherapy), diuretics and tranquilizers. A dose of 250 mg is reported to be effective in 80% of the cases. Waters (1957) noticed an increased incidence of premenstrual tension in the third decade of life which he believes to be correlated with the frequency of luteal insufficiency at that age. A single injection of 125 mg of 17α-hydroxyprogesterone caproate caused complete cessation of symptoms in three quarters of thirty cases and improvement in three (treatment during three cycles). Inhibition of ovulations appears at least temporarily to eliminate the symptoms of premenstrual tension. Drill (1966), citing six authors, states that premenstrual tension decreased during the cyclic use of Enovid (Binks *et al.*, 1962) or Conovid E (Pullen, 1962), Ortho-Novum (Goldzieher *et al.*, 1962), Anovlar (Mears and Grant, 1962; Bockner, 1963) or Provest (Gould, 1963).

7. PRURITUS VULVAE

Since the etiology of pruritus vulvae communis is usually unknown and no generally reliable treatment has been found, progesterone or its derivatives may be tried in serious cases.

Besold (1950) found that refractory cases often responded rapidly to progesterone and he therefore strongly recommends giving it a trial.

8. SKIN DISEASES

Acne

The various forms of acne (*A. vulgaris, A. cystica, A. rosacea* and *A. seborrhoica* in women) appear to respond surprisingly well to the cyclic administration (between days 14 to 18) of 125 mg of 17α-hydroxyprogesterone caproate. Baker (1959) reported on seventy-six women, aged 15–36, 80% of whom were markedly improved or cured by treatment of 2 to 8 months duration.

A favorable influence of an oral progestational compound (allylestrenol) on preovulatory and premenstrual acne, when given at the appropriate time of the cycle, was reported by Amann (1965). An influence of the administration of progesterone or its derivatives on the activity of sebaceous glands in the rat has been demonstrated by de Groot *et al.* (1965). The minimal response dose was 10 mg/100 g bodyweight.

Sclerodermia

In recent years sclerodermia has been thought to be caused by the formation of antibodies against collagen. Though such a mechanism has not been proven, the number of studies on the antigenicity of collagen fractions is increasing. For literature see Korting *et al.* (1964), Holzmann *et al.* (1964).

Sclerodermia, like acne in women, is often cycle-dependent and a connection with ovarian hormones is worth studying.

Holzmann *et al.* (1965) obtained good results in sclerodermia by injections of 17α-hydroxyprogesterone caproate in weekly doses of 100–250 mg. They observed an increase of hydroxy-prolin excretion (which in patients with progressive sclerodermia is usually within the normal range) and consider this to be an essential effect of progesterone.

Shelley *et al.* (1964) saw a good result of the same treatment in a case described as chronic and extensive distinctive vesiculobullous eruption in a young woman, resembling dermatitis herpetiformis clinically and erythema multiforme histologically. They believe that they were dealing with an auto-immune phenomenon, elicited by endogenous progesterone which was eliminated by an ovulation inhibiting drug.

9. STERILITY

Among the causes of sterility amenable to progesterone therapy, insufficiency of the corpus luteum ranks high. Tyler (1957) reported that in twenty-five out of forty-nine patients suffering from this form of sterility he saw pregnancies after two injections of 187 mg of 17α-hydroxyprogesterone caproate, the first given 2 days after ovulation and the second 7 to 10 days later.

10. SURGICAL REMOVAL OF CORPUS LUTEUM

This operation requires substitution treatment not only when it has been performed during the first 4 months of pregnancy but also when it is followed by uterine bleeding, the result of inadequate endometrial development.

Rauscher (1958) gave single injections of 125 mg of 17α-hydroxyprogesterone caproate together with 10 mg of estradiol benzoate or 250 mg of the gestagen with 20 mg of the estrogen, in order to postpone the withdrawal bleeding which follows 2 to 5 days after the surgical removal of a corpus luteum. The larger dose delayed bleeding for 10 to 13 days. The author considers this test as a reliable measure for the efficacy and the duration of action of a depot-gestagen. The results were essentially the same as those obtained by Ober (1957) with a dose of 200 mg of progesterone plus 10 mg of estradiol monobenzoate in a suspension of crystals, administered 24–27 days after ovariectomy.

Rauscher's studies show that 250 mg of 17α-hydroxyprogesterone caproate, together with 20 mg of estradiol benzoate, represent a complete substitution for the endometrial effect of the corpus luteum.

11. UTERINE HYPOPLASIA

Uterine hypoplasia stands out among genital dysplasias not only as being the cause of menstrual disturbances and sterility or infertility but also because it is to some extent amenable to hormonal therapy. Treatment with estrogens and gestagens stimulates growth of the uterus but the result is all

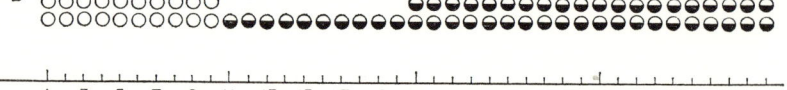

Fig. 5. Pharmacological pseudopregnancy. From Staemmler (1965).  Depot estrogen. ○ orally active estrogen. ◓ tablet of estrogen + gestagen.

too often transient and high hopes are not warranted. The best effect may be expected from the pharmacological induction of pseudopregnancy. A dosage schedule as proposed by Staemmler (1965) is shown in Fig. 5. For further information see Bengtsson et al. (1966), Courrier (1950), Dapunt (1965), Hohlweg and Reifenstuhl (1965), Hofhansl (1961), Igarashi et al. (1965), Käser (1959), Migliavacca (1960), Pschyrembel (1964), Rock et al. (1957), Ufer (1956).

MISCELLANEOUS CLINICAL USES

Arthritis

Because of the fact that women suffering from rheumatoid arthritis may show striking remissions during pregnancy Gorlitzer et al. (1953) treated sixty-six patients (forty-three women and twenty-three men) with injections of long-acting progesterone (combined with isoniazide). Results were very satisfactory. Positive reports were also published by Kyle and Crain (1950), Duthie (1951), Kersley (1955). Most of these observations date from pre-cortisone days.

Cholecystopathies

Aldercreutz (1953), starting from the fact that cholecystopathies are more frequent among women than among men and that the corpus luteum hormone may lower the tone of certain smooth muscles, gave progesterone therapy in cases of biliary dyskinesias and in the postcholecystectomy syndrome. A dosage of 10 mg once to twice weekly gave convincing results. Similar results were reported by Laszló and Görgey (1960) who treated 250 patients with posthepatitic or postcholecystectomy complaints caused by biliary dyskinesias.

B. THERAPEUTIC APPLICATION IN THE PREGNANT WOMAN

The effects of progesterone on the endometrium, in particular on the formation of the decidua and its maintenance during early pregnancy, are of course well known. (For a review of the literature see Semm, 1965.) It is less clear to what extent it could be of use in the treatment of imminent abortion. The problems connected with the influence of progesterone on the myometrium have been covered in Chapters 5, 6 and 24. For the equally relevant questions regarding blood levels see Chapter 22.

In attempting to use progesterone or a progestational drug as a compensation for an assumed or proven deficiency in pregnancy, one will have to take into account the quantities of progesterone normally produced. According to Zander and Münstermann (1956) the mean daily production in the 11th week of pregnancy is 29 mg and in the 18th week 41 mg. During the last weeks of pregnancy 190 to 280 mg progesterone per 24 hours are passing from the placenta into the maternal organism, 75 mg into the fetus. More recently Zander (1967) gave values from 200 to more than 550 mg per 24 hours as secretion rates during the last trimester of pregnancy.

Not only when abortion is imminent may a pregnancy be considered to be endangered. Some concern will be justified in those cases also where the pregnancy has been preceded by one or more abortions, or by a prolonged period of treatment for sterility and those complicated by some general disease of the mother. Contamin (1961) gives progesterone and vitamin E prophylactically during the entire duration of pregnancy for a great variety of indications.

Any prophylactic treatment of abortion becomes problematical if one considers that 25–60% of all early abortions are attributed to malformation of the embryo or degenerative changes of the trophoblast. Disturbances of trophoblast development are considered to be the cause of spontaneous abortions in the following percentages:

        25–90% (Thomsen, 1957)
        35%   (Käser, 1953 a,b)
        27%   (Rauscher, 1964)

Morphological changes in the chorionic villi are particularly frequent. Amongst the many causes sperm deficiencies; exogenous damage before or after conception; deficiencies of certain hormones, vitamins or oxygen; hypoplasia of the uterus; and psychological factors may play a role. Late abortions may be due to anomalies of the uterus, cervical insufficiency, fibromyomas, polyposis, severe anomalies of uterine position (such as a fixed retroflection), etc.

A study by Rauscher (1964) may be cited as an example to illustrate the merits (or worthlessness?) of hormonal treatment in incipient abortion (uterine bleeding in early pregnancy). Out of 221 patients, 61 aborted and 160 carried to term. In 60 of the abortions there was some abnormality of the conceptus. Altogether 170 patients received hormonal treatment and of these 44 aborted (with oval abnormalities). This is summarized in Table 1.

TABLE 1.

	Abortions	Term
Treated	44 (27%)	126 (73%)
Untreated	17 (33%)	34 (66%)
Total	61	160

Pregnanediol excretion values were considered by some authors to be important parameters in judging the chances of success of progesterone therapy. Thus Guterman (1953) reported that of sixteen women with threatened abortion and subnormal pregnanediol values, the untreated group had eight abortions and one retention while in the progesterone treated group there were five retentions and two abortions. However, these encouraging observations were not borne out by later studies and 13 years later Zander (1967) concluded that pregnanediol excretion values do not permit any prognosis as to the outcome of a pregnancy in a woman with a record of habitual abortion. This conclusion was based on, *inter alia*, a double-blind study by Shearman and Garrett (1963) who found an 80% salvage rate both in the group treated with 17α-hydroxyprogesterone caproate and in the placebo group.

For the treatment of *habitual* abortions Tyler (1957) recommended 17α-hydroxyprogesterone caproate in weekly doses of 250-375 mg, combined with 5 mg of estradiol valerate, to begin before conception.

Plotz (1960) recommended doses of 50–100 mg of the same compound 3 to 5 times per week or 500 mg once a week. A woman with a history of seven miscarriages was treated with 500 mg of the drug per week. Though pregnanediol excretion in the urine remained low she delivered a normal baby.

Reifenstein (1958) tried to evaluate the results of prophylactic treatment with 17α-hydroxyprogesterone caproate by comparing the results of forty-five authors. These studies comprised 253 women who had had 1085 pregnancies but had delivered only 131 live infants. They were classified in four groups:

I. women with at least three abortions;
II. women whose last pregnancy had ended in abortion;
III. women with primary habitual abortion;
IV. women with secondary habitual abortion (at least three).

Total doses of the drug varied between 1.0 and 31.5 g, duration of treatment between 4 and 34 weeks. The number of women delivering live children after the pregnancies so treated, as compared with those in all previous pregnancies, were as follows:

Group I: 62 out of 89 = 69.7% as against 13.4%
Group II: 56 out of 82 = 68.3% as against 11.3%
Group III: 36 out of 56 = 64.3% as against 0%
Group IV: 20 out of 26 = 76% as against 28.7%

Reifenstein thus calculated that the percentage of salvaged pregnancies in the treated group was roughly 4 times that in the previous pregnancies without hormonal protection and he finds his results comparable to those of Davis and Plotz (1957). At present the usual intramuscular dose of 17-α-hydroxyprogesterone caproate is 250 to 500 mg once a week.

The question regarding the efficacy of progesterone and its substitutes in the prevention of abortion (habitual or incipient) has not been disposed of statistically. Roland (1965), in his book on progestagen therapy, pictures the situation by saying: "It is obviously very difficult to assess the results of therapy in habitual abortion, especially if Goldzieher (1964) is correct in maintaining that the spontaneous salvage rate in patients with low pregnanediol levels is of the order of 80 percent."

Zander (1967), who himself has made such fundamental contributions to our knowledge of the physiological importance of progesterone, finds himself unable to prove its therapeutic value in cases of threatened or habitual abortion—all the more since these terms are used with respect to very heterogeneous groups of patients. He does, however, employ injections of 500 mg of 17α-hydroxyprogesterone caproate every 5 days in cases of clearly increased uterine contractility, for a period of 20 to 30 days. He shortens the intervals between injections in the second trimester of pregnancy or when symptoms become alarming.

The difficulties of evaluation are even greater when, instead of progesterone or its nearest relatives, the long-acting esters of 17α-hydroxyprogesterone, the many orally active synthetic compounds, are considered. As was discussed in Chapter 28, these substances vary greatly in their pharmacological activities, including their ability to maintain pregnancy in castrated animals. As animal studies may serve as a guide for initial clinical studies, a first selection of drugs could be and has been made on that basis. There is, however, the additional problem of new pharmacological properties cropping up in new molecules, which may be harmful to the fetus, e.g. by causing masculinization in a female embryo. Such incidents have been described. The mechanism by which these genital abnormalities are produced is not sufficiently understood. It is not necessarily correlated with an androgenic effect demonstrable after administration to normal infantile or castrated rats.

Masculinized baby girls have been born to mothers who received diethylstilbestrol in large doses. The authors Bongiovanni *et al.* (1959) assume that an influence of the synthetic estrogen on the fetal adrenal was instrumental in bringing this change about. One year earlier Wilkins *et al.* (1958) had published twenty-one cases of fetal masculinization. In fifteen cases the mothers had been given ethisterone during pregnancy, in four cases progesterone combined with stilbestrol or methyltestosterone and in two cases no hormonal treatment. Ethisterone has been known for a long time to be quite androgenic. Norethisterone and norethynodrel have been described as causes of fetal masculinization in eight cases and in one respectively (Grumbach *et al.*, 1959).

Since these reports appeared the pharmaceutical companies have been paying great attention to the androgenicity of new compounds and to their capacity of causing intrauterine masculinization. A number of progestational substances have been found to be free from these properties in animal experiments and have so far not been reported to have caused genital malformations in the human.

Since the statistical evaluation of the efficacy of hormonal drugs in preventing abortion in the human is as difficult as we have described, other approaches are highly desirable and have been sought.

We have studied an enzyme which appears to be specific for pregnancy since it has so far only been found in the maternal blood during gestation, the 3.4.1? serum-oxytocinase (Dittmar and Semm, 1967; Semm, 1957, 1958, 1963, 1965; Semm and Wiendl, 1962; Semm and Bernhard, 1963; Waidl and Semm, 1960; Werle and Semm, 1956). We know a good deal about the occurrence of this enzyme under normal and pathological

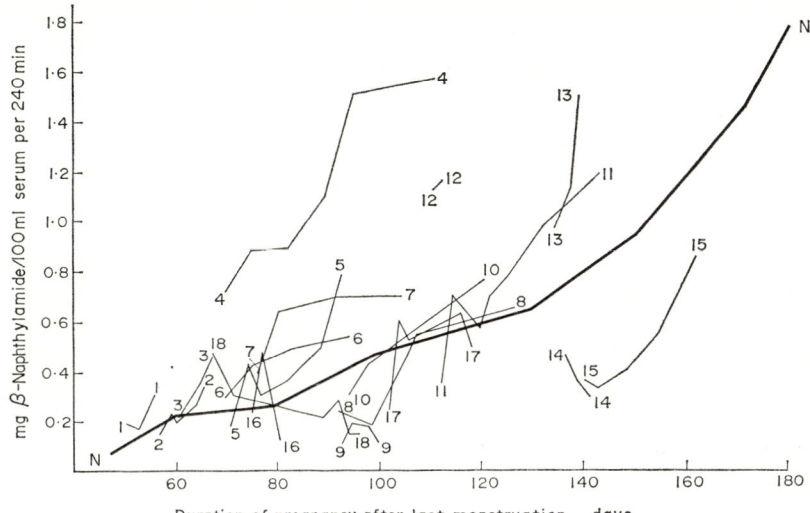

FIG. 6. Changes of serum levels of oxytocinase in cases of imminent abortion after injection of 17α-hydroxyprogesterone caproate. Cases 9 and 14 aborted. From Semm (1964).

conditions (Semm, 1960). In cases of threatened abortion its level is generally decreased. When 17α-hydroxyprogesterone caproate was given to these patients and pregnancy was maintained, we observed a regular increase in serum oxytocinase (Fig. 6). It is, of course, impossible to say whether this biochemical change was in some way responsible for the preservation of pregnancy or merely caused by it. We have seen a similar rise in oxytocinase after the oral administration of allylestrenol (Gestanon®) in doses of 5 mg 5 times a day to healthy pregnant women and to patients with threatened abortion. This observation, together with those of Szontágh and his group, indicating an increase in estriol and pregnanediol excretion after the administration of allylestrenol, has been interpreted as a kind of "placentotropic" effect.

Szontágh et al. (1963) studied the influence of allylestrenol (and other steroids) "in healthy women in the 8th to 12th week of pregnancy, prior to therapeutic abortion". In oral doses of 15 mg daily the drug (Gestanon®) was reported to stimulate significantly the excretion of HCG and particularly of estriol, as well as of pregnanediol, in comparison with two pretreatment values, the increases becoming apparent after 2 days of treatment.

Szontágh and Sas (1965), in further commenting on their findings, state that of the compounds tested only allylestrenol significantly increases the excretion of estriol and pregnanediol which is attributed to a *stimulating* effect on the placental syncytium. Clearly such an effect, if confirmed, would deserve great medical interest. The fact that it was observed in healthy women makes one speculate on its bearing on the conditions prevailing in pathological cases of threatened abortion. In the last paper quoted the authors describe five such cases, three of which are reported to have been successful, two as failures. We have somewhat elaborated on these reports because of the interest presented by the approach of the Hungarian investigators and because of the publicity given to them. The clinical experience of the group (salvage of pregnancies regardless of steroid excretion), as reported by Sas *et al.* (1965), comprised eighty-one women with *habitual* abortion, treated prophylactically with 5 to 10 mg of Gestanon® per day or therapeutically (when bleeding) with 15 mg; 12.4% of the women aborted notwithstanding the treatment. The authors consider the method superior to others. This conclusion is essentially in agreement with those of Borglin (1962), Borglin and Eliasson (1962) and others.

C. THE TREATMENT OF PRECOCIOUS PUBERTY

In 1962 Kupperman and Epstein in a preliminary report described their observations on five girls (4 to 10 years) and two boys (11 to 12 years) treated for precocious puberty with medroxyprogesterone acetate (MAP, Depo-Provera®).

Already in 1953 Lawson Wilkins, the great endocrinologist in the field of pediatrics, wrote: "The possibility remains that some steroid or other chemical structurally related to the sex hormones may be found capable of inhibiting the secretion of pituitary gonadotropin while causing little or no estrogenic or androgenic manifestations." The description by Glenn *et al.* (1959) of the inhibiting effect of MAP on the gonads and adrenals of rats (see Chapter 28) pointed to the possible usefulness of this compound in the way Wilkins (1953) had visualized.

The following papers are reporting on the use of this progestational compound in children with idiopathic precocious puberty, whose number is indicated:

Kupperman and Epstein (1962)	5 girls	2 boys
Hahn *et al.* (1964)	5 girls	
Lemli *et al.* (1964)	3 girls	
Surti (1965)	1 girl	
Thamdrup (1965)	3 girls	1 boy
Laron and Rumney (1965)	3 girls	3 boys

Zimprich and Gupta (1965)	2 girls	1 boy
Schoen (1966)		3 boys
Kaplan et al. (1968)	17 girls	4 boys
Rifkind et al. (1969)	3 girls	1 boy
Mathews et al. (1970)	6 girls	1 boy

In all these cases the injectable, long-acting form of MAP was the only therapy used, though three of the five girls reported on by Hahn et al. (1964) had had the oral form for some time before (2.5 to 7.5 mg per day). The parenteral dosage in all reports varied between 100 and 200 mg every other week, with few exceptions. Only one other drug, norethisterone (Norlutin®), was used in one patient by Thamdrup (10 mg daily for 2 years) and although this was apparently effective the author preferred the parenteral depot-treatment with MAP.

The biggest series, as can be seen, is that described by Kaplan et al. (Los Angeles) and their conclusions are in very good agreement with the other reports. They define sexual precocity as development of secondary sexual characteristics in girls before the age of 7 and in boys before the age of 8.8 years. The restriction "idiopathic" of course excludes those cases where sexual precocity is caused by tumors in the brain and related conditions. (See the report on ninety-six cases by Sigurjonsdottir and Hayles, 1968.)

In the report by Kaplan et al. (1968) the age at which the first signs of prococious puberty appeared varied between 1 month and 6 years in girls and 1 to 2 years in boys. The symptoms had existed for periods up to 5 years before treatment began, but in some cases this was started as soon as the first signs were discovered. The treatment at the time of reporting had been continued for an average of $2\frac{1}{2}$ and a maximum of $4\frac{1}{2}$ years.

Ten out of seventeen girls had regular vaginal bleedings and these ceased in every case. Breast-size increased during treatment in three girls, decreased in eight and remained unchanged in three.

As to growth and accelerated epiphysial maturation, expressed as predicted adult height, there was no change in the girls and an increase from 152 to 166.4 cm in the boys, but the authors consider the number of male patients too small to draw conclusions. In the girls regular menses did not appear on termination of treatment and this "amenorrhea" lasted for 16 months in one patient but her age at the time of reappearance of menses is not mentioned. The authors conclude that "arrest of menstruation in infants and preschool children is the most useful objective attained by this form of therapy".

Other authors concur, some considering decrease in breast-size as equally important. Pubic hair does not as a rule disappear. The precocious maturation of the epiphysial zones which limits adult height was practically not influenced in the majority of patients—"the most serious and the only permanent handicap these children suffer" (Hahn et al., 1964), though Schoen (1966) observed a retardation of skeletal maturation in one boy in whom treatment was started early and Mathews et al. (1970) even found "dramatic retardation" in a child in which treatment was begun at the age of 16 months. The same could be said of two of Zimprich and Gupta's patients, particularly the boy.

The number of boys in all these reports is much smaller than that of girls and although a regression of sexual precocity is regularly found, this is more difficult to assess than the symptoms in the girls.

Since medroxyprogesterone acetate is an adrenal inhibitor, attention is called to the investigation by Mathews et al. (1970) who studied pituitary-adrenal function in ten children (eight girls and two boys), three of whom had organic lesions in the CNS. They had weekly injections of 100 mg MAP (except one girl who had 150 mg weekly). Parameters studied were plasma 17-hydroxycorticosteroids before and after ACTH infusions (25 I.U. over a 4-hour period) and response to a metyrapone test. The authors concluded that the drug had a mild suppressive effect on pituitary-adrenal function without causing clinical symptoms of hypo-adrenocorticism even during periods of stress and with rapid return to normal on discontinuation of the drug.

MAP as discussed in Chapters 28 and 31 has in itself corticosteroid-like properties which, while accounting for the mild suppression of ACTH secretion, might make up for a certain amount of cortisol deficiency. Therefore its possible effect on growth of children deserves consideration.

As to the mechanism of action it is noteworthy that Rifkind et al. (1969) found gonadotropins depressed by MAP in only two out of four patients with idiopathic precocious puberty, using separate bio-assays for FSH and LH and radioimmuno-assays in addition, on pools of urine. They quote five sources for their statement that "after single 24 hour urinary gonadotropin measurements made before and at various times during treatment with medroxyprogesterone acetate some investigators have reported decreases and others have reported either no effect or increases of gonadotropin excretion". It cannot be said at the present time that the development of idiopathic precocious puberty is consistently accompanied by increased gonadotrophin excretion, nor that efficacy of MAP therapy depends on its decrease.

In summary it appears that of the various progestational compounds only medroxyprogesterone acetate (as i.m. depot) has been tested on a reasonably large scale and found to arrest various symptoms of idiopathic precocious puberty in most cases, but premature epiphysial maturation only in a minority of them.

REFERENCES

ADLERCREUTZ, E. (1953) Corpus luteum hormone in the treatment of biliary dyskinesia and especially of the post cholecystectomy syndrome. *Acta Med. Scand. (Stockh.)* **145:** 15–19.
AEPPLI, H. and HERRMANN, V. (1954) Allergische Reaktion auf Progesteron. *Schweiz. Med. Wschr.* **84:** 1366–1367.
ALDER, R. M. and KRIEGER, V. I. (1957) Hormonal therapy and the significance of the pregnanediol excretion test in recurrent abortion. *Med. J. Aust.* **44:** 122–133.
ALEMANY, R. V. and HERNANDEZ, R. G. (1952) Pregnanediol in the treatment of asthma. *Rev. Clin. Espan.* **46:** 168–170.
ALVAREZ, R. R. and SEAHLE (1954) Amenorrhea. *J. Amer. Med. Ass.* **156:** 582–585.
AMANN, W. (1965) Änderung im Verhalten der Akne vulgaris bei hormonell beeinflußten menstruellem Zyklus (II. Mitteilung). *Z. Haut- u. Geschl.-Kr.* **38:** 246–247.
ANDERSON, D. G. (1965) Management of advanced endometrial adenocarcinoma with medroxyprogesterone acetate. *Amer. J. Obstet. Gynec.* **92:** 87–99.
ANDREOLI, C. (1955) Sulla terapia della minaccia d'aborto con una sospensione microcristallina di progesterone-estrogeni. *Minerva Ginec.* **4:** 214–217.
ANDREWS, M. C., ANDREWS, W. C. and STRAUSS, A. F. (1959) Effects of progestin-induced pseudopregnancy on endometriosis: Clinical and microscopic studies. *Amer. J. Obstet. Gynec.* **78:** 776–785.
ANTOINE, T. (1963) Orale Gestagentherapie. *Münch. Med. Wschr.* **105:** 1513–1517.
ARRIGHI, L. (1964) Clinica y tratamento de las metrorrhagias funcionales de la adolescencia. *Orient. Med.* **601:** 102.
ARTNER, J. (1965) Das prämenstruelle Syndrom. *Zbl. Gynäk.* **87:** 145–162.
ASHITAKA, Y. (1955) Studies on the prediction of abnormalities of pregnancy (threatened abortion) by the urine color reaction and its treatment. *Med. J. Osaka Univ.* **6:** 261.
AYDAR, C. and GREENBLATT, R. (1964) 6α-Dehydro-retroprogesterone (Duphaston) an interesting progesterone-like compound. *Int. J. Fertil. Steril.* **9:** 585–595.
BAANDERS-VAN HALEWIJN, E. A. (1962) Constitutionele en erfelijke aspecten van het endometriumcarcinoom. Thesis Utrecht.
BAANDERS-VAN HALEWIJN, E. A., DE WAARD, F., MASTBOOM, J. L., TONKES, E. and MEINSMA, L. (1963) Konstitutionelle und erbliche Aspekte des Endometriumkarzinoms. *Z. Geburtsh. Gynäk.* **161:** 77–93.
BACIGALUPO, G. (1961) Zum Problem Mastopathie–Mammakarzinom. *M. Kurse ärztl. Fortbildg.* **11:** 168–174.
BACKER, M. H. (1962) Isopregnenone (Duphaston): A new progestational agent *Obstet. Gynec.* **19:** 724–729.
BAKER, K. C. (1959) Treatment of persistent acne in women with 17-α-hydroxy-progesterone caproate. *J. Invest. Dermat. (Baltimore)* **31:** 247–250.
BAKER, W. S., BANCROFT, E. C., LYNDA, E. W. and LEHMAN, J. J. (1955) Value of urinary pregnanediol determinations as indication of or the use of progesterone in treatment of threatened abortion. *Amer. J. Obstet. Gynec.* **69:** 405–414.
BALINA, P. A. (1962) Una experiencia con tratamiento prolongado de noresteroides en la endometriosis. *Orient. Med.* **497:** 96–102.

BARNES, A. C. and ROTHSCHILD, S. (1953) Experimental use of intravenously administered progesterone in advanced cases of cervical carcinoma. *Obstet. Gynec.* **1**: 147–155.

BARNES, L. W. (1958) Urinary excretion of pregnanediol after intravenous administration of progesterone in threatened abortion. *Amer. J. Obstet. Gynec.* **75**: 53–59.

BAUMGARTEN, K. (1963) "Librium" und "Valium" in der Schwangerschaft und unter der Geburt. *Wien. Klin. Wschr.* **75**: 263–270.

BAYER, R. (1964) Die Behandlung der Endometriose bei Frauen im Fertilitätsalter. Konservative Operation, Androgen-Gestagenkombinationen. *Zbl. Gynäk.* **86**: 537–548.

BÉCLÈRE, CL. (1962) Dutriple dosage hormonal des gonadotrophines, des oestrogènes et du prégnandiol et du triple traitement hormonal éventuel dans le traitement des avortements récidivants. *Bull. Fed. Gynèc. Obstét.* **14**: 124–127.

BEGGS, J. A. (1952). Herpes gestationis treated with testosterone. *Can. Med. Assoc. J.* **67**: 52–54.

BEHRENS, H. (1957) Follikelhormon und Corpuscarzinom des Uterus. *Geburtsh. Frauenheilk.* **17**: 1126–1135.

BENGTSSON, L. PH. (1959) Beziehungen zwischen Progesteron, Pregnandiol und Erhaltung der menschlichen Schwangerschaft. *Arch. Gynäk.* **193**: 338–339.

BENGTSSON, L. PH. (1962a) Endocrine factors in labour. *Acta Obstet. Gynec. Scand.* **41**: Suppl. 1, 87–116.

BENGTSSON, L. PH. (1962a) Experiments on the suppressive effect of a synthetic gestagen on the activity of the pregnant human uterus. *Acta Obstet. Gynec. Scand.* **41**: 124–144.

BENGTSSON, L. PH. and CSAPO, A. I. (1962) Oxytocin response, withdrawal and reinforcement of defense mechanism of the human uterus at midpregnancy. *Amer. J. Obstet. Gynec.* **83**: 1083–1093.

BENGTSSON, L. PH. and FUCHS, F. (1962) Endocrine factors in certain pathological conditions of pregnancy and labour. *Acta Obstet. Gynec. Scand.* **41**: Suppl. 1, 117–143.

BENGTSSON, L. PH. (1963) Experiments on the endocrine control of the pregnant uterus. *Bull. Soc. Roy, Belge Gynec. Obstet.* **33**: 467–475.

BENGTSSON, L. PH. et al. (1966) The effects of oestrogen and gestagen on the non-pregnant human uterus. *J. Obstet. Gynaec. (Brit. Cwlth.)* **73**: 273–281.

BENJAMIN, F. and CASPER, D. J. (1966) Alterations in carbohydrate metabolism induced by progesterone in case of endometrial carcinoma and hyperplasia. *Amer. J. Obstet. Gynec.* **94**: 991–996.

BENJAMIN, F. and ROMNEY, S. L. (1964). Disturbed carbohydrate metabolism in endometrial carcinoma, *Cancer* **17**: 386–390.

BELL, E. I. and LORAINE, J. A. (1965) Effect of dydrogesterone on hormone excretion in patients with dysmenorrhea. *Lancet* **1**: 403–406.

BERGER, M. and NEUWEILER, W. (1962) Relaxation und Sedation des menschlichen Uterus. *Geburtsh. Frauenheilk.* **22**: 1275–1277.

BERGSJÖ, P. (1965) Progesterone and progestional compounds in the treatment of advanced endometrial carcinoma. *Acta Endocr. (Kbh.)* **49**: 412–426.

BERNARD, J. (1955) La prophylaxie endocrinienne de l'avortement spontané: Evolution des idées et tendances actuelles. *Ann. d'Endocr.* **16**: 315–333.

BERNARD, I. Y MALGOUYAT (1955) Contribucion endocrina en la profilaxis del aborto espontaneo. *Ann. Endocr. (Paris)* **6**: 863–872.

BESOLD, F. (1950) Heilung des Pruritus vulvae mit Gelbkörperhormon. *Münch. Med. Wschr.* **92**: 883–885.

BEYL, G. (1959) Praktische und klinische Erfahrungen mit "hormonaler Curettage". *Medizinische* **11**: 205–206.

BICKENBACH, W. (1953) Herpes labialis menstruationis. *Dtsch. Med. Wschr.* **78**: 647.
BICKENBACH, W. and DÖRING, G. K. (1959) *Die Sterilität der Frau.* Verlag Georg Thieme, Stuttgart.
BINKS, R., CAMBOURN, P. and PAPWORTH, R. A. (1962). Preliminary report of a clinical trial of oral norethynodrel for fertility control. *Med. J. Australia* **1**: 716.
BISHOP, P. M. F. (1961) A new oral progestogen in the treatment of dysemnorrhea. *Proc. Roy. Soc. Med.* **54**: 752–754.
BOCKNER, V. (1963) The contraceptive pill: a clinical evaluation of its longterm use. *Med. J. Australia* **50**: 809–812.
BOLCK, F. (1960) Die Pathologie des Uterusmyoms. *Arch. Gynäk.* **195**: 167–177.
BOLTE, A. (1961) Zur hormonalen Behandlung der drohenden Fehlgeburt. *Fortschr. Med.* **79**: 305.
BONGIOVANNI, A. M., DI GEORGE, A. M. and GRUMBACH, M. M. (1959) Masculinization of the female infant associated with estrogenic therapy alone during gestation: four cases. *J. Clin. Endocr.* **19**: 1004–1010.
BORGLIN, N. E. (1956) The excretion of pregnanediol in the urine in threatened abortion. *Acta Endocr. (Kbh.)* **22**: 49–54.
BORGLIN, N. E. (1962) Resultats du traitement par l'allylestrénol dans la menace d'avortement et l'avortement habitual. *Gynéc. Obstét.* **61**: 493–506.
BORGLIN, N. E. and ELIASSON, G. (1962) Analysis of the pregnancy-maintaining effect of allylestrenol in threatened and habitual abortion. *Fertil. Steril.* **13**: 411–420.
BORGLIN, N. E. and WOLBERT, B. (1957). The prognostic value of histaminase and pregnanediol determination in threatening abortion. *Acta Obstet. Gynec. Scand.* **36**: 382–397.
BORGLIN, N. E., THEANDER, G. and WEHLIN, L. (1965) Roentgenographic observations on the effect of pseudopregnancy in endometriosis. *J. Obstet. Gynaec. (Brit. Cwlth.)* **72**: 544–556.
BORTH, R., GSELL, M. and DE WATTEVILLE, H. (1954) Thérapeutique par la progestérone dans les menaces d'avortement et avortement répétés. *Acta Endocr. (Kbh.)* **17**: 22–30.
BORTH, R. and STAMM, O. (1958) Pregnandiol- und Oestriolausscheidung im Urin bei Geburtsbeginn. *Geburtsh. Frauenheilk.* **178**: 600–604.
BOSCHANN, H. W. (1955) Klinische Erfahrungen mit 17-alpha-oxyprogesteron-17-capronat. *Geburtsh. Frauenheilk.* **15**: 1070–1081.
BOSCHANN, H. W. (1958) Observations on the role of progestational agents in human gynecologic disorders and pregnancy complications. *Ann. New York Acad. Sci.* **71**: 727–752.
BOTELLA LLUSIA, J. (1958) Über die Ursachen der Fehlgeburt. *Berl. Med.* **9**: 131–137.
BOTELLA LLUSIA, J. (1962) Insuficiencia progestacional y aborto. *Acta ginec. (Madrid)* **13**: 201–213.
BOTELLA LLUSIA, J. and MARIN BONACHERA, E. (1961) El aborto ignorado en mujeres aparamente estériles. (Un nuevo sindrome de infertilidad humana). *Acta Ginec. (Madrid)* **12**: 433–443.
BOVERI, J. L. (1962) El 17 capronate 17a-hidroxiprogesterona en el tratamiente de la amenaza de aborto y del aborto habitual. *Obstet. y Ginec. Lat. Amer.* **20**: 670–673.
BRACHO LEON, J. (1963) Sobre un caso de una paciente con embarazo a termino despues de seis abortos consecutivos, tratada con el capronato de 17 alfa-hidroxiprogesterona. *Risquez* **5**: 31–34.
BRADSHAW, T. E. T. and JESSOP, W. J. E. (1953) The urinary excretion of oestrogens and pregnanediol at the end of pregnancy, during labour and during early puerperium. *J. Endocr.* **9**: 427–439.
BREITNER, J. (1955). Quantitative-chemische Untersuchungen über die Östrogenausscheidung bei der Frau and ihre Bedeutung für die Physiologie und Pathologie der Schwangerschaft und des Cyclus. *Arch. Gynäk.* **185**: 258–298.

BRET, A. J. and BOUJNAH (1955) Prophylaxie de l'avortement et de l'interruption prématurée de la grossesse. Surveillance biologique, biochimique et cytologique. *Sem. Hop.* **31**: 2947–2955.

BRUINSMA, A. H. and DE WAARD, F. (1959). Oestrogenic activity at menopausal age in women with diabetes mellitus ("Diabète gras"). *Acta Endocr. (Kbh.)* **32**: 233–242.

BRONSTEIN, S., PLAINS, M., GRATER, W., JACOBSON, C., ORENTREICH, N. and APPLEZWEIG, N. (1966) Human and animal anti-inflammatory activity of an acetamide of progesterone. *Arch. Dermat.* **93**: 114–118.

BRUNO, R. O. (1961) Tratamiento hormonal en las amenazas de aborto de causa endocrina. *Sem. Med. B. Aires* **119**: 736–740.

BRUNTSCH, K. H. (1960) Zur Behandlung der Fehlgeburt. *Dtsch. Med. J.* **11**: 433–436.

BUCHHOLTZ, R. (1959) Gonadotropinausscheidung beim Menschen. *Geburtsh. Frauenheilk.* **19**: 851–858.

BUSCHBECK, H. (1962) Über die Behandlungsversuche bei therapieresistenter Amenorrhoe. *Geburtsh. Frauenheilk.* **22**: 818–830.

BÜTTNER, W. and TRAPPMANN, R. (1940) Der Einfluß von Progesteron auf die Ausscheidung des gonadotropen Hormons im Harn von Frauen außerhalb der Geschlechtsreife. *Arch. Gynäk.* **170**: 413–421.

BYGDEMAN, M. and ELIASSON, R. (1964) Effect of progesterone and oestrone on the motility and reactivity of the pregnant human myometrium *in vitro*. *J. Repr. Fertil.* **7**: 47–52.

CAROL, W. and MÜLLER, W. (1964). Beitrag zur Klinik der Adnexendometriose. *Z. Geburtsh. Gynäk.* **162**: 185–194.

CARTER, B. (1962) Treatment of endometriosis. *J. Obstet. Gynaec. Brit. Cwlth.* **69**: 783–789.

CASTELAZO AYALA, L. (1953) Valor comparativo del dietilestilbestrol y la progesterona a dosis altas, en el tratamiento de la amenaza de aborto. *Ginec. Obstet. Méx.* **8**: 167–170.

CASTELAZO AYALA, L. *et al.* (1959). Effectos del capronato de 17-alfa-oxyprogesterona en 100 casos de amenaza de aborto. *Ginec. Obstet. Méx.* **14**: 249–251.

CHALMERS, J. A. (1962) Treatment of endometriosis with anovlar. *J. Obstet. Gynaec. Brit. Cwlth.* **69**: 801–803.

CHARTIER, M., CORDIER, P. and CORNU, C. (1966). Traitement de l'endométriose par le SH 513 et le SH 639. *Gynéc. Prat.* **17**: 259–263.

CLARK, S. L. and GREENBLATT, R. B. (1957) The effect of progestional agents in human gynecologic and adrenal disorders. New York Academy of Sciences, October 1957.

COHEN, A. M. (1964) De Behandeling van endometriose met synthetische progestative Stoffen. Thesis (Amsterdam).

COHEN, M. R. and HANKIN, H. (1959) The inadequate luteal phase. *Int. J. Fertil.* **4**: 58–65.

COMAS FUNALLET, J. (1958) La insuficiencia del cuerpo luteo como causa de abortos de repeticon. *Acta ginec. (Madrid)* **9**: 257–260.

CONTAMIN, R. (1959) L'accouchement préparé par la synergie vitamine E-progesterone. *Thérapie* **14**: 907–911.

CONTAMIN, R. (1961) Die vorbereitete Entbindung. *Arch. Gynäk.* **195**: 395–402.

CONTAMIN, R., MOULIN, CL. and LORILLOU, J.-S. (1961) L'importance de la gynécologie en obstétrique. *Gaz. Méd. Fr.* **68**: 2007–2014.

CONTE, J. C. (1961) Treatment of threatened abortion with progesterone. New forms of application. *Dia. Med. B. Aires* **33**: 1136–1138.

CROMER, J. K. (1965) Endometriosis of the colon (sigmoid, recto-sigmoid and rectovaginal septum). *Sth. Med. J.* **58**: 807–815.

CROOKE, A. C. and BUTT, W. R. (1953) *Proceedings Society Study of Fertility* 1953, pp. 87–96.

COURRIER, R. (1950) Interaction between estrogens and progesterone. *Vitamins and Hormones* **8**: 179–183.
CROWLEY, C. G. and MACDONALD, J. (1965) Delalutin and oestrogens for the treatment of advanced mammary carcinoma in the post-menopausal women. *Cancer* **18**: 436–445.
CROWLEY, L. G., DEMETRIOU, J. A., KOTIN, P., DONOVAN, A. J. and KUSHINSKI, ST. (1965) Excretion patterns of urinary metabolites of estradiol-4-C^{14} in post-menopausal women with benign and malignant desease of the breast. *Cancer Res.* **25**: 371–376.
CROWSON, L. B., WINER, B. A. and NOYES, R. W. (1965) Evaluation of a new progestin. *Obstet. Gynec.* **67**: 349–355.
CULLEN, J. H., BRUM, V. C. and REIDT, W. V. (1959) The respiratory effects of progesterone in several pulmonary emphysema. *Amer. J. Med.* **27**: 551–557.
CUNNINGHAM, K. and LANG, W. (1962) Result of a blind clinical trial conducted on 50 cases of hormonal mastopathy. *Med. J. Aust.* **49**: 341–344.
CURCHOD, A. (1970) Traitement hormonal du Cancer de l'endomètre et de ses metastases. *Schweiz. Z. Gynäk, Geburtsh.* **1**, 69–87.
CURWEN, S. (1963) The value of norethisterone acetate in the treatment of advanced carcinoma of the breast. *Clin. Radiol.* **16**: 445–446.
DALSGAARD-NIELSEN, T. (1965) Profylaktisk behandling of migraene med et myt progesteronderivat. *Nordisk Medicin* **74**: 713–736.
DAPUNT, O. (1965) Erfahrungen mit der therapeutischen amenorrhoe. *Zbl. Gynäk.* **87**: 896–903.
DAURIA, P. (1960) The hormone treatment of secondary amenorrhea of short duration. *Sem. Med. (B. Aires)* **117**: 1777–1778.
DAVIS, M. E. (1958) Premenstrual tension. *Med. Clin. N. Amer.* **42**: 257–262.
DAVIS, M. E. (1960) Persönliche Mitteilung zit. aus Plotz, E. J. (1960) Die Behandlung habitueller Fehlgeburten mit Gestagenen. *Med. Welt* **41**: 2134–2138.
DAVIS, M. E. and PLOTZ, E. J. (1957) The metabolism of progesterone and its clinical use in pregnancy. *Rec. Progr. Hormone Res.* **13**: 347–388.
DAVIS, M. E. and WIED, G. L. (1957) Long-acting progestation agents. *Geburtsh. Frauenheilk.* **17**: 916–928.
DAVIS, M. E., PLOTZ, E., LUPU, I. and EJARQUE, P. M. (1959) The metabolism of progesterone and its related compounds in human pregnancy. *Fertil. Steril.* **11**: 18–48.
DE GROOT, C. A., V.D. LELY, M. A. and KOOIJ, R. (1965) The effect of progesterone on the sebaceous glands of the rat. *Brit. J. Dermatol.* **77**: 617–621.
DEKANIĆ-MILOSEVIĆ, V. and IVANCEVIĆ-CUDIĆ, ST. (1954) Hormonale Therapie des Abortus imminens. *Med. Pregl.* **1**: 28–35.
DESAULLES, P. A. (1958) Die Entwicklung auf dem Gebiet der gestagenen Steroide. *Geburtsh. Frauenheilk.* **18**: 667–672.
DESPHANDE, G. N., TURNER, A. K. and SOMMERVILLE I. F. (1960) Plasma progesterone and pregnanediol in human pregnancy, during labour and post-partum. *J. Obstet. Gynaec. (Brit. Emp).* **67**: 954–961.
D'INCERTI BONINI, L. (1964) Trattamento endocrino dell'adenocarcinoma endometriale. *Ann. Ostet. Ginec.* **86**: 1–64.
DICZFALUSY, E. (1962) Endocrinology of the foetus. *Acta Obstet. Gynec. Scand.* **41**: Suppl. 1, 45–85.
DITTMAR, F. W. and SEMM, K. (1967) Geburtseinleitung mit einem Serum-Oxytocinase resistenten Oxytocin-Analogon. *Z. Geburtsh. Gynäk.* **166**: 197–200.
DÖRING, G. K. (1959) Relative Corpus-luteum Insuffizienz. *Dtsch. Med. Wschr.* **84**: 489–491.
DOMINGUEZ VILAR, E. and CABALLERO-GORDO, A. (1962) Concepto actual de la etiologia, diagnostico y prevencion del aborto habitual. *Acta Ginec. (Madrid)* **13**: 331–343.

DRILL, V. A. (1966) *Oral Contraceptives*. The Blakiston Division, McGraw-Hill Book Co., New York.
DUJOVICH, A. (1960) Estado actual del tratamiento de la endometriosis. *Prensa Med. Argent.* **47**: 3002–3005.
DURHAM, W. D. (1961) Progestational steroid requirements for inducing and maintaining decidua in women. *Fertil. Steril.* **12**: 45–54.
DUTHIE, J. J. R. (1951) Fundamental treatment of rheumatoid arthritis. *Practitioner* **166**: 22–32.
ELERT, R. (1957) Die Behandlung des Abortus imminens. *Dtsch. Med. Wschr.* **82**: 2104–2107.
ERB, H., KELLER, M. and HAUSER, G. A. (1962) Östrogen- und Pregnandiolausscheidung bei hypotensiver Gestose. *Zbl. Gynäk.* **84**: 474–480.
EZÉS, H. (1957) Prophylaxie des avortements involontaires a répétition. *Concours Méd.* **79**: 5189–5194.
FERIN, J. (1957) La méthyloestrénolone (Norméthandrolone), nouvelle substance progestogène, active par la voie perlinguale. *Geburtsh. Frauenheilk.* **17**: 10–24.
FERIN, J. (1964). Hypooestrogenic amenorrhoae and/or sterility induced by lynestrenol. *Int. J. Fertil.* **9**: 29–34.
FINKE, L. (1959) Der habituelle Abort. *Med. Klin.* **54**: 28–31.
FINKE, L. (1963) Die Bedeutung der Endometriose. *Med. Klin.* **58**: 421–425.
FOIX, A. (1961) Tratamiento hormonal de la amenaza de aborto de causa endocrina. *Prensa Med. Argent.* **48**: 1178–1187.
FOIX, A., BRUNO, R. and VIGGIANO, CH. (1961) Tratamiento de la amenaza de aborto con la progesterona endovenosa. *Dia. Méd.* **53**: 1629–1632.
FOLEY, J. and WILSON, A. C. (1958) Treatment of habitual abortion. *Brit. Med. J.* **5104**: 1103–1104.
FOLEY, J. (1963) The use of intramuscular progesterone in pregnancy with special reference to vaginal aplasia. *J. Obstet. Gynaec. (Brit. Cwlth.)* **70**: 429–436.
FRICK, H. C. (1965) Progestational drugs in the management of endometrial cancer. *Metabolism* **14**: 348–355.
FRIES, K. (1962) Die Prognose der "juvenilen Metropathie" auf lange Sicht. *Geburtsh. Frauenheilk.* **22**: 511–521.
FROEWIS, J. and LEEB, H. (1960) Die Therapie der funktionellen Blutungen mit dem neuen Gestagen. *Wien. Klin. Wschr.* **72**: 881–886.
FUCHS, F. (1962) Endocrine factors in the maintenance of pregnancy. *Acta Obstet. Gynec. Scand.* **41**: Suppl. 1, 7–44.
FUCHS, F. and STAKEMANN, G. (1960) Treatment of threatened prematurity with large doses of progesterone. *Amer. J. Obstet. Gynaec.* **79**: 172–176.
GARRETT, W. J. (1959) A theory of uterine action. *J. Obstet. Gynaec. (Brit. Empire)* **66**: 927–938.
GAUTRY, J. P., DARBEL, A., CABANNES, R., CARDONC, H. and JAHIER, J. (1961) Etude statistique de 279 grossesses biologiquement anormales. *Gynec. et Obstet.* **60**: 479–505.
GEIPEL, K. and V. LÖHR, G. W. (1963) Thrombozythopathien in der Menarche. *Med. Welt.* **52**: 2678–2685.
GELLER, J., VOLK, H. and LEWIN, M. (1961) Objective remission of metastatic breast carcinoma in a male who received 17-a-hydroxyprogesterone caproate (delalutin). *Cancer Chemother. Rep.* **14**: 77–81.
GIESEN, W. and PAULI, H. (1959) Beitrag zur kombinierten Hormontherapie bei habituellem Abortus. *Zbl. Gynäk.* **81**: 1922–1926.
GITSCH, E. (1956) Zur Behandlung des Abortus imminens mit Sexualhormonen. *Wien. Klin. Wschr.* **68**: 370–373.

GITSCH, E. (1957) Laparotomie und intrauterine Gravidität. *Wien. Klin. Wschr.* **69**: 348–350.
GITSCH, E. (1964) Die Amenorrhoe, *Wien. Klin. Wschr.* **76**: 673–680.
GLENN, E. M., RICHARDSON, S. L. and BOWMAN, B. J. (1959) Biologic activity of 6-alphamethyl compounds corresponding to progesterone, 17-alpha-hydroxy-progesterone acetate and compound S. *Metabolism* **8**: 265–285.
GOLDZIEHER, J. W. (1957) Lack of androgenicity of 17-hydroxyprogesterone or its 17-capronate ester. *J. Clin. Endocrinol.* **17**: 323–325.
GOLDZIEHER, J. W. (1964) Double-blind trial of progestin in habitual abortion. *J. Amer. Med. Ass.* **188**: 651–654.
GOLDZIEHER, J. W. and BENIGNO, B. B. (1958) The treatment of threatened and recurrent abortion. A critical review. *Amer. J. Obstet. Gynec.* **75**: 1202–1214.
GOLDZIEHER, J. W., MOSES, L. E. and ELLIS, L. T. (1962) Studies of Norethindrone in contraception. *J. Amer. Med. Ass.* **180**: 359–361.
GONZALES CUESTA, A. (1962) Progestágenes como causa de aborto diferido. *E. Medico* **12**: 41–44.
GOODMAN, A. L. (1946) Progesterone therapy in uterine fibroyoma. *J. Clin. Endocr.* **6**: 405–408.
GORLITZER, V. MUNDY, V. and FRIEDL, W. (1953) Die Behandlung der Arthritis mit Corpus luteum. *Med. Klin.* **48**: 1333–1334.
GOULD, J. (1963) Control of ovulation with Provest. *Int. J. Fertil.* **8**: 737–741.
GRANT, A. (1961) The non-surgical treatment of endometriosis by progestogens. *Med. J. Aust.* **48**: 936–938.
GRASSET, J. (1955) L'avortement endocrinien existe-t-il? *Rev. Med. Moyen-Orient.* **12**: 161–163.
GRAY, L. A. (1965) Endometriosis of the bowel: treatment by excision or castration. *Southern Med. J.* **58**: 815–822.
GREEN, R. (1962) Water retention in migraine. *Proc. Roy. Soc. Med.* **55**: 196–171.
GREENBLATT, R. B. (1963) Amenorrhea and the endocrine disorders. *J. Int. Fertil. Gynec. Obstet.* **1**: 94–97.
GREENBLATT, R. B. and JUNGCK, E. C. (1958) Delay of menstruation with norethindrone an orally given progestational compound. *J. Amer. Med. Ass.* **166**: 1461–1463.
GREENBLATT, R. B. and SCARPA-SMITH, C. J. (1959) Nymphomania in postmenopausal women. *J. Amer. Geriat. Soc.* **7**: 339–342.
GREENBLATT, R. B. and ROSE, F. D. (1962) Delay of menses: test of progestational efficiency in induction of pseudo-pregnancy. *Obstet. Gynec.* **19**: 730–735.
GREGOIRE, L., FONTAINE, J. and NICOLAS, A. (1963) Traitement de l'endométriose par la lynestrénol. *Bull. Soc. Roy. Belge Gynéc. Obstét.* **35**: 153–157.
GRUMBACH, M. M., DUCHARME, J. R. and MOLOSHOK, R. E. C. (1959) On the fetal masculinizing action of certain oral progestins. *J. Clin. Endocr.* **19**: 1369–1380.
GUIOT, G., LEVY, J., AUQUIER, L. and COMOY, C. (1965) Sciatique par endométriose. La sciatique cataméniale. *Press. Méd.* **73**: 1397–1398.
GUTERMAN, H. S. (1953) Progesterone metabolism in the human female: its significance in relation to reproduction. *Rec. Progr. Hormone Res.* **8**: 293–331.
GYÖRY, G. and LÁSZLO, J. (1965) Über die Anwendung von Gestagenen bei Entzündungen im kleinen Becken. *Zbl. Gynäk.* **87**: 171–172.
HAHN, H. B., HAYLES, A. B. and ALBERT, A. (1964) Medroxyprogesterone and constitutional precocious puberty. *Mayo Clin. Proc.* **39**: 182–190.
HALLER, J. (1965) Karzinomprophylaxe mit Gestagen. *Selecta* **7**: 122.
HALLER, J. (1968) *Ovulationshemmung durch Hormone.* 2. Auflage, Georg Thieme Verlag, Stuttgart.
HAMADA, H. (1965) Functional uterine bleeding. *Bull. Osaka Med.*
HARTL, H. (1959) Neues aus der Geburtshilfe 1958. *Landarzt* **35**: 681–686.

HAUSER, G. A. et al. (1960) Juvenile Blutungen. *Therap. Umschau* **17**: 299.
HAYDEN, G. E. (1958) Progesterone-induced withdrawal bleeding as a simple physiologic test for pregnancy. *Amer. J. Obstet. Gynec.* **76**: 271–278.
HEBER, K. R. (1964) The treatment of acroparaesthesia with progesterone. *Med. J. Aust.* **51**: 272–274.
HECHT-LUCARI, G. (1965) Antioestrogene und antiandrogene Effekte gewisser oral wirksamer Gestagene. *Geburtsh. Frauenheilk.* **25**: 620–623.
HECKMANN, B. (1965) Zur Wirkung von Norhydroxyprogesteronkapronat auf das Adenocarcinom des Corpus uteri in der Gewebekultur. *Dtsch. Med. Wschr.* **90**: 2328–2330.
HEISS, H. (1954) Das Adrenalin in der Behandlung des Abortus imminens. *Zbl. Gynäk.* **76**: 1727–1736.
HELPAP, B. (1963) Zur Behandlung der Endometriose mit Äthinyl-nortestosteronazetat. *Geburtsh. Frauenheilk.* **23**: 539–544.
HENDRICKS, CH. H. (1964) A new technique for the study of motility in the non-pregnant human uterus. *J. Obstet. Gynaec. Brit. Cwlth.* **71**: 712–715.
HENZL, M., HORSKÝ, J., PREŚL, J. and JIRASEK, J. (1962) Zum Mechanismus der hämostatischen Wirkung des 16-α-Äthinyl-19-nor-testosterons. *Arch. Gynäk.* **196**: 425–434.
HEROLD, K. (1962) Blutungen in der Schwangerschaft, unter der Geburt und im Wochenbett, ihre Ursachen und ihre Behandlung. *Landarzt* **38**: 983–987.
HERRMANN, U. (1958) Zur Behandlung des drohenden Abortes und der Frühgeburt. *Therap. Umschau* **15**: 138.
HERRMANN, U. and GEISER, P. (1957) Neuere Erkenntnisse in der Diagnostik und Behandlung des Abortus imminens. *Z. Geburtsh. Gynäk.* **148**: 199–216.
HERTIG, A. (1964) Gestational hyperplasia of endometrium. *Lab. Invest.* **13**: 1153–1157.
HERTZ, R. and CRONER, J. K. (1952) Progesterone and carcinoma of the cervix. *J. Amer. Med. Ass.* **154**: 1114–1117.
HILLEMANNS, H. G. (1965) Karzinomprophylaxe mit Gestagenen. *Selecta* **7**: 1227.
HOCHSTÄDT, B., LANGE, W. and SPIRA, M. (1960) Vaginal cytology as a guide to the treatment of habitual abortion. *J. Obstet. Gynaec. (Brit. Empire)* **67**: 102–109.
HODGKINSON, C. P. and IGNA, J. (1958) High potency progestational agents in human pregnancy. *Ann. N.Y. Acad. Sci.* **71**: 753–758.
HODGKINSON, C. P., IGNA, J. and BUKSAVIDI, A. P. (1958) High potency progesterone drugs and threatened abortion. *Amer. J. Obstet. Gynec.* **76**: 279–287.
HÖRMANN, G. (1960) Behandlung der Fehlgeburt. *Therapiewoche* **10**: 294–296.
HOFF, F. and BAYER, R. (1954) Ovarialhormone und Uterusmotilität. *Z. Geburtsh. Gynäk.* **144**: Beilageheft.
HOFFMANN, F. and v. LÁM, L. (1948) Über die Progesteronbildung im Zyklus und in der Schwangerschaft. *Zbl. Gynäk.* **70**: 1177–1184.
HOFFMANN, FR. and UHDE, G. (1955a) Über die Bedeutung des Progesteronstoffwechsels für die Auslösung der Geburtsvorgänge. *Zbl. Gynäk.* **77**: 1909–1913.
HOFFMANN, FR. and UHDE, G. (1955b) Über den Progesterongehalt des Blutes im uterinen und im fetalen Kreislauf. bei der schwangeren Frau. *Arch. Gynäk.* **185**: 469–475.
HOFHANSL, W. and BAUMGARTEN, K. (1960) Die Behandlung des Abortus imminens mit Gestagenen. *Wien. Klin. Wschr.* **72**: 853–856.
HOFHANSL, W. (1961) Die therapeutische Pseudogravidität. *Zbl. Gynäk.* **83**: 113–119.
HOFMANN, D. (1966) Einige Betrachtungen zum Krankheitsbild der Endometriose. *Med. Welt* **17**: 1024–1030.
HOHLWEG, W. V. and REIFENSTUHL, G. (1965) Langzeitbehandlung mit Hormonen in der Gynäkologie. *Wien. Klin. Wschr.* **77**: 878–881.
HOLLSTEIN, K. (1958) Das Schicksal der Frucht nach drohendem Abortus. *Zbl. Gynäk.* **80**: 16–21.

HOLZMANN, H., KORTING, G. W. and MORCHES, B. (1965) Zur Therapie der Sklerodermie mit Gestagenen. *Hautarzt* **16:** 546–458.
HOLZMANN, H., KORTING, G. W., HAMMERSTEIN, F., STECHER, K. H., DURRUTI, M., IWANGOFF, P. and KÜHN, K. (1964) Quantitative Bestimmung der einzelnen Kollagenfraktionen der Haut nach Anwendung von Resochin und Progesteron. *Naturwissensch.* **51:** 310–318.
HUGGINS, C. (1958) Hormonabhängige Geschwülste. *Klin. Welt* **36:** 1102–1106.
HUSSLEIN, H. (1964) Die moderne Gestagentherapie. *Wien. Med. Wschr.* **114:** 726–729.
HUSSLEIN, H. and HOFHANSL, W. (1959) Möglichkeiten der Menstruationsverschiebung. *Wien. Klin. Wschr.* **71:** 821–823.
HVIDT, W. (1962) Gestagene Behandlung einer Endometriose des Kolon. *Dan. Med. Bull.* **9:** 152–156.
IGARASHI, M. (1957) Rebound phenomenon of the women ovarian function and its therapeutic application in female sterility. *Fertil. Steril.* **8:** 302–306.
IGARASHI, M., MATSUMOTO, S. and HOSAKA, H. (1965) Further studies on the rebound phenomenon of ovarian function. *Fertil. Steril.* **16:** 257–268.
JACOBSON, B. D. (1960) Abortion: Its prediction and management. Critical evaluation of newer progestational agents and clinical report on their use in more than 1000 patients, based on observations of cervical mucus. *Fertil. Steril.* **11:** 399–413.
JADRESIC, A., AGUILO, J., SAAVEDRA, R., RAMIREZ, H., HERREROS, M. and MATUS, A. (1961) Determination of phenolsteroids and pregnanediol in normal pregnancy and in habitual abortion. *Rev. Chil. Obstet. Ginec.* **26:** 363–384.
JAILER, J. W., GOLD, J. J., VAN DE WIELE, R. and LIEBMANN, S. (1955) 17α-Hydroxyprogesterone and 21-desoxyhydrocortisone; their metabolism and possible role in congenital adrenal virilism. *J. Clin. Invest.* **34:** 1639–1644.
JANN, R. (1956) Zur Frage der Nachbehandlung der glandulär-cystischen Hyperplasie. *Schweiz. Med. Wschr.* **86:** 1221–1223.
JASSIN, A. et al. (1962) The use of intravenous progesterone in threatened abortion. *Dia. Med.* **34:** 1816–1817.
JAVERT, C. T. (1954) Results of treatment in 100 patients. *Obstet. Gynec.* **3:** 420–423.
JAYLE, M.-F. and ROBEY, N. (1962) Intérèt du dosage du prégnandiol et des phénolstéroides pour le diagnostic et le traitement des avortements récidivants d'origine hormonales. *Presse Méd.* **70:** 1193–1196.
JELLE, B. (1962) Progesterone in the treatment of advanced malignant tumors of breast, ovary and uterus. *Brit. Med. J. Cancer* **2:** 209–213.
JONES, H. O. and BREWER, J. J. (1941). A study of the ovaries and endometriums of patients with fundal carcinomas. *Amer. J. Obstet. Gynec.* **42:** 207–217.
JOOSSE, L. A. (1961) Endometriosis externa. *Ned. T. Geneesk.* **105:** 561–565.
JUNG, H. (1964) Untersuchungen zur Wirkungsquantität von Valium am Uterus. *Fortschr. Geburtsh. Gynäk.* **19:** 70–76.
JUNG, H. (1964) Experimentelle Ergebnisse zur Wirksamkeit der Gestagen-Behandlung bei gestörter Schwangerschaft. *Med. Mitt. (Schering)* **25:** 11–19.
JUNKMANN, K. (1954) Über protrahiert wirksame Gestagene. *Arch. Exper. Path. Pharmakol.* **223:** 243–249.
KAPLAN, S. A., LING, S. M., and IRANI, N. G. (1968) Idiopathic isosexual precocity. Therapy with medroxyprogesterone. *Amer. J. Dis. Child.* **116:** 591–598.
KÄSER, O. (1953a) Studien an menschlichen Aborteiern mit besonderer Berücksichtigung der frühen Fehlbildungen und ihrer Ursachen (I. Mitteilung). *Schweiz. Med. Wschr.* **79:** 509–513.
KÄSER, O. (1953b) Studien an menschlien Aborteiern mit besonderer Berücksichtigung der frühen Fehlbildungen und ihrer Ursachen (II. Mitteilung), die Fehler oder Molen und ihre hormonale Aktivität. *Schweiz. Med. Wschr.* **79:** 780, 803, 1050 1079.

KÄSER, O. (1958) Amenorrhoe. *Dtsch. Med. Wschr.* **83**: 1461–1468.
KÄSER, O. (1959) Die therapeutische Pseudogravidität. *Geburtsh. Frauenheilk.* **19**: 593–604.
KÄSER, O. (1962) Über die chronischen Kreuz- und Unterleibsschmerzen bei der Frau. *Hippokrates* **33**: 977–981.
KAISER, R. (1957) Über die progestative Wirkung von 19-Nortestosteronverbindungen bei oraler Verabreichung. *Geburtsh. Frauenheilk.* **17**: 24–37.
KAISER, R. (1958) Die Wirkung von Gestagenen beim Corpus-Carcinom. *Arch. Gynäk.* **193**: 196–199.
KAISER, R. (1962) Zur frühzeitigen Abortusprophylaxe mit Gestagen-Östrogen-Kombinationen. *Geburtsh. Frauenheilk.* **22**: 906–909.
KAISER, R. and EICHSTÄDTER, A. (1955) Das Unterscheidungsverhältnis Östriol: Pregnandiol in Cyclus und Schwangerschaft. *Arch. Gynäk.* **185**: 726–738.
KAISER, R. and WILL, J. (1953) Das Verhalten der Ovarialhormone bei der Übertragung. *Arch. Gynäk.* **184**: 159–180.
KAMAL, J. (1955) Prolonged progesterone therapy in habitual abortion. *Ber. Ges. Gynäk. Geburtsh.* **56**: 198.
KARLSON, ST. et al. (1959) Behandling vid hotande abort och förtidsbörd. *Nordisk. Med.* **61**: 750–754.
KARLSON, ST. (1959) The influence of seminal fluid on the motility of the non-pregnant human uterus. *Acta Obstet. Gynec. Scand.* **38**: 503–521.
KARNAKY, K. J. (1965) Atrophic and senile vagino-perineal disorders: new treatment with an estrogen-progesterone vaginal cream. *J. Amer. Geriat. Soc.* **13**: 820–827.
KAUFMANN, C. (1933) Echte Menstruation bei einer kastrierten Frau durch Zufuhr von Ovarialhormonen. *Zbl. Gynäk.* **42**: 42–56.
KAUFMANN, C. (1953) Corpus luteum. *Arch. Gynäk.* 264–275.
KAUFMANN, C. (1961) Zur Therapie mit Keimdrüsenhormonen. *Dtsch. Med. Wschr.* **86**: 1577–1581.
KAUFMANN, C., WESTPHAL, U. and ZANDER, J. (1951) Untersuchungen über die biologische Bedeutung der Ausschedidungsprodukte des Gelbkörperhormons. *Arch. Gynäk.* **179**: 247–299.
KAUFMANN, C., WEBER, M. and ZANDER, J. (1959) Das Problem der hormonalen Behandlung drohender Fehlgeburten. *Dtsch. Med. Wschr.* **84**: 347–350.
KEIL, CH. (1953) Chitraines por hyperfolliculine. *Rev. Méd. Liege* **8**: 521–522.
KERSLEY, G. D. (1955) Symposium on rheumatic disorders; rheumatoid disease. *Clin. J.* **79**: 85–90.
KINNUNEN, O. and MUSTAKALLIO, M. (1952) Kinkantisiin hiittyvän migreenin hoidosta keltaranhasvalnisteilla. *Duodecim (Helsinki)* **68**: 282–287.
KISTNER, R. W. (1958a) Conservative treatment of endometriosis. *Postgrad. Med.* **24**: 282–287.
KISTNER, R. W. (1958b) The use of newer progestins in the treatment of endometriosis. *Amer. J. Obstet. Gynec.* **75**: 264–278.
KISTNER, R. W. (1959) The treatment of endometriosis by inducing pseudopregnancy with ovarian hormones. *Fertil. Steril.* **10**: 539–556.
KISTNER, R. W. (1960). The use of steroidal substances in endometriosis. *Clin. Pharmacol. Therap.* **1**: 525–537.
KISTNER, R. W. (1961) Newer progestins in the treatment of endometriosis. *Int. J. Fertil.* **6**: 1–14.
KISTNER, R. W. (1962) Infertility with endometriosis. A plan of therapy. *Fertil. Steril.* **13**: 237–245.
KISTNER, R. W. (1965) The effects of new synthetic progestogens on endometriosis in the human female. *Fertil. Steril.* **16**: 61–80.

KISTNER, R. W. and BAGINSKI, S. (1961) Observations on the use of 17-alpha-hydroxyprogesterone caproate on primary metastatic endometrial carcinoma. *Surg. Forum* **12**: 424–426.

KISTNER, R. W., GRIFFITHS, C. T. and CRAIG, J. M. (1965) Use of progestional agents in the management of endometrial cancer. *Cancer* **18**: 1563–1579.

KLEIBEL, F. and BECKER, J. (1960) Die funktionelle Hypophysektomie mit Äthinyl-Nortestosteron bei 130 klinischen Fällen. In: *Adv. Abstracts of Short Communications First International Congress of Endocrinology*, p. 935. Fuchs, F. (Ed.). Periodica, Copenhagen.

KNEER, M. (1957) Der habituelle Abort. *Dtsch. Med. Wschr.* 1059–1061.

KÖHLER, V. and WALSCH, E. (1951) Reflexerythem, ovarieller Zyklus und Gravidität. *Ärztl. Wschr.* **6**: 344.

KÖNIG, W. (1958) Aufgaben und Grundlagen einer Schwangerenberatung. *Mittl. Österr. Sanitätsverw.* **59**: 1.

KOHLER, R. (1949) Corpus luteum Hormon bei Asthma bronchiale. *Med. Klin.* **44**: 469–471.

KOLSTAD, P. (1964) Endometriosen og ens behandling. *Tidsskr. Norske Laegeforen.* **84**: 1684–1685.

KORTE, W. (1963) Histologie, Diagnose und Therapie der Endometriose. *Ärztl. Mittl. (Köln)* **60**: 883–890.

KORTING, G. W., HOLZMANN, H. and KÜHN, K. (1964) Biochemische Bindegewebsuntersuchungen in Analogie zum Sklerodermie-Problem. *Med. Welt* **34**: 1751–1756.

KOTTMEIER, H. L. (1962) Erfahrungen mit Progesteron in Fällen von Korpuskarzinom. *Geburtsh. Frauenheilk.* **23**: 1070–1072.

KRATER, J. E. (1960) Die hormonelle Behandlung des Gebärmutterfibroms. *Obstet. si. Ginec.* **7**: 73–76.

KRÄUBIG, H. and GELLER, H.-F. (1954) Die neuzeitliche Behandlung der gefährdeten Schwangerschaft. *Med. Klin.* **53**: 1948–1954.

KUPPERMAN, H. S. and EPSTEIN, J. A. (1962) Medroxyprogesterone acetate in the treatment of constitutional sexual precocity. *J. Clin. Endocr.* **22**, 456–458.

KYLE, L. H. and CRAIN, D. J. (1950) Clinical and metabolic effects of progesterone and anhydrohydroxyprogesterone in rheumatoid arthritis. *J. Amer. Med. Ass.* **143**: 1518.

LACNY, J. (1962) Cyclic progestational therapy of amenorrhea. *Can. Med. Ass. J.* **86**: 931–933.

LANDAU, R. L., EHRLICH, E. and HUGGINS, C. (1962) Estradiol benzoate and progesterone in advanced human breast cancer. *J. Amer. Med. Ass.* **182**: 632–636.

LAROCHE, G., SIMONNET, H. and BOMPARD, E. (1937) Influence de la progésterone sur l'elimination urinaire des principes gonadotropes. *Compt. Rend. Soc. de Biol.* **126**: 1159–1160.

LARON, Z. and RUMNEY, G. (1965) Treatment of precocious sexual development by medroxyprogesterone acetate. *Acta Endocr. (Kbh.)* Suppl. **101**: 27.

LÁSZLO, B. and GÖRGEY, E. (1960) Die Behandlung biliärer Dyskinesien mit Gelbkörper-Hormon. *Münch. Med. Wschr.* **102**: 231–234.

LAURITZEN, C. (1957) Die Wirkung des Äthinylnortestosterons auf die Basaltemperatur in der Schwangershaft. *Geburtsh. Frauenheilk.* **17**: 807–812.

LAURITZEN, C. (1966) Untersuchungen zur biologischen Aktivität von Progesterol-20-alpha- und 20beta. *Geburtsh. Frauenheilk.* **26**: 611–616.

LAURITZEN, C. and LEHMANN, W. D. (1964) Pregnandiolbestimmung im Plasma vor, während und nach der Entbindung. *Z. Geburtsh. Gynäk.* **162**: 159–173.

LAURITZEN, C. and LEHMANN, W. D. (1965) Der Einfluß natürlicher und synthetischer Gestagene auf die Ausscheidung von Choriongonadotropin im Harn. *Endokrinologie* **48**: 170–180.

LAX, H. (1956) Bedeutung der Plazentahormone für die Entstehung und Verlauf der Toxikose. *Z. Geburtsh. Gynäk.* **145**: 113–158.

LAX, H. (1961) Über die Behandlung der Endometriose mit Androgenen und Gestagenen. *Zbl. Gynäk.* **83**: 524–531.

LAX, H. (1965) Karzinomprophylaxe mit Gestagenen. *Selecta* **7**: 1229.

LEBHERZ, TH. B. and FOBES, D. C. (1961) Management of endometriosis with nor-progesterone. *Amer. J. Obstet. Gynec.* **81**: 102–110.

LEIMDÖRFER, A., NOVAK, J. and PORGES, O. (1912) Kohlensäurespannung des Blutes in der Gravidität. *Z. Klin. Med.* **75**: 301.

LEINZINGER, E. (1959) Hormontherapie der funktionellen Blutungen. *Medizinische* **52**: 2553–2556.

LEMLI, L., ARON, M., and SMITH, D. W. (1964) The action of Depo-Proversa in 3 girls with idiopathic isosexual precocity: decrease in estrogen effect without urinary gonadotropin reduction. *J. Ped.* **65,**: 888–894.

LEVIT, E. J., NODINE, J. H. and PERLOFF, W. H. (1957) Progesteron-induced porphyria. *Amer. J. Med.* **22**: 831–833.

LIPSCHÜTZ, A. (1950) *Steroid Hormones and Tumors.* Williams & Wilkins, Baltimore.

LIPSCHÜTZ, A. and IGLESIAS, R. (1938) Multiples tumeurs utérines et extragénitales provoquées par la benzoate d'oestradiol. *Compt. Rend. Soc. Biol.* **129**: 519–524.

LOJODICE, G., VENTO, R. and DE CELLO, C. (1964) Pseudoermafroditiemo feminile probabilmente indotto da un progestimico sommninstrabile per via intramuscolare: il 17-a-hidrossiprogesterone capronato. *Minerva Pechiatr.* **16**: 946–950.

LÜTGE, P.-K. (1957) Über die Erfolge der Therapie des drohenden Abortes. *Z. Ärztl. Fortbild.* **51**: 490–491.

LYON, R. A. (1946) Pregnandiol excretion at onset of labor. *Amer. J. Obstet. Gynec.* **51**: 403-410.

MACDONALD, R. R. and SHARMAN, A. (1959) Cervical mucus in early pregnancy. *Int. J. Fertil.* **4**: 338–346.

MACDONALD, R. R. (1963) Cervical mucus and the management of abortion. *J. Obstet. Gynaec. (Brit. Cwlth.)* **70**: 580–593.

MACDONALD, R. R. (1965) Norethynodrel and mestranol (Enovid) in the prevention of recurrent abortion. *Lancet* **II**: 623.

MACH, S. (1965) Die Blasenendometriose und ihre Behandlung an der Universitäts-Frauenklinik Berlin 1941–1963. *Z. Urol.* **58**: 573–578.

MARDONES, E., IGLESIAS, R. and LIPSCHÜTZ, A. (1953) Vergleich über die antifibromatogene Wirkung von Progesteron und Delta-11-Dehydroprogesteron. *Experientia* **9**: 303–304.

MARKLE, J. (1950) *Menstruation and its Disorders.* Angle, Springfield.

MASTERS, W. H., MAZE, L. W. and GILPATRICK, T. W. (1957) Etiological approach to habitual abortion. *Amer. J. Obstet. Gynec.* **73**: 1022–1034.

MATSUMOTO, S. and WATANABE, M. (1958) Kombinierte Östrogen-Progesteron-Behandlung mit Depothormonen. *Zbl. Gynäk.* **80**: 1997–2007.

MATHEWS, J. H., ABRAMS, C. A. L., and MORISHIMA, A. (1970) Pituitary-adrenal function in ten patients receiving medroxyprogesterone acetate for true precocious puberty. *J. Clin. Endocr.* **30**: 653–658.

MAUVAIS-JARVIS, P. and DECOURT, J. (1964) L'inhibition ovarienne therapeutique par les progestatits de synthèse. *Sem. Hop.* **40**: 2659–2669.

MEARS, E. (1967) Side effects of oral contraception. In: *Proceedings of the Fifth World Congress on Fertility and Sterility*, pp. 1005–1010. International Congress Series 133, Excerpta Med. Foundation, Amsterdam–New York.

MEARS, E. and GRANT, E. C. G. (1962) "Anovlar" as an oral contraceptive. *Brit. Med. J.* **2**: 75–79.

MEERHOFF, M. (1962) Progesteron in der Migränebehandlung. *Rev. Assoc. Méd. Argent.* **76**: 59–63.
MEHRING, W. (1961) Notfälle in der Gynäkologie. *Landarzt* **37**: 1376–1383.
MERGER, R., LÉVY, J., BÉJAT, G. and MELCHIOR, J. (1954) Interruption prématurée spontanée de la grossesse d'origine endocrinienne test cytologique de l'évolution et de controle du traitement. *Presse Med.* **62**: 925–927.
MERGER, R. *et al.* (1961) Jugement sur la valeur de la cytologie vagina le dans la surveillance de la maladie abortive. *Bull. Géd. Gynéc. Franc.* **13**: 136–147.
MEY, R. (1959) Über Geburtsverlauf und kindliche Mißbildungen nach drohender Fehlgeburt. *Med. Klin.* **54**: 54–64.
MEYERHOFF, K. H., BROWN, W. H. and DIOFFI, L. A. (1962) The use of 17-alphahydroxyprogesterone caproate to maintain pregnancy. *Curr. Ther. Res.* **4**: 499–505.
MIGLIAVACCA, A. (1960) The treatment of uterine hypoplasia by production of pseudopregnancy using the new progestogenic steroids. *Ann. Ostet. Gynec.* **82**: 490–493.
MIKULICZ-RADECKI, F.V. (1954). Appendicitis während der Schwangerschaft. *Med. Klin.* **49**: 1644–1649.
MILLS, W. G. (1962) A treatment for recurrent endometriosis. *J. Obstet. Gynaec. (Brit. Emp.)* **69**: 795–798.
MIXON, T. and HAMMOND, P.O. (1961) Response of fibromyoma to a progestin. *Amer. J. Obstet. Gynec.* **82**: 754–760.
MONZO, O. Z. (1960) Experiences en el tratiamento de la amenorrea. *J. Med. B. Aires* **116**: 390–392.
MORGAN, J., HACKET, W. R. and HUNT, T. (1960) The place of progesterone in the treatment of abortion. *J. Obstet. Gynaec. (Brit. Emp.)* **67**: 323–324.
MOSLER, K. H. (1964) Über den Einfluß von Progesteron auf die Motilität des menschlichen Uterusmuskels. *Naunyn- Schmiedeberg's Arch. Exp. Path. Pharmak.* **247**: 322–323.
MÜLLER, C. (1956) Der habituelle Abort. *Praxis* **45**: 213.
MÜLLER, C. (1963) Zum Problem der bioelektrischen Wehenregistrierung. *Schweiz. Med. Wschr.* **83**: 1145–1146.
MÜLLER, D. (1962) Die wichtigsten chirurgischen Komplikationen im Bauchraum während der Schwangerschaft. *Münch. Med. Wschr.* **104**: 791–724.
MURRAY, E. G. and RAMELLA, J. E. (1961) Resultado de la terapeutica hormonal en la endometriosis. *Undecimo Congreso Argentino de Obstetricia y Ginecologica* 22.– 27.10.1961, p. 685.
NAPP, J. H. (1962) Die zystisch-glanduläre Hyperplasie des Endometrium. *Tägl. Praxis* **3**: 119–128.
NAPP, J. H., TONGUC, M. and KARAALILER, S. (1960) Die Östrogen- und Pregnandiolausscheidung vor, während und nach der Geburt. *Arch. Gynäk.* **194**: 1–12.
NARIK, G. and ROCKENSCHAUB, A. (1951) Die Formen des Hyperöstrinismus und deren Behandlung mit Gelbkörperhormon. *Zbl. Gynäk.* **20**: 1607–1613.
NEVINNY-STICKEL, J. (1962) Die Bedeutung des Gestagen-Effektes auf das Endometrium für die Behandlung der Endometriose. *Geburtsh. und Frauenheilk.* **22**: 689.
NIEDERHOFER, M. and PUCK, A. (1953) Hat das Follikelhormon eine Bedeutung für den Geburtstermin? *Med. Klin.* **48**: 72–75.
NOVAK, E. R. and HOGE, A. F. (1958) Endometriosis of the lower genital tract. *Obstet. Gynec.* **12**: 687–693.
OBER, K. G. (1953) Die Behandlung der unzulänglichen Keimdrüsenfunktion. In: Seitz, L. and Amreich, A., *Biologie und Pathologie des Weibes*, II. Aufl. Band II, pp. 726–848.
OBER, K. G. (1957a) *Klinik der inneren Sekretion.* Springer-Verlag, Berlin–Heidelberg, 1957.

OBER, K. G. (1957b) Die Anwendung der Sexualhormone in der Gynäkologie. *Geburtsh. Frauenheilk.* **17:** 610–627.
OBER, K. G., KLEIN, I. and WEBER, M. (1954) Zur Frage der Progesteronbehandlung. Experimentelle Untersuchungen mit dem Hooker-Forbes-Test und klinische Beobachtungen mit Kristallsuspensionen. *Arch. Gynäk.* **184:** 543–616.
O'DRISCOLL, D. T. (1959) Secondary habitual abortion. *J. Obstet. Gynaec.* (*Brit. Emp.*) **66:** 457–561.
PALMER, R. (1964) Celioscopic study of women treated with cyclic norethisterone for endometriosis. *Int. J. Fertil.* **9:** 121–122.
PALMER, R. and ROBEL, J. (1960) Intérét clinique du dosage concomitant du prégnandiol des phénolstériodes et des 17-cétostéroides chez les femmes sujettes aux avortements du 1er trimestre. *Cah. Coll. Med. Hop.* **1:** 551–555.
PARKER, A. S., JR. (1960) The premenstrual tension syndrome. *Med. Clin. N. Amer.* **44:** 339–348.
PASETTO, N. (1958) Sul problema della terapia ormonale estroluteinica nella minaccia d'aborto. *Minerva Med.* **49:** 2342–2345.
PASI, P. L. M. *et al.* (1962) Amanaza de aborto—tratamiento. *Obstet. Ginec. lat. Amer.* **20:** 308–711.
PEARLMAN, W. H. (1957) Steroid hormone levels in relation to steroid hormone production. II. Circulating. *Ciba Found. Coll. Endocrinology* **11:** 233–237.
PEZZALI, M. (1962) Il trattamento ormonale della minaccia di parto prematuro. *Quad. Clin. Ostet. Ginec.* **17:** 341–348.
PIAUX, G., ROBEY, M. and SIMONNET, H. (1953) Nouvelle recherches sur les anomalies des steroides sexuels dans l'avortement endocrinien. *Gynec. Obstet.* **52:** 441–473.
PINCUS, G., ROCK, J., GARCIA, C. R., RICE-WRAY, E., PANIAGUA, M. and RODRIGUEZ, J. (1958) Fertility control with oral medication. *Amer. J. Obstet. Gynec.* **75:** 1333–1346.
PION, R. J. CONRAD and WOLF, J. (1966) Pregnenolone sulfate, an efficient precursor for the placental production of progesterone. *J. Clin. Endocr.* **26:** 225–226.
PLOTZ, J. (1950) Die Bedeutung des Progesterons bei der Entstehung und Behandlung der Fehlgeburt. *Arch. Gynäk.* **178:** 212–215.
PLOTZ, J., DAVIS, E. and EJARQUE, M. E. (1959) Untersuchungen des Hormonstoffwechsels beim Chorionepitheliom. *Arch. Gynäk.* **193:** 317–322.
PLOTZ, J. (1959) Untersuchungen mit markierten Gestagenen. In: *Mitteilungen der Schering A.G.* Berlin/West, **20:** 1–11.
PLOTZ, J. (1960) Die Behandlung habitueller Fehlgeburten mit Gestagenen. *Med. Welt* **41:** 2134–2138.
POSSE, N. (1958) The motility pattern of the nonpregnant uterus. Studies *in vivo* of the motility of the human uterus during and after the reproductive period. *Acta Obstet. Gynec. Scand.* **37:** Suppl. 2.
POTS, P. (1955) Zur Progesteronbehandlung funktioneller Blutungen. *Zbl. Gynäk.* **77:** 1754–1759.
POTS, P. (1958) Gestagen-Depotwirkung von Äthinylnortestosteronänanthat. *Geburtsh. Frauenheilk.* **18:** 673–676.
PRILL, H. J. (1957) Die Behandlung gynäkologisch funktioneller Blutungen durch die sogenannte hormonelle Curettage. *Münch Med. Wschr.* **99:** 944–945.
PRILL, H. J. (1959) Über die Durchblutung des Uterus. Die medikamentöse Beeinflussung der Uterusdurchblutung. *Z. Geburtsh. Gynäk.* **152:** 180–202.
PSCHYREMBEL, W. (1964) *Praktische Gynäkologie.* De Gruyter Verlag, Berlin.
PSLACHEWSKI, K. (1961) High doses of progesterone in the therapy of preinvasive-carcinoma of the uterus cervix. *Ginek Pol.* **32:** 609–613.
PUCK, A. and POLENZ, B. (1963) Beobachtungen einer Nabelendometrios während eines Zyklus unter der Behandlung mit 17α-Aethinyl Oestrenol. *Geburtsh. Frauenheilk.* **23:** 809–813.

PUJOHL, J. M. (1960) Treatment of certain amenorrheas with delayed action hormone-therapy. *Gaz. Med. Franc.* **67**: 117–119.
PULLEN, D. (1962) Convoid E as an oral contraceptive. *Brit. Med. J.* **2**: 1016–1019.
RANDALL, C. L., HALL, D. W. and BIRTSCH, P. K. (1955) Pregnancies observed in likely-to-abort patient with or without hormone therapy before or after conception. *Amer. J. Obstet. Gynec.* **69**: 643–656.
RAURAMO, L. and BATJA, U. (1961) Intravenous use of methergin and oxytocin in the third stage of labour. *Ann. Chir. Gynaec. Fenn.* **50**: 172–178.
RAUSCHER, H. (1958) Zur Substitution der Gelbkörperwirkung durch 17α-Oxy-Progesteron-Capronat. *Zbl. Gynäk.* **80**: 312–317.
RAUSCHER, H. (1964) Personal communication.
RAUSCHER, H. and KOFLER, E. (1958) Wirkungserwartung, Zeitpunkt des Eintritts und Dauer der Blutung nach Verabreichung des Depotgestagens 17α-Oxy-Progesteron-Capronat. *Geburtsh. Frauenheilk.* **18**: 766–770.
RAUSCHER, H. and ROMBERG, G. (1956) Erfolgreiche Behandlung funktioneller gynäkologischer Blutungen durch einmalige Verabreichung in Öl gelöster Östrogen-Gestagen-Kombination. *Zbl. Gynäk.* **78**: 2002–2010.
RAWLINGS, W. J. and KRIEGER, V. I. (1958) Studies in the prevention of recurrent abortion due to corpus luteum deficiency. *Med. J. Aust.* **45**: 561–566, 572–575.
RAWLINGS, W. J. and KRIEGER, V. I. (1959a) Long-acting progesterone preparations and orally administered "Primolut N" in the treatment of habitual abortion. *Med. J. Aust.* **46**: 428–436.
RAWLINGS, W. J. and KRIEGER, V. I. (1959b) 17-alpha-hydroxyprogesterone and virilism of adrenogenital syndrome associated with congenital adrenocortical hyperplasia. *J. Clin. Endocr.* **16**: 1262–1275.
REIFENSTEIN, E. C. (1958) Clinical use of 17-α-hydroxy-progesterone 17-n-caproate in habitual abortion. *Ann. N.Y. Acad. Sci.* **71**: 762–765.
REIFENSTEIN, E. C., ORATT, TH.E., HARTZEL, K. A. and SHAFER, W. B. (1965) Artificial menstrual cycles induced in ovulating women by monthly injection of progestogen-estrogen. *Fertil. and Steril.* **16**: 652–664.
REIFFENSTUHL, G. and MAYER, H. G. K. (1962) Die Bedeutung von Librium für die Relaxation des menschlichen Uterus. *Wien. Med. Wschr.* **112**: 608–610.
RICHTER, K. (1964) Die Bedeutung der vaginalen Operation bei der Behandlung der Endometriosis externa. *Zbl. Gynäk.* **87**: 1750–1757.
RIFKIND, A. B., KULIN, H. E., CARGILLE, C. M., RAYFORD, P. C. and ROSS, G. T. (1969) Suppression of urinary excretion of luteinizing hormone (LH) and follicle stimulating hormone (FSH) by medroxyprogesterone acetate. *J. Clin. Endocr.* **29**: 506–513.
RIISFELDT, O. (1942) Progesteron bei Mastopathia cystica. *Nord. Med.* **42**: 1892–1895.
RIVA, H. L., WILSON, H. and KAWASAKI, D. M. (1961) Effect of norethynodrel on endometriosis. *Amer. J. Obstet. Gynec.* **82**: 109–118.
RIVA, H. L., KAWASAKI, D. M. and MESSINGER, A. (1962) Further experience with norethynodrel in treatment of endometriosis. *Obstet. Gynec.* **19**: 111–117.
ROBEY, M. (1958) Les Hémorragies utérines fonctionelles. *Presse Méd.* **66**: 1313–1315.
ROCK, J., GARCIA, R. and PINCUS, G. (1957) Synthetic progestine in the normal human menstrual cycle. *Recent Progr. Hormone Res.* **13**: 323–346.
ROTHSCHILD, J. (1957) *J. Clin. Endocrinol.* **17**: 754–261.
ROLAND, M. (1965) *Progestogen Therapy*, p. 74. Charles C. Thomas, Springfield, Ill.
RUA, I. J. (1961) Aborto habitual. *Órientacion Méd.* **10**: 320–326.
RUST, W. (1956) Die Auslösung der Ovulation durch Progesteron bei den verschiedenen Formen des anovulatorischen Cyclus. *Zbl. Gynäk.* **78**: 1363–1369.

SACK, H. and HANDRICK H. (1956) Zur Ätiologie und Therapie der Migräne beim weiblichen Geschlecht. *Dt. Med. Wschr.* **81**: 1841–1846.
SALOMON, Y. (1964) Progestoides de synthese en gynecologie. *Gaz. Méd. Franc.* **71**: 3089–3104.
SAS, M., RAPCSÁK, V. and OROJAN, J. (1965) Untersuchungen über die Wirksamkeit des Allylösternol in der Behandlung wiederholten Abortus. *Zbl. Gynäk.* **87**: 1544–1548.
SCHLÖSSER, W. (1958) Klinische Erfahrungen mit 17-α-oxy-Progesteron-Kapronat und Östradiolbenzoat. *Med. Klin.* **53**: 1182–1184.
SCHMIDT-MATTHIESEN, H. (1963) *Das Hormonelle Menschliche Endometrium.* Verlag Georg Thieme, Stuttgart.
SCHMIDT-MATTHIESEN, H. and WELLERS, H. (1968) Zur Gestagentherapie fortgeschrittener Korpuskarzinome. *Geburtsh. Frauenheilk.* **28**: 417–427.
SCHOEN, E. J. (1966) Treatment of idiopathic precocious puberty in boys. *J. Clin. Endocr.* **26**: 363–370.
SCHWARTZ, H. A. and SEFGAR, G. (1957) Progesterone in anovulatory uterine bleeding. *Fertil. Steril.* **8**: 103–109.
SCHWARTZ, H. A. and HUTCHERSON, W. P. (1961) Hormone in early or suspect pregnancy. *Southern Med. J. (Bham. Ala.)* **54**: 80–84.
SCHWARTZ, H. A. and POWELL, W. (1961) Hormones in early or suspect pregnancy. *Southern Med. J. (Bham. Ala.)* **54**: 80–84.
SCOTT, R. B. and WHARTON, L. R. (1962) Effects of progesterone and norethindrone on experimental endometriosis in monkeys. *Amer. J. Obstet. Gynec.* **84**: 867–875.
SEMM, K. (1957) Der Abbau von synthetischem Oxytocin. *Die Naturwissenschaften* **44**: 424–425.
SEMM, K. (1958a) Oxytocin und Wehen. *Fortschr. Geburtsh. Gynäk.* **2**: 81–88.
SEMM, K. (1958b) Die Bildungsstätte der Serum-Oxytocinase. *Arch. Gynäk.* **191**: 57–64.
SEMM, K. (1960) Das Wehenproblem mit besonderer Berückischitgung des Oxytocin-Oxytocinase-Haushaltes. *Z. Geburtsh. Gynäk.* **154**: Beilageheft.
SEMM, K. (1963a) Nachweis der Serum-Oxytocinase in normalen und pathologischen Placentagewebe. *Arch. Gynäk.* **198**: 149–151.
SEMM, K. (1963b) Die Serum-Oxytocinase-Aktivität in der Plazenta. *Arch. Gynäk.* **199**: 265–270.
SEMM, K. (1965a) Anstieg der Serum-Oxytocinase-Aktivität im Blut nach 17α-Hydroxyprogesteronkapronat oder Allylöstrenol-Zufuhr. *Arch. Gynäk.* **202**: 459–461.
SEMM, K. (1965b) Fermente, Hormone und Vitamine in der Geburtshilfe. In: Schwalm, H. and Döderlein, G., *Klinik der Frauenheilkunde und Geburtshilfe,* Bd. IV, pp. 121–299. Verlag Urban & Schwarzenberg, München, Berlin-Wien.
SEMM, K. and BERNHARD, J. (1963) Zur Diagnostik des placentaren Stoffwechsels durch die Serum-Oxytocinase Bestimmung im mütterlichen Blut. *Arch. Gynäk.* **199**: 271–278.
SEMM, K. and WAIDL, E. (1962) Histochemische Untersuchungen über die Serum-Oxytocinase-Bildung im menschlichen Trophoblasten. *Z. Geburtsh. Gynäk.* **158**: 165–171.
SEMM, K. and WIENDL, H. J. (1962) Über Oxytocin inaktivierende Gewebeextrakte. *Zbl. Gynäk.* **84**: 1669–1674.
SHEARMAN, R. P. and GARRETT, W. J. (1963) Double-blind-study of effect of 17-α-hydroxyprogesterone caproate on abortion rate. *Brit. Med. J.* **5326**: 292–295.
SHELLEY, W. B., PREUCEL, R. W. and SPOONT, ST. S. (1964) Autoimmune progesterone dermatitis. *J. Amer. Med. Ass.* **190**: 35–38.
SHORT, R. V. (1958a) Progesterone in blood. I. The chemical determination of progesterone in peripheral blood. *J. Endocr. (London)* **16**: 415–425.
SHORT, R. V. (1958b) Progesterone in blood. II. Progesterone in the peripheral blood of pregnant cows. *J. Endocr. (London)* **16**: 426–428.

SHORT, R. V. (1960) Blood progesterone levels in relation to parturition. *J. Reprod. Fertil.* **1**: 61–70.
SIGURJONSDOTTIR, T. J. and HAYLES, A. B. (1968) Precocious puberty. A report of 96 cases. *Amer. J. Dis. Child.* **115**: 309–320.
SILSON, J. E. (1962) Prenenolone acetate, a dermatologically active steroid. *J. Soc. Cosmetic. Chemists* **13**: 129–139.
SIMONNET, H., PIAUX, G. and ROBEY, M. (1954) Les anomalies des stéroides sexuels dans l'avortement endocrinien. *Gynéc. Obstét.* **53**: 78–94.
SKOV JENSEN, T. and LASS, F. (1965) Progestogenbehandling af metastaserende cancer corporis uteri. *Ugeskr. Laeg.* **127**: 1294–1297.
SMITH, R. A. and ALBERT, A. (1955) Effects of estrogen on urinary gonadotropin. *Proc. Staff Meet. Mayo-Clinic* **30**: 617–620.
SNAITH, L. (1962) Long-term progestogen therapy in endometriosis. *J. Obstet. Gynaec. (Brit. Emp.)* **69**: 799–800.
SOIVA, K. and CASTRÉN, O. (1963) The conservative treatment of endometriosis with lynestrenol. *Ann. Chir. Gynaec. Fenn.* **52**: 376–382.
SOIVA, K. and CASTRÉN, O. (1964) Clinical observations on the effect of lynestrenol on endometriosis and ovarian function. *Int. J. Fertil.* **9**: 253–255.
STAEMMLER, H.-J. (1962) Graviditätsprophylaxe, Amenorrhoe, Schwanger. schaftsblutungen und die neuen Gestagene. *Dtsch. Med. J.* **13**: 134–135.
STAEMMLER, H.-J. (1963) Klinik des hypoplastischen Ovariums. *Arch. Gynäk.* **198**: 377–393.
STAEMMLER, H.-J. (1964) *Die gestörte Regelung der Ovarialfunktion*, Springer-Verlag, Berlin–Göttingen–Heidelberg.
STAEMMLER, H.-J. (1965) *Grundriß der Gynäkologischen Endokrinologie.* Verlag Georg Thieme, Stuttgart.
STEINKAMM, E. (1951) Mitteilung über extragenitale Wirkungen von Progesteron. *Med. Klin.* **7**: 211–212.
STOLL, P. and RUMMEL, H. R. (1964) Pathologische Anatomie und Klinik der Stroma-Endometriose. *Geburtsh. Frauenheilk.* **24**: 902–915.
SURTI, N. R. (1965) Treatment of constitutional precocious puberty with medroxyprogesterone acetate. *Proc. Roy. Soc. Med.* **58**: 123–124.
SWYER, G. I. M. (1960) Progestogens and their clinical uses. *Brit. Med. J. (Brit. Emp.)* **5166**: 48–49, 121–123.
SWYER, G. I. M. (1962) Gestagene Steroide und ihre klinische Anwendung. *Fortschr. Pharmazie* **1**: 25–29.
SZONTÁGH, F. E. and SAS, M. (1965) Recherches sur l'influence de l'Allyloestrénol sur la sécrétion placentaire de stéroides. *Grenoble Médico. Chirurgical* **3**: 5–11.
SZONTÁGH, F. E., SAS, M., TRAUB, A., KOVÁCS, L., BÁRDOCZY, A. and SZEREDAY, Z. (1963) The influence of different norsteroids on the hormone excretion and on the histomorphologic pattern in the trophoblast in early pregnancy. *Gynaecologia (Basel)* **156**: 369–379.
TACHEZY, R. (1951) Asthma bronchique et hormone du corps jaune. *Schweiz. Med. Wschr.* **81**: 1180–1183.
TAPFER, S. (1959) Follikelhormon als Wehenmittel. *Bibl. Gynaec. (Basel)* **20**: 162–168.
THAMDRUP, E. (1965) Trials with progestational agents on the treatment of precocious puberty. *Acta Endocr. (Kbh.)*, Suppl. **101**: 28.
THOMAS, H. H. (1958) Dysfunctional uterine bleeding. A simplified one injection treatment using long-acting ovarian steroids. *Southern Med. J. (Bham. Ala.)* **51**: 1266–1269.
THOMAS, H. H. (1960) Conservative treatment of endometriosis. Use of long-acting ovarian steroid hormones. *Obstet. Gynec.* **15**: 498–503.

THOMSEN, K. (1957) Zur Ätiologie und Therapie der Spontanaborte. *Therapiewoche* **7**: 477–480.

TIMONEN, S. and GÖLTNER, E. (1959) Die Bedeutung der vaginalen Hormonzytologie und der Pregnandiolausscheidung für die Prognose des Abortus imminens. *Zbl. Gynäk.* **81**: 1263–1274.

TYLER, E. T. (1957) The use of a new long-acting progestational compound (17-alpha-hydroxyprogesterone-caproate) in infertility and habitual abortion. *Studies on Fertility*, Vol. 8. R. G. Harrison, Springfield, Ill.

UFER, J. (1956) Hochkonzentrierte Progesteron-Östrogen-Therapie bei Hypogenitalismus. *Proc. II. World Congress on Fertility and Sterility*, Vol. I, pp. 363–372. Neapel, 1958.

UFER, J. (1959) Fortschritte in der gynäkologischen Endokrinologie. *Geburtsh. Frauenheilk.* **20**: 999.

UFER, J. (1961) Therapie mit der durch Sexualhormone erzielten "Pseudograviditäť". *Münch. Med. Wschr.* **103**: 1982–1986.

UFER, J. (1966) *Hormontherapie in der Frauenheilkunde*. De Gruyter Verlag, Berlin.

UHER, J., JIRASEK, J. E. and CERNOCH, A. (1965) On the activity of 16-methylen-6-dehydro-17-a-acetoxyoprogesterone (NDAP) on the human fetus. *Gynaecologia (Basel)* **159**: 377–383.

UPTON, R. D. (1962) The conservative management of endometriosis. *Med. J. Austr.* **49**: 15–19.

VARGA, A. and HENRICKSEN, E. (1965) Histologic observations on the effect of 17-α-hydroxyprogesterone-17-n-caproate on endometrial carcinoma. *Obstet. Gynec.* **26**: 656–664.

DE WAARD, F. (1958) On the aetiology of endometrial carcinoma. *Acta Endocr. (Kbh.)* **29**: 279–294.

DE WAARD, F. and OETTLÉ, A. G. (1965) A cytological survey of post-menopausal estrus in Africa. *Cancer* **18**: 450–459.

DE WAARD, F. and SCHWARZ, F. (1964) Weight reduction and postmenopausal estrogenic effect. *Acta Cytol. (Philad.)* **8**: 449–453.

WAIDL, E. and SEMM, K. (1960) Der Beginn der hypothalamischen Neurosekretion in der Fetalzeit. *Arch. Gynäk.* **192**: 269–276.

WASCHKE, G. (1960) Östrogenfreie Behandlung der durch Zyklusfunktionsstörungen bedingten Dauerblutungen mit Mindestdosen von Primolut N und Äthinyl-nortestosteronazetat. *Zbl. Gynäk.* **82**: 1721–1732.

WATERS, H. W. (1957) Delalutin for premenstrual tension. *J. Med. Ass. (Ala.)* **50**: 3–4.

WERLE, E. and SEMM, K. (1956) Über die Oxytocinase des Schwangerenblutes. *Arch. Gynäk.* **187**: 449–457.

WILBRAND, U., PORATH, CH., MATTHAES, P. and JASTER, R. (1959) Der Einfluß der Ovarialsteroide auf die Funktion des Atemzentrums. *Arch. Gynäk.* **193**: 507–531.

WILKINS, L. (1953) The need for an inhibitor of gonadotropin. *J. Clin. Endocr.* **13**: 738–741.

WILKINS, L. (1960) Masculinization of female fetus due to the use of orally given progestins. *J. Amer. Med. Ass.* **17**: 1028–1032.

WILKINS, L., JONES, H. W., HOLMAN, G. H. and STEMPFEL, R. S. (1958) Masculinization of the female fetus associated with administration of oral and intramuscular progestins during gestation: non-adrenal female pseudohermaphrodism. *J. Clin. Endocr.* **18**: 559–585.

WILL, I. (1961) Die schwangerschaftserhaltende Wirkung der Gestagene und ihr Einfluß auf die Frucht. *Z. Geburtsh. Gynäk., Beilageheft* **157**: 113–116.

WILLIAMS, B. F. P. (1962) Conservative treatment of endometriosis with progestin therapy. *Amer. J. Obstet. Gynec.* **83**: 715–719.

WILSON, R. A. (1962) The roles of estrogen and progesterone in breast and genital cancer. *J. Amer. Med. Ass.* **182**: 327–331.
WILSON, R. N. (1955) Habitual abortion. Hormonal physiology and a suggested endocrine treatment for selected patients. *Amer. J. Obstet. Gynec.* **69**: 614–628.
WINTER, G. F. and POTS, P. (1956) Morphologische Untersuchungen über die medikamentöse Transformation des Endometriums. *Z. Geburtsh. Gynäk.* **147**: 44–51.
WINTER, G. F. and PANKOW, M. (1959) Zur Kritik der hormonalen Behandlung des Abortus imminens. *Zbl. Gynäk.* **81**: 830–841.
WOLF, W. (1942) Die Behandlung der drohenden Fehl- und Frühgeburt durch i.v. Injektionen von Progesteron (Lutocyclin i.v.). *Münch. Med. Wschr.* **89**: 914–916.
WOOD, C., ELSTEIN, M. and PINKERTON, J. H. M. (1963) The effect of progestogens upon uterine activity. *J. Obstet. Gynaec. (Brit. Cwlth.)* **70**: 839–846.
WRIGHT, H. L. et al. (1959) Fetal salvage with a long acting progestogen: hormonal protection in a poor-risk pregnancy. *Amer. Pract.* **10**: 1544–1546.
WRIGHT, ST. W. (1962) Endometriosis. *J. Obstet. Gynaec. (Brit. Cwlth.)* **69**: 804–805.
ZANDER, J. (1952a) Die C_{21}-Steroide, ihr Verhalten im Organismus und Nachweis. *Klin. Wschr.* **30**: 873–882.
ZANDER, J. (1952b) Über die Ausscheidung der C_{21}-Glucuronide (Pregnandiolkomplex) nach kontinuierlicher Zufuhr hoher Progesterondosen. (Beitrag zur Frage des Progesteronverbrauchs in der Schwangerschaft.) *Klin. Wschr.* **30**: 312–315.
ZANDER, J. (1957) Die Gestagen-wirksamen Hormone im Organismus. *Geburtsh. Frauenheilk.* **17**: 876–895.
ZANDER, J. (1963) Die Hormonbildung der Plazenta und ihre Bedeutung für die Frucht. *Arch. Gynäk.* **198**: 113–127.
ZANDER, J. (1967) Die bedrohte Schwangerschaft: Die Behandlung der bedrohten Schwangershaft. *Arch. Gynäk.* **204**: 92–109.
ZANDER, J. and MÜNSTERMANN, A. M. (1956). Progesteron im menschlichen Blut und Geweben. III. Progesteron in der Plazenta, in der Uterusschleimhaut und im Fruchtwasser. *Klin. Wschr.* **34**: 944–953.
ZANDER, J., WIEST, W. G. and OBER, K. G. (1962) Klinische, histologische und biochemische Beobachtungen bei polycystischen Ovarien mit gleichzeitiger adenomatöser atypischer Hyperplasie des Endometriums. *Arch. Gynäk.* **196**: 481–503.
ZIMMER, F. (1960) Das Erregungssystem des Uterus. *Arch. Gynäk.* **192**: 492–500.
ZIMMERMAN, R. (1942) Behandlung des Asthma bronchiale mit Follikelhormon. *Dtsch. Med. Wschr.* **42**: 1033–1034.
ZIMMERMAN, H. (1949) Behandlung der Migräne mit Corpus-luteum Hormon. *Med. Klin.* **48**: 835–836.
ZIMPRICH, H. and GUPTA, D. (1965) Zur Therapie der idiopathischen Pubertas praecox. I. Teil: Klinische Studien. *Helv. Paediat. Acta*, **20**: 446–455.
ZIZINE, L. (1951) Asthma und endokrin-genitale Störungen. *Belg. T. Geneesk.* **2**: 15.
ZORN, H. (1958) Zur Behandlung funktioneller Blutungen mit 17-a-Hydroxyprogesteronkapronat. *Geburtsh. Frauenheilk.* **18**: 924–933.
ZORN, H. (1959) Behandlung funktioneller Blutungen mit 17-alpha-aethinyl-19-nortestosteron-acetat. *Med. Klin.* **54**: 1399–1401.

SUBSECTION III

THE ANTIFERTILITY EFFECTS OF ESTROGENS, PROGESTATIONAL COMPOUNDS AND COMBINATIONS OF THESE

CHAPTER 33

ESTROGENS AS ANTIFERTILITY AGENTS

Fred A. Kincl

Biological Concepts Inc., New York

A. ANALYSIS OF EFFECTS TO BE CONSIDERED

I. INTRODUCTION

The antifertility activity of phenolic steroids is surveyed in this report, along with a discussion of non-steroidal estrogens.

Of the steroid hormones, estrogens are quantitatively the most active; whereas milligram quantities of cortisol, testosterone and progesterone are needed to produce their respective endocrine effects in experimental animals, only micrograms of estradiol-17β produce the desired physiological response.

In contrast with synthetic progestational agents, where substitutions on different carbon atoms of the steroid molecule have been found to potentiate the endocrine activity, this is generally not the case with phenolic steroids. Practically any substitution introduced into the estrogen molecule decreases the activity of the parent compound. 17α-Alkynyl substitutions which give rise to estrogenic compounds having high oral potency constitute a notable exception. The organic chemist has thus not been fortunate in synthesizing a variety of highly active synthetic estrogens, and at the present time the only synthetic steroids that have found wide clinical use are 17α-ethynyl estradiol (17α-ethynyl-1,3,5(10)-estratrien-3,17β-diol) and its 3-methyl ether (mestranol, 3-methoxy-17α-ethynyl-1,3,5(10)-estratrien-17β-ol).

Estrogens have been shown to interfere with almost all of the processes of reproduction in the female. They inhibit maturation and transport of ova, influence and interfere with implantation and, in sufficiently high doses, arrest embryonic development and cause fetal death. These antifertility effects are reversible, and, depending upon the dosage used and the duration of administration, the animals regain their ability to reproduce after varying periods of time. A different situation is seen in newborn animals. Estrogens administered shortly after birth may produce in the mature individual infertility, which appears to be irreversible.

2. CONCENTRATION IN TISSUES

Jensen and Jacobson (1962) studied specific binding sites of estradiol (estradiol-17β) and demonstrated that it accumulates selectively in the uterus and in the vagina. Furthermore, they showed that estrone was not *per se* active and that enzymatic reduction to estradiol was a requisite to physiological effect. The original findings were later confirmed by Roy *et al.* (1964) and by Eisenfeld and Axelrod (1965), who also demonstrated that estradiol is selectively bound by the anterior pituitary. Michael (1965) reported that specific neurons in the hypothalamus (the optic region and septum) would concentrate estrogenic compounds. The accumulation of labeled estradiol in peripheral organs and in the central nervous system appears to be independent of age or sex, but male sex peripheral organs (testes and the prostate) do not concentrate labeled estradiol (Eisenfeld and Axelrod, 1966).

3. ACTIVITY IN IMMATURE AND ADULT MAMMALS

(a) Hypothalamo-pituitary axis and the gonad

Although estrogen treatment of short duration may result in a stimulation of LH output by the pituitary (Hohlweg, 1934; Lane and Hisaw, 1934; Hisaw *et al.*, 1934; Hohlweg and Chamorro, 1937; Swelheim, 1965), when given in high enough amounts it inhibits the synthesis and/or release of gonadotrophins; the growth of the gonads is arrested. Meyer *et al.* (1930, 1932) found that estrone causes ovarian atrophy, and Kraus (1930) and Moore and Price (1932) demonstrated gonadal atrophy in males following estrone injection and showed that this could be prevented by administration of exogenous gonadotrophins. Similar repair of gonadal functions by exogenous gonadotrophins in females inhibited with estrogens has been reported by Noble (1938).

1. *Hypothalamo-pituitary axis.* The importance of the central nervous system in ovulation was demonstrated in 1932 by Hohlweg and Junkmann and confirmed in 1938 by Westman and Jacobsohn. Both groups found that, in immature female rats, pituitary stalk section prevented corpus luteum formation induced by a single injection of estrogen. The area of the

brain involved in the regulatory action is the posterior median eminence-basal tuberal region of the hypothalamus (Flerkó, 1957). Implantation of estradiol in this area results in ovarian atrophy (Davidson and Sawyer, 1961) and decrease in luteinizing hormone levels in plasma and the pituitary (Kanematsu and Sawyer, 1964). However, these studies do not exclude a direct effect of estrogens on the puitary.

Prolonged treatment causes characteristic changes in pituitary histology, degranulation of the basophils, and acidophils and chromophobes, many of which are enlarged (Hohlweg, 1934). Enlargement of the pituitary gland in rats and mice under the influence of estrogens was reported by Noble (1938) and Deanesly (1939). That the pituitary gland is larger in females, compared to males, has already been noted by Evans and Simpson in 1929.

Haterius and Nelson (1932) noted that histological changes in the pituitaries of castrated male rats could be prevented or, if already present, reversed by ovarian transplants. Nelson (1934) demonstrated disappearance of castration cells and increase in the number of chromophobes by estrone administration in cryptorchid rats. In a similar study, Schoeller et al. (1936) used daily dosages of 0.15 mcg in females to achieve the same effect.

Bogdanove (1963) prevented castration changes in contiguous cells of the anterior pituitary by steroid implants. Lisk (1965) prevented pregnancy in virgin female rats by estradiol. He reported, however, that implants of similar "size" were more active if placed in the arcuate or mammillary region of the hypothalamus. Döcke and Dörner (1965) concluded from their studies on ovulation induction by estradiol benzoate implants in immature females that although the anterior hypothalamus is necessary for the positive feed-back mechanism, the anterior pituitary may be the main site of action of estrogens.

It is, therefore, likely that estrogens influence not only the secretion of gonadotrophin-releasing factors in the hypothalamus, but also directly inhibit the synthesis and/or release of gonadotrophins from the pituitary. Instead of viewing these two areas as *two independently working units*, the hypophyseal and diencephalic systems, they should from the functional point of view be looked upon as, in effect, *one unit*, as suggested by Borell et al. (1947, 1948). They found that, in normal rats, estradiol benzoate increased ^{32}P turnover in both the adenohypophysis and tuber cinereum, but in hypophysectomized rats it had no effect (Borell and Westman, 1949).

Assays measuring the suppression of pituitary gonadotrophin content have been developed (Saunders and Drill, 1958). However, most of the data on pituitary inhibiting effect of estrogens had been accumulated from indirect assays in the parabiotic rat. Meyer and Hertz (1937), using the parabiotic rat technique, found that a larger dose of estrogens, or of androgens, is needed to inhibit male rats than female rats. Biddulph et al. (1940) repeated the test with estradiol and estriol, and reported the same difference (Table 1) and also noted that, in females, the dose of estrogen needed to inhibit the pituitary function may well be below the dose needed to provoke estrus reactions in the peripheral tissues (Byrnes and Meyer, 1951).

TABLE 1. MINIMUM DAILY DOSES OF ESTROGENS NEEDED TO INHIBIT CASTRATION-INDUCED HYPERSECRETION OF GONADOTROPHIN

Steroid	Males (mcg)	Females (mcg)
Estradiol	0.15	0.025
Estrone	1.0	0.20
Estriol	10	1.5

Data from Meyer and Hertz (1937) and Biddulph et al. (1940).

Dorfman and Dorfman (1963) confirmed the claim by Meyer and co-workers (*loc. cit.*) that the parabiotic rat assay can be used for quantitative measurements. They used estrone by subcutaneous injection as the standard and reported the useful range to be between 0.5 and 2.5 mcg total dose in a 10-day test with a precision of a λ value of 0.3.

2. *The ovary.* The atrophy of the gonads observed in animals treated with estrogens is the result of inhibitory action on the production of follicle-stimulating hormone. The effects on luteinizing hormone release are less clear. In some specific circumstances, estrogens were observed to have a stimulatory effect (above, p. 348). Additional evidence was provided by several groups: in immature, hypophysectomized rats, implants of stilbestrol (average daily release 130 to 170 mcg) or of estradiol dipropionate (40 to 63 mcg) prevented ovarian atrophy and increased the response of the ovarian follicle to pregnant mare's serum (Pencharz, 1940). Furthermore, ovogenesis in the rodent may be estrogen-dependent. Cell division in the germinal epithelium of mice is highest during late estrus and lowest during diestrus (Bullough, 1946). Small doses of estrogen may help to maintain corpora lutea. This has been shown in rats by Selye et al. (1935),

in rabbits by Allen and Heckel (1936) and in hypophysectomized animals by Greep (1940). Swelheim (1965) noted an increase of luteinizing hormone levels in the plasma following an injection of 50 mcg of estradiol benzoate. Thus, the assumption that estrogens in some manner provide a luteinizing stimulus to the pituitary is widely accepted. Nevertheless, this hypothesis has been questioned by some (Greep and Jones, 1950).

If estrogens are given to immature animals at a sufficiently advanced stage of life, the development of the ovary is arrested, it remains small and the follicles do not ripen. When the treatment is stopped, the ovary becomes functional, estrus cycles appear and the animals are able to reproduce (Selye et al., 1935). Byrnes and Meyer (1951) tested graded doses of estradiol (0.002 mcg to 0.05 mcg) injected daily for 10 days in 30-day-old rats, examined the ovaries for corpora lutea and follicles and assayed the pituitaries in intact, 21-day-old rats. They report a daily dose of 0.0075 mcg as inhibitory. Shipley (1962) studied the inhibition of luteinization in immature rats and found that 10 mcg of estradiol valerate in a single injection into 21-, 24-, 27-, 30- and 33-day-old rats inhibited luteinization. The treatment was not effective if injected at the age of 35 days or later.

Transitory ovarian atrophy is also observed in adult animals. Estrogens injected in the early part of the cycle of monkeys significantly postpone the next expected ovulation (Ball and Hartman, 1939) and cause atresia of vesicular follicles (Gillman, 1942). Greenwald (1965a) studied the effect of a single injection of stilbestrol (0.25 mg) in the hamster and found that this dose induced follicular atresia, but did not interfere with the release of ovulating hormone at the end of the estrus cycle.

References to ovarian atrophy in rats and mice produced by estrogens are numerous. A few have already been cited; others are included in Section B. The atrophy is usually accompanied by inhibition of follicular growth and of sex-dependent tissue (uterus, vaginal lining, etc.). There is at present no evidence indicating that estrogens may directly inhibit the function of the ovary. This subject has been studied by Krähenbühl and Desaulles (1964) and Rudel and Kincl (1966) in immature hypophysectomized rats, in which ovulation was induced by exogenously administered gonadotrophins (Table 2).

3. *The testes.* As with the ovary, the atrophic effect of repeated injections of estrogens is due to their influence in decreasing the synthesis and/or release of gonadotrophins by the pituitary. Simultaneous administration of exogenous gonadotrophins, or androgens, prevents this atrophy (Moore and Price, 1932).

In immature rats, the inhibitory action is manifested by failure of the

TABLE 2. FAILURE OF VARIOUS ESTROGENS TO BLOCK OVULATION IN GONADO-
TROPHIN-STIMULATED IMMATURE HYPOPHYSECTOMIZED RATS

Treatment	Total dose used	Age of rats (days)	Gonadotrophin stimulation	Reference
Estradiol	0.02 mg	22	PMS/HCG	Rudel and Kincl (1966)
	0.2 mg	22	PMS/HCG	Rudel and Kincl (1966)
	6 mg/kg	30	FSH/LH	Krähenbühl and Desaulles (1964)
	0.002 mg	30	PMS/HCG	Rudel and Kincl (1966)
	0.02 mg	30	PMS/HCG	Rudel and Kincl (1966)
Estrone	20 mg/kg	30	PMS/HCG	Krähenbühl and Desaulles (1964)
Mestranol	0.01 mg	30	PMS/HCG	Rudel and Kincl (1966)
	0.05 mg	30	PMS/HCG	Rudel and Kincl (1966)
	0.25 mg	30	PMS/HCG	Rudel and Kincl (1966)

testes to descend and by azoospermia (Ludwig, 1950) and decrease in pituitary gonadotrophin content (Golding and Ramirez, 1928; Greep and Jones, 1950). In young cats, on the other hand, estrogens produce no deleterious effect (Starkey and Leathem, 1939). An inhibitory effect of a single injection of estradiol benzoate in producing testicular atrophy in immature animals belonging to several species is shown in Table 3 (Leathem and Wolf, 1955).

In adult animals, estrogens produce marked testicular involution, the maturation wave is disrupted, spermatozoa, spermatids and spermatocytes are absent (Ludwig, 1950), but mitosis of spermatogonia is not arrested

TABLE 3. INHIBITORY EFFECT OF A SINGLE INJECTION
OF ESTRADIOL BENZOATE IN PRODUCING TESTICULAR
INVOLUTION IN SEVERAL SPECIES

Species	Dose (mcg)	% Involution
Mouse	10	20
	25	45
Rat	100	70
Hamster	35	77
Guinea pig	166	56
Rabbit	250	21
	2500	71

Data from Leathem and Wolf (1955).

(Spencer et al., 1931). Following short treatment, Leydig cells become atrophic and may revert to fibroblasts. Prolonged treatment may cause multiplication and swelling of Leydig cells, deposition of lipid material in germinal epithelium, decrease in glycogen and testicular hyperplasia (Burrows, 1937). The atrophy may proceed so that only the Sertoli cells remain in the tubules, but even these may disappear with the induction of peritubular hyalinization and sclerosis. The inhibitory effect of estrogen in males is reversible. In rats treated with estradiol or stilbestrol, regeneration begins in about 2 weeks and is completed within 6 weeks (Lynch, 1952).

Quantitative studies on the effect of a synthetic estrogen, mestranol, given either orally or by subcutaneous injection to rats, were reported by Patanelli and Nelson (1959). The effect of treatment was judged by measuring total pituitary gonadotrophin content, the weights of the testes, seminal vesicles, prostate, and epididymis, and histological evaluation. Given orally, a daily dose of 0.005 mg was moderately effective, and 0.02 mg was markedly active. When injected, the potency was increased about twofold.

Testicular atrophy following stilbestrol therapy has been observed in bulls (Ferrara et al., 1953) and boars (Wallace, 1949). In guinea pigs, estrogens may affect the Leydig cells directly; in hypophysectomized animals; they become atrophic and the seminiferous epithelium is damaged (Marescaux, 1950).

As stated above, testicular atrophy is due to the suppression of stimulation by gonadotrophins. This also results in the decrease in endogenous androgen production which leads to the atrophy of sex-dependent tissues, involution of the epithelium and loss of secretory activity. Involution of sex-dependent tissues has been used as a measure of gonadotrophin inhibitory effect by Beyler and Potts (1957) who studied the dosages of estradiol, estradiol benzoate and estrone necessary to effect a 50% and 100% castration atrophy of seminal vesicles and ventral prostate of mature male rats. McGinty and Djerassi (1958) reported on the effect of estrone and mestranol in a similar test.

(b) Effects on ova and zygote transport

The transport of fertilized ova through the oviduct depends on a proper progesterone/estrogen balance (see Chapter 7). Studies describing acceleration (or retention) of ova induced by exogenous estrogens are numerous. These include the studies in rabbits by Corner (1928), Allen and Corner (1929), Burdick and Pincus (1935), Pincus and Kirsch (1936), Whitney and Burdick (1938), Greenwald (1959, 1961) and Noyes et al. (1959); and in mice and rats by Burdick and Pincus (1935), Whitney and Burdick (1936, 1939), Burdick and Whitney (1938), Burdick et al. (1942), Banik and Pincus (1964), and Rudel and Kincl (1966). Typical results of such experiments are shown in Table 4. Egg transport in the rat is retarded by ovariectomy, as well as by daily injections of 1 mcg of estradiol benzoate (Rudel and Kincl, 1966). Ovariectomy performed 4 to 6 hours after ovulation had no influence on zygote movement in the oviducts for the first 32 hours. After that time, the zygotes remained in the ovarian and central segments and began to disintegrate. Estradiol benzoate administered to intact rats produced not only a delay in zygote transport, but also created an environment hostile to their survival.

Banik and Pincus (1964), in work with rats, found that the number of ova was markedly decreased or nil within 24 hours after injection of estradiol (20–250 mcg). Deanesly (1963) observed expulsion of eggs in the guinea pig injected with 5 mcg of estradiol benzoate. Greenwald (1965b) used estradiol cyclopentyl propionate (ECP) in rabbits and reported that a dose of 25 mcg caused accelerated ova movement, whereas a tenfold increase in the dose resulted in retention. A more detailed study in several laboratory species was published by Greenwald in 1967. In all, ova were trapped at the ampullary-isthmic region. In guinea pigs, a dose of 50 mcg accelerated transport of ova, whereas a dose of 250 mcg caused tube locking. The same

TABLE 4. INFLUENCE OF ESTRADIOL ON OVA TRANSPORT IN MATED ADULT RATS

Treatment	No. of rats	Time after ovulation (hr)	Total number of recovered ova per group (range)[b]			
			Ovarian segment	Central segment	Uterine segment	Uterine horn
0	6	32	22 (0–5)	28 (0–5)	1 (0–1)	0
		56	3 (0–3)	6 (0–4)	24 (0–6)	1 (0–1)
		80	0	15 (0–4)	38 (0–8)	0
		104	0	0	3[a] (0–3)	30 (0–5)
Ovariecto-mized	6	32	10 (0–7)	22[a] (0–5)	3 (0–3)	[a]
		56	1[a] (0–1)	15[a] (0–5)	17 (0–6)	0
		80	[a]	18[a] (0–5)	0	0
Estradiol	4	8	30 (0–7)	2 (0–2)	0	0
		32	8 (0–8)	9 (0–4)	2[a]	0
		56	0	0	[a]	0

[a] Disintegrating cells present; numbers not included.
[b] Individual observations of number of ova per animal.
From Rudel and Kincl (1966).

dose also caused tube locking in hamsters. In mice 0.1 mcg caused moderate ova retention at the utero-tubal junction, whereas a dose of 1 mcg caused ova retention at the ampullary-isthmic junction. In rats, a dose of 10 mcg apparently caused an acceleration of the ova.

Similar studies were reported by Hafez (1962) and Chang and Yanagimachi (1965) in rabbits. These data are summarized in Table 5.

TABLE 5. INFLUENCE OF HORMONAL TREATMENT ON OVA TRANSPORT IN VARIOUS SPECIES

Species	Treatment	Dose (mcg)	Influence on ova transport	Reference
Rabbits	Estradiol	4	Retention	Hafez (1962)
	Estrone	36	Retention	Hafez (1962)
	Estradiol	5	Retention	Greenwald (1959)
	ECP	25	Acceleration	Greenwald (1967)
		100	Retention	Greenwald (1967)
		500	Retention	Chang and Yanagimachi (1965)
Rats	EB	1	Retention	Rudel and Kincl (1966)
	Estradiol	20	Acceleration	Banik and Pincus (1964)
	ECP	10	Acceleration	Greenwald (1967)
Mice	ECP	0.1–1	Retention	Greenwald (1967)
Hamsters	ECP	250	Retention	Greenwald (1967)
Guinea pigs	EB	5	Acceleration	Deanesly (1963)
	ECP	50	Acceleration	Greenwald (1967)
		250	Retention	Greenwald (1967)

EB—estradiol benzoate.
ECP—estradiol cyclopentyl propionate.

The effect of a synthetic estrogen, ethynyl estradiol, fed to rabbits on days 1, 2 and 3 after ovulation, was studied by Chang (1966). This treatment caused acceleration of ova movement. The effect of a single oral dose of this estrogen given to rabbits 24 hours after ovulation was described by Chang and Harper (1966). A dose of 0.02 to 10 mg produced an irregular, accelerated pattern, and decrease in the percentage of eggs recovered (Fig. 1). In this study, the oviduct was arbitrarily divided into eight segments, and the position of ova in each segment was recorded (Harper et al., 1960).

A combined effect of different estrogens on ova transport and blastocyst development was described by Chang and Harper (1966). They used artificially inseminated rabbits in which ovulation was induced by an i.v.

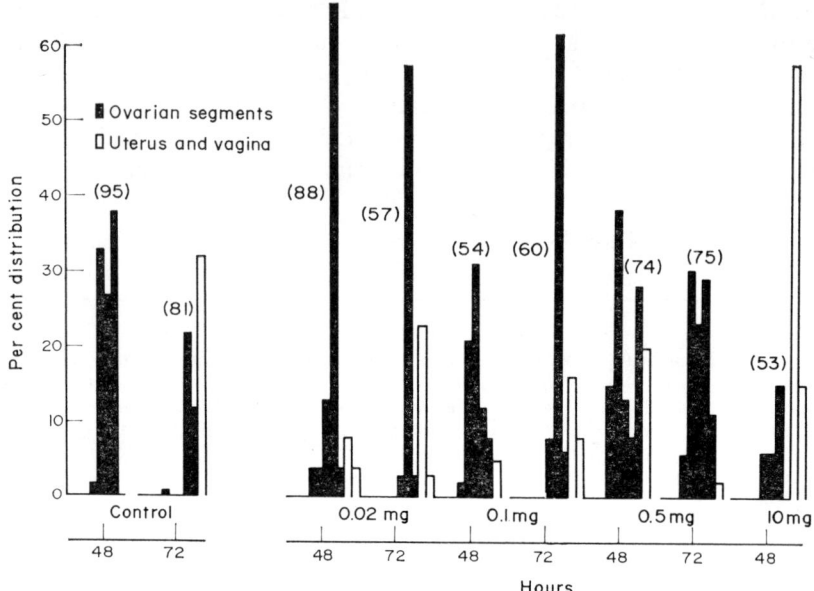

Fig. 1. The influence of a single oral dose of ethynyl estradiol on transport of ova in rabbits. From Chang and Harper (1966). Figures in parentheses: percentage of recovered eggs.

injection of human chorionic gonadotrophin (HCG). Various estrogens were given orally for 3 days, beginning 24 hours after insemination. The effect, expressed as ED_{50}, was calculated from the ratio between normal blastocysts recovered and the number of corpora lutea present. Table 6 summarizes the findings.

Direct evidence for the lethal effect of estrogens was provided by

TABLE 6. EFFECTIVENESS OF VARIOUS ORALLY ADMINISTERED ESTROGENS IN INHIBITING BLASTOCYST DEVELOPMENT IN THE RABBIT

Estrogen	ED_{50} (mg/day)
Estradiol	<0.1
Estrone	0.048
Ethynyl estradiol	0.012
Estradiol cyclopentyl propionate	0.160
Stilbestrol	0.135

From Chang and Harper (1966).

Ketchel and Pincus (1964). They incubated fertilized rabbits' ova in calcium-free Ringer's solution containing 5% rabbit serum and found that a short incubation (5 min) had no effect. When the incubation period was prolonged to 24 hours, a concentration of 1 mg/ml stilbestrol was lethal. Daniel and Cowan (1966) cultured fertilized rabbit ova and reported that mestranol at a concentration of 5 mcg/ml caused retardation of ova cleavage. A concentration of 25 mcg/ml was inhibitory. Ethynyl estradiol was more active. Fragmentation occurred at a concentration of 5 mcg/ml and inhibition at a dose of 10 mcg/ml.

(c) *Effects on the uterus*

1. *Implantation.* Preparation of the uterus for implantation, the transformation and differentiation of the endometrial stroma into decidual tissue, and nidation of the blastocyst are the direct result of estrogen-progesterone synergism (Krehbiel, 1941; Weichert, 1942; Bloch, 1948), though in some species, such as the hamster, high doses of progesterone may be sufficient for implantation. Although the actual nature of nidation and decidual tissue formation remains obscure, exogenous estrogens are found to be effective agents in blocking this process.

That estrogens may interfere with implantation was suggested by Parkes and Bellerby (1926) and Smith (1926) and confirmed by several others (Parkes *et al.*, 1938; Dreisbach, 1959; Edgren and Shipley, 1961). Insight into the estrogen requirements needed for implantation has been obtained by Psychoyos and Courrier (1962) who achieved implantation in ovariectomized, progesterone-treated rats with 0.1 mcg of estradiol. Nutting and Meyer (1964) using the same system caused implantation with 0.3 mcg of estrone in the presence of 4000 mcg of progesterone; a dose of 10 mcg/day prevented nidation. Psychoyos (1966) reported that the dissolution of the zona pellucida in the rat is estrogen-dependent. Martin (1963) found that in intact mice, 0.15 mcg of estradiol given daily on days 4, 5, and 6 of pregnancy resulted in fetal death. Stone and Emmens (1964a) inhibited pregnancy by 1.6 to 2.5 mcg of estradiol and found the greatest effect when they gave it about 72 hours after mating. The same sensitivity in rats was reported by Dreisbach (1959).

2. *Deciduoma formation.* Stone and Emmens (1964a) reported that the dose of estradiol (0.02 mcg) needed to inhibit deciduoma formation in mice was much smaller than that needed to interrupt pregnancy. In rats, 0.04 mcg of estradiol was inhibitory (Stone and Emmens, 1964b). Estriol was active at a dose of 4 mg, compared with 0.4 mg of progesterone in mice when a decidual response was provoked by histamine (Miyake *et al.*, 1963).

3. *Uterine biochemistry.* The influence of ovarian hormones on the chemical constituents of the uterine washings of the rat and rabbit was studied by Heap and Lemming (1962). In spayed rabbits, estradiol benzoate (0.1 mcg/3 days) caused increased sodium, potassium, total nitrogen and carbohydrate content above that seen in controls. Bialy and Pincus (1962) measured the inhibition of the uterine carbonic anhydrase in immature rats, and found that a daily dose of 0.05 mcg of estradiol given for 4 days was active. The response of the enzyme to estrogen treatment was rapid. Within 6 hours after injecting 0.1 mcg there was a significant decrease in uterine carbonic anhydrase concentration. In contrast, enzyme levels were found to be increased in mice following estrogen administration (Ogawa and Pincus, 1962). The results of a systematic study of a number of phenolic steroids, using carbonic anhydrase inhibition in rabbit uteri studied against a standard dose of 2 mg of progesterone, are given in Table 7 (Pincus and Bialy, 1963).

TABLE 7. DOSES OF VARIOUS PHENOLIC STEROIDS WHICH PRODUCED SIGNIFICANT INHIBITION OF RABBIT UTERINE CARBONIC ANHYDRASE ACTIVITY

Steroid	Dose range studied (mg)	Minimal active dose (mcg)
Estradiol	0.0025–0.25	2.5
Estrone	0.0025–0.25	2.5
Estriol	0.0025–0.25	2.5
Stilbestrol	0.0025–0.25	2.5
Estradiol dibenzoate	1–10	5000
1-Hydroxy estradiol	0.1–10	400
1-Hydroxy estradiol triacetate	0.025–10	125
1,3-Diacetoxy-16α-hydroxy-1,3,5(10)-estratrien-17-one	5–10	5000
1,4-Diacetoxy-1,3,5(10)-estratrien-17-one	0.5–10	2000
18-Norestrone 3-methyl ether	5–9	9000
1ξ-Thiomethyl-1,3,5(10)-estratrien-17-one	0.025–10	125

Data from Pincus and Bialy (1963).

4. *The cervix.* It has been well established, especially from human studies, that during the follicular phase cervical mucus is copious, thin and watery and presents an optimum environment for sperm penetration. There are no published records of studies on the effect of phenolic steroids

TABLE 8. CONDITIONS USED BY VARIOUS INVESTIGATORS TO PRODUCE STERILITY BY INJECTING ESTROGENIC HORMONES TO NEONATAL ANIMALS

Steroid used	Type of Treatment	Daily dose (mcg)	Total dose (mcg)	Reference
Females				
Estradiol dipropionate	Mice; from birth for 38 days, 3 times weekly	6	38	Wilson (1943)
Estradiol benzoate	Mice; from birth for 5 days	5	25	Takasugi and Bern (1962)
Estrone	Rats; from birth for 5 days	25	125	Arai (1964a)
Estradiol dipropionate	Mice; injected on day 10	10	10	Merklin (1953)
Estradiol dipropionate	Mice; injected on day 5	10	10	Leathem (1956)
Estradiol benzoate	Rats; injected on day 5	5	5	Gorski (1963)
Males				
Estrone	Rats; from birth for 20 to 40 days	12.5	250–500	Takasugi (1954)
	Rats; from birth for 30 days	25–100	1750	Arai (1964b)
Estradiol benzoate	Rats; from birth for 60 days	10–40	1800	Steinberger and Duckett (1965)
	Rats; injected on day 5	30	30	Kincl et al. (1963)
	Guinea pigs; injected on day 1	120	120	Kincl and Folch-Pi (1963)
Mestranol	Mice; injected on day 5	1	1	Rudel and Kincl (1966)

on the composition and physical properties of the cervical mucus during the estrus phase.

The dilatation or softening of the uterine cervix towards the end of pregnancy appears to be under the influence of estrogen–progesterone–relaxin hormonal control. Under some specific conditions, estrogens may be able to prevent dilatation. In the sow, estrogen treatment was reported to constrict the uterine cervix (Smith and Nalbandov, 1958). In the rat 50 mcg of estradiol cyclopentyl propionate caused a decrease of cervix dilatability (Kroc et al., 1959).

4. ACTIVITY IN NEONATAL MAMMALS

It has been stated in Chapter 11 that administration of estrogens to neonatal animals produces permanent sterility when they reach reproductive age. In rats and mice repeated injections of estradiol beginning on the first day after birth, or a single injection within the first 10 days of life, were used to produce sterility (Table 8).

In females short-term treatment produces atrophic, non-luteinized ovaries, and the vaginal epithelium is constantly cornified, but if the injections are repeated for longer periods (30 days) vaginal cornification may not take place (see Takasugi, 1954). Male animals develop azoospermia, the maturation wave is destroyed and endogenous androgen production is decreased (Kincl et al., 1963). The changes seen in the testes

TABLE 9. COMPARATIVE INHIBITORY ACTIVITY OF VARIOUS STEROIDS INJECTED INTO FIVE-DAY-OLD RATS

Steroid	Minimum effective dose (mcg)	
	Male	Female
Rats		
Mestranol	0.1	0.1
Ethynyl estradiol	1	1
Estradiol benzoate	30	30
Estriol	100	100
Estradiol	120	120
17-Deoxyestrone	100	100
Estrone	1000	1000
Estradiol-3-methyl ether	500	500
3-Deoxyestrone	1000	1000

Data from Kincl et al. (1965) and Rudel and Kincl (1966).

depend on the dose used and may range from the absence of free sperm in the lumen to complete absence of spermatids and spermatogonia (Maqueo and Kincl, 1964). In the pituitaries the numbers of basophils and acidophils are reduced, but chromophobes and castration cells increase (Kawashima and Takewaki, 1966; Maqueo et al., 1966; Presl et al., 1966). This permanent sterilizing effect is also produced by other estrogens (Table 9) and is seen not only in mice and rats, but also in guinea pigs and the Coturnix quail (Table 10).

TABLE 10. STERILIZING EFFECTIVENESS OF VARIOUS STEROIDS IN MALES AND FEMALES OF VARIOUS SPECIES

Steroid	Species	Day of administration	Effective dose (mcg)
Mestranol	Rat	5	0.1
	Mice	5	0.1
	Coturnix quail	1	50
Estradiol benzoate	Rat	5	30
	Guinea pig	1	120

Data from: Kincl and Folch-Pi (1963), Kincl et al. (1965), Kincl and Sickles (1966).

The mechanism of action by which estrogens produce permanent sterility when injected into neonatal animals is not yet clear. These compounds may interfere with the differentiation of the hypothalamic centers which in later life are destined to control the gonadal function as was proposed for testosterone–propionate-sterilized females (Harris and Levine, 1965). However, it may be that steroids administered to neonatal mammals decrease the sensitivity of gonads towards circulating gonadotrophins or provoke some other reaction of, as yet unrecognized, etiology, which leads to decreased or abnormal steroidogenesis in the gonads (Kincl, 1967).

5. ACTIVITY IN NON-MAMMALIAN VERTEBRATES

No systematic studies have been made on antifertility effects of estrogens in lower vertebrates. Research is concerned mainly with sex differentiation and sex reversal. These striking effects of transforming testes into ovaries, or to "intersexual" forms, have been described for many species of amphibians (Burns, 1961). The experiments of Foote (1940) are illustrative: addition of estrone or estradiol dipropionate in concentration of 500 mcg/l to tank water in which axolotls (*Ambystoma tigrinum*) are being raised results in sex reversal, formation of ovotestes and increased growth of Mullerian ducts. In the lizard *Anolis*, administration of estradiol results in atrophy of the testes, and to a lesser degree of ovaries (Evans and Clapp, 1940). Similar results were reported with estrone implants in adult male *Sceloporus* (Forbes, 1941). In the fish (*Platypoecilius*) estradiol benzoate inhibited the growth of ovaries and testes (Tavolga, 1949).

Birds

The effect of estradiol (1500 to 3000 r.u.) or of estrone (0.5 to 1 mg) injected into brown leghorn eggs between day 3 and day 5 of incubation was studied by Domm (1939). In males this treatment produced atrophy of the right testes (the left testes developed as ovotestes), in some cases retention and development of oviducts and development of "female-type" plumage. Gaarenstroom (1939) injected 300 mcg of estradiol benzoate into white leghorn eggs on the 2nd day of incubation and found that this dose produced a modification of the testes to a pseudo-ovary, followed by a transition to an ovotestis.

Kincl and Sickles (1966) used the Coturnix quail to study the effect of mestranol. Three different experimental approaches were used: (1) steroid dissolved in oil injected into fertile eggs on day 12 of incubation, (2) fertile eggs dipped into a solution of steroid in dimethyl sulfoxide, (3) quail chicks were injected with steroid on the day of hatching. In all cases, there was a marked reduction in egg laying when the birds matured (Table 11). The males were apparently not affected by the treatment; testes were comparable to controls in weight and histology. Riddle and Tange (1928) studied the effect of estrogens in adult pigeons and reported that they caused atrophy of the gonads. In young cockerels, estrogens inhibit gonadotrophin secretion; the testes are atrophic and the combs are smaller, indicating that endogenous androgen production is decreased (Breneman, 1953). This may be also achieved by topical application of 75 mcg of estradiol to 3-day-old cockerels (Boas and Ludwig, 1950).

B. DATA FOR INDIVIDUAL COMPOUNDS

As has been shown in Section A, the antifertility action of estrogens was recognized many years ago. Research in recent years has contributed only marginally to our knowledge of the basic principles involved. It was orientated mainly to collecting quantitative information on the antifertility activity of a number of estrogens.

TABLE 11. EGG-LAYING PERFORMANCE OF COTURNIX QUAIL TREATED WITH MESTRANOL

Treatment	Dose (mcg)	Average no. eggs/female	Age first eggs laid
Injected on day 12 of incubation	10	2.4	67 days
	50	0	
Immersed in DMSO solution day 15 of incubation	0.01%	6.6	46 days
	0.1%	1.0	57 days
	1.0%	0	
Injected into 1-day-old chicks	10	4.9	41 days
	50	1.3	43 days
	250	0	
Untreated controls	0	8.1	43 days

Data from Kincl and Sickles (1966), Kincl et al. (1967).

1. GENERAL FERTILITY STUDIES IN THE FEMALE

Edgren and Shipley (1961) have studied the effect of a single injection of estrone in interrupting pregnancy in rats during the first 10 days postinsemination. Saunders (1965) used estradiol (Table 12). Both groups confirmed that the most sensitive period is on the 3rd day during the period of tubal passage.

Schofield (1962) measured the effect of estradiol on the oxytocin threshold of the myometrium during pregnancy. Higher dosages were necessary to interrupt pregnancy towards the end.

TABLE 12. INTERRUPTION OF PREGNANCY IN RATS BY A SINGLE INJECTION OF ESTRONE OR ESTRADIOL

Day of injection	Estrone ED_{50} (mcg)	Estradiol effective dose (1 mcg/kg)
1	13	50
2	17	50
3	4.2	20
4		20
5	45	100
6		500
7	> 140	1000
8		500
9		100
10	140	> 5000

From Edgren and Shipley (1961) and Saunders (1965).

TABLE 13. ANTIFERTILITY ACTIVITY OF ESTRADIOL AND ESTRONE IN RATS AND MICE

Steroid	Species	Type of treatment	Effective dose (mcg)	Reference
Estradiol	Rats	1 injection locally day 4	ED_{50} 1.53	Emmens and Finn (1962)
		1 injection SC day 4	ED_{50} 53	Emmens and Finn (1962)
		7 injections beginning day 3	ED_{75} 3/kg/day	Desaulles and Krähenbühl (1964)
	Mice	1 injection locally day 4	ED_{50} 0.46 × 10^{-3}	Emmens and Finn (1962)
		1 injection SC day 4	ED_{50} 1.2	Emmens and Finn (1962)
		3 injections beginning day 1	0.05/day	Martin (1963)
		3 injections beginning day 4	0.15/day	Martin (1963)
Estrone	Rats	3 injections beginning day 1	10/kg/day	Saunders (1965)
		7 injections beginning day 3	20/kg/day	Desaulles and Krähenbühl (1964)

General antifertility activities of estradiol and estrone reported by several investigators are summarized in Table 13. Emmens and Finn (1962) and Desaulles and Krähenbühl (1964) began the treatment on day 4 and on day 3 post-insemination respectively, and measured inhibition of implantation. Saunders (1965) began the treatment on day 1 of pregnancy and measured the inhibition of tubal transport.

TABLE 14. ANTIFERTILITY ACTITITY OF VARIOUS ESTROGENS IN THE RODENT

Species	Compound	Route of administration	Effective dose (mcg)	Reference
Rats	Estriol	Subcutaneous	250/kg/day	Desaulles and Krähenbühl (1964)
		Oral	30	Peterson and Edgren (1965)
	Ethynyl estradiol	Subcutaneous	4/kg/day	Desaulles and Krähenbühl (1964)
		Oral	5/kg/day	Watnick et al. (1964)
	Mestranol	Subcutaneous	150/kg/day	Desaulles and Krähenbühl (1964)
			20/kg/day	Saunders (1965)
		Oral	50/kg/day	Saunders (1965)
			20	Kincl and Dorfman (1965)
	Methoxyestradiol	Subcutaneous	150/kg/day	Desaulles and Krähenbühl (1964)
Mice	16α-Chloro-1,3,5(10)-estratrien-17-one	Subcutaneous	< 1000/day	Emmens (1965)
	3-Methoxy-16α-methyl-1,3,5(10)-estratrien-16β, 17β-diol		< 100/day	Emmens (1965)
	3-Methoxy-16α-methyl-16β-hydroxy-1,3,5(10)-estratrien-17-one		> 1000	Emmens (1965)
	Estradiol	Subcutaneous	30/day	Emmens (1962)
Rabbits	Ethynyl estradiol		12/day	Chang and Harper (1966)
	Estrone	Gavage	135/day	Chang and Harper (1966)
	Estradiol cyclopentyl propionate		160/day	Chang and Harper (1966)
	Estradiol		> 500/day	Chang and Harper (1966)

Table 14 summarizes the activity of several phenolic steroids tested in general antifertility assays. Peterson and Edgren (1965) gave the test compound for 30 days and measured not only the fertility index, but also the effect on mating behavior. Besides several synthetic progestational agents, testosterone and progesterone were included in the study (effective doses 300 and 100 mcg, respectively). Watnick *et al.* (1964) gave ethynyl estradiol for 12 or 45 days to mature female rats housed, during the study, with fertile males. A daily dose of 0.005 mg/kg/day inhibited pregnancy in 50% of the test animals. A tenfold dose (50 mcg/kg/day) was inhibitory in all the animals.

Emmens (1962) found that 30 mcg of estradiol was equally effective in decreasing the number of implants in pregnant rabbits, whether it was given from day 5 to day 7, or from day 7 to day 9. Chang and Harper (1966) studied the oral activity of various estrogens given orally on days 1, 2, and 3 after insemination on ova development.

Falconi and Ercoli (1963) fed mestranol and ethynyl estradiol 3-cyclopentyl ether to adult female rats for 30 days. The antifertility effect was

TABLE 15. ANTIFERTILITY EFFECTS OF PHENOLIC STEROIDS IN A SUBCUTANEOUS INJECTION ASSAY

Steroid	Daily dose range (mcg)	Relative antifertility activity	Estrogenic activity[a]
Estradiol		100	100
Mestranol	1 to 25	13	10
3-Methoxy-17β-cyanoethoxy-1,3,5(10)-estratrien	0.1 to 100	9	2
3-Acetoxy-6,7-dichloro-1,3,5(10)-estratrien-17-one	3 to 30	3	
1,3,5(10)-Estratrien-17β-ol	10 to 1000	2	2
3-Methoxy-17α-fluoro-1,3,5(10)-estratrien	300 to 3000	0.3	0.05
1,3,5(10)-Estratrien-17-one	50 to 1000	0.2	0.7
1-Methyl-3-acetoxy-1,3,5(10),6-estratetraen-17-one	1000	0.03	0.001
2-Methyl estradiol	2000	0.02	15
3-Methoxy-17β-methoxyformyl-1,3,5(10)-estratrien	100 to 1000	0.02	8
4-Allylestradiol	1000	0.05	
2,4-Diallylestradiol	3000	0.02	

[a] Mouse uterotrophic assay.
Data from Kincl and Dorfman (1965).

determined by percentage of rats with normal or inhibited estrous cycles, number of matings and deliveries. Mestranol at daily doses of 4.65 and 9.3 mcg was not active, whereas the 3-cyclopentyl analogue was inhibitory at the same doses. It was noted that in both experiments estrus cycles were inhibited in a large percentage of rats.

Kincl and Dorfman (1965) gave test compounds for 7 days beginning on the day of proestrus. On day 9 of the test implantation sites were counted. Estrogenic activity measured in the uterotrophic test was included for comparative purposes. Comparative activities of phenolic steroids given by subcutaneous injection are listed in Table 15, those by gavage in Table 16. Morris and van Wagenen (1967) achieved placental separation, loss of decidua, vacuolization, degeneration of the endometrium and fetal death in rabbits. Test compounds were effective whether given between days 5–7, 9–11 or 17–19 post-insemination. Effective dosages were 0.02 mg/kg/day for estradiol, 0.02–0.05 mg for mestranol and ethynyl estradiol, and 0.15–1.5 mg for stilbestrol.

The same investigators also reported that stilbestrol (1 to 25 mg) or estradiol (10 mg) given orally for 6 days following positive mating prevented pregnancy in Rhesus monkeys (*Macaca mulatta*).

For human studies see Chapter 34, p. 391.

TABLE 16. ANTIFERTILITY ACTIVITY OF PHENOLIC STEROIDS IN AN ORAL ASSAY

Steroid	Daily dose range (mcg)	Relative antifertility activity	Estrogenic activity[a]
Mestranol		100	100
3-Methoxy-17β-cyanoethoxy-1,3,5(10)-estratrien	0.5 to 270	600	8
Estradiol-17β-tetrahydropyranyl ether	10 to 1000	200	160
Estradiol	1 to 25	150	300
Estradiol-3,17β-bis-tetrahydropyranyl ether	1 to 450	100	3
17α-Ethynylestradiol-3,17-bis tetrahydropyranyl ether	10 to 90	75	33
17α-Ethynyl-1,3,5(10)-estratrien-17β-ol	2 to 1000	50	5
17β-(2′-Hydroxy)-ethoxy-1,3,5(10)-estratrien-3-methoxy	30 to 300	33	6
1,3,5(10)-Estratrien-3-ol	100 to 900	15	0.2
1,3,5(10)-Estratrien-17-one	100 to 1000	5	1

[a] Mouse uterotrophic assay.
Data from Kincl and Dorfman (1965).

2. INHIBITION OF OVULATION

(a) Inhibition of induced ovulation

Kincl and Dorfman (1963) found that in the adult mated rabbit, a single subcutaneous dose of 0.05 mg of mestranol reduced from 8 to 4.7 the average number of ovulations. Increasing the dose to 0.5 mg, however, did not result in complete inhibition. A similar decrease, but not complete inhibition, was seen when mestranol was given by gavage.

Purshottam et al. (1961) induced superovulation in 20-day-old mice by injecting pregnant mares' serum gonadotrophin (PMS), followed 42–43 hours later by an injection of human chorionic gonadotrophin (HCG). The number of shed ova was counted and used as the endpoint to evaluate the effect. Estrone (1 mg) and mestranol (0.05 mg), given for 2 days, were reported to reduce significantly the number of shed ova. Comparable results (Table 17) were obtained by Rudel and Kincl (1966) who

TABLE 17. FAILURE OF ESTRADIOL AND MESTRANOL TO BLOCK OVULATION IN PMS-HCG STIMULATED HYPOPHYSECTOMIZED RATS

Treatment[a]	Total dose (mcg)	Ovarian response[b]	Average no. of ova ± S.E.
30-day-old rats:			
0	0	33/35	27.3 ± 3.5
Estradiol	0.002	10/11	20.8 ± 6.2
	0.02	12/12	28.0 ± 3.8
Mestranol	0.01	8/8	15.9 ± 2.9
	0.05	7/7	29.1 ± 8.4
	0.25	8/8	11.5 ± 4.2
22-day-old rats:			
0	0	4/7	18.4 ± 7.9
Estradiol	0.02	5/6	18.7 ± 4.9
	0.2	6/6	25.0 ± 3.7

[a] Subcutaneous injection.
[b] Ovarian response: (number of ovulating rats)/(total number of rats).
Data from Rudel and Kincl (1966).

induced ovulation by PMS-HCG in 22-day or 30-day-old hypophysectomized animals. It should be stressed, however, that the inhibition of superstimulated ovaries was not complete, but only partial. Hence, estradiol, estrone, or mestranol in relatively high doses did not inhibit directly the ovarian function.

(b) *Suppression of ovulation in spontaneously ovulating animals*

It is generally less common to use adult rats or mice in antiovulation tests, because of the necessity to predict with fair accuracy the time of ovulation. Desaulles and Krähenbühl (1964) using regularly 4-day cycling rats, began the administration on the day of met-estrus and continued for 3 days. The number of ova was counted, a dose-response curve plotted, and the dose which inhibited ovulation in 75% of the animals was taken as effective. The active dose of estradiol was 42 mcg/kg/day. Relative potencies of other estrogens compared with estradiol are shown in Table 18.

TABLE 18. COMPARATIVE ACTIVITY OF VARIOUS STEROIDS IN INHIBITING NIDATION, OVULATION AND GONADOTROPHIN RELEASE IN THE RAT

Steroid	Relative potency		
	Anti-nidation	Anti-ovulation	Anti-gonadotrophin[a] release
Estradiol	100	100	100
Estrone	70	150	30
Estriol	12	15	10
Ethynyl estradiol	70	170	300

[a] Measured in the parabiotic rat.
Data from Desaulles and Krähenbühl (1964).

Greenwald (1965c) gave a single injection of various estrogens to hamsters at met-estrus, killed the animals 5 days later and judged the effect by microscopic evaluation of the ovaries. He reports that estradiol prevented ovulation by inducing atresia in the developing follicles and that esterification markedly increased the activity of the parent steriod (Table 19).

TABLE 19. EFFECT OF VARIOUS ESTROGENS ON FOLLICLE DEVELOPMENT IN THE HAMSTER

Steroid	Dose range used (mcg)	Total no. of animals	Effective dose (mcg)
Estradiol	10–250	10	250
Estradiol benzoate	10–25	10	10
Estradiol cyclopentyl propionate	10–25	10	10
Estrone	100–500	9	500
Conjugated estrogens (Premarin)	400–5000	12	> 5000
Diethylstilbestrol	100–2500	13	250

Data from Greenwald (1965c).

3. ACTIVITY IN THE PARABIOTIC RAT

The use of the parabiotic rat technique to measure inhibition of gonadotrophin hypersecretion after castration has already been discussed in Section A. This section only summarizes the activity of estrogens as reported by various investigators. As originally reported by Meyer and coworkers (see Biddulph et al., 1940; Byrnes and Meyer, 1951), many investigators confirmed that estrogens inhibit gonadotrophin secretion at doses that do not stimulate uterine growth.

Activities of numerous ring A phenolic steroids studied by Kincl et al. 1964) are summarized in Table 20. The test compounds were injected

TABLE 20. RELATIVE POTENCY OF VARIOUS STEROIDS ASSAYED BY SUBCUTANEOUS INJECTION IN INTACT FEMALE-OVARIECTOMIZED PARABIOTIC PAIR

Compound	Relative potency	
	Gonadotrophin inhibition	Uterotrophic
Ethynyl estradiol	100	300
Ethynyl estradiol 3-methyl ether	20	20
Estrone	10	20
1,3,5(10)-Estratrien-3-ol	3	0.2
3-Methoxy-17β-cyanoethoxy-1,3,5 (10)-estratriene	3	1
17α-Methyl-1,3,5(10)-estratrien-17β-ol	0.5	0.5
1,3,5(10)-Estratrien-17-one	0.1	0.1
17α-Ethynyl-1,3,5(10)-estratrien-17β-ol	0.2	0.6
1-Methyl-3-acetoxy-1,3,5(10)- 6-estratetraene-17-one	0.01	0.01
3,6α-Diacetoxy-4-methylacetoxy-1, 6,5(10)-estratrien-17-one	0.01	0.01
3-Acetoxy-4-methylacetoxy-1,3,5(10) 6-estratetraene-17-one	0.01	0.01

subcutaneously, once daily for 10 days. Estrogens are usually more active when injected than when given by gavage. This is illustrated in Table 21 in which are compared the effective daily doses of three compounds given by both routes (Rudel and Kincl, 1966).

4. NON-STEROIDAL ESTROGENS

A number of non-steroidal compounds related to stilbestrol, triphenylethanol, 2,3-diphenyl indenes and 3,4-diphenylcoumarines (Fig. 2) were

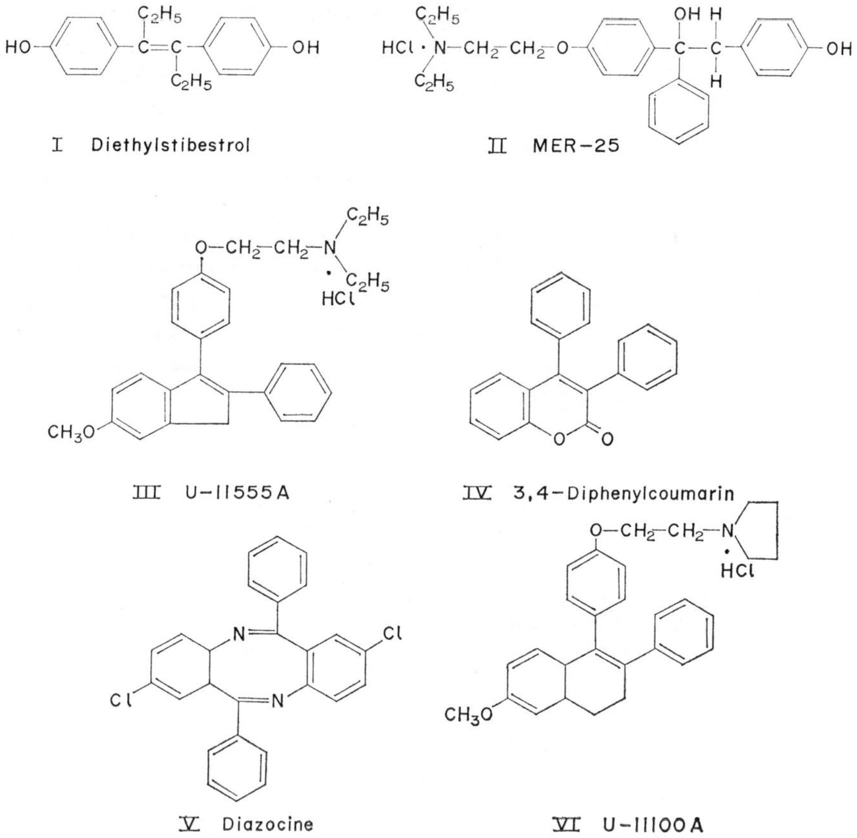

FIG. 2. Non-steroidal estrogens.

TABLE 21. COMPARISON OF GONADOTROPHIN INHIBITORY ACTIVITY OF THREE ESTROGENS GIVEN BY INJECTION OR ORALLY

Steroid	Effective daily dose (mcg)	
	Oral	Subcutaneous
Mestranol	0.1	0.05
Ethynyl estradiol	0.1	0.01
Estradiol	1.0	0.01

From Rudel and Kincl (1966).

reported as active antifertility agents in the rodents. With the exception of strong estrogens related to stilbestrol which act by inhibiting the synthesis and/or release of gonadotrophins by the pituitary, these substances may act as anti-estrogens. In general, these compounds exhibit a low degree of estrogenic (uterotrophic) activity, and higher dosages inhibit the stimulating effect of estrone or estradiol. Thus, their antifertility effects appear to be related to their anti-estrogenic activity.

Austin and Bruce (1956) added stilbestrol (diethylstilbestrol) (I) to drinking water of female rats and mice prior to cohabitation with males. Within 36 hours after finding sperm in the vaginal smears the females were killed, the Fallopian tubes examined for the presence of ova, and the ovaries examined microscopically to confirm the occurrence or absence of ovulation. This treatment inhibited ovulation in both species, but sperm penetration of ova was affected only slightly (Table 22).

TABLE 22. OVULATION AND SPERMATOZOON PENETRATION IN RATS AND MICE ON DIFFERENT LEVELS OF STILBESTROL INTAKE

Stilbestrol (mcg/day)[a]	No. of animals	Mean no. of ovulated eggs	% penetrated eggs
Mice			
0	19	9.7	75
0.08	16	9.7	92
0.08	20	8.9	86
2.3	19	6.7	25
5.6	18	3.0	100
Rats			
0	12	11.4	91
1.0	7	10.9	91
2.6	10	9.3	100
8.5	14	7.5	100
22.0	6	0	0
65.0	9	0	0

[a] Given in 7 to 14 days.
Data from Austin and Bruce (1956).

Antifertility activity of a triphenyl ethanol derivative, MER-25 [1-(p-2-diethylaminoethoxyphenyl)-1-phenyl-2-p-methoxyphenyl(II)], was reported in 1958 by Segal and Nelson, Lerner et al., and Chang. Oral treatment in a single or repeated dose (25 mg/kg) in rats affected ova development during

TABLE 23. INFLUENCE OF SUBSTITUTION IN STILBESTROL MOLECULE ON ESTROGENIC AND ANTIFERTILITY ACTIVITY IN MICE[a]

$$\text{}_5H_2C \diagdown N-C_2H_4O-\bigcirc-\underset{C\ \ D}{\overset{A\ \ \ B}{C\underset{Y}{=}C}}-\bigcirc-R$$

Compound	Substituent						MED$_{50}$ (daily dose, mcg)		
	A	B	C	D	Y	R	Estrogenic	Antifertility day 1 to 3	day 4 to 6
MRL-41		Cl	Ph*		=		100	100	100
MER-25	OH	H	Ph*	H	—	—OCH$_3$	Inactive	1000	1000
MRL-37	H	H	Ph*	H	—	—OCH$_3$	Inactive	800	1600

[a] Subcutaneous injection.
* Ph = phenyl group.
Data from Emmens (1965).

Y represents a single bond or a double bond as shown in the table.

TABLE 24. INFLUENCE OF SUBSTITUTION IN STILBESTROL MOLECULE ON ESTROGENIC AND ANTIFERTILITY ACTIVITY[a]

Parent Compound $HO-\bigcirc-\underset{C\ \ D}{\overset{A\ \ B}{C\underset{Y}{=}C}}-\bigcirc-OH$

Y represents a single bond or a double bond, as shown in the Table.

Substituent					MED$_{50}$ (daily dose, mcg)		
A	B	C	D	Y	Estrogenic	Antifertility Day 1 to 3	Day 4 to 6
C$_2$H$_5$	C$_2$H$_5$			=	0.2	0.3	0.3
CH$_3$	CH$_3$			=	60	90	30
CH$_3$			H	=	1200	Inactive	
C$_2$H$_5$			H	=	500		70
n-C$_3$H$_7$			H	=	500		70
CH$_3$	CH$_3$	H	H	—	20		<1.0
CH$_3$	H	H	CH$_3$	—		Inactive	
C$_2$H$_5$	CH$_3$	H	H	—	1.0	0.8	0.8
C$_2$H$_5$	CH$_3$	H	H	—	>50	50	50
C$_2$H$_5$	H	H	H	—	Inactive		
C≡N	C$_2$H$_5$	H	H	—	>1000[a]	100[b]	200 mg/kg[b] 100/kg[b]
C≡N	C$_2$H$_5$			=		100[b]	
COCH$_3$	C$_2$H$_5$	H	H	—		5/kg[a]	
C≡N	H	H	C$_2$H$_5$	—		1000/kg[a]	

[a] From Pincus et al. (1964) in rats.
[b] From Saunders and Rorig (1964) in rats.
All other from Emmens (1965) in mice.

tubal passage, but not decidual development. A closely related derivative, chloramiphene (MRL-37; 1-[-p-(β-diethylaminoethoxy)phenyl]-1-phenyl-2-(p-methoxyphenyl)-ethane) was active at a dose of 0.1 mg/kg day in parabiotic rats, and inhibited fertility in the adult animals (Holtkamp et al., 1960; Segal and Nelson, 1961). Barnes and Meyer (1962) studied the oral activity of clomiphene (MRL-41; 1-[p-(β-diethylaminoethoxy)-phenyl]-1,2-diphenyl-2-chloroethylene) in pregnant rats. A dose of 2.5 mg/kg and 20 mg/kg respectively inhibited the passage of ova, and implantation. When given during days 8 to 12 of pregnancy, the treatment caused embryonic death. In a later study Schlough and Meyer (1965) reported that the lower dosage inhibited estrone-induced implantation. Blastocyst development, however, is probably not affected (Staples, 1966). The influence of structural modification on biological activity is seen from

TABLE 25. INFLUENCE OF SUBSTITUTION IN 2,3-DIPHENYLINDENE MOLECULE ON ANTI-FERTILITY ACTIVITY IN RATS

A	B	R	HX	Effective dose, (mg/day)[a]
		$CH_2CH_2N(C_2H_5)_2$	$HClO_4$	0.5 (U-11555A)
6-OCH_3		CH_2CH_2N (piperidine)	HCl	0.025
6-OCH_3		CH_2CH_2N (pyrrolidine)	HCl	0.1
6-OCH_3		CH_2CH_2N (morpholine-like)	HCl	0.1
6-OCH_3		$CH_2CH_2N(C_2H_5)_2$	HCl	0.1
6-OCH_3	m-OCH_3	$CH_2CH_2N(C_2H_5)_2$	HCl	2
6-OCH_3	p-OCH_3	$CH_2CH_2N(C_2H_5)_2$	HI	0.5
5-OCH_3		$CH_2CH_2N(C_2H_5)_2$	HCl	0.5
5,6-diOCH_3		$CH_2CH_2N(C_2H_5)_2$	HCl	2
	p-OCH_3	$CH_2CH_2N(C_2H_5)_2$	HCl	0.5

[a] Oral administration for 7 days; 100% inhibition of pregnancy.
Data from Lednicer et al. (1965a)

TABLE 26. INFLUENCE OF SUBSTITUTION IN 3,4-DICOUMARINE MOLECULE ON ANTIFERTILITY ACTIVITY IN RATS

Parent compound

Substitution			Effective dose (mg/day)[a]
A	B	C	
OAc	H	OCH$_3$	0.1
OAc	H	H	0.1
OH	H	OCH$_3$	10
H	OAc	OCH$_3$	10
OCH$_2$CH$_2$N(C$_2$H$_5$)$_2$	H	OCH$_3$	>10
H	OCH$_2$CH$_2$N(C$_2$H$_5$)$_2$	OCH$_3$	>10

[a] Subcutaneous injection, 7-day administration.
Data from Lednicer et al. (1965b).

Tables 23 and 24. Additional studies on the activity of these compounds were reported by Emmens et al. (1964), Pincus et al. (1964), Saunders and Rorig (1964), Roy et al. (1964), and Emmens (1965). Antifertility activity of non-steroidal compounds, chemically unrelated to those described above, was reported as follows:

(a) 2,3-Diphenylindenes (Duncan and Lyster, 1963; Lednicer et al., 1965a). Table 25 shows the influence of different substitutions on antifertility activity. A typical example is 2-[-p-(6-methoxy-2-phenylindene-3-yl)phenoxy]-triethylamine hydrochloride (U-11555A) (III) which is an active antifertility agent in several species (Duncan et al., 1962).
(b) 3,4-Diphenylcoumarines (IV) by Lednicer et al. (1965b) (Table 26).
(c) Diazocine (2,8-dichloro-6,12-diphenyldibenzo [b,f] [1,5] diazocine) (V) by Duncan et al. (1965).
(d) 3,4-Dihydronaphthalenes and 1,2,3,4-tetrahydro-1-naphthols by Lednicer et al. (1967).

Of this series 6-methoxy-1,2-diphenyl-[1-p-ethoxypyrrolidine]-3,4-dihydronaphthalene hydrochloride (U-11100A) (VI) was studied in detail,

Pregnancy inhibition was achieved by oral dose of 2.5 mcg/kg in rats, guinea pigs and rabbits (Duncan et al., 1963). Measured by vaginal smears, (VI) is a weak estrogen in mice and rats; the MED_{50} is 500 mcg and 50 to 100 mcg respectively (Emmens and Martin, 1965). Table 27 shows the activity of several other compounds. Two other examples of structure-activity relationship are shown in Table 28.

TABLE 27. INFLUENCE OF SUBSTITUTION IN 3,4-DIHYDRONAPHTHALENE MOLECULE ON ANTIFERTIILTY ACTIVITY IN RATS

Parent compound

R	Effective dose (mg/day)[a]	
—OCH$_2$CH$_2$ N⟨ ⟩ · HCl	0.005	U-11100A
—CH$_2$ N⟨ ⟩ · HCl	10	
—CH$_2$CH$_2$ N⟨ ⟩ · HCl	0.05	
—CH$_2$CH$_2$CH$_2$ N⟨ ⟩ · HCl	0.005	
—OCH$_2$CH$_2$ N(C$_2$H$_5$)$_2$ · HCl	0.05	

[a] Oral administration for 7 days; 100% inhibition of pregnancy.
From Lednicer et al. (1967).

Activity of yet another weak estrogen, phloretin, [β-(p-hydroxyphenyl)-2,4,6-trihydroxypropiolone] was described by Lerner et al. (1963) and Deanesly (1963). Administered on days 1 to 4 after mating, it decreased pregnancies by 40%.

TABLE 28. INFLUENCE OF SUBSTITUTION IN 1,2,3,4-TETRAHYDRO-, AND 3,4-DIHYDRONAPHTHALENES ON ANTIFERTILITY ACTIVITY IN RATS

Parent compounds, effective dose, mg/day[a]

R		
3-pyridyl	0.01	0.1
4-pyridyl	0.05	0.1

REFERENCES

ALLEN, W. M. and CORNER, G. W. (1929) Physiology of the corpus luteum. III. Normal growth and implantation of embryos after early ablation of the ovaries, under the influence of extracts of corpus luteum. *Amer. J. Physiol.* **88**: 340.

ALLEN, W. M. and HECKEL, G. P. (1936) The effect of continued injections of progestin and combinations of oestrin and progestin on the endometrium of castrated rabbits. *Anat. Rec.* **64**: Abstr. 2.

ARAI, Y. (1964a) Changes in the hypothalamic-pituitary system after ovariectomy in persistent estrous and diestrous rats. *J. Fac. Sci.* **10**: 369–379.

ARAI, Y. (1964b) Long-lasting effects of early post-natal treatment with estrogen on pituitary-gonadal system in male rats. *Endocr. Jap.* **11**: 153–158.

AUSTIN, C. R. and BRUCE, H. M. (1956) Effect of continuous oestrogen administration on oestrus, ovulation and fertilization in rats and mice. *J. Endocr.* **13**: 376–383.

BALL, J. and HARTMAN, C. G. (1939) A case of delayed ovulation after estrin administration in the intact monkey. *Proc. Soc. Exp. Biol. (N.Y.)* **40**: 629–631.

BANIK, U. K. and PINCUS, G. (1964) Estrogens and transport of ova in the rat. *Proc. Soc. Exp. Biol. (N.Y.)* **116**: 1032–1034.

BARNES, L. E. and MEYER, R. K. (1962) Effects of ethanoxytriephetol MRL-37 and clomiphene on reproduction in rats. *Fertil. Steril.* **13**: 472–480.

BEYLER, A. L. and POTTS, G. O. (1957) The effects of ethynylandrostenediol 3-cyclopentyl propionate on the reproductive tract of male and female rats. *Endocrinology* **60**: 519–531.

BIALY, G. and PINCUS, G. (1962) Effects of estrogen and progestin on the uterine carbonic anhydrase of immature rats. *Endocrinology* **70**: 781–785.

BIDDULPH, C., MEYER, R. K. and GUMBRECK, L. G. (1940) The influence of estriol, estradiol and progesterone on the secretion of gonadotropic hormones in parabiotic rats. *Endocrinology* **26**: 280–284.

BLOCH, S. (1948) Zum Problem der Nidationsverzögerung bei der säugenden Maus. *Bull. schweiz. Akad. Med. Wiss.* **4**: 309–332.

BOAS, N. F. and LUDWIG, A. W. (1950) The mechanism of estrogen inhibition of comb growth in the cockerel, with histologic observations. *Endocrinology* **46**: 299–306.

BOGDANOVE, E. M. (1963) Direct gonad-pituitary feed-back: an analysis of effects of intracranial estrogenic depots on gonadotropin secretion. *Endocrinology* **73**: 696–712.

BORELL, U. and WESTMAN, A. (1949) The effect of oestrogen on the phosphate turnover in the hypophyseal-diencephalic system. *Acta Endocr. (Kbh.)* **3**: 111–118.

BORELL, U., WESTMAN, A. and ÖRSTROM, Å. (1947) Studies on the functions of the hypophyseal-diencephalic system and of the ovaries by means of radio-active phosphorus. *Gynaecologia (Basel)* **123**: 185–200.

BORELL, U., WESTMAN, A. and ÖRSTROM, Å. (1948) The phosphate metabolism in the hypophyseal-diencephalic system and ovaries of rats determined by means of P^{32}. *Acta Physiol. Scand.* **15**: 245–253.

BRENEMAN, W. R. (1953) The effect of gonadal hormones alone and in combination with pregnant mares' serum on the pituitary, gonad, and comb of white leghorn cockerels. *Anat. Rec.* **117**: 533–534.

BULLOUGH, N. S. (1946) Mitotic activity in the adult female mouse (*Mus musculus* L.). A study of its relation to the oestrus cycle in normal and abnormal conditions. *Phil. Trans. Roy. Soc.*, ser. B, **231**: 453–516.

BURDICK, H. O. and PINCUS, G. (1935) The effect of oestrin injections upon the developing ova of mice and rabbits. *Amer. J. Physiol.* **111**: 201–208.

BURDICK, H. O. and WHITNEY, R. (1938) Fate of ova accelerated in their rate of passage through the Fallopian tubes of mice by massive injections of Progynon B. *Endocrinology*, **22**: 631.

BURDICK, H. O., WHITNEY, R. and EMERSON, B. (1942) Observations on the transport of tubal ova. *Endocrinology* **31**: 100–108.

BURNS, R. K. (1961) Role of hormones in the differentiation of sex. In: *Sex and Internal Secretions*, pp. 91–95. Young, W. C. and Corner, G. W. (Eds.). The Williams & Wilkins Co., Baltimore, Maryland.

BURROWS, H. (1937) Oestrogens, Chap. 4. In: *Biological Action of Sex Hormones*, Cambridge Univ. Press.

BYRNES, W. W. and MEYER, R. K. (1951) Effect of physiological amounts of estrogen in the secretion of follicle stimulating and luteinizing hormones. *Endocrinology* **49**: 449–460.

CHANG, M. C. (1958) Capacitation of rabbit spermatozoa in the uterus with special reference to the reproductive phases of the female. *Endocrinology* **63**: 619–628.

CHANG, M. C. (1966) Effects of oral administration of medroxyprogesterone acetate and ethynyl estradiol on the transportation and development of rabbit eggs. *Endocrinology* **79**: 939–948.

CHANG, M. C. (1966) Transport of eggs from the Fallopian tube to the uterus as a function of oestrogen. *Nature* **212**: 1048–1049.

CHANG, M. C. and HARPER, M. J. K. (1966) Effect of estrogens and other compounds as oral antifertility agents on the development of rabbit ova and hamster embryos. *Fertil. Steril.* **16**: 281–291.

CHANG, M. C. and HARPER, M. J. K. (1966) The effect of ethynyl estradiol in egg transport and development in the rabbit. *Endocrinology* **78**: 860–872.

CORNER, G. W. (1928) Physiology of the corpus luteum. I. The effect of very early ablation of the corpus luteum upon embryos and uterus. *Amer. J. Physiol.* **86**: 74.

DANIEL, J. C. and COWAN, M. L. (1966) Effects of some steroids in oral contraceptives on the cleavage of rabbit eggs *in vitro*. *J. Endocr.* **35**: 155–160.

DAVIDSON, J. M. and SAWYER, C. H. (1961) Effects of localized intracerebral implantation of oestrogen on reproductive function in the female rabbit. *Acta Endocr. (Kbh.)* **37**: 385–393.

DEANESLY, R. (1939) Depression of hypophyseal activity by the implantation of tablets of estrone and estradiol. *J. Endocr.* **1**: 36–48.

DEANESLY, R. (1963) Further observations on the effects of oestradiol on tubal eggs and implantation in the guinea pig. *J. Reprod. Fertil.* **5**: 49–57.

DESAULLES, P. A. and KRÄHENBÜHL, C. (1964) Comparison of the antifertility and sex hormonal activities of sex hormones and their derivatives. *Acta Endocr. (Kbh.)* **47**: 444–456.

DÖCKE, F. and DÖRNER, G. (1965) The mechanism of the induction of ovulation by oestrogens. *J. Endocr.* **33**: 491–499.
DOMM, L. V. (1939) Intersexuality in adult brown Leghorn male as result of estrogenic treatment during early embryonic life. *Proc. Soc. Exp. Biol. (N.Y.)* **42**: 310–312.
DORFMAN, R. I. and DORFMAN, A. S. (1963) Pituitary gonadotropic inhibitory action of estrone in parabiotic rats. *Endocrinology* **72**: 115–116.
DREISBACH, R. H. (1959) The effects of steroid sex hormones on pregnant rats. *J. Endocr.* **18**: 271–277.
DUNCAN, G. W. and LYSTER, S. C. (1963) Effect of a diphenylindene derivative (U-11555A) on blastocyst survival *in utero. Fertil. Steril.* **14**: 565–571.
DUNCAN, G. W., STUCKI, J. C., LYSTER, S. C. and LEDNICER, D. (1962) An orally effective mammalian antifertility agent. *Proc. Soc. Exp. Biol. (N.Y.)* **109**: 163–166.
DUNCAN, G. W., LYSTER, S. C., CLARK, J. J. and LEDNICER, D. (1963) Antifertility activities of two diphenyl-dihydronaphthalene derivatives. *Proc. Soc. Exp. Biol. (N.Y.)* **112**: 439–441.
DUNCAN, G. W., LYSTER, S. C. and WRIGHT, J. B. (1965) Reproductive mechanism influenced by Diazocine. *Proc. Soc. Exp. Biol. (N.Y.)* **120**: 725–728.
EDGREN, R. A. and SHIPLEY, G. C. (1961) A qualitative study of the termination of pregnancy in rats with estrone. *Fertil. Steril.* **12**: 178–181.
EISENFELD, A. J. and AXELROD, J. (1965) Selectivity of estrogen distribution in tissues. *J. Pharmacol. Exp. Ther.* **150**: 469–475.
EISENFELD, A. J. and AXELROD, J. (1966) Effect of steroid hormones, ovariectomy, estrogen pretreatment, sex and immaturity on the distribution of ^{3}H-estradiol. *Endocrinology* **79**: 38–42.
EMMENS, C. W. (1962) Action of oestrogens and anti-oestrogens on early pregnancy in the rabbit. *J. Reprod. Fertil.* **3**: 246–249.
EMMENS, C. W. (1965) Oestrogenic, anti-oestrogenic and anti-fertility activities of various compounds. *J. Reprod. Fertil.* **9**: 277–283.
EMMENS, C. W. and FINN, C. A. (1962) Local and parenteral action of oestrogens and anti-oestrogens on early pregnancy in the rat and mouse. *J. Reprod. Fertil.* **3**: 239–245.
EMMENS, C. W. and MARTIN, L. (1965) Biological activities of U11100A. *J. Reprod. Fertil.* **9**: 269–275.
EMMENS, C. W., COX, R. I. and MARTIN, L. (1964) The oestrogenic and anti-oestrogenic activity of compounds related to diethylstilbestrol. *Acta Endocr. (Kbh.) suppl.* **90**: 61–70.
ERICSSON, R. J. and BAKER, V. F. (1966) Transport of oestrogens in semen to the female rat during mating and its effect on fertility. *J. Reprod. Fertil.* **12**: 381–384.
EVANS, L. T. and CLAPP, M. L. (1940) The effects of ovarian hormones and seasons in *Anolis carolinensis*. II. The genital system. *Anat. Rec.* **77**: 57–75.
EVANS, H. M. and SIMPSON, M. E. (1929) A sex difference in the hormone content of the anterior hypophysis of the rat. *Amer. J. Physiol.* **89**: 375–378.
FALCONI, G. and ERCOLI, A. (1963) 3-Cyclopentyl ether of 17α-ethynylestradiol: A potent anti-gonadotrophic and contraceptive agent in rodents. *Experientia (Basel)* **XIX,** 249,
FERRARA, B., ROSATI, P. and CONSOLI, G. (1953) Azione degli stilbenici sul testiculo; ricerche sperimentali in ovis aries. *Boll. Soc. ital. Biol. sper.* **29**: 66.
FLERKÓ, B. (1957) Le role des structures hypothalamiques sous l'action inhibitrice de la folliculine sur la sécrétion de l'hormone folliculo-stimuline. *Arch. Anat. Micr. Morph. Exp.* **46**: 159–172.
FOOTE, C. L. (1940) Response of gonads and gonaducts of ambystoma larvae to treatment with sex hormones. *Proc. Soc. Exp. Biol. (N.Y.)* **43**: 519–523.

FORBES, T. R. (1941) Observations on the urogenital anatomy of the adult male lizard, *Sceloporus*, and on the action of implanted pellets of testosterone and of estrone. *J. Morph.* **68**: 31–69.
GAARENSTROOM, J. H. (1939) Effect of diethylstilbestrol on sex. *Acta Brev. Neerl. Physiol.* **9**: 13–14.
GILLMAN, J. (1942) Temporary ovarian damage produced in baboons by single administration of estradiol benzoate and progesterone in the first part of the cycle. *Endocrinology* **30**: 61–70.
GOLDING, G. T. and RAMIREZ, F. T. (1928) Ovarian and placental hormone effects in normal, immature albino rats. *Endocrinology* **12**: 804–812.
GORSKI, R. A. (1963) Modification of ovulatory mechanisms by postnatal administration of estrogen to the rat. *Amer. J. Physiol.* **205**: 842–844.
GREENWALD, G. S. (1959) Tubal transport of ova in the rabbit. *Anat. Rec.* **133**: 386.
GREENWALD, G. S. (1961) A study of the transport of ova through the rabbit oviduct. *Fertil. Steril.* **12**: 82.
GREENWALD, G. S. (1961) The antifertility effects in pregnant rats of a single injection of estradiol cyclopentyl propionate. *Endocrinology* **69**: 1068–1073.
GREENWALD, G. S. (1965a) The effect of a single injection of diethystilbestrol or progesterone on the hamster ovary. *J. Endocr.* **33**: 13–23.
GREENWALD, G. S. (1965b) A study of the transport of ova through the rabbit oviduct. *Fertil. Steril.* **12**: 80–95.
GREENWALD, G. S. (1965c) Anti-ovulatory potency of various steroids determined by single injection into female hamsters. *J. Endocr.* **33**: 25–32.
GREENWALD, G. S. (1967) Species differences in egg transport in response to exogenous estrogens. *Anat. Res.* **157**: 163–172.
GREEP, R. O. (1940) Changes in the corpora lutea of rabbits following hysterectomy during pregnancy. *Anat. Rec.*, Suppl. **76**: 25.
GREEP, R. O. and JONES, C. I. (1950) Steroid control of pituitary function. *Recent Progr. Hormone Res.* **5**: 197–254.
HAFEZ, E. S. E. (1962) Endocrine control of reception, transport, development and loss of rabbit ova. *J. Reprod. Fertil.* **3**: 14–25.
HARPER, M. J. K., BENNETT, J. P., BOURSNELL, J. C. and ROWSON, L. E. (1960) An autoradiographic method for the study of egg transport in the rabbit Fallopian tube. *J. Reprod. Fertil.* **1**: 249.
HARRIS, G. W. and LEVINE, S. (1965) Sexual differentiation of the brain and its experimental control. *J. Physiol.* **181**: 379–400.
HATERIUS, H. O. and NELSON, W. O. (1932) Experimental studies of the anterior pituitary. 1. The influence of ovarian implants on the castration cell type in the male rat pituitary. *J. Exp. Zool.* **61**: 175–180.
HEAP, R. B. and LEMMING, G. E. (1962) The influence of ovarian hormones on some chemical constituents of the uterine washing of the rat and rabbit. *J. Endocr.* **25**: 57–68.
HOHLWEG, W. (1934) Veränderungen des Hypophysenvorderlappens und des Ovariums nach Behandlung mit grossen Dosen von Follikelhormon. *Klin. Wschr.* **13**: 92–95.
HOHLWEG, W. and CHAMORRO, A. (1937) Uber die luteinisierende Wirkung des Follikelhormons durch Beinflussung der luteogenen Hypophysenvorderlappensekretion. *Klin. Wschr.* **16**: 196–197.
HOHLWEG, W. and JUNKMANN, K. (1932) Die hormonal—nervöse Regulierung der Funktion des Hypophysenvorderlappens. *Klin. Wschr.* **11**: 321–323.
HOLTKAMP, D. E., GRESLIN, J. G., ROOT, C. A. and LERNER, L. J. (1960) Gonadotrophin inhibiting and antifecundity effects of chloramiphene. *Proc. Soc. Exp. Biol. (N.Y.)* **105**: 197–201.

JENSEN, E. V. and JACOBSON, H. I. (1962) Basic guides to the mechanism of estrogen action. *Recent Progr. Hormone Res.* **18**: 387–414.

KANEMATSU, S. and SAWYER, C. H. (1964) Effects of hypothalamic and hypophysial estrogen implants on pituitary and plasma LH in ovariectomized rabbits. *Endocrinology* **75**: 579–585.

KAWASHIMA, S. and TAKEWAKI, K. (1966) Basophils and erythyrosinophils in the anterior hypophysis of steroid sterilized female rats. *Annot. Zool. Japoneses* **39**: 23–29.

KETCHEL, M. M. and PINCUS, G. (1964) *In vitro* exposure of rabbit ova to estrogens. *Proc. Soc. Exp. Biol. (N.Y.)* **115**: 419–421.

KINCL, F. A. (1967) Effects of steroids in neonatal animals. Possible relationships to immune reactions. *Excerpta Med. Internat. Congress Series* **132**: 1028–1032.

KINCL, F. A. and DORFMAN, R. I. (1963) Anti-ovulatory activity of steroids in the adult oestrus rabbit. *Acta Endocr. (Kbh.)* Suppl. **42**: 73.

KINCL, F. A. and DORFMAN, R. I. (1965) Antifertility activity of various steroids in the female rat. *J. Reprod. Fertil.* **10**: 105–113.

KINCL, F. A. and FOLCH-PI, A. (1963) Efecto del tratamiento con esteroides en el cuyo. *Ciencia (Mex.)* **22**: 209–211.

KINCL, F. A. and SICKLES, J. S. (1966) Inhibition of sexual development in birds with steroid hormones. Abstracts of meeting of the Mexican Endocrine Society, Istapan de la Sal, Mexico, pp. 265–272. See also *Gen. Comp. Endocr.* **9**: 401–405 (1967).

KINCL, F. A., BIRCH, A. J. and DORFMAN, R. I. (1964) Pituitary gonadotropic inhibitory activity of various steroids in ovariectomized-intact female rats in parabiosis. *Proc. Soc. Exp. Biol. (N.Y.)* **117**: 549–552.

KINCL, F. A., FOLCH-PI, A. and HERRERA LASSO, L. (1963) Effect of estradiol benzoate treatment in the newborn male rat. *Endocrinology* **72**: 966–968.

KINCL, F. A., FOLCH-PI, A., MAQUEO, M., HERRERA LASSO, L., ORIOL, A. and DORFMAN, R. I. (1965) Inhibition of sexual development in male and female rats treated with various steroids at the age of five days. *Acta Endocr. (Kbh.)* **49**: 195–206.

KRAUS, E. J. (1930) The effect of prolan (Aschheim-Zondek) upon the male sex-organs. *Klin. Wschr.* **9**: 1493–1495.

KRÄHENBÜHL, C. and DESAULLES, P. A. (1964) The action of sex hormones on gonadotrophin-induced ovulation in hypophysectomized prepuberal rats. *Acta Endocr. (Kbh.)* **47**: 457–465.

KREHBIEL, R. H. (1941) The effects of Theelin on delayed implantation in the pregnant lactating rat. *Anat. Rec.* **81**: 381–392.

KROC, R. L., STEINETZ, B. G. and BEACH, V. L. (1959) The effects of estrogen, progestogens and relaxin in pregnant and non-pregnant laboratory rodents. *Ann. N.Y. Acad. Sci.* **75**: 942.

LANE, C. E. and HISAW, F. L. (1934) The follicular apparatus of the ovary of the immature rat and some of the factors which influence it. *Anat. Rec.*, Suppl. **60**: 52.

LEATHEM, J. (1956) The influence of steroids on prepubertal animals. *Proc. IIIrd Int. Congr. Animal Reprod.*, Cambridge, 25th–30th June.

LEATHEM, J. H. and WOLF, R. C. (1955) The varying effects of sex hormones in mammals In: *Physiology of Reproduction. Mem. Soc. Endocr.* **4**: 220–236.

LEDNICER, D., BABCOCK, J. C., MARLATT, P. E., LYSTER, S. C. and DUNCAN, G. W. (1965a) Mammalian antifertility agents. I. Derivatives of 2,3-diphenylindenes. *J. Med. Chem.* **8**: 52–57.

LEDNICER, D., LYSTER, S. C. and DUNCAN, G. W. (1965b) Mammalian antifertility agents. II. Basic ethers of 3,4-diphenylcoumarines. *J. Med. Chem.* **8**: 725–726.

LEDNICER, D., LYSTER, S. C. and DUNCAN, G. W. (1967) Mammalian antifertility agents. IV. Basic 3,4-dihydronaphthalenes and 1,2,3,4-tetrahydro-1 naphthols. *J. Med. Chem.* **10**: 78–84.

LERNER, L. J., HOLTHAUS, F. J., JR and THOMPSON, C. R. (1958) A non-steroidal estrogen antagonist 1-(*p*-2-diethylaminoethoxyphenyl)-1-phenyl-2-*p*-methoxyphenyl ethanol. *Endocrinology* **63**: 295–301.

LERNER, L. J., TURKHEIMER, A. R. and BORMAN, A. (1963) Phloretin, a weak estrogen and estrogen antagonist. *Proc. Soc. Exp. Biol. (N.Y.)* **114**: 115–117.

LISK, R. D. (1965) Reproductive capacity and behavioural oestrus in the rat bearing hypothalamic implants of sex steroids. *Acta Endocr. (Kbh.)* **48**: 209–219.

LUDWIG, D. J. (1950) The effect of androgen on spermatogenesis. *Endocrinology* **46**: 453–481.

LYNCH, K. M., JR. (1952) Recovery of the rat testis following estrogen therapy. *Ann. N.Y. Acad. Sci.* **55**: 734.

MCGINTY, D. A. and DJERASSI, C. (1958) Some chemical and biological properties of 19-nor-17α-ethynyl-testosterone. *Ann. N.Y. Acad. Sci.* **71**: 500–514.

MAQUEO, M. and KINCL, F. A. (1964) Testicular histomorphology of young rats treated with oestradiol-17β benzoate. *Acta Endocr. (Kbh.)* **46**: 25–30.

MAQUEO, M., BURT, A. and KINCL, F. A. (1966) Pituitary histology of rats treated neonatally with steroid hormones. *Acta Endocr. (Kbh.)* **53**: 438–442.

MARESCAUX, J. (1950) Mecanisme d'action de la folliculine sur le testicule chez le cobaye. *C.R. Soc. Biol. (Paris)* **144**: 1102.

MARTIN, L. (1963) Interactions between oestradiol and progestogens in the uterus of the mouse. *J. Endocr.* **26**: 31–39.

MERKLIN, R. J. (1953) Reproductive performance of female mice treated prepubertally with a single injection of estradiol dipropionate. *Endocrinology* **53**: 342–343.

MEYER, R. K. and HERTZ, R. (1937) Effect of oestrone on secretion of gonadotropic complex as evidenced by parabiotic rats. *Ann. J. Physiol.* **120**: 232–237.

MEYER, R. K., LEONARD, S. L., HISAW, F. L. and MARTIN, S. J. (1930) Effect of oestrin on gonad-stimulating power of the hypophysis. *Proc. Soc. Exp. Biol. (N.Y.)* **27**: 702–704.

MICHAEL, R. P. (1965) Oestrogens in the central nervous system. *Brit. Med. Bull.* **21**: 87–90.

MIYAKE, T., KAKUSHI, H. and HARA, K. (1963) Deciduomatogenic and anti-deciduomatogenic activity in steroids. *Steroids* **2**: 749–763.

MOORE, C. R. and PRICE, D. (1932) Gonad hormone functions and the reciprocal influence between gonads and hypophysis with its bearing on the problem of sex-hormone antagonism. *Amer. J. Anat.* **50**: 13–17.

MORRIS, J. M. and VAN WAGENEN, G. (1967) Compounds interfering with ovum implantation and development. III. The role of estrogens. *Amer. J. Obst. Gynec.* **96**: 804–813.

NOBLE, R. L. (1938) Effect of synthetic estrogenic substances on the body growth and endocrine organs of the rat. *Lancet* **ii**: 192–195.

NELSON, W. O. (1934) Effect of oestrin and gonadotropic hormone injections upon hypophysis of the adult rat. *Proc. Soc. Exp. Biol. (N.Y.)* **32**: 452–454.

NOYES, R. W., ADAMS, C. E. and WALTON, A. (1959) The transport of ova in relation to the dosage of oestrogen in ovariectomized rabbits. *J. Endocr.* **18**: 108–117.

NUTTING, E. F. and MEYER, R. K. (1964) Effect of oestrone on the delay of nidation, implantation and foetal survival in ovariectomized rats. *J. Endocr.* **29**: 235–242.

OGAWA, Y. and PINCUS, G. (1962) Estrogen effects on the carbonic anhydrase content of mouse uteri. *Endocrinology* **70**: 359–364.

PARKES, A. S. and BELLERBY, C. W. (1926) Studies on the internal secretions of the ovary. II. The effects of injection of the oestrus-producing hormone during pregnancy. *J. Physiol.* **62**: 145–155.

PARKES, A. S., DODDS, E. C. and NOBLE, R. L. (1938) Interruption of early pregnancy by means of orally active oestrogens. *Brit. Med. J.* **2**: 557–559.

PATANELLI, D. J. and NELSON, W. O. (1959) The effect of certain 19-nor steroids and related compounds on spermatogenesis in male rats. *Arch. Anat. Micr. Morph. Exp.* **48:** 199–222.

PENCHARZ, R. I. (1940) Effect of estrogens and androgens alone and in combination with chorionic gonadotropin on ovary of hypophysectomized rat. *Science* **91:** 554–555.

PETERSON, D. L. and EDGREN, R. A. (1965) The effect of various steroids on mating behavior, fertility and fecundity of rats. *Int. J. Fertil.* **10:** 327–332.

PINCUS, G. and BIALY, G. (1963) Carbonic anhydrase in steroid-responsive tissues. *Recent Progr. Hormone Res.* **19:** 201–250.

PINCUS, G. and KIRSCH, R. E. (1936) The sterility in rabbits produced by injection of oestrone and related compounds. *Amer. J. Physiol.* **115:** 219–228.

PINCUS, G., BANIK, U. K. and JACQUES, J. (1964) Further studies on implantation inhibitors. *Steroids* **4:** 657–676.

PRESL, J., JIRÁSEK, J., HORSKÝ, J. and HENZL, M. (1966) Effect of early postnatal oestrogen administration on pituitary cytology in the adult female rat. *J. Endocr.* **34:** 409–410.

PSYCHOYOS, A. (1966) Influence of oestrogen on the loss of the zona pellucida in the rat. *Nature* **211:** 864.

PSYCHOYOS, A. and COURRIER, M. R. (1962) Le déterminisme de l'ovoimplantation. *C.R. Acad. Sci. (Paris)* **255:** 775–777.

PURSHOTTAM, N., MASON, M. M. and PINCUS, G. (1961) Induced ovulation in the mouse and the measurement of its inhibition. *Fertil. and Steril.* **12:** 346–352.

RIDDLE, O. and TANGE, M. (1928) The physiology of reproduction in birds. XXV. The action of the ovarian and placental hormone in the pigeon. *Amer. J. Physiol.* **87:** 97–109.

ROY, S., MAHESH, V. B. and GREENBLATT, R. B. (1964) Effects of clomiphene on the physiology of reproduction in the rat. II. Its oestrogenic and anti-oestrogenic action. *Acta Endocr. (Kbh.)* **47:** 657–668.

RUDEL, H. W. and KINCL, F. A. (1966) The biology of anti-fertility steroids. *Acta Endocr. (Kbh.).* **51:** Suppl. 105.

SAUNDERS, F. J. (1965) Effects on the course of pregnancy of norethynodrel with mestranol (Enovid®) administered to rats during early pregnancy. *Endocrinology* **77:** 873–878.

SAUNDERS, F. J. and DRILL, V. A. (1958) Some biological activities of 17-ethynyl and 17-alkyl derivatives of 17-hydroxy estrenones. *Ann. N.Y. Acad. Sci.* **71:** 516–530.

SAUNDERS, F. J. and RORIG, K. (1964) Separation of antifertility and classic estrogenic effects. *Fertil. Steril.* **15:** 202–205.

SCHLOUGH, J. S. and MEYER, R. K. (1965) Effect of antiestrogens on estrogen-induced ova implantation in the ovariectomized rat. *Fertil. Steril.* **16:** 106–112.

SCHOELLER, W., DOHRN, M. and HOHLWEG, W. (1936) The superiority of the female sex hormone to the male sex hormone in its action on the male and female hypophysis. *Klin. Wschr.* **15:** 1907–1908.

SCHOFIELD, B. M. (1962) The effect of injected oestrogen on pregnancy in the rabbit. *J. Endocr.* **25:** 95–100.

SEGAL, S. J. and NELSON, W. O. (1958) An orally active compound with antifertility effects in rats. *Proc. Soc. Exp. Biol. (N.Y.)* **98:** 431–436.

SEGAL, S. J. and NELSON, W. O. (1961) Antifertility activity of chloramiphene. *Anat. Rec.* **139:** 273 (Abst.).

SELYE, H., COLLIP, J. B. and THOMPSON, D. L. (1935) Age factor in responsiveness to gonadotropic hormones. II. Effect of estrin on ovaries and adrenals. *Proc. Soc. Exp. Biol. (N.Y.)* **32:** 1377–81.

SHIPLEY, E. G. (1962) Anti-gonadotropic steroids, inhibition of ovulation and mating, Chap. 5. In: *Methods in Hormone Research*. Dorfman, R. I. (Ed.). Academic Press, New York.

SMITH, J. C. and NALBANDOV, A. V. (1958) The role of hormones in the relaxation of uterine portion of the cervix in swine. *Amer. J. Vet. Res.* **19**: 15.

SMITH, M. G. (1926) On the interruption of pregnancy in the rat by the injection of ovarian follicular extracts. *Bull. Johns Hopkins Hosp.* **39**: 203–214.

SPENCER, J., GUSTAVSON, R. G. and D'AMOUR, F. E. (1931) Effects of estrin injections on the growth curve of young rats. *Proc. Soc. Exp. Biol. (N.Y.)* **28**: 500–501.

STAPLES, R. E. (1966) Effect of clomiphene on blastocyst nidation in the rat. *Endocrinology* **78**: 82–86.

STARKEY, W. F. and LEATHEM, J. H. (1939) Action of estrone on sexual organs of immature male cats. *Anat. Rec.* **75**: 85.

STEINBERGER, E. and DUCKETT, G. E. (1965) Effect of estrogen or testosterone on maintenance of spermatogenesis in the rat. *Endocrinology* **76**: 1184–1189.

STONE, G. M. and EMMENS, C. W. (1964a) The action of oestradiol and dimethyl stilbestrol on early pregnancy and deciduoma formation in the mouse. *J. Endocr.* **29**: 137–145.

STONE, G. M. and EMMENS, C. W. (1964b) The effect of oestrogens and anti-oestrogens on deciduoma formation in the rat. *J. Endocr.* **29**: 147–157.

SWELHEIM, T. (1965) The influence of a single high dose of oestradiol benzoate on the ICSH-content in the serum of gonadectomized male and female rats. *Acta Endocr. (Kbh.)* **49**: 231–238.

TAKASUGI, N. (1954) Veränderungen der hypophysären, gonadotropen Aktivität der reifen, weiblichen Ratten, denen von Geburt an zwei gemischten Arten von hormonischen Steroiden injiziert wurden. *J. Fac. Sci. (Tokyo) Imp. Univ. Sec. IV*, **7**: 153–159.

TAKASUGI, N. and BERN, H. A. (1962) Crystals and concretions in the vaginae of persistent-estrus mice. *Proc. Soc. Exp. Biol. (N.Y.)* **109**: 622–624.

TAVOLGA, M. C. (1949) Differential effects of estradiol, estradiol benzoate and pregnenolone on *Platypoecilius maculatus*. *Zoologica* **34**: 215–237.

THOMSON, J. L. (1968) Effect of two non-steroidal antifertility agents on pregnancy in mice. *J. Reprod. Fertil.* **15**: 223–231.

WALLACE, C. (1949). The effects of castration and stilbestrol treatment on the semen production of the boar. *J. Endocr.* **6**: 205.

WATNICK, A. S., GIBSON, J., VINEGRA, M. and TOLKSDORF, S. (1964) Ethynyl estradiol: a potent orally active contraceptive in rats. *Proc. Soc. Exp. Biol. (N.Y.)* **116**: 343–347.

WEICHERT, C. K. (1942) The experimental control of prolonged pregnancy in the lactating rat by means of estrogens. *Anat. Rec.* **83**: 1–17.

WESTMAN, A. and JACOBSOHN, D. (1938) Endokrinologische Untersuchungen an Ratten mit durchtrenntem Hypophysenstiel. III. Uber die luteinisierende Wirkung des Follikelhormons. *Acta Obstet. Gynec. Scand.* **18**: 115–123.

WHITNEY, R. and BURDICK, H. O. (1936) Tube locking of ova by oestrogenic substances. *Endocrinology* **20**: 643–647.

WHITNEY, R. and BURDICK, H. O. (1938) Acceleration of the rate of passage of fertilized ova through the Fallopian tubes of rabbits by massive injections of progynon-B. *Endocrinology* **22**: 639.

WHITNEY, R. and BURDICK, H. O. (1939) Effect of massive doses of an estrogen on ova transport in ovariectomized mice. *Endocrinology* **24**: 45–49.

WILSON, J. G. (1943) Reproductive capacity of adult female rats treated prepubertally with estrogenic hormone. *Anat. Rec.* **86**: 341–359.

CHAPTER 34

ORAL CONTRACEPTIVES. HUMAN FERTILITY STUDIES AND SIDE EFFECTS

Harry W. Rudel and Fred A. Kincl

Biological Concepts Inc., New York

A. HUMAN FERTILITY STUDIES

1. INTRODUCTION

Although the development of oral contraceptives coincided with public awareness of a world-wide population explosion, this method of control has not been applied to areas of great need. Rather, it is in the sophisticated societies of Europe and America, where contraceptive practices are well established, that the oral contraceptives find increasing acceptance. Consequently, as the physician assumes his role in family planning, these methods have greater importance in his pharmacologic armamentarium than in a public health program sponsored for the underprivileged.

Reviewed here is the current status of hormonal agents used clinically in fertility control. In many instances, the reviewers were faced with the difficulty of selecting references for statements made. There is no lack of publications in the oral-contraceptive field but observations are not always made under similar conditions or evaluated by acceptable statistical methods. Since the development of these drugs was done mostly in the United States and Great Britain, overwhelmingly these reports have their origins there.

2. GENERAL PRINCIPLES

Regulation of reproductive function by hormones is not a very recent idea. About a quarter of a century ago, Sturgis and Albright (1940), using estrogens, proposed the basic concept of ovulation suppression and suggested that estrogens might provide symptomatic relief of dysmenorrhea. Shortly thereafter, Lyon (1943) demonstrated that ethynyl estradiol

0.05 mg, given orally from day 4 or 5 to day 25 of the menstrual cycle, inhibited ovulation and temporarily controlled symptoms of intractable primary dysmenorrhea. However, it was generally accepted that the estrogens allowed for "pituitary escape", and therefore failed to consistently control ovulation. Thus, in the earlier research, their value as antifertility agents was overlooked. Unfortunately, this belief was not based upon direct studies on ovulation, but rather on the more obtuse observation that the symptoms of dysmenorrhea recurred while patients were still receiving cyclic stilbestrol therapy.

Later, when Pincus and his group turned their attention to fertility control, they undertook studies first with progesterone and, later, with certain synthetic progestogens. Makepeace *et al.* (1937) and later Pincus and Chang (1953) had shown that progesterone inhibited ovulation in rabbits. In the first clinical studies, progesterone in large oral daily doses was antiovulatory in humans but failed to give adequate cycle control (Pincus, 1956).

Shortly thereafter, Pincus *et al.* (1956) showed that two 19-nor progestogens,* norethynodrel and norethindrone, both containing an estrogen contaminant (mestranol), inhibited ovulation in the rabbit. Later, Pincus and Rock (1958) demonstrated ovulation suppression in women with combinations of the same estrogen and progestogens. This became so well established as a method of contraception that the estrogen–progestogen mixture is almost synonymous with oral contraception. Today there are a number of combination products differing as to chemical composition, absolute quantity and proportion of ingredients.

In early studies, ovulation suppression was stressed as the mechanism of fertility control, and, in this respect, the action of progestogens was emphasized. Recognizing that the earlier work did not clearly define the extent of effectiveness of the estrogens in fertility control, Rudel and Martinez-Manautou (1964) and Rudel and Martinez-Manautou (1967) demonstrated that both mestranol and the closely related ethynyl estradiol are capable of consistently inhibiting ovulation from cycle to cycle and, as a sole agent, successfully controlled fertility in limited clinical studies. However, the addition of a progestogen to the last few days of estrogen therapy in each cycle was found to be a more acceptable method since it provided regular withdrawal bleeding. This is the so-called sequential method of contraception.

In sequential therapy, mestranol or ethynyl estradiol must be given in

* Throughout this paper the term progestogen is used to describe compounds having progesterone-like action.

sufficient amounts to suppress ovulation, as this is the only antifertility mechanism operating.

In the "classic pill" (estrogen–progestogen mixtures), the estrogen generally has been used in amounts which regularly inhibit ovulation. The progestogen must be given in amounts which counterbalance the estrogen effects on the endometrium and cervical mucus to gain full advantage of the contraceptive effect of progestogens. These quantities may be enough to inhibit ovulation also.

Although estrogens inhibit ovulation, they produce a proliferative endometrium, an endometrial state which can support pregnancy if there is subsequent ovulation. In addition, under the influence of estrogens, the cervical mucus becomes thin, watery and copious—an excellent environment for good spermatozoal motility and penetration. On the other hand, progestogens have an effect counter to the estrogens; they inactivate the glandular endometrium, and produce a thick, tenacious cervical mucus (cf. p. 265). The effect of varying estrogen–progestogen ratios on tubal motility and egg transport has not been evaluated in women.

Subsequently, it was shown that these progestational effects on the endometrium and cervical mucus could be obtained with doses of progestogens lower than were required to suppress ovulation (Rudel *et al.*, 1965). These smaller doses were also shown to have antifertility properties. Thus, by selecting a suitably small dose of a progestogen to be given on a continuous non-cyclic basis, fertility may be controlled without inhibiting ovulation and, at the same time, permitting normal menstrual cycling. Notwithstanding, the combination of progestogen and estrogen, on the basis of effectiveness, remains the superior method, apparently because it relies upon ovulation suppression as well as antifertility effects peripheral to the ovary.

As we have shown (see above), estrogens *per se* have definite contraceptive potential, but because of certain disadvantages, have not been developed as a method. Currently, three methods of fertility control have evolved, as follows:

1. Cyclic combined estrogen–progestogen.
2. Sequential estrogen and progestogen.
3. Non-cyclic continuous progestogen.

Contraceptive protection with any one of these methods is greater than mechanical techniques.

Although the pendulum of research interest in conception control has swung from progestogens in high doses to combinations of estrogens and progestogens to estrogens and back to progestogens in microgram doses, hormonal fertility control is still a compromise between effectiveness and side effects. One principle must be followed in hormonal contraception—a minimal physiological insult should be imposed in creating this temporary state of infertility. This can be achieved with the smallest possible effective dose of a drug with the smallest number of non-essential interferences with other systems and organs of the body not related to the primary site of the contraceptive action.

3. MECHANISM OF ANTIFERTILITY EFFECTS

In the light of present knowledge, oral contraception is not synonymous with antiovulation. It has been shown from animal experiments that gonadal hormones act by inhibiting the hypothalamic–pituitary axis, tubal transport and nidation (see Chapters 16, 17, and 28). In women, the concentration of plasma LH and, to a lesser extent, FSH rise sharply at mid-cycle. In women using ovulation-inhibiting steroid contraceptives the mid-cycle peak in LH secretion is abolished. In some instances with non-sequential preparations and also possibly dependent on the dose and treatment duration used, both the early follicular phase elevation of serum FSH as well as the mid-cycle LH and FSH peak can be abolished. Other preparations, notably sequential preparations containing an estrogen for 15 days followed by 5 days of an estrogen–progestogen combination, may suppress the early rise in serum FSH levels and the mid-cycle FSH peak and induce erratic peaks in the levels of serum LH. In addition, the effect on the endometrium and cervix uteri may also be of importance. Ovulation suppression, with the progestogen–estrogen mixtures, is the principle method of blocking fertility and probably the sole mechanism involved in the sequential technique. However, it is considerably less important in the low-dose continuous progestogen method. Techniques are adequate to determine ovulation suppression in women but are lacking in sophistication to define the site of action. These techniques are the histologic picture of endometrium, direct visualization of the ovary, excretion pattern of urinary pregnanediol and estrogens, urinary gonadotrophins, and measurements of plasma LH and progesterone. Additional information can be had from basal temperature variations, vaginal cytology and cervical mucus examination.

(a) *Estrogens*

Martinez-Manautou and Rudel (1966) studied a series of synthetic and natural estrogens including mestranol, ethynyl estradiol, stilbestrol,

TABLE 1. ANTIOVULATORY ACTIVITY OF SEVERAL ESTROGENS

Compound	Dose	No. of cases	No. of cycles	Ovulatory cycles
Ethynyl estradiol	20 mcg	10	20	2
	50 mcg	20	40	1*
Ethynyl estradiol 3-methyl ether	20 mcg	10	20	2
	80 mcg	18	60	1
Estradiol	1 mg	4	11	5
	2 mg	10	18	7
	5 mg	10	24	3
Estriol	5 mg	5	7	6
Premarin	1.25 mg	10	18	12
	3.75 mg	15	17	1
Stilbestrol	5 mg	6	12	1
Total		128	247	41

* Secretory endometrium one patient in 12th cycle.

estradiol, estriol, and conjugated estrogens (Table 1). The compounds were given for 20 days beginning on day 5 of the cycle. Urinary pregnanediol determinations were performed on a sample collected between days 19 and 21, using the method of Goldzieher and Nakamura (1962). In this method, a value of 1.2 mg for 24 hours is indicative of ovulation. Biopsies were taken at the end of the treatment cycle. Mestranol 0.08 mg and ethynyl estradiol 0.05 mg gave the most consistent inhibition of ovulation. Jackson *et al.* (1968) obtained inhibition of ovulation in ten out of thirteen patients on 0.05 mg of ethynyl estradiol daily. A daily dose of 0.1 mg produced ovulation inhibition in all the patients studied.

Ovulation suppression with mestranol has also been demonstrated by direct culdoscopic visualization of the ovary (Table 2; Rudel and Martinez-Manautou, 1967).

Studies of urinary gonadotrophin excretion patterns in patients on estrogen therapy have been limited. Vorys *et al.* (1965) determined FSH by the Steelman-Pohley method and LH by the ovarian ascorbic acid depletion method. Conjugated estrogens, ethynyl estradiol and mestranol were studied. Conjugated estrogens in doses of 0.625 to 3.75 mg daily throughout the cycle failed to influence their measurement of FSH. On the other hand, LH excretion patterns were irregular on the higher doses. Ethynyl estradiol 0.05 mg and mestranol 0.08 mg daily decreased FSH excretion. The effect on LH excretion was less clear. The authors suggested that these

TABLE 2. SUPPRESSION OF OVULATION WITH SEQUENTIAL THERAPY
(Mestranol, 0.08 mg/day for 11 days. Mestranol, 0.08 mg, plus chlormadinone 1.0 mg/day for 10 days)

Cycle no.	No. of patients	Culdoscopy	Pregnanediol	Endometrial biopsy
	Pre-treatment control			
1	9	Follicular maturation Corpora lutea	Average level 1.89 mg	Secretory endometrium day 24
	1	No ovarian activity No follicular maturation	Average level 0.33 mg	Proliferative endometrium
	Treatment sequential			
2–4	10	No follicular maturation No corpora lutea	Average level 0.25 mg	Secretory endometrium day 19 (artificial cycle)
	Post-treatment control			
5	10	Follicular maturation Corpora lutea	Average level 1.95 mg	Secretory endometrium day 23

two agents may have stimulated LH production. Their work with conjugated estrogens is in contrast to data published by Rosemberg and Engel (1960) who reported that human hypophyseal gonadotrophin excretions were significantly reduced by daily doses of 2.5 and 5.0 mg of conjugated estrogen. In another study, Stevens and Vorys (1964) and Stevens *et al.* (1968) used graded doses of mestranol (0.1, 0.08, 0.06 mg) and reported that repeated cyclic administration of mestranol suppressed both FSH and LH excretion. Interestingly, a dose of 0.01 mg of mestranol per day had a stimulatory effect on both FSH and LH excretion. Buchholz *et al.* (1964) using ethynyl estradiol 0.06 mg clearly showed a suppression of the cyclic pregnanediol and estrogen excretion and decrease in total urinary gonadotrophin. They also noted monophasic basal temperature curves. Schmidt-Elmendorff and Kopera (1966) reported that a progestogen (lynestrenol, 5 mg per day) inhibited LH excretion. In a combination with mestranol (Lyndiol 2.5) it also decreased FSH excretion.

Nevinny-Stickel (1964) examined basal temperatures in seventeen patients receiving 0.05 to 0.1 mg of mestranol and found that these doses inhibited ovulation. In some of the cycles, ovulation was deferred until the time when medication was withdrawn.* We believe that this might account for some of the method failures with sequential therapy. This will be fully discussed in Section 4a.

In general estrogens, except for the suppression of the pituitary–gonadal axis, are not used as antifertility agents in women. Few investigators recommended the use of estrogens postcoitally to inhibit pregnancy "morning-after pill" (Morris and van Wagenen, 1966; Haspels, 1969). It was presumed that, similarly to what was observed in laboratory animals, high doses of estrogens given postcoitally might interfere with ova transport, or nidation; and preliminary results of clinical studies, usually limited to rape cases, were indicative of contraceptive effect. The usual dose used was 25–50 mg of stilbestrol, or 2–5 mg of ethynyl estradiol started within 48 hours of coitus. More recently, Haspels (personal communication to the Section Editor) has surveyed 800 cases in whom an estrogen had been administered for 5 days postcoitum and only two pregnancies had occurred. These two failures led to a change in the recommendation to the effect that the drug (3–5 mg of ethynylestradiol,

---

* Nevinny-Stickel has also studied 17α-acetoxyprogesterone, 1,2α-methylene-6-chloro-6-dehydro-17α acetoxyprogesterone, 16α-methyl-6-chloro-6-dehydro-17α-acetoxy progesterone, 9α-fluoro-11-hydroxy-16-methylene-17α-acetoxyprogesterone, 16α-allylestrenol, 19-nor-17α-acetoxyprogesterone plus ethynyl estradiol, norethisterone acetate plus ethynyl estradiol.

not 2–5) should be taken within 36 (not 48) hours and perhaps 24 hours postcoitum.

On the other hand, Bačić et al. (1970) found that no abortion is produced in women in whom estrogen treatment is started 32 to 48 days following the first day of the last menstrual period and they suggest that its efficiency as a postcoital contraceptive may be limited to a relatively short period following ovulation and prior to implantation.

(b) *Progestogens*

As in the case with the estrogens, the progestogens also inhibit ovulation, but unlike the estrogens, they produce possibly additional antifertility changes in the endometrium and in the cervical mucus. Taymor and Klibanoff (1962), Taymor (1964), Rudel (1964), Nevinny-Stickel (1964), Rudel et al. (1965), Loraine et al. (1965), Schmidt-Elmendorff and Kopera (1966) have reported on the antiovulatory effect of progestogens using as indices pregnanediol or gonadotrophin excretion and direct ovarian examination. Their data are summarized in Table 3. From this table it is

TABLE 3. ANTIOVULATORY EFFECT OF PROGESTOGENS

Compound studied	Effective dose (mg)	End-point	Reference
Norethindrone acetate	2	Total gonadotrophins, pregnanediol	Loraine et al. (1965)
	2.5	Pregnanediol; LH	Taymor (1964)
	2.5	Pregnanediol	Taymor and Klibanoff (1962)
Norethindrone	2.5	Pregnanediol	Rudel and Kincl (1966)
	0.5	Pregnanediol	Rudel and Kincl (1966)
	0.5	Plasma progesterone, urinary LH, pregnanediol and estrogens	Larsson-Cohn et al. (1970b)
Norethynodrel	2.5	Pregnanediol	Rudel et al. (1965)
Ethinyldiol diacetate	2.0	LH	Vorys et al. (1965)
Chlormadione acetate	1–2	Pregnanediol	Nevinny-Stickel (1964)
	1–4	Pregnanediol	Rudel and Kincl (1966)
Lynestrenol	5.0	Pregnanediol, LH	Schmidt-Elmendorff and Kopera (1966)

clear that the progestogens commonly used in oral contraceptive mixtures are capable, in themselves, of inhibiting ovulation. That the inhibition is mainly due to suppression of mid-cycle LH peak follows from the work of Taymor (1964), Brown et al. (1964, 1966) and McCormick et al. (1968). During short-term therapy, FSH excretion appears not to be affected (Brown et al., 1962). Stevens et al. (1968) found a variable suppression of both FSH and LH in patients treated with 2 mg of chlormadinone acetate daily. There are no data with more prolonged cyclic treatment. This is unfortunate since there is indirect evidence indicating that follicular development may persist for up to 2 months (Starup and Østergaard, 1966). It was found that ovulation could be stimulated with human chorionic gonadotrophin in patients treated for 2 months, but it was not possible in patients receiving such therapy for more than two cycles.

Ovulation suppression by progestogens is dose dependent. Chlormadinone acetate 2 or 4 mg daily was inhibitory in most cases and the antiovulatory effect of 4 mg differed significantly from 1 mg ($p = 0.05$) (Rudel and Kincl, 1966). Chlormadinone acetate in daily doses of 0.5 mg failed to inhibit ovulation in up to 92% of the patients treated as seen by direct observation of the ovary, endometrial biopsy and urinary pregnanediol excretion patterns (Martinez-Manautou et al., 1967). Measurements of plasma progesterone and the urinary excretion of LH, pregnanediol and total estrogens support the findings that ovulation is inhibited only infrequently with a dose of 0.5 mg daily (Diczfalusy et al., 1969; Orr and Elstein, 1969; Larsson-Cohn et al., 1970c). Norethindrone is similar in this respect to chlormadinone acetate although it would appear to be more potent. The incidence of ovulation suppression does not differ from 0.5 mg and 10.0 mg of norethindrone, whereas 0.1 mg daily inhibited ovulation in only three of twelve women. Suppression of urinary pregnanediol excretion and endometrial biopsies were used to judge treatment effect (Rudel, 1967). Larsson-Cohn et al. (1970a, b) assessed the inhibitory activity of 0.3 mg and 0.5 mg daily dose of norethindrone in several patients. Daily determinations of plasma level of progesterone and the urinary excretion of LH, total estrogens and pregnanediol were the endpoints. All the patients receiving a dose of 0.3 mg showed signs of luteal activity, but the levels of progesterone and pregnanediol were lower than during the corresponding control cycles. Estrogen excretion was not affected. A daily dose of 0.5 mg resulted in abolished mid-cycle LH peak but basal LH excretion remained apparently normal. Diczfalusy et al. (1969) found complete suppression of urinary excretion of LH, pregnanediol and estrogens in patients receiving 2.5 mg daily.

In addition to inhibiting ovulation, progestogens may suppress the estrogen-controlled endometrial glandular development when given from the beginning of the cycle for 20 or more days. Rudel et al. (1967) have shown that this effect, which they call antiestrogenic, is directly proportional to the dose of the progestogen used. In their assay measuring the relative antiestrogenic potency of progestogens, norethindrone was found to be about 3 times as potent as chlormadinone acetate even though chlormadinone acetate is 5 times more active than norethindrone from the standpoint of inducing secretory activity in the preformed glands. This confirms the non-parallelism of antiestrogenic and progestational activity seen earlier in animal tests (Dorfman and Kincl, 1963). The endometrial antiestrogenic assay is useful in selecting the dose of progestogen in progestogen–estrogen combination products. Originally, this was based upon the secretory potency of the progestogen. We now believe that inhibition of glandular proliferation is more important. It has been generally accepted that endometrial inactivation would adversely affect nidation, though this has not been proven in the human. In animals, at any rate (see Chapter 6), it is essential that the endometrium be in phase with the ovary. It is true that nidation is able to take place outside the uterus under conditions quite different from those offered by a secretory endometrium, but whether this indicates that it would be equally possible inside the uterus in an out-of-phase endometrium is an unanswered question. We personally hold the opinion that these endometrial changes are important to antifertility action but that they may be influencing reproductive function prior to fertilization perhaps through such mechanism as capacitation.

Antiestrogenic activity may determine the dose of progestogen useful for the suppression of hyperplastic endometria and perhaps even for the hormonal management of dysmenorrhea. It is also important in selecting the upper limit of practical dosage for the continuous progestogen method of contraception.

Progestogens cause a thickening in the consistency of the cervical mucus usually associated with a decreased motility of spermatozoa when visualized postcoitally. This has been seen with doses of chlormadinone acetate which are less than those required to inhibit endometrial development or ovulation (Rudel et al., 1965; Rudel and Martinez-Manautou, 1967). It is not known to what degree these changes in the cervical mucus are hostile to fertility. No definitive study has been made to see if spermatozoa are physically trapped, in part or in toto, in this viscid mucus or if they are biochemically modified.

(c) *Progestogen–estrogen combination*

A number of authors have reported that the combination of estrogens and progestogens inhibits ovulation using such end-points as pregnanediol excretion, direct visualization of the ovaries, total gonadotrophins, the inhibition of the mid-cycle rise of LH and endometrial biopsies. Since almost all of these agents produce a basal temperature rise due to their progestogen component, this end-point has not been utilized for the determination of ovulation suppression. Inhibition of urinary pregnanediol excretion with combined progestogen–estrogen therapy has been studied by Pincus (1959), Brown *et al.* (1962), and Goldzieher *et al.* (1962, 1964).

Fresh corpora lutea in the ovary have been shown to be absent in women treated with these compounds by Rock *et al.* (1957), Matsumoto *et al.* (1960), Lauweryns and Ferin (1964) and Ryan *et al.* (1964).

Feldman and Carter (1960), Martin and Cunningham (1961), Buchholz *et al.* (1962, 1964), Lin *et al.* (1964), Taymor (1964) and Starup (1966) all found decreases in total urinary gonadotrophin excretion in such patients. Inhibition of LH output has been demonstrated by the use of immunological assay methods (Brown *et al.*, 1964; Wide *et al.*, 1965; Orr and Elstein, 1969). On the other hand, Matsumoto *et al.* (1960), Rosemberg and Engel (1960), Albert and Smith (1961), Brown and Billewicz (1962) and Loraine *et al.* (1965) could not detect any decrease in urinary gonadotrophin. According to Diczfalusy (1965) the reason for these conflicting results lies in the very nature of the biological test employed. The end-points used to estimate total gonadotrophins respond to both FSH and LH. Furthermore, no correlation is possible in assays where different strains of animals react differently to the same FSH/LH ratios. Thus, if LH, but not FSH, output is inhibited, one strain more sensitive to LH may indicate a decreased output of "total gonadotrophins", whereas estimation in animals more sensitive to FSH could show unchanged urinary gonadotrophin levels.

Another explanation may lie in the experimental design used by several investigators. Starup (1966) found that in patients using a combination of megestrol acetate and mestranol, a marked suppression of gonadotrophins occurred after 20 to 60 days of treatment. This observation has been extended by Starup and Østergaard (1966), who found that human chorionic gonadotrophin alone was able to stimulate ovulation during the first 2 months of therapy with megestrol acetate and ethynyl estradiol. After 2 months of therapy, only a combination of PMS plus human chorionic gonadotrophin was able to evoke ovulation. This clearly demonstrates that the ovarian follicle may persist for 60 days and be responsive to luteinizing hormone or its equivalent during that time. After this, the follicle regresses and the ovary requires stimulation with FSH as well as chorionic gonadotrophin or LH to produce follicular development and ovulation. Thus, it may be that one would not see suppression of total gonadotrophin excretion in the first cycle of treatment.

Direct ovarian inhibition by progestogens or estrogens would appear unimportant in ovulation suppression, even though Loraine *et al.* (1965) and Staemmler (1964) failed to show inhibition of total urinary gonadotrophin excretion with norethindrone acetate and suggested that these agents inhibit ovulation at the ovarian level rather than at the pituitary–hypothalamic axis. Also, Lunenfeld *et al.* (1963) and Hecht-Lucari (1964) reported suppressed ovarian reaction to HCG. Subsequently, work by Johannison *et al.* (1965) showed conclusively that the ovary under treatment with combination preparations would respond to human hypophysial (HHG) or menopausal gonadotrophin (HMG) followed by human chorionic gonadotrophin (HCG). It should be pointed out that this experiment does not rule out a reduction in ovarian sensitivity since there has never been established a human ovarian response curve to varying doses of HHG or HMG and HCG. The interaction of the combination of estrogens and the progestogens on the hypothalamic–pituitary axis and their eventual effect on ovulation suppression has not been studied quantitatively. It is not known whether these agents maintain their separate actions on the hypothalamus and pituitary or whether they have synergistic or antagonistic effects.

Interaction between progestogen and estrogen can be demonstrated at both the endometrial and cervical mucus levels. We have shown (Maqueo *et al.*, 1963) that in general the progestational component of these mixtures predominates in its effect in the endometrium, producing an inactive glandular state. However, as progestogen dosage is reduced, the estrogen effect becomes more obvious and may actually predominate over the progestogen (Rudel *et al.*, 1965).

The same type of interaction is also manifested in the cervical mucus. Again, if the progestational component is reduced in the combination agent, the estrogenic effect will prevail. Jackson (1963) has shown that the cervical mucus has an estrogenic quality being plentiful with motile spermatozoa in patients receiving norethynodrel 5 mg plus mestranol 0.75 mg or norethynodrel 2.5 mg plus mestranol 0.1 mg. Similar observations were made by Greenblatt (1961) and Jackson (1961). If the full contraceptive potential of the combination products is to be realized, the antiestrogenic action of the progestogen must prevail over the estrogen component at all reproductive endorgans distal to the ovary.

4. DATA ON INDIVIDUAL PREPARATIONS

This section summarizes data on individual preparations. In so far as was possible, information on effectiveness has been taken from aggregate data given in manufacturers' reports (package inserts). Only when such information was not readily available, individual reports from various investigating groups were included separately. Composition of various contraceptive agents presently used is listed in Tables 4a and 4b.*

(a) Effectiveness

It is generally agreed that hormonal methods offer the most complete control of fertility of any method to date. Fertility may be expressed as an index or rate of pregnancy per 100 woman years of exposure (Pearl, 1932). This is calculated by determining the number of pregnancies in a given population, preferably over a 1-year period of exposure, multiplying this by 1200 and dividing it by the woman months of observation. This may be expressed as follows:

$$P.R. = \frac{N_p \times 1200}{N_w \times M_e}$$

where
- P.R. = pregnancy rate,
- N_p = number of pregnancies,
- N_w = number of women,
- M_e = number of months of exposure.

The unprotected rate varies with given populations, but it is thought to be between 70 and 100 (Tietze *et al.*, 1950). The authors point out that these figures are based upon observation in the total population, including postpuerperal amenorrheic and lactating women. Further, a population made up of couples practicing contraception retains its high fecundity since it is not subjected to losses of more fecund couples by spontaneous pregnancy. There is, in this group, a chance of conception per month of 0.26, or one in four. Therefore, the use of pregnancy rates of 70–100 as a basis of comparison may not adequately express the clinical effectiveness of a contraceptive method.

* Compiled in 1968 and modified as of August 1971; trade names given may not cover all the various preparations sold throughout the world.

TABLE 4a. Composition of Various Steroid Contraceptives

Abbreviations: EE = ethynyl estradiol; MEE = mestranol.
When the manufacturer uses various names for identical preparations in different countries only those used in most countries are given.

Tablet composition (mg)		No. tablets in package	Firm	Product name
Progestogen	Estrogen			
Chlormadinone acetate (2)	MEE (0.05)	21	Polfa (Poland)	Femigen
Chlormadinone acetate (3)	MEE (0.1)	21	Bracco (Italy)	Gestamestrol
		20	Jenapharm (E. Germany)	Ovosisten
		21	Merrell (U.S.A.)	Nogestin
Ethynodiol diacetate (0.5)	EE (0.05)	21	Searle (U.S.A.)	Ovulen 0.5/50
Ethynodiol diacetate (0.5)	MEE (0.1)	21	Searle (U.S.A.)	Ovulen 0.5 } also available with 7 placebos
Ethynodiol diacetate (1)	EE (0.05)	21	Searle (U.S.A.)	Ovulen 1/50
Ethynodiol diacetate (1)	MEE (0.1)	21	Ferran (Spain)	Ovulen 21
Ethynodiol diacetate (1)	MEE (0.08)	21	Searle (U.S.A.)	Prandiol
Ethynodiol diacetate (2)	MEE (0.1)	20	Areana (Austria)	Ovulen
Ethynodiol diacetate (1)	MEE (0.1)	21(?)	Richter (Hungary)	Alfames
		21	Farmila (Italy)	Bisecurin
		20	Serono (Italy)	Etinodiene
Lynestrenol (1)	MEE (0.1)	22	Organon (Holland)	Luteolas
		22	Ciba (Switzerland)	Ovostat
				Anacyclin 101, Microcyclin (also available with 6 placebos)
Lynestrenol (2.5)	EE (0.05)	22	Organon (Holland)	Lyndiol (new formula), Minilyn
Lynestrenol (2.5)	MEE (0.075)	22	Organon (Holland)	Lyndiol 2.5†, Ovariostat
		20	Ciba (Switzerland)	Noracicline 22, Anacyclin 22
Lynestrenol (5	MEE (0.15)	22	Organon (Holland)	Lyndiol (old formula)
		20	Ciba (Switzerland)	Anacyclin, Noracycline
Medroxyprogesterone acetate (2)	EE (0.075)	20	Farmitalia (Italy)	Estrofarlutal
		20	Proquifar (Brazil)	Ciclofarlutal
		20	Majer-Meyer (Brazil)	Ciclobon
Medroxyprogesterone acetate (4)	EE (0.06)	20	Farmochimico (Italy)	Aliben
Medroxyprogesterone acetate (5)	EE (0.05)	20	Farmitalia (Italy)	Ciclofarlutal
		20(?)	Farmila (Italy)	Regulene
Medroxyprogesterone acetate (10)	EE (0.05)	21	Ikapharm (Israel)	Nogest
		20	Leo (Denmark)	Gestovex
		20	Lovens (Sweden)	Protex
		20	Upjohn (U.S.A.)	Provest, Provestral
Megestrol acetate (2)	EE (0.1)	21	BDH (U.K.)	Nuvacon, Volidan-V
		21	Carlo Erba (Italy)	Nofer
		21	Glaxo (U.K.)	Co-Ervonum

† Replaced by Lyndiol (new formula), simply called syndiol as of May 1972.

Contraceptives: Human Fertility Studies and Side Effects

Compound (mg)	Estrogen	Refs	Manufacturer (Country)	Trade names
Megestrol acetate (4)	EE (0.05)	20, 21	BDH (U.K.)	Volidan (−21), Volplan, Voldys
		21	Novo (Denmark)	Planovin, Neo-Delpregnin
		20	Herbrand (W. Germany)	Agenoral
		21	Teva (Israel)	Anova
		21	Maggioni (Italy)	Arnile
		21	Yamanouchi (Japan)	Noval
		20	Glaxo (U.K.)	Ovucal
		21	Inibsa (Spain)	Ovulsin
		20	Lepetit (Italy)	Plamiden
		21	Meiji Seika (Japan)	Sapilon
			Weimer (W. Germany)	Weradys
Megestrol acetate (5)	MEE (0.1)	20, 21	Novo (Denmark)	Delpregnin
Norethisterone (0.5)	MEE (0.1)	21	Ortho (U.S.A.)	Ortho-Novum 0.5, Novulon 0.5 } (also with 7 placebos)
Norethisterone (1)	MEE (0.05)	20, 21	Syntex (U.S.A.)	Norinyl-1
		20, 21	Ortho (U.S.A.)	Ortho-Novum 1/50
		21	Atral (Portugal)	Anogenil
		21	Grémy-Longuet (France)	Nor-50
		20	Shionogi (Japan)	Norluten D1
		21	Recordati (Italy)	Regovar 1
Norethisterone (1)	MEE (0.08)	20, 21	Ortho (U.S.A.)	Ortho-Novum 1/80 } (also with 7 placebos)
		21	Syntex (U.S.A.)	Norinyl 1/80
		21	Ortho (U.S.A.)	Conlunett-21
Norethisterone (1)	MEE (0.1)	21		Ortho-Novum 1/100
		21		Oralestrin 1
Norethisterone (2)	EE (0.05)	21	Lääke (Finland)	Econ
Norethisterone (2)	MEE (0.1)	20, 21	Ortho (U.S.A.)	Ortho-Novum 2, Novulon
		20, 21	Syntex (U.S.A.)	Norinyl 2 (also with 7 placebos)
		21	Astra (Sweden)	Conluten
		20	Hormona (Mexico)	Noralestrin, Noralutin E, Oralestrin
		20	Shionogi (Japan)	Norluten D2
		21	Vita (Spain)	Ovulen novum
		20	Westmont (Philippines)	Ovutrol
		20	DAK (Denmark)	Plan
Norethisterone (3)	MEE (0.1)	21	Teikoku Zoki (Japan)	Sophia-C
Norethisterone (5)	MEE (0.05)	20	Orma (Italy)	Trofinor
Norethisterone (5)	MEE (0.075)	21	Shionogi (Japan)	Norluten D
Norethisterone acetate (0.5)	EE (0.05)	20, 21	Ortho (U.S.A.)	Ortho-Novum 5
Norethisterone acetate (1)	EE (0.05)	20, 21	Gutis (Costa Rica)	Proter
			Parke-Davis (U.S.A.)	Orlest, Norlestrin 1 (also with 7 placebos) (also with 7 iron tabs.)
			Schering (W. Germany)	Anovlar 1, Minovlar, Milli-Anovlar (also with 7 placebos)
Norethisterone acetate (2.5)	EE (0.05)	20, 21	Parke-Davis (U.S.A.)	Etalontin, Norlestrin, Orlestrin (also with 7 placebos) (also with 7 iron tabs.)

(continued overleaf)

TABLE 4a—cont.

Tablet composition (mg)		No. tablets in package	Firm	Product name
Progestogen	Estrogen			
Norethisterone acetate (3)	EE (0.05)	21	Schering (W. Germany)	Anovlar 3, Gynovlar
Norethisterone acetate (4)	EE (0.05)	20, 21	Schering (W. Germany)	Anovlar
Norethisterone acetate (4)	MEE (0.1)	21	Vita (Spain)	Ovulen 3 S
Norethynodrel (2.5)	EE (0.05)	21	Roussel (France)	Sinovaryl
Norethynodrel (2.5)	MEE (0.1)	20, 21	Searle (U.S.A.)	Conovid-E, Enavid-E
		21	Cimex (Pakistan)	Anoryol
		20	Lafar (El Salvador)	Cicolfar
		20	Valeas (Italy)	Elan
		20	Richter (Hungary)	Infecundin
		21	Chinoin (Mexico)	Kebal
		21	Desbergers (Canada)	Novinol
		22	Adam (Australia)	Oralyn 22
		21	Fher (Spain)	Ovarion
		20, 21	Roussel (France)	Previson
		25	Farbar (Mexico)	Sin-Conse
Norethynodrel (3)	MEE (0.075)	21	Rendell (U.K.)	Norolen
Norethynodrel (4.925)	MEE (0.075)	20	Byla (France)	Enidrel
Norethynodrel (5)	MEE (0.075)	20	Waco (Argentina)	Regulador
		20	Searle (U.S.A.)	Conovid, Enavid
		20	Infan (Mexico)	Neo-Andril
		20	SAM (Italy)	Norigen
i-Norgestrel (0.25)	EE (0.05)	21	Wyeth (U.S.A.)	Stediril-d, Nordiol
d,l-Norgestrel (0.5)	EE (0.05)	21	Schering (W. Germany)	Neogynon
		21	Wyeth (U.S.A.)	Ovral, Stediril
		21	Schering (W. Germany)	Eugynon, Primovlar
		21	Fontoura (Brazil)	Anfertil
		21	Recip (Sweden)	Follinyl
		21	Ido (Denmark)	Gentrol
Norgestrienone (0.5)	EE (0.05)	21	Roussel (France)	Miniplanor
Norgestrienone (2)	EE (0.05)	21	Roussel (France)	Planor
Quingestanol acetate (0.5)	EE (0.05)	21	Apothkernes Lab. (Norway)	Piloval
		21	Warner-Chilcott (U.S.A.)	Riglovis
Superlutin (5)		21	Vister (Italy)	Reglovis
Vinylestrenolone (1)	MEE (0.1)	20	Spofa (Czechoslovakia)	Antigest
Vinylestrenolone (2.5)	EE (0.1)	21	Richter (Italy)	Vestaline-1
Vinylestrenolone (5)	EE (0.1)	21	Richter (Italy)	Vestaline M
	EE (0.075)	20	Richter (Italy)	Vestaline

(also with 7 placebos)
Note: Eugynon-28 starts on day 1 of the menstrual cycle

Products containing chlormadinone acetate were withdrawn by most manufacturers from most markets. Products listed here were commercially available at least in some countries at the time of composing this table.

Contraceptives: Human Fertility Studies and Side Effects 401

TABLE 4b

Sequentials: first course begins on day (—) of menstrual cycle

Compounds	Number of tablets	Firm	Product name
MEE (0.1) / Chlormadinone acetate (1.5) — MEE (0.1)	14 / 7	Lilly (U.S.A.)	C-quens 21, Sequens 21 (day 5)
EE (0.05) / Chlormadinone acetate (2) — EE (0.05)	11 / 10	Latino (Spain) (Syntex)	Normotonal (day 5)
MEE (0.08) / Chlormadinone acetate (2) — MEE (0.08)	15 / 5	Roussel (France)	Menol (day 5)
	15 / 5	Lilly (U.S.A.)	C-quens, Sequens (day 5)
MEE (0.08) / Chlormadinone acetate (2) — MEE (0.08)	16 / 5	Syntex (U.S.A.) / Warner-Chilcott (U.S.A.)	Secuentex, Alternyl (day 5) / Lutoral (day 5)
Chlormadinone acetate (2) — MEE (0.08)	15 / 5	Lääke (Finland)	Sekvecon (day 5)
Chlormadinone acetate (2) — MEE (0.08)	6 / 15	Syntex (U.S.A.)	Secuentex 21 (day 5) (also + 7 placebos)
Chlormadinone acetate (2) — MEE (0.08)	11 / 10	Syntex (U.S.A.)	Sequental (day 5)
EE (0.1) / Dimethisterone (25)	16 / 5	Recordati (Italy) (Syntex) / Teva (Israel) / Warner-Chilcott (U.S.A.)	Fisiosequil (day 5) / Madinon-S (day 5) / Syncrocept (day 5)
	16 / 5	Mead Johnson (U.S.A.)	Oracon, Ovin (day 5) (also + 7 placebos)
MEE (0.1) / Ethynodiol diacetate (0.5) — MEE (0.08)	11 / 10	British Drug Houses (U.K.)	Secrovin (day 5)
Ethynodiol diacetate (1) — MEE (0.08)	14 / 7	Searle (U.S.A.)	Miniquen (day 5)
Hydroxyprogesterone acetate (100?) MEE (0.08)	16 / 5	Elea (Argentina)	Evelea (day 5)
Medroxyprogesterone acetate (10) MEE (0.08)	15 / 5 + 7 placebos	Gador (Argentina)	Hormolidin (day 5)
EE (0.025) / Medroxyprogesterone acetate (10) — EE (0.1)	5 / 7	Gador (Argentina)	Lidestan (day 5)
MEE (0.08)	14 / 7	Upjohn (U.S.A.)	Verafem (day 1)
Lynestrenol (2.5) / EE (0.1)	7 / 15	Organon (Holland)	Ovanon (day 1)
Megestrol acetate (1) — MEE (0.075)	16 / 5	Novo (Denmark)	Novoquens, Menoquens (day 5)
EE (0.1) / Megestrol acetate (5) — EE (0.1) / Megestrol acetate (0.1) — EE (0.1) / Megestrol acetate (1)	16 / 5 / 16 / 7 + 5 placebos	British Drug Houses (U.K.) / Glaxo (U.K.) / Mead Johnson (U.S.A.) / British Drug Houses (U.K.)	Serial 28 (day 5) (+ 7 placebos) / Ovisec (day 5) (+ 7 placebos) / Ovex (day 5) / Serial C (day 3)
MEE (0.05) / Norethisterone (1) — MEE (0.05)	14 / 7	Novo (Denmark) / Asta/Lappe (W. Germany) / Glaxo (U.K.) / Mavi (Mexico)	Kombiquens (day 3) / Oraconal (day 3) / Tri-Ervonum (day 3) / Mestronil (day 5)

TABLE 4b—cont.

Compounds	Number of tablets	Firm	Product name
MEE (0.08) Norethisterone (1) MEE (0.08)	14 7	Hormona (Mexico)	Norace-1 (day 5)
MEE (0.08) Norethisterone (2) MEE (0.08)	14 7	Syntex (U.S.A.)	Norquen (day 5)
MEE (0.08) Norethisterone (2)	14 6	Ortho (U.S.A.)	Novulon "S", Ortho-Novum SQ (day 5)
MEE (0.08)	15	Syntex (U.S.A.)	Norquen 21 (day 5) (also + 7 placebos)
Norethisterone (2) MEE (0.08) MEE (0.08) Norethisterone (2	6 14 7	Hormona (Mexico)	Norace, Frenogest (day 5)
		Ortho (U.S.A.)	Ortho-Novum SQ/21 (day 5)
MEE (0.1) Norethisterone (2) EE (0.1)	14 7 6	Ortho (U.S.A.)	Ortho-Novin SQ (day 5)
Norethisterone (5) MEE (0.1)	15	Grémy-Longuet (France)	Norquential (day 5)
Norethynodrel (2.5) MEE (0.1)	16 5	London Rubber (U.K.)	Feminor 21 (day 5)
Norethynodrel (5) MEE (0.075)	15 5	London Rubber (U.K.)	Feminor Sequential (day 5)
Superlutin 7 MEE (0.075)	15 5	Spofa (Czechoslovakia)	Antigest-B (day ?)
Luteal supplementation products: Chlormadinone acetate (0.5)	35, 42 28, 35 35 42 35	Syntex (U.S.A.) Merck (W. Germany) G. Ramon (Argentina) Dexter (Argentina) Astra/Syntex (Sweden) Ortho (U.S.A.)	Normenon, Retex Nonstop, Urbal Fraslan Cero Concludag, Mini-P Micro-Nor, Micro-Novum
Norethisterone (0.3) Norethisterone (0.35)			
Unidose products: Ethynodiol diacetate (8) quinestrol (5)	1 package-form	Elea (Argentina)	Soluna
Injectable products: Dihydroxyprogesterone acetophenide (75) Estradiol enanthate (10)	1 amp. 1 ml	Nezel (Spain)	Ova-Repos
Dihydroxyprogesterone acetophenide (150) Estradiol enanthate (10)	1 amp. 1 ml	Europharma (Spain)	Topasel
Dihydroxyprogesterone acetophenide (150) Estradiol benzoate (?) (10)	1 amp. 3 ml	Promeco (Mexico) Recalcine (Chile) Emyfar (Spain) Andrade (Portugal)	Perlutal Agurin Primyfar Cicnor
Hydroxyprogesterone caproate (250) Estradiol cyclopentyl propionate (5)	1 amp. 1 ml	Mavi (Mexico)	Sinbios
Hydroxyprogesterone caproate (250) Estradiol valerate (10) Estradiol benzoate (1)	1 amp. 3 ml	Reuffer (Mexico)	Sin-Ol
Medroxyprogesterone acetate (150)	1 amp. 3 ml	Upjohn (U.S.A.) Farmitalia (Italy)	Depo-Provera, Depo-Clinovir Farlutal depot

The Pearl formula combines individuals with short and long durations of use and fails to take into account the duration of contraceptive practice in each individual. This defect may be overcome by using the "life table technique" which shows the size of decreasing population at risk and the percentage of patients protected from unplanned pregnancy during each successive 6-month period of continuous use. The cumulative per cent protected, which is the cumulative multiplication of all preceding percentages, is usually used to express the effectiveness (Potter, 1966; Tietze and Lewit, 1968).

If pregnancy rate is calculated on the basis of the total number of pregnancies for the exposure period not excluding those patients who missed tablets, the resulting index is called *use effectiveness*. Pregnancy rates for 100 woman years for several non-hormonal methods of contraception are as follows (data from: (a) Westoff *et al.*, 1961; (b) Baunach and Baunach, 1964).

Condom	13.8[a]; 14[b]
Diaphragm	14.4[a]; 12[b]
Withdrawal	16.8[a]; 18[b]
Rhythm	38.5[a];
Douche	40.8[a]; 31[b]

The use-effectiveness pregnancy rate for the Lippes Loop, perhaps the most widely used intra-uterine device, is 2.9. This includes pregnancies occurring with the device *in situ* as well as those occurring after unnoticed expulsion (WHO Report, 1966). For the several combination oral-contraceptive agents, the reported use effectiveness varies from 0 to 3.1 (Table 5). From the data represented in this table it would appear that drugs containing norethindrone have lower pregnancy rates than those containing norethynodrel, although one has to bear in mind that they were obtained at different times and by different investigators. It is suggested that the higher antiestrogenic activity of norethindrone compared with that for norethynodrel as is also shown in animal experiments (see Chapter 28) may be a factor in bringing about such a difference. Sequential therapy has a lower use effectiveness pregnancy rate (Table 6) attributed by some investigators to method failure (Mendel and Brannon, 1968). The continuous progestogen method has a pregnancy rate of about 2 to 3.

In addition to use effectiveness the continuation rate is of importance in assessing the impact of oral contraceptives on population growth. Although detailed data are not available several reports indicate that the dropout

TABLE 5. PREGNANCY RATES WITH COMBINED ORAL CONTRACEPTIVES

Progestogen	Dose (mg)	Oestrogen dose (mg)	No. of cycles	Pregnancy rate	Reference
Norethynodrel	10	0.15	9472	2.8	Pincus (1964)
			10,402	2.6	Garcia and Pincus (1964)
	5	0.075	18,949	0.95	Pincus (1964)
			13,741	0.9	Garcia and Pincus (1964)
			3267	0.73	Mears (1964)
	2.5	0.1	2613	1.4	Pincus (1964)
			1278	3.1	Garcia and Pincus (1964)
			2718	0.88	Mears (1964)
Norethindrone	10	0.06	16,808	0.71	Tyler et al. (1964)
			12,543	0.6	Goldzieher and Rice-Wray (1966)
			8812	0.6	Goldzieher and Rice-Wray (1966)
	2	0.1	3902	0.0	Tyler et al. (1964)
			3464	0.3	Goldzieher and Rice-Wray (1966)
			2953	0.0	Goldzieher and Rice-Wray (1966)
	1	0.05	51,544	0.02	Greaney et al. (1968)
Norethindrone acetate	4	0.05	2093	0.0	Mears (1964)
			13,652	0.0	Goldzieher and Rice-Wray (1966)
			11,107	0.76	Kirchhoff and Haller (1964)
Lynestrenol	5.0	0.15	876	1.4	Turpeinen (1964)
	5.0	0.15	9496	0.0	Kopera et al. (1964)
	2.5	0.075	2695	0.46	Goldzieher and Rice-Wray (1966)
	2.5	0.075	4913	0.0	Moses et al. (1969)
Norgestrel	0.5	0.05	49,683	0.0–0.27	Laurie and Lewis (1968)
Ethynodiol diacetate	1	0.1	9931	0.0	Andrews et al. (1966)
			8457	0.43	Holmstrom (1965)

rate may be high. The results of the 1965 National Fertility Study indicate that in the United States one-third of the women who had been taking oral contraceptives since 1960 had discontinued by the autumn of 1965; 80%

TABLE 6. PREGNANCY RATES WITH SEQUENTIAL ORAL CONTRACEPTIVES

Preparation*	No. of cycles	Pregnancy rate	Reference
C-Quens†	201,938	0.96	Goldzieher et al. (1968)
Oracon	57,492	0.23	Sturtevant and Wait (1970)
Ortho-Novum SQ	13,941	<0.1	Tyler et al. (1966)
	2091	0.0	Andrews et al. (1966)
Ovanon	1087	0.0	Rice-Wray et al. (1968)

* See Table 4b for composition.
† Withdrawn from U.S. market in October 1970.

of these had discontinued because of "side effects" connected with the therapy (Westoff and Ryder, 1968). In Asia the dropout rate may be even higher. Mehra et al. (1970) report that cumulative discontinuation per 100 users after 12 months of use was from 28.9 to 52.9% in India, 58.0% in Taiwan, 43.2% in Puerto Rico, 92.4% in Turkey and 24.3% in Ceylon. In Korea the rate was from 40.0 to 57.8% after 6 months of use.

In much of the oral-contraceptive literature, great emphasis is placed upon patient failure or patients missing tablets, and these women are usually excluded from the calculation of the pregnancy rate. This may be unjustified in considering overall effectiveness of a given method since the physician is interested in patients' ability to follow a treatment schedule as well as in the optimal use of the agent in protecting patients from pregnancy. It is difficult to attribute pregnancy to a patient failure if one or two tablets are missed during a cycle, particularly where multiple mechanisms are operating as in combined progestogen–estrogen therapy. As was reported previously (loc. cit.), Starup and Østergaard showed that during the first one or two cycles of treatment, a residual follicle may respond to luteinizing hormone stimulation and ovulate. Thus, tablets missing could be a factor in early cycles of use, but less so in subsequent cycles when the follicles are no longer responsive to luteinizing hormone alone, but require both follicle stimulating as well as luteinizing hormone for full development and ovulation.

If ovulation suppression is the sole mechanism of fertility control, withdrawal of the suppressive agent could allow for follicular development and ovulation by pituitary-gonadotrophin release, resulting in a high pregnancy potential. This may be an important consideration in the method of handling intermenstrual bleeding or failure of withdrawal bleeding. In the former case, some investigators advise the patient to discontinue medication if intermenstrual bleeding occurs in the quantity of a normal menstrual period, to wait for 5 days and begin therapy again. This may actually leave the patient unprotected and allow for an ovulation to occur during the course of medication withdrawal. Similarly, ovulation may ensue if there is a failure of menses after a treatment course, and the patient waits for the menses to occur. For this reason, it is advisable to wait no more than 7 days between tablet courses.

In 1970 two important developments took place. Because of the established relationship between oral contraceptives and thromboembolic diseases, both the British and U.S. regulatory agencies recommended prescriptions of products containing 0.075 mg of "estrogens" or less. In October 1970 chlormadinone acetate with mestranol (C-Quens) and medroxy-progesterone acetate in combination with ethynyl estradiol (Provest) were withdrawn from U.S. markets since chronic toxicity studies in beagles have shown an increased incidence of mammary nodules (Anonymous, 1970; this is discussed in more detail in Section B9). See also Chapter 28, Subsection 24.2).

(b) Literature on combined therapy

Comparative studies on various preparations were reported by Tyler and Olson (1959), Korn (1961), Rice-Wray (1963), Rice-Wray *et al.*, (1963), Satterthwaite (1964) and Mears (1966).

Following is a brief summary on individual preparations, in alphabetical order (for their composition, see Table 4a). Arbitrarily, studies on less than 100 patients were not included in references listed.

Anovlar (Schering A.G., Berlin). No pregnancies were reported in approximately 11,000 cycles, representing about 1700 patients (Bockner, 1963; Devenish-Meares, 1965; Mears, 1963; Rice-Wray *et al.*, 1966, and Schlegelmilch, 1964). Experience in Taiwan has been reported by Lee *et al.*, 1966.

Antigest A (Spofa, Prague, Czechoslovakia). Šterba (1966) reported seventeen pregnancies in 877 patients for a total of 5107 cycles. Of these, ten were attributed to patient failure and seven presumably to the failure of the therapy (Šterba *et al.*, 1965).

Enovid (G. D. Searle & Co., Chicago, Illinois). Reported effectiveness is 0.0 to 1.2. This information is based on studies summarized by Drill (1966) which involved about 11,000 women for a total of about 89,000 cycles (Drill, 1966).

Enovid-E or Conovid (G. D. Searle & Co., Chicago, Illinois). Pregnancy rates from 0.0 to 4.5 (more than 1400 patients and approximately 12,000 cycles) were reported (Drill, 1966).

Lyndiol. Two preparations are available (N.V. Organon, Oss, Holland). Pregnancy rate of 1.4 for the combination containing 5 mg of lynestrenol and 0.15 mg mestranol was reported by Kopera *et al.* (1964) and Turpeinen (1964), who studied a total of 10,372 cycles (2181 patients). A report on the cooperative study on the second perparation (2.5 mg of lynestrenol with 0.075 mg of mestranol) was presented by Strade (1966). A total of 1741 patients was treated for 20,014 cycles. Accidental pregnancies occurred in nineteen women, but eighteen were ascribed to tablet omissions. Moses *et al.* (1969) reported no pregnancies in 268 patients treated for 4913 cycles.

Norinyl 2 (Syntex Laboratories, Inc., Palo Alto, California; also licensed as *Ortho-Novum* to Ortho Pharmaceutical Corp., Raritan, New Jersey). In addition to already listed reports (Table 5) the following studies are of interest: Hutcherson *et al.*, 1963; Rice-Wray, 1963; Rice-Wray *et al.*, 1963; Ringrose and Douglas, 1963; Behrman, 1964; Crocker and Stitt, 1964; Francis, 1964; Matthews, 1964; Merritt, 1964; Newland *et al.*, 1964; Rovinsky, 1964; Tyler, 1964; and Wilson *et al.*, 1967. This preparation is remarkably effective. No pregnancies were reported.

Norinyl 1 (Syntex Laboratories, Inc., Palo Alto, California; also licensed as *Ortho-Novum* 1 to Ortho Pharmaceutical Corp., Raritan, New Jersey). Two preparations are available, one containing 0.05 mg of mestranol, and one 0.08 mg of the same estrogen. The latter is identified as Norinyl 1 + 80. Both are quite effective. Greaney *et al.* (1968) report one pregnancy (probably patient failure) in 51,544 cycles of treatment.

Norlestrin (Parke-Davis and Co., Detroit, Michigan). Two preparations are available, one containing 2.5 mg of norethindrone acetate and 0.05 mg of ethynyl estradiol and one containing 1 mg of the acetate and 0.5 mg of the estrogen. No published reports are available concerning either preparation.

Ovral (Wyeth Laboratories, Philadelphia, Pennsylvania). Results of extensive clinical trials were summarized by Laurie and Lewis (1968, table 5). Five pregnancies, attributed to patient failures, were reported during 49,683 cycles of use. Rice-Wray *et al.* (1968) reported no pregnancies in a smaller study (300 patients, 3175 cycles). Andelman *et al.* (1968) reported three pregnancies attributed to patient failure in 2505 women who completed a total of 24,752 cycles.

Ovulen (G. D. Searle and Co., Chicago, Illinois). Original reports were published by Pincus (1963), Andrews and Andrews (1964), Satterthwaite (1964), and Holmstrom (1965). Subsequent to these, additional reports confirmed the efficacy of this preparation (Andrews *et al.*, 1966; Dahlberg, 1966; Heber, 1968; Holmstrom, 1965; and Puddy, 1967).

Provest (The Upjohn Company, Kalamazoo, Michigan). This preparation has found limited use apparently because of unfavorable effects on menstruation. No unwanted pregnancies were reported by Dingle (1963), Hass (1963), Livingston (1963), Moghissi *et al.* (1963), Sobrero (1963), and Eichner (1964). Recently this product has been withdrawn from the United States market because of the development of breast nodules in beagle dogs.

Volidan (British Drug Houses, Ltd., London, England). Mears (1964) reported one pregnancy (attributed to patient failure) in 178 patients (2100 cycles). Dehejia *et al.* (1967) reported three unwanted pregnancies (patient failure) in a study involving 341 women (2223 cycles).

(*c*) *Sequential therapy*

In the section on estrogens, it was demonstrated that mestranol and the closely related ethynyl estradiol inhibit ovulation when given in a cyclic fashion for 20 days of the month beginning on day 5 of menstruation. It was recognized that the addition of progestogen to the last 5 to 10 days of the estrogen therapy would create a maturation and secretory change in the exogenously produced proliferative endometrium, thereby ensuring a more consistent withdrawal bleeding. This was suggested as a possible method for hormonal fertility control (Rudel and Martinez-Manautou, 1964). The effectiveness of the method in large-scale clinical trials has been demonstrated by Goldzieher *et al.* (1963, 1964). Aydar and Greenblatt, in 1961, used a similar type of preparation containing ethynyl estradiol 0.1 mg as the estrogen for the treatment of dysmenorrhea in fourteen patients for forty courses of therapy. They reported that inhibition of ovulation was successful in these patients, but did not suggest the use of such a method for contraceptive purposes.

This method of oral contraception became known as the sequential therapy. At present, the therapy consists of 15 days' administration of 80–100 mcg of an estrogen, followed by a 5- to 6-day administration of combined estrogen and progestogen. Some investigators (Liggins, 1967; Kamal *et al.*, 1968; Laurie and Lewis, 1968; and Di Saia *et al.*, 1968) recommended the addition of seven placebo tablets to provide the patient with a continuous supply ("a package strip"). Several commercial preparations are available. As already stated, the estrogen must be given in sufficient quantity to inhibit ovulation, the progestogen only in amounts to provoke withdrawal bleeding. Few investigators (Liggins, 1967; Rovinsky, 1968) claimed increased effectiveness by varying the composition of the combined pills, but these reports remain unconfirmed by other studies at this time.

There have been comments on sequential therapy being more physiological than combined estrogen–progestogen contraceptive therapy. It should be noted that any method which inhibits ovulation and pituitary–gonadal function, whether it be estrogen or combinations of estrogen and progestogen, is truly not physiological. This use of the expression "physiological" came about from the fact that, with combined medication, the endometrium was inactive or suppressed following 20 days of therapy. On the other hand, with sequential therapy the endometrium, in the majority of cases, had the appearance of a day-17 or day-19 secretory endometrium, reflecting the 5 or 6 days of progestogen therapy following estrogen priming. Since the estrogen is given for about two-thirds of the cycle unopposed by progestogen, the benefit of the contraceptive effect of the progestogen given throughout the cycle is absent.

Data on individual preparations are summarized below (see also Table 6 and Table 4b for preparation composition). Comparative data on several preparations were given by Balin *et al.* (1969).

Antigest B (Spofa, Prague, Czechoslovakia). Šterba (1966) reported one pregnancy in an aggregate group of 576 patients (a total of 1890 cycles).

C-Quens (Eli Lilly, Indianapolis, Indiana). Large-scale trials in a total of 14,353 cycles in 1486 patients were reported by Goldzieher *et al.*, (1963 and 1964) and Parkinson *et al.* (1966). Goldzieher and Maas (1965) summarized findings of several groups of investigators and reported pregnancy incidence of 1.3 in over 6000 patients representing more than 81,000 cycles. Recently this product has been withdrawn from the United States market because of the development of breast nodules in beagle dogs.

Oracon (Mead Johnson Laboratories, Evansville, Indiana). Young *et al.* (1965) reported one pregnancy, suspected to be a drug failure, in 410 patients (6038 cycles). The results of extensive clinical trials based on evaluation of 5952 patients and 57,492 cycles were reported by Sturtevant and Wait in 1970. There were thirty-seven unplanned pregnancies, or a use effectiveness of 0.77. Of these twenty-six patients admitted failure to follow directions or "method failure" rate of 0.23.

Ortho-Novum SQ (Ortho Pharmaceutical Corporation, Raritan, New Jersey). Newland *et al.* (1966) and Tyler *et al.* (1966) reported two pregnancies in 1038 patients representing 13,941 cycles. Andrews *et al.* (1966) have seen no pregnancy in 294 patients (2091 cycles).

Ovanon (N.V. Organon, Oss, Holland). In this "normophasic" regimen 0.08 mg of mestranol, given for only 7 days, is followed by a combination of 0.075 mg of mestranol and 2.5 mg of lynestrenol, given for 15 days. Rice-Wray *et al.* (1968) reported no pregnancies in 122 women (1087 cycles). Results of a smaller study (99 patients) were reported by Durandeau (1968); apparently, the therapy was fully effective. Everse and Esselink (1970) reported on 857 patients (7066 cycles) with no pregnancy.

Other Preparations

Megestrol acetate (British Drug Houses, Ltd.; Mead Johnson Laboratories) has been used by several investigators. Suran (1967) used 0.1 mg of ethynyl estradiol (16 tablets), followed by a combination of megestrol acetate (5 mg, or 2 mg) and 0.1 mg of the same estrogen (5 tablets). One pregnancy was reported in 208 patients (3240 cycles), i.e. overall pregnancy rate of 0.37. Kamal *et al.* (1968) used a similar sequential preparation, except that the dose of the progestational agent was reduced to 1 mg. Two pregnancies were reported in seventy women (722 cycles). Liggins (1967), on the other hand, used 4 mg of megestrol acetate in a sequential therapy combined either with 0.075 mg, or 0.05 mg of ethynyl estradiol. Estrogen therapy (0.075 mg of ethynyl estradiol) was the same for both. He reported a high pregnancy rate of 6.9 for the first preparation, and even a higher rate, 15.4, for the second. Rozin *et al.* (1966) reported sequential therapy (143 women, 1274 cycles) using mestranol (0.1 mg) and 17α-acetoxy progesterone (100 mg). They report with this preparation a successful inhibition of fertility throughout the period of treatment, which was from 6 to 12 months.

Ethynodiol diacetate (0.5 mg) and ethynyl estradiol (0.1 mg) were used by Shah (1968); the estrogen was given for 10 days, followed by a combined pill, also given for 10 days. No pregnancy was reported in a total of 3000 cycles.

Anagestone, 3-desoxyacetoxymethyl progesterone (6α-methyl-17α-acetoxy-4-pregnen-20-one), was used by Rovinsky (1968). Mestranol (0.08 mg) was given for 16 days, followed by a combination of mestranol and 1 mg or 2 mg of the progestogen. The author reports a pregnancy rate of 1.76 (230 patients, 1362 cycles) for the first preparation, and a rate of 0.25 (444 patients, 4755 cycles) for the second. Wamsteker (1968) described yet another sequential regimen consisting of 0.05 mg of ethynyl estradiol from day 5 through day 14 followed by a combination of the estrogen and 1 mg norethindrone acetate for 11 days. Incidence of pregnancy was reported to be 0.45, and overall incidence of "side effects" not improved (e.g. breakthrough bleeding and spotting 5.2%, nausea 2.0%, weight gain 38%). These data are based on the observation of 964 women who completed a total of 7917 cycles.

(d) Continuous progestogen method

With chlormadinone acetate, the idea of a sensitivity differential was found between dosage and the degree of inhibition of cervical mucus, endometrium and pituitary–ovarian axis (Rudel et al., 1965). In these early studies it was demonstrated that this steroid given without interruption to allow for withdrawal bleeding provided contraceptive protection. Since menses occurred in most patients it was believed that ovulation was not inhibited. Most marked changes were seen in the quality of cervical mucus.

Differences between control cycles and treatment cycles as regards amount, spinnbarkeit, viscosity, transparency and ferning were seen at all dose levels of chlormadinone acetate given in doses of 0.05, 0.1, 0.2, 0.3, 0.4, and 0.5 mg daily; a dose of 0.4 mg produced a near maximal inhibitory change in cervical mucus (Table 7); Gregoire and Ustay (1969) confirmed these findings. The contraceptive efficacy of progestogen therapy in continuous daily doses was likewise dose dependent (Table 8). In these early trials, a dose of 0.5 mg apparently produced a satisfactory antifertility effect (Rudel, 1967).

A dose of 0.5 mg was selected for expanded studies in 945 non-lactating, highly fertile women under 36 years of age (Martinez-Manautou et al., 1967). In 8091 cycles representing 8108 woman months of experience (over 200 patients have been on therapy for 13 months), there were fourteen pregnancies, of which thirteen were associated with a failure to take the medication regularly. The pregnancy rate adjusted for these patient failures is 0.15. The use-effectiveness pregnancy rate, in which all pregnancies are considered, is 2.1. This is similar to results of similar trials with other drugs reported recently (Table 9). It is of interest to note that for one progestogen, megestrol acetate, contraceptive activity was very poor when a conventional tablet was used. This was markedly improved when an oil solution in peanut oil in soft gelatine capsules was substituted for tablets

TABLE 7. PHYSICAL PROPERTIES OF CERVICAL MUCUS IN PATIENTS RECEIVING VARIOUS DOSES OF CHLORMADINONE ACETATE

No. of patients	Dose (mcg)	Amount		Aspect		Viscosity*		Spinnbarkeit		Ferning	
		Normal	Decrease	Transparent	Opaque	Normal	Increase	Normal	Decrease	Normal	Decrease
10	50	3	7	5	5	5	5	8	2	7	3
6	100	2	4	4	2	2	2	3	3	3	3
9	200	1	8	3	6	2	7	3	6	4	5
10	300	0	10	1	9	2	8	3	7	4	6
10	400	0	10	0	10	0	10	0	10	3	7
10	500	0	10	0	10	0	10	0	10	2	8

* Estimated.

TABLE 8. CONTRACEPTIVE EFFECTIVENESS OF VARIOUS DOSES OF CHLORMADINONE ACETATE AND NORETHINDRONE GIVEN CONTINUOUSLY

Dose (mg)	No. of patients	No. of cycles	No. of pregnancies	Pearl's index
Chlormadinone acetate				
0.10	73	164	28	205
0.25	274	2168	22	12.1
0.30	190	1449	11	9.1
0.40	237	1861	8	5.1
0.50	1196	6212	10	1.9
Norethindrone				
0.05	110	384	13	40.6
0.10	146	402	11	32.8
0.20	296	2192	17	9.3
0.25	215	646	3	5.5
0.30	405	2328	7	3.6
0.50	66	329	0	0
1.0	21	66	0	0

(Avendaño et al., 1970). This indicates that this steroid in oil solution may be absorbed by intestinal lacteals and have a different metabolic fate and distribution than when given in aqueous suspension (a tablet) which is presumably absorbed directly into the gastro-intestinal capillary and portal circulatory system.

TABLE 9. PREGNANCY RATES WITH CONTINUOUS PROGESTOGEN ORAL CONTRACEPTIVES

Compound used	Daily dose (mg)	No. of cycles	Pearl index of effectiveness
Chlormadinone acetate*	0.5	8091	2.1[a]
Megestrol acetate	0.5†	599	1.0[b]
	0.5	1290	14.0[b]
Norgestrel	0.05	1500	0.8[c]

* Withdrawn from U.S. market in October 1970.
† In oil solution (soft gelatin capsule).
[a] Martinez-Manautou et al. (1967).
[b] Avendaño et al. (1970).
[c] Foss (1968).

The basis of the antifertility effect seen with continuous progestogen therapy still remains obscure. Results of progesterone plasma determinations and excretion values of urinary gonadotrophins, pregnanediol and

TABLE 10. ENDOMETRIAL RESPONSE

Dose (mg)	Secretory (%)	Irregular secretory (%)	Irregular (%)	Inactive (%)	Proliferative (%)	Total no. of biopsies
Chlormadinone acetate						
0.25	59.4	29.6	4.9	1.2	4.9	81
0.50	30.2	35.1	17.3	6.0	11.4	202
Norethindrone						
0.2	40.0	36.0	6.3	4.6	13.1	175
0.3	30.3	32.4	14.1	13.1	10.1	99
Megestrol acetate						
0.25	39.6	37.5	14.6	0	3.3	48
0.50	39.1	52.2	6.5	0	2.2	46
0.50 (oil)	24.0	60.0	0.0	4	12.0	24

estrogens indicate that in the majority of patients ovulation is not inhibited.

In some patients the mid-cycle LH peak appears to be abolished (Diczfalusy et al., 1969; Orr and Elstein, 1969; Larsson-Cohn et al., 1970c).

The absence of an interference with the temporal sequence of gonadal hormone production is reflected in the high percentage of normal secretory and irregular secretory endometria found in patients in the large clinical trials (Table 10). Culdoscopic visualization of the ovary and ovarian biopsies demonstrating corpora lutea also imply normal gonadal function. Despite this apparent lack of ovarian function suppression a relatively high incidence of breakthrough bleeding may occur especially in the first few months of therapy (cf. also van Leusden, 1969; Roth et al., 1969; Avendaño et al., 1970). The possibility of a depressed hormone production by the corpora lutea is discussed in Chapter 31 (p. 279).

The results of cervical mucus studies correlate well with the antifertility effect of chlormadinone acetate, but failure of spermatozoal recovery from the reproductive tract must be demonstrated before one can be certain that mucus changes are able to block penetration. Lastly, studies of tubal and endometrial secretion, capacitation of spermatozoa, egg or blastocyst transport and tubal and uterine motility are needed for an ultimate understanding of this fertility interruption with continuous progestogens therapy.

The research with chlormadinone acetate given orally shows that the continuous dosages progestogen program, as outlined, may form a basis for an acceptable method for certain societies. We believe the ultimate goal should be a parenteral material lasting many months. It is believed that ease of administration of a contraceptive agent, coupled with a minimal modification of menstrual function, is more important than complete effectiveness to the ultimate acceptance of any method for population control in the developing nations.

(e) Other methods

Injections of various long-acting steroids have been used. Although this chapter is dealing with *oral* contraceptives, it has been found convenient to include a short section on those injectables.

Deladroxate®, the acetophenide of 16α-17α-dihydroxyprogesterone combined with estradiol enanthate, was studied at different dose levels, administered in 1-monthly injection, by Rutherford et al. (1964). Ovulation was regularly inhibited but resumption of cycles after treatment was unpredictable. Side effects included prolonged menstrual flow, breast discomfort and reduced libido. Arnold et al. (1967) reported on a small series with encouraging results. Haller (1968), quoting three further reports and his own observations, states that it is generally possible to maintain a fair control of menstrual cycles. The contraceptive activity appeared to be reliable. Pupkin et al. (1970) observed 518 women in Chile for 6992 woman months and found the regimen satisfactory to over 75% of them.

Medroxyprogesterone acetate (Depo-Provera®) was used in a dose of 150 mg without added estrogen as a single injection every 3 months by a number of investigators. Haller (1968) quoting Zañartu et al. (1966) and Tyler (1967) stresses contraceptive reliability of the method and also the severe disturbance of the cycles and the occurrence of long-lasting anovulatory periods following termination of treatment. Essentially similar findings were reported by Tyler (1970), Pupkin et al. (1970), McDaniel and Zelenik (1970; field trial in Thailand), Rubio and González (1970), Harnecker et al. (1970), and Zartman (1970). Mishell et al. (1970), apart from clinical observations (including persistence of contraceptive effectiveness as long as one year after the last injection), have also shown that during treatment serum LH- and FSH- peaks are suppressed, endometria become thin and atrophic and cervical mucus scanty and viscid.

These authors conclude that at present it would seem best that this method of contraception be limited to those women who have already completed their families.

Other investigators advocated a less frequent exposure to oral dosages. Coutinho and de Souza (1968) found that a combination of norgestrel (0.5 mg) and ethynyl estradiol (0.05 mg) could be given on alternate days to obtain contraceptive protection. Greenblatt (1967) explored a single dose of a long-acting oral estrogen, quinestrol (ethynyl estradiol 3-cyclopentyl ether, 2–5 mg), in combination with different oral progestogens. He reported that if given on day 25, withdrawal bleeding usually occurred after 72 hours. Contraceptive protection was obtained for the following cycle, but the number of patients used was small.

A similar approach, in a larger group, was reported by Maqueo-Topete et al. (1968). This group used a combination of 2 mg quinestrol and 5 mg quingestanol acetate (norethindrone acetate cyclopentyl enol ether). A total of 2673 cycles (259 women) was studied; four pregnancies were reported, i.e. the overall pregnancy rate was 2.0. Larranaga and Berman (1970) tested this preparation in 303 patients (2493 cycles). Four patients became pregnant, all during the first month of treatment, a rate of 1.9 per 100 woman years.

A single dose of quinestrol, 2 mg, was reputed to inhibit ovulation in 60% of patients (Arronet et al., 1969). A single dose of 0.8 mg of quingestanol acetate taken less than 24 hours after coitus provided good contraceptive protection to 200 patients studied for 1004 cycles. A single dose of 0.5 mg taken similarly was less effective, the rate being 6.5 per 100 women years (Rubio et al., 1970).

B. OTHER (AND SIDE) EFFECTS OF ORAL CONTRACEPTIVE DRUGS

The effects of oral contraceptives, other than the desired temporary fertility control, are considered as side effects. These may include undesirable effects on menstrual cycles and the breast, though these are in part due to hormonal action of the gonadal steroids on primary target organs. Other effects reflect the action of these agents on endocrine systems unrelated to reproduction, on parenchymal organs, and other tissues. A wide variety of side effects or oral contraceptives has been described including delayed menses, amenorrhea, spotting, headache, nausea, vomiting, gastric distress, pelvic cramps, feeling of abdominal fullness, nervousness, anxiety, depression, dizziness, leg cramps, breast tenderness, breast enlargement, unusual fatigue, backache, hirsutism, acne, urticaria, chloasma, weight gain, weight loss, and changes in libido. These have been reviewed repeatedly (Drill, 1966; Garcia, 1968; Haller, 1969). A detailed review of the metabolic effects has been recently published (Salhanick et al., 1969).

1. REPRODUCTIVE ORGANS AND BREASTS

(a) Ovary

Under the influence of drugs which inhibit ovulation, morphological changes in the ovaries must, of course, be expected. They are discussed in the present context with a view to the possibility of irreversible or otherwise harmful effects. A number of investigators have observed the ovary during laparotomy or by culdoscopy and have seen an absence of follicles and corpora lutea (Section A3). These inhibitory effects on the ovary would appear to be indirect through the hypothalamic–pituitary suppression of gonadotrophin and it has been shown by Johannison et al. (1965) and Starup (1966) that ovaries under the influence of oral contraceptives can respond to gonadotrophin stimulation. Pincus (1965) found no indication of ovarian damage in women treated with norethynodrel and mestranol combination. He studied the density of follicles per mm^2 and the percentage of atretic follicles in various age groups and reported that these were similar in treated and untreated patients. In older Enovid users (28- to 42-year-old group) oocyte density was actually higher (0.31 ± 0.07 follicles per mm^2) as compared to control (0.09 ± 0.03 follicles per mm^2). This may be due simply to a reduction of ovarian mass and not a real increase in the amount of primordial follicles. Ryan *et al.* (1964) described the ovaries of eighteen patients undergoing hysterectomy after cyclic norethynodrel 5.0 plus mestranol 0.075 mg for 20 days' cycles. Patients were treated for up to 2 years. He saw no corpora lutea; a normal number of primordial ova were believed to be present without actual count in all patients. Inactive cystic and atretic follicles were present in almost all of the patients. In patients on medication for more than 1 year, local cortical condensation of the stroma was present to some degree in about half of the cases. This, the author felt, was impermanent and regenerated after cessation of therapy. Diddle *et al.* (1966) reported that ovaries of three oral-contraceptive users were characterized generally by the presence of atretic follicles and complete absence of formation of corpora lutea in two patients; few primordial follicles were seen. The capsules had a thickness seen in sclerotic ovaries. Zussman *et al.* (1967) examined the ovaries from ten patients treated from one to three cycles with norethindrone 2 mg plus mestranol 0.1 mg. They found an increased fibrosis involving the stromal and subcapsular tissue, numerous cysts, hypervascularity, degeneration of germinating follicles and decreased luteinization. Plate (1968) studied the ovaries of eleven women who used Lyndiol 2.5, Orthonovum, Planovin, Anovlar or Gynovlar 21 during four to forty cycles. He found thickening of tunica albuginea and a moderate to severe fibrosis of the stroma in seven women. These changes were no longer visible in six patients who had discontinued oral contraception some time before and therefore they are considered as reversible in most cases. Lauweryns and Ferin (1964) and Linthorst (1966) also described ovaries of oral-contraceptive users but did not comment on ovarian fibrosis. The significance of the histological findings is not clear at the present; it should be noted here that thickening of tunica albuginea has been described during normal pregnancy (Maqueo and Goldzieher, 1966).

Sanchez-Rivera *et al.* (1968) reported a study involving thirty women treated for two to four cycles with various preparations. Mestranol (0.15 mg daily) inhibited consistently the formation of corpora lutea, but not follicle maturation; similar results were obtained with 5-mg daily dose of a progestational agent 17α-acetoxy-19 norprogesterone (17α-acetoxy-19 nor-4-pregnene-3,20-dione). A second progestational agent studied, 6,17α-dimethyl-6-dehydroprogesterone (6,17α-dimethyl-4,6-pregnadiene-3,20-dione), had a very weak and uncertain effect. Only in two of five patients studied (daily dose 10 mg) were corpora lutea present. Two combined preparations were studied: one, containing ethynodiol diacetate, 1 mg, and mestranol,

0.15 mg, and another, containing 5 mg of lynestrenol plus 0.15 mg of mestranol. In all patients but one the ovaries were atrophied, the number of mature follicles was reduced, or they were completely absent. Corpora lutea were not present.

These results would indicate that, in the majority of cases, the ovarian function was completely inhibited. In most cases, such changes are likely to be transient, as demonstrated by the return to fertility after discontinuance of oral-contraceptive therapy (*see below*).

(b) *Endometrium*

The histologic appearance of the endometrium may vary with the type of steroid regimen employed, although prolonged administration tends to diminish these differences (Rice-Wray *et al.*, 1963; Roland *et al.*, 1964). Maqueo-Topete *et al.* (1963) have documented the changes in the endometrium produced by progestogen–estrogen combinations. Early in the course of treatment secretory changes occur which progress to glandular suppression (cf. also Waidl *et al.*, 1968). Varying amounts of pseudodecidual changes and stromal edema are also seen. Goldzieher *et al.* (1962) have reported that the endometria of patients treated a year or less with norethindrone and mestranol may return to a normal histological state after withdrawal of treatment. In those treated from twelve to twenty-five cycles, there were some residual changes consisting of a lag in endometrial development and a persistence of glandular regression for the initial post-treatment cycles.

Sequential therapy produces secretory changes resembling the appearance of a normal day 18 or 19 endometrium (Maqueo-Topete *et al.*, 1963). However, a small percentage of biopsies shows no progestational conversion of the estrogen-induced proliferative endometrium.

With low dose continuous chlormadinone acetate treatment, Martinez-Manautou *et al.* (1967) have reported that approximately one-third of patients have normal datable secretory endometria, 11% have proliferative endometria and the remainder reveal varying degrees of glandular suppression.

Endometrial changes may be related to complaints regarding menstrual cycle behavior. Due to the suppression of endometrial development with the combined products, a number of women report scanty menstrual flow. This is in contrast to patients on sequential therapy where the flow resembles that of a normal menstrual period. Prolonged periods of amenorrhea following cessation of treatment may result.

Histochemical studies of endometria have shown that changes occur in enzymatic activity during treatment (see also Chapter 23). Acid and alkaline phosphatases and DPN diaphorase, which are hormone-dependent, are greatly reduced. Alterations are demonstrable in activity of many enzymes, as carbonic anhydrase, uterine peroxidase, β-glucuronidase, succinic dehydrogenase, lactic dehydrogenase, and several other enzymes (Townsend *et al.*, 1965; Flowers *et al.*, 1966; Connell *et al.*, 1967).

(*c*) *Amenorrhea*

The "silent period", or the intermedication amenorrhea which represents a failure of the endometrium to respond to hormonal withdrawal, is of great importance to the patient. The reasons for this are not established but may depend upon intensity of endometrial suppression occasionally seen with the combined agents, or it may reflect quantitatively inadequate hormonal withdrawal. The latter is perhaps the basis of missed bleeding episodes of sequential therapy. The monthly bleeding period is a natural sign that conception has not occurred. A failure of menses creates apprehension on the part of the patient. With combined therapy it is unlikely that this represents a pregnancy, particularly if the patient has taken all of her medication. However, if the patient has failed to follow the therapeutic regime, or if she has had two consecutive periods of amenorrhea, she should be investigated for pregnancy. The incidence of missed menstruation, defined as failure to bleed within 7 days of the last tablet taken, is shown in Table 11.

Persistent amenorrhea following cessation of therapy has also been described. Whitelaw *et. al.* (1966) reported on twenty-four women given medroxyprogesterone acetate parenterally, sixteen cases receiving norethynodrel plus mestranol orally and one case norethindrone with mestranol. All had a complication of either amenorrhea or irregular cycling following cessation of therapy. Endometrial pictures varied from atrophic to proliferative. Amenorrhea with medroxyprogesterone and with norethynodrel and mestranol has persisted up to 1 year. Whitelaw quoted a number of personal communications from other physicians in the United States reporting similar experiences. Lamb (1966) reports on a study of 145 patients. In this group, six developed prolonged amenorrhea following injections of medroxyprogesterone acetate, with the duration from 3 to 9 months. He points out that the incidence of amenorrhea in patients on oral contraceptives is quite low, and one would need a large series of patients to describe the relative risk of amenorrhea in a treated population. On the other hand, the incidence in patients receiving injected medroxyprogesterone is significant. Reports of other investigators are included in subsection (*l*), p. 426.

TABLE 11. FAILURE OF CYCLIC WITHDRAWAL BLEEDING* WITH CONTRACEPTIVE AGENTS

Preparation	Overall percentage	Number of cycles studied	Reference
Chlormadinone acetate (2 mg, sequential)	2.6		(a)
Dimethisterone (25 mg, sequential)	1.0		(a)
Ethynodiol diacetate (1 mg)	0.2		(a)
Lynestrenol (5 mg)	4.7	7257	Dukes et al. (1963)
(2.5 mg)	1.3	20,014	Strade (1966)
Medroxyprogesterone acetate (10 mg)	4.0		(a)
Norethindrone (1 mg)	6.3		(a)
(1 + 80)	1.4		(a)
(2 mg)	0.1		(a)
Norethindrone acetate (4 mg)	1.9	7186	(b)
Norethynodrel (5 mg)	2.0	3267	Mears (1964)
(2.5 mg)	1.5	10,097	(b)
Norgestrel (0.5 mg)	0.7	49,683	Laurie and Lewis (1968)
Superlutin (5 mg)	5.0	5107	Šterba (1966)

* Misnamed amenorrhea by manufacturers. Not to be confused by amenorrhea upon cessation of therapy.

(a) Data obtained from information supplied by the manufacturer to the United States Food and Drug Administration.

(b) Average values from Drill (1966).

(d) Intermenstrual bleeding

Intermenstrual bleeding has been reported with all products—combined, sequential or continuous progestogen. It has the greatest incidence in the first cycle of treatment and decreases in subsequent cycles. It appears to be less frequent with sequential therapy than with combined or continuous. There is a significantly higher incidence with derivatives of 17α-acetoxy progesterone than with those of estrane.

It is the opinion of many that intermenstrual bleeding should not be treated and the women be instructed to continue taking medication in the same manner throughout the period of bleeding until their treatment course has been completed. This is in contrast to earlier methods of management in which dosage was doubled or the patient was instructed to stop medication and allow for a menstrual period to develop. This procedure may unduly expose the patient to unwanted pregnancy because there is no assurance that ovulation may not occur during the period of no treatment. This is particularly true if the interruption of treatment occurs early in the cycle.

TABLE 12. INCIDENCE OF INTERMENSTRUAL BLEEDING FOR VARIOUS PREPARATIONS

Preparation	Percentage of breakthrough bleeding				Reference
	Cycles			All cycles studied	
	1	2	6		
Chlormadinone acetate (2 mg, sequential)	7.0	5.0			(a)
Dimethisterone (25 mg, sequential)	4.4	2.2			(a)
Ethynodiol diacetate (1 mg)	14.2	7.7			(a)
Lynestrenol (5 mg)			2.9		(b)
(2.5 mg)				3.5	Strade (1966)
Medroxyprogesterone acetate (10 mg)	20.5	16.1		3.4	(a)
Norethindrone (1 mg)	13.3	8.1	4.4		(a)
(2 mg)	12.1	6.1	2.2		(a)
(2 mg, sequential)	6.3	3.4	2.7		(a)
(1 + 80)	4.0	2.4	2.2		(a)
Norethindrone acetate (4 mg)	14.4	8.3		0.7	(b)
(2.5 mg)				5.4	(b)
Norethynodrel (5 mg)	11.0			6.2	(b)
2.5 mg)	20.3			11.3	(b)
(2.5 mg)	13.6	10.9	8.9		(a)
Norgestrel	2.6			1.3	Laurie and Lewis (1968)

(a) Data obtained from information supplied by the manufacturer to the United States Food and Drug Administration.
(b) Average values from Drill (1966).

The incidence of intermenstrual bleeding (including both "spotting" and bleeding) for several preparations is included in Table 12.

(e) Cervix

During the normal menstrual cycle the cervical mucus undergoes well-known changes in the amount and physiochemical properties (see Chapters 22 and 30). These cyclic changes are abolished in patients on oral-contraceptive therapy (see above, p. 411). Predominance of progestational effect will produce a viscous mucus hostile to penetration and migration of spermatozoa (Moghissi, 1966; Martinez-Manautou *et al.*, 1967; Bowman, 1968). The α-amylase content is increased more markedly after combined than after sequential therapy, but glycogen content of the ectocervix remains within normal limits (Gregoire *et al.*, 1967). Mucorrhea due to estrogen stimulation of cervical mucus production has been described as a side effect with sequential therapy (Andrews *et al.*, 1966).

Oral contraceptives may increase the frequency of cervical erosion. Morphological changes may include hypersecretion and hyperplasia of the cervical glands, stromal edema, and softening may be the main features (Maqueo *et al.*, 1966; Taylor *et al.*, 1967). Fibrin thrombi formation in the capillaries and arterioles were noted in about 50% of the biopsy specimens in one study (Gall *et al.*, 1969).

(f) Fibromyomata

There have been reports of enlargement and development of edema and degenerative changes in fibromyomata, similar to changes seen in pregnancy, during treatment with progestogen–estrogen mixtures given continuously and in considerably larger doses than those used in contraceptive regimes. Goldzieher *et al.* (1966) have shown that norethindrone (estrogen-free), 2.0 mg daily, failed to produce any gross or histological change in myomata, whereas increasing the progestational effect by giving larger doses of medrogestone (estrogen-free), 25.0 mg daily for 14 to 21 days, produced more intense changes in myomata than seen during pregnancy. However, there was no evidence of cellular proliferation. Upon cessation of therapy, fibrosis and hylanization developed. The authors believe that these changes are independent of uterine enlargement and do not need estrogen for their production. If this is the case, it would seem likely that progestogen–estrogen mixtures used in relatively small contraceptive doses would have little effect on myomata.

(g) *Vagina*

Wied *et al.* (1966), comparing the cytological records of a group of 1628 patients receiving oral contraceptives of the progestogen–estrogen type for at least 1 year, with a 19,325-case control group, found a significant difference between the observed bacterial flora in the contraceptive group and the expected flora, based upon observations in the control group. There was a decrease in B. vag. Döderlein, an increase in coccoid bacteria and an increase in both fungi and trichomonads. According to the authors, these findings may be only remotely or not at all connected to medication. However, others have suggested that there may be a causal relationship between progestogen–estrogen contraceptives and vulvovaginal candidiasis. Yaffee and Grots (1965) reported the first four cases of vaginal candidiasis in patients receiving norethynodrel and mestranol. This was followed by another report involving thirteen patients (Porter and Lyle, 1966). Three of these patients had to stop the use of the oral contraceptive before they became responsive to local nystatin therapy. The authors had not seen vaginal candidiasis with sequential therapy at the time of the report. An editorial in the *Journal of the American Medical Associates* (1966) also suggests that sequential therapy may be preferred in these patients. Cotteral (1966) similarly observed the development of candidiasis in fourteen women receiving norethynodrel and mestranol contraceptives, two of whom required cessation of oral contraceptives before the vaginitis was controlled by nystatin therapy.

(h) *Pelvic vasculature*

Myometrial hypertrophy, dilation of sinusoids, and edema are recognized effects of hormonal contraceptives. There have been reports on congestion and increased vascularity of tissues noted during pelvic surgery when oral contraceptives were not discontinued for a sufficient period of time prior to operation. Ryan *et al.* (1964), in a study of women undergoing hysterectomy on norethynodrel–mestranol therapy, noted three incidences of pelvic thrombi, two in ovarian veins and one in the uterine vein. Since these were uncontrolled random observations, the interpretation of the finding would require larger series with adequate controls. Kaufman and Boatwright (1967) studied the pelvic venous systems in a group of women before and during oral contraceptive therapy with norethindrone 2.0 mg and mestranol 0.1 mg. Using radiographic contrast techniques, they failed to find any evidence of venous dilatation or pelvic congestion. However, they suggested that additional studies be performed, preferably using cinemato-radiographic methods, before the effects of oral progestogen–estrogen contraceptives on the pelvic veins could definitely be ruled out.

(*i*) *Breasts*

Changes in the size of the breasts have been attributed to oral-contraceptive agents, but this has not been documented by controlled observations. On the other hand, there seems to be a relationship between the use of hormonal contraceptives and the symptom of breast tenderness.

(*j*) *Lactation*

Initially it was thought that hormonal contraceptive therapy would no jeopardize milk production provided lactation had been established Semm and Dittmar (1965) reported that Lyndiol (2.5 mg) did not influence the onset of lactation, or amount of milk flow, during a 10-day observation period. It is now apparent that this must not be generalized. Kora (1969) reported that the amount of lactation, and infants' weight gains, were reduced by maternal use of a combination of ethynodial diacetate, 1 mg, and mestranol, 0.1 mg. Pincus (1965) presented data indicating that lactation tends to be diminished with higher doses of Enovid. Kaern (1967) found measurable diminution in the quantity of milk in mothers on Norinyl-1. When oral-contraceptive therapy is begun immediately postpartum and is continued long enough, lactation can actually be inhibited. A double-blind controlled study, using complete inhibition of lactation as the end-point, was reported by Rudel (1963). Lactation was completely inhibited within 30 to 60 days when contraceptive therapy was begun in the immediate postpartum period in contrast to a placebo group where lactation was apparently normal (Table 13).

TABLE 13. INFLUENCE OF VARIOUS CONTRACEPTIVE PREPARATIONS ON LACTATION

Preparation used	No. of patients	No. of patients with diminished flow*
Placebo	15	0
Mestranol, 80 mcg	13	6
Ethynyl estradiol, 50 mcg	16	7
Norethynodrel, 2.5 mg plus mestranol, 100 mcg	11	4
Norethindrone, 2 mg plus mestranol, 100 mcg	14	11
Norethindrone acetate, 2.5 mg plus mestranol, 50 mcg	8	3
Lynestrenol, 5 mg plus mestranol, 100 mcg	15	7

* Within 30 to 60 days after beginning medication.

It was reported that radioactive norethynodrel was excreted in breast milk (Pincus et al., 1966; Laumas et al., 1967). The excretion in the milk of the components of Lyndiol, lynestrenol and mestranol, labeled with 4-^{14}C, were studied by Van der Molen et al. (1969) and Wijmenga and Van der Molen (1969) respectively. It was found that of a 5 mg Lyndiol tablet 0.022–0.088% of the radioactivity of lynestrenol and 0.0002–0.013% of mestranol were found in the milk within 4 to 5 days. It was calculated that in the order of 1 mcg of lynestrenol and 0.03–0.06 mcg of mestranol (or metabolites) might be excreted in 100 ml of milk.

(k) *Galactorrhea*

Gregg (1966) has reported a case of galactorrhea developing in a young woman taking up to four tablets daily of norethynodrel 5.0 mg and mestranol 0.75 mg. This was associated with areolar pigmentation and multiple fibroadenomas in the breast. Lloyd (1967) has seen four cases of galactorrhea associated with oral-contraceptive therapy. He states that in these cases, in order to see milk, it must be manually expressed from the breast.

(l) *Return of fertility*

After cessation of oral-contraceptive therapy ovulation resumes in most cases in 4 to 8 weeks. Pituitary and ovarian function is recovered first; the endometrium may require as long as 3 months to regain its normal histologic appearance and enzymatic activity (Flowers et al., 1966). In few women, however, long-term amenorrhea may persist (Lamb, 1966; Bell and Loraine, 1967; Dodek and Kotz, 1967; Dunn, 1967; Bowman, 1968; Horowitz et al., 1968; McGregor, 1968; Shearman, 1968a). These patients usually require treatment with clomiphene, human menopausal gonadotrophins or human chorionic gonadotrophins. Once established, ovulation appears to continue spontaneously (Shearman, 1968b; Homesley and Goss, 1970).

Most clinical investigators report that after discontinuation of oral contraceptives most women conceive "promptly". Yet, such statements are not supported by valid statistical information. If evaluation to assess return of fertility among those who discontinued is based on the percentage of women who conceived, it neglects the duration of follow-up. If the distribution of pregnancies by number of months required for conception is used, the percentage of women who did not conceive is neglected. If conception rates per 100 woman-years of exposure are used it fails to take into account that the conception rate declines with age (Corfman, 1969). There have also been reports beginning with that of Pincus et al. (1959)

that fertility is actually enhanced after stopping oral-contraceptive medication. Since such findings are most likely based upon studies done in fecund women and may be an expression of their inherent fertility, such data cannot be evaluated with fairness. Data of several investigators showing the incidence of elective pregnancy in the first six months after cessation of oral-contraceptive therapy are summarized in Table 14.

TABLE 14. SUBSEQUENT FERTILITY IN USERS OF ORAL CONTRACEPTIVES

Total no. of patients	Percent pregnant patients				Reference
	Months when pregnancy occurred				
	1	2	3	6	
41	66				Goldzieher et al. (1962)
241	27	37		19	Satterthwaite and Gamble (1962)
208	41	17	12	15	Rice-Wray et al. (1965)
85		68			Morris (1965)
75			66	25	Banks et al. (1965)
108	38	22			Mears (1965)

At this time the concern that fertility may become impaired in oral-contraceptive users cannot be substantiated. The occasional isolated reports on infertility cannot be evaluated with fairness since the overall population of the users that desired to become pregnant is still very small. For the same reason, it is also doubtful whether the increased fertility rate claimed by various investigators will be borne out when larger groups of patients will be available for comparative purposes.

2. OTHER ENDOCRINE ORGANS

(a) *Adrenal cortex*

Estrogens are known to increase transcortin levels in the plasma. As a result binding of plasma cortisol is increased and its clearance from the plasma is decreased. Increases in protein bound cortisol has been reported in patients on estrogen–progestogen combinations (Layne et al., 1962; Wallach et al., 1963; Metcalf and Beaven, 1963; Dodek et al., 1965). This results in decreased excretion of cortisol metabolites (Layne et al., 1962) and clearance rate from peripheral plasma (Dodek et al., 1965). Wallach et al. (1963) and Leach and Margulis (1965) measured urinary excretion of

17-keto and 17-hydroxy steroids and considered that the adrenal gland responds normally to ACTH stimulation. Starup *et al.* (1966) found a normal response to metopirone® and ACTH in patients treated with a combination of megestrol acetate and mestranol but a decreased excretion of 17-ketogenic and 17-ketosteroids believed to be due to the increased plasma levels of protein bound cortisol. Leach and Margulis (1965) found a suppression in response to metopirone® in patients receiving norethindrone acetate with ethynyl estradiol. Similar results have been reported by Mestman *et al.* (1968) in women who received norethindrone plus mestranol for periods ranging from 6 to 25 months. They also found that the pituitary–adrenal response to bacterial pyrogen was normal. The investigators believe that these agents will not affect the pituitary–adrenal response to stressful situations in spite of the impaired response to metopirone®. There is also no evidence that these agents will affect the pituitary–adrenal response to stressful situations, such as surgical procedure or other stresses. For a discussion of the influence of progestogens on adrenal functions in the human see Chapter 31, p. 288.

If adrenal function studies are contemplated hormonal contraceptives containing estrogens should be discontinued for 6 weeks prior to tests.

Increased secretion rate of aldosterone has been observed in some patients treated with norethynodrel and mestranol (Layne *et al.*, 1962).

(b) Thyroid

Protein bound iodine is known to increase during pregnancy. Similarly an increase has been seen in both females and males with estrogen therapy and has been noted with estrogen containing oral-contraceptive agents (Hollander *et al.*, 1963; Beaton, 1964; Florsheim and Faircloth, 1964; Larsson-Cohn, 1965a). This is due to the effect of estrogen in increasing thyroxin binding globulin. Other investigators (Walser *et al.*, 1964; Satterthwaite, 1964) report no change. Fisher *et al.* (1966) in a study of norethynodrel and mestranol combinations concluded that this contraceptive did not alter thyroxin utilization rate or cause increased TSH secretion. Irizarry *et al.* (1966) found that there was no significant difference in the average values of radioactive iodine uptake by the thyroid between women receiving either norethynodrel 2.5 or 5.0 mg plus mestranol 0.1 or 0.075 mg respectively and those of a control group. In a study lasting 3 months, comparable results were obtained with the subjects acting as their own controls. An exception to this was the group receiving ethynodiol diacetate 2.0 mg and mestranol 0.1 mg. However, according to the authors this difference was within the limits of normal variation for euthyroid patients and consequently was of no clinical significance. Other investigators reported that the basal metabolic rate, cholesterol levels, ^{131}I and concentrations of "free" thyroxine remain within normal range (Goolden et al., 1967). Also, a normal response of the thyroid gland to small doses of TSH is maintained (Margulis and Leach, 1966). Development of thyroid adenomas, hyperthyroidism, and hypothyroidism have not been reported.

Within 2 to 4 months after cessation of treatment, thyroid function tests return to normal (Winikoff and Taylor, 1966). If thyroid endocrinology is to be studied in a patient receiving oral contraceptives of the combined or sequential type, the drug must be discontinued for a prior period of 6 weeks so that apparent abnormal values do not result in thyroid function studies.

(c) *Pituitary gland*

The effects on gonadotrophin excretion and/or release and the return of hypothalamo–pituitary–gonadotrophin function following cessation of contraception was discussed. There are, at present, no studies on pituitary histology.

(d) *Carbohydrate and lipid metabolism*

Glucose tolerance may be diminished in women taking oral-contraceptive drugs. The abnormality is usually more pronounced with the oral than with the intravenous test and is more severe in women predisposed to diabetes and in those with latent or overt disease. In non-diabetic subjects increased insulinogenesis is observed following both short-term and long-term use of oral contraceptives and again the effects are more pronounced with combined than with sequential regimens. In long-term use, the tendency is for glucose tolerance to return to normal while insulin levels remain elevated, suggesting that hyperinsulinism may serve as a compensatory mechanism for maintaining glucose homeostasis. Similar findings of abnormal glucose tolerance test are seen in gravid women (Benjamin and Cooper, 1967). One estrogen, mestranol, was reported to cause a decrease in glucose tolerance (Javier *et al.*, 1968; Beck, 1969) but only minor changes were seen after the use of this drug for 6 months by Spellacy (1969).

In a random study of oral-contraceptive users, Gershberg *et al.* (1964) found that 10% of the women tested had elevated fasting levels of blood glucose. Following glucose tolerance testing, abnormally high levels in 20% for the first hour and 46% for the second hour were seen. This incidence of abnormal glucose tolerance was greater in women with a family history of diabetes. The authors suggested this change may be related to similar findings seen during pregnancy in prediabetic women. In contrast, Peterson et al. (1966), evaluating glucose metabolism in women receiving norethynodrel or ethynodiol diacetate combined with mestranol, found only one woman of the sixty-one observed who had an elevated fasting glucose level. However, following a glucose meal, fifteen patients (24%) had elevated levels at 1 hour with twelve of them exceeding diabetic levels. Twenty-one (34%) were increased at the 2-hour reading and 16% of these were greater than diabetic levels. By the third hour, nine women (14%) still showed elevation in plasma glucose.

Both oral and intravenous glucose tolerance were studied by Wynn and Doar (1966a) in 105 women given progestogen–estrogen contraceptive mixtures for more than 3 months. Approximately 80% of these patients received combinations of ethynodiol diacetate and mestranol; the remaining group was divided between users of norethynodrel and mestranol or norethindrone acetate and ethynyl estradiol. Eighteen per cent of the oral and 15% of the intravenous glucose-tolerance tests were abnormal. However, unlike the experience of Gershberg et al. (1964), the mean plasma glucose was unchanged. An increase in the level of fasting non-esterified fatty acid and blood pyruvate was also observed. The authors liken these changes to those seen in steroid diabetes.

In a group of twenty-five healthy women given norethynodrel 9.85 mg plus mestranol 0.15 mg for 19 days, Spellacy and Carlson (1966) also found abnormally elevated and delayed intravenous glucose-tolerance tests when compared to their control test. There also was a significant elevation in the plasma insulin values during the contraceptive treatment period. Subsequently Spellacy et al. (1967a) showed that mean values for intravenous glucose tolerance test were not altered from control values in a group of thirty-two women receiving norethynodrel 5.0 mg plus mestranol 0.075 mg cyclically for a 6-month period. However, there was significant elevation in plasma insulin levels both during the fasting state and after the intravenous glucose stimulus. The degree of elevation could not be correlated with either familial history of diabetes melitus or the subject's weight change while taking the drug. Similar results were obtained in thirty-five women who for 6 months received a sequential contraceptive containing mestranol 0.08 mg daily for 15 days followed by chlormadinone 2.0 mg plus mestranol 0.08 mg for 5 days (Spellacy et al., 1968). In contrast to these results Starup et al. (1968) failed to find a significant change in fasting blood glucose, the k-value in the intravenous glucose tolerance test, fasting serum insulin and the response in serum insulin after an intravenous glucose stimulus, in twenty-seven non-diabetic women receiving megestrol acetate

5.0 mg plus mestranol 0.1 mg cyclically for 1 year. The one diabetic woman in the study showed a significant increase in fasting blood glucose and a slight decrease in the k-value during treatment but her insulin dose was not changed.

These findings support the concept that increased insulinogenesis is essential for prevention of hyperglycemia in subjects receiving steroid contraceptives. In non-diabetic patients contraceptive-induced hyperglycemia is accompanied not only by increased secretion of insulin but also by a significant increase in resistance to insulin. This raises the question whether pancreatic islet cells can sustain hyperactivity during long-term use of steroid contraceptives.

The mechanism of this interference in carbohydrate metabolism has not been completely elucidated. However, both Wynn and Doar (1966a) and Spellacy and Carlson (1966) suggest that these changes may be subsequent to an increase in circulating levels of free fatty acid which could impair glucose assimilation and pyruvate oxidation. The latter groups considered that this could produce a relative resistance to insulin action and an increase in plasma insulin levels. Wynn and Doar (1966a) liken the changes in plasma pyruvate and glucose levels seen in oral-contraceptive users to those seen in patients receiving glucocorticoids or having Cushing's disease. Similar elevations of blood pyruvate occurred in women receiving estrogen alone (Doar *et al.*, 1969). Seng *et al.* (1969) found slight but significant increases in the levels of ketone bodies, pyruvate, triglycerides, in women on Lyndiol 2.5 (2.5 mg lynestrenol and 75 mcg of mestranol) but all values stayed within normal limits. It is interesting that cortisol failed to evolve an additional increase in plasma glucose levels following a glucose meal in a group of postmenopausal women treated with estrogens (Buchler and Warren, 1966). More recently di Paola *et al.* (1968) studied prednisone–oral-glucose tolerance in a group of 161 women who variously received mestranol combined with norethindrone, ethynyl estradiol combined with norethindrone, mestranol combined with chlormadinone acetate and norethindrone acetate. In this test the subjects are given two doses of prednisone, 10.0 mg, 8 and 2 hours prior to the glucose tolerance test. They found that only those patients who received mestranol had a highly significant percentage of abnormal prednisone responses.

The role of both the pituitary–adrenal axis and growth hormone, as a mediator of these changes in glucose metabolism, has still to be determined. Spellacy *et al.* (1967b) have shown that human growth hormone levels were elevated during the fasting state and following an insulin stimulus in a group of twenty-six normal women taking a combination of norethynodrel

5.0 mg plus mestranol 0.075 mg for a 3-month period. Elevations of growth hormone levels were also seen after 2 years of therapy but they were significantly different from the control values only at the 2- and 3-hour time period following the insulin stimulus (Spellacy et al., 1969).

These changes in growth hormones are consistent with reports that show non-esterified fatty acid levels are higher in subjects receiving either estrogen alone or in oral contraceptives. The study of the long-term effect of the estrogen-containing oral contraceptives must be continued. If this condition is at all akin to gestational diabetes, then the possibility of non-gestational diabetes developing in these women at a later time cannot be neglected. In addition, even asymptomatic or chemical diabetes is associated with an increased incidence of vascular complications.

Since progestogens antagonize the peripheral action of estrogens on the reproductive organs (Rudel et al., 1965; Rudel, 1967), the question has been raised as to possible interference with estrogenic effects on other systems. This may not be the case as far as thyroid binding globulin or transcortin are concerned, as the estrogen-induced increase in these factors prevail with the use of progestogen–estrogen mixtures. On the other hand, Wynn and Doar (1966b) have shown that serum triglyceride, cholesterol and low-density and very low-density lipoprotein levels are elevated in women receiving a variety of combination estrogen–progestogen oral contraceptives. These changes resemble the serum lipid and lipoprotein patterns seen in males. This was also shown by an increase in the mean atherogenic index and a reduction in the mean S_f 0–12 lipoproteins.

In a later paper (Wynn and Doar, 1969), the same authors report that no significant increases in fasting serum cholesterol were seen in a longitudinal study of a group of sixty-eight women using one of eight contraceptive tablets though a fall of these values was observed in another group when drug-treatment was discontinued. Increases in triglyceride levels were seen in 97% of the first group but were above the normal level only in 18%.

Seng et al. (1969) in their study on Lyndiol 2.5 found no significant changes in lipoproteins. Gershberg et al. (1968) have reported that 61% of a group of thirty-nine women treated for more than 10 months with norethynodrel 5.0 mg plus mestranol 0.075 mg had serum triglyceride levels greater than 110 mg/100 ml. The authors speculate that this may be due to an alteration in liver function. The same group (Zorrilla et al., 1968) have reported a severe hypertriglyceridemia developing in a woman taking sequential mestranol and chlormadinone acetate and a diabetic man taking mestranol. The levels reached 1948 mg and 1240 mg/100 ml, respectively, in a period of 2 months. Changes in serum cholesterol paralleled the triglyceride change but were not as great. Both patients had moderately elevated serum triglyceride before therapy. Plasma insulin was also increased in response to glucose stimulus during the pretreatment period.

3. LIVER FUNCTION

Many symptom-free women on oral contraceptives show changes in liver function tests. The severity of changes and the number of patients responding are dose dependent. It has been suggested that hormonal steroids produce their effects through modifying permeability of the liver cells rather than by causing parenchymal cell damage (Roman and Hecker, 1968). One group has described changes (altered shape, increase in size and presence of paracrystalline inclusions) in the mitochondria of patients on oral contraceptives from 12 to 36 months but failed to find a correlation between mitochondrial changes and liver function tests (Perez et al., 1969).

Most commonly observed changes are: retention of sulfobromophthalein (BSP) in the liver; fall in plasma amino acid levels; and elevation of transaminase values. In addition, oral contraceptives affect enzyme systems other than those already mentioned: increases in activity of β-glucuronidase, isocitrate dehydrogenase and ceruloplasminoxidase levels and decreases in activity of lactic dehydrogenase and alkaline phosphatase may occur.

Abnormally high BSP retention with 17-alkyl 19-norprogestogens has been reported by several investigators (Borglin, 1965; Larsson-Cohn, 1965b; Eisalo et al., 1965; Kleiner et al., 1965). Allan and Tyler (1967), in studies with norethindrone, have found that the incidence of abnormal BSP retention is directly related to the dose of this 17-alkylated progestogen, being highest with the 10 mg dose. The frequency in patients receiving 1 mg was comparable to the control group.

The mechanism of the retention has been studied with both the anabolic (Heaney and Whedon, 1958) and the progestational compounds. Scherb et al. (1963) have demonstrated that the interference is not in the ability of the liver to take up and store BSP but in the rate limiting phenomena of conjugation and/or transport which can be expressed functionally as a transport maximum (T_m). Kleiner et al. (1965) showed that BSP T_m is decreased in patients receiving norethynodrel on a cyclic basis, and with larger doses of the progestogen given within interruption, there was a further decrease in the T_m of BSP.

The significance of these changes in BSP excretion has yet to be determined. Allan and Tyler (1967) have pointed out that, as the length of treatment with contraceptive steroids increases, the number of patients having abnormal retention may decrease. Further, Kleiner et al. (1965) reported that the BSP T_m returns to pretreatment levels upon cessation of therapy. These observations would tend to support the conclusion that contraceptive agents containing 17-alkyl progestogens were producing no anatomic or serious functional change in hepatic cells.

Jaundice occurs in about one woman in 10,000 on oral contraceptives (Ockner and Davidson, 1967) particularly in patients having a familial or personal history of icterus or pruritus gravidarum (Larsson-Cohn and Strenram, 1965; Holzbach and Sanders, 1965; Thulin and Nermark, 1966; Larsson-Cohn, 1967). The patients have a typical history of nausea, malaise, and itching followed by clinical jaundice including production of dark urine. Liver-function tests show increased levels of bilirubin and moderately elevated levels of transaminases. Liver biopsies show canalicular and hepatico-cellular bile stasis. Liver tests in most patients with this condition revert to normal within several weeks after the cessation of therapy. In a few, however, abnormal liver-function tests may persist for longer periods.

Studies in the experimental animals, and results with continuous progestogen contraception where jaundice is rarely seen, implicate the estrogenic component in impairment of bile transport (Stoll et al., 1966). Studies on liver function during normal pregnancy and ethynyl-estradiol therapy led Kreek (1969) to the conclusion that an increased sensitivity of the hepatic excretory mechanisms to endogenous or exogenous estrogen may be the primary defect in those patients who have had cholestasis of pregnancy and are abnormally responsive to challenge. Larsson-Cohn (1967) has suggested that there might be an hereditary factor in explaining the higher incidence of idiopathic jaundice of pregnancy in Scandinavian populations. It is interesting that United States and British investigators have not generally found an increase in serum transaminase, nor have they reported as great an incidence of BSP retention in patients using oral contraceptives as have the Scandinavian investigators. These differences might have, as a basis, the same conditions which are responsible for the different incidences of icterus gravidarum in these areas.

Oral contraceptive drugs have been shown to affect other enzymes. Increases in β-glucuronidase and isocitrate dehydrogenase and decreases in activity of lactic dehydrogenase and alkaline phosphatase were reported (Pulkkinen and Willman, 1967). Estrogens have been implicated in observed increases in ceruloplasmin-oxidase levels (Carruthers et al., 1966; Shokeir, 1968), progestogens in the glutamic oxalacetic transaminase levels

(Stoll et al., 1966). Increased aminolevulinic acid (ALA) synthetase levels, an enzyme that participates in the production of heme, as well as urinary coproporphyrin has also been noted in a significant proportion of women (Burton et al., 1967). Oral contraceptives are known to alter liver capacity to transform various drugs to biologically inactive substances. The effects of hormonal steroids on drug detoxification may not reside solely in the enzyme-inducing potency of these drugs. Steroids are known to serve as substrates for the microsomal drug-metabolizing enzyme system in the liver, and could, therefore, compete with various exogenous substances for oxidative transformation by the enzyme system.

4. THROMBOSIS, EMBOLISM AND BLOOD COAGULABILITY

There have been a number of reports on the occurrence of thromboembolic disease in women taking oral-contraceptive agents which in some cases ended in death. Venous thrombosis, embolism of pulmonary artery and cerebrovascular occlusions were reported. A summary of these reports will be found in the review by Tausk (1969).

Prior to 1967 less attention was given to these isolated reports. It was pointed out that deaths from idiopathic thromboembolic disease also occur in women of reproductive age not using oral contraceptives (Cahal, 1965). Indeed in 1969 the Advisory Committee on Obstetrics and Gynecology, United States Food and Drug Administration concluded, "the data derived from mortality statistics are not adequate to confirm or refute the role of oral contraceptives in thromboembolic disease. They do, however, suggest that if oral contraceptives act as a cause, they do so very infrequently relative to the number of users."

Beginning in 1967, however, there have appeared several reports, all from Britain, which strongly indicated a relationship between the use of oral contraceptives and the risk of thromboembolic disease (Inman and Vessey, 1968; Doll et al., 1969). The findings of the British investigators may be summarized as follows: (1) in the absence of other predisposing causes the risk of developing venous thrombosis or pulmonary embolism is increased approximately eightfold in women who are taking an oral contraceptive and (2) no relation was found between the use of oral contraceptives and death from coronary thrombosis, but there was a relation with death from pulmonary embolism or infarction. The data which formed the basis of the conclusions are summarized in Table 15.

The results of the British studies led the United States Food and Drug Administration to order the following change of labeling for the oral contraceptives: "The physician should be alert to the earliest manifestations of thrombotic disorders (thrombophlebitis, cerebrovascular disorders, pulmonary embolism, and retinal thrombosis). Should any of these occur or be suspected, the drug should be discontinued immediately."

TABLE 15. DEATHS DUE TO THROMBOEMBOLIC DISORDERS IN WOMEN USING ORAL CONTRACEPTIVES COMPARED WITH DEATHS FROM THE SAME CAUSES IN NON-USERS

Category	Mortality rates per 100,000		Hospitalization rates (morbidity) per 100,000 Age 20–44
	Age 20–34	Age 35–44	
Users	1.5	3.9	47
Non-users	0.2	0.5	5

In 1969 the Advisory Committee to the United States Food and Drug Administration made public the results of a retrospective study by Sartwell *et al.* of cases of thromboembolism and equally matched controls in five large cities. The subjects were women of reproductive age who were discharged alive over a 3-year period from forty-three teaching hospitals. The controls were women admitted to the same hospitals in the same 6-month period matched by race, age, marital status, parity, residence, and hospital-pay status. Most cases had thrombophlebitis, pulmonary embolism, or both: a few had cerebral or retinovascular disease. The report concluded that "the risk of thromboembolism to a woman using hormonal contraceptives was 4.4 times that of the non-user. The risk was higher for users of sequential products." The excess risk did not persist after cessation of use, nor did prolonged continuation of use enhance the risk. As already noted, no striking differences were seen among contraceptive products except for increased risk associated with the use of sequential therapy.

In 1970 Inman *et al.* published a report to the Committee on Safety of Drugs in England, based on a statistical analysis of the incidence of thromboembolism associated with the use of different contraceptive preparations. For each of the preparations available on the market in the United Kingdom, Sweden and Denmark the sales were estimated and the number of expected cases of thromboembolism (as a share of the sum total recorded for the country) were compared with the number actually observed. In this way a ratio of observed to expected "was established and a positive correlation was found between the dose of estrogen and the risk of pulmonary embolism, deep vein thrombosis, cerebral thrombosis, and coronary thrombosis in the United Kingdom. A similar association was found for venous thrombosis and pulmonary embolism in Sweden and Denmark. The Committee on Safety of Drugs (1970) published a statement to the effect that of five products which contain 150 or 100 mcg of estrogens (mestranol or ethynylestradiol) all but one carried a substantial excess of observed reports", whereas in five of seven preparations which contained 75 or 50 mcg, there was a substantial deficit. Although there were some notable exceptions (Conovid E, containing 100 mcg mestranol had a ratio of O/E of 0.59) the committee felt it necessary to issue a warning against the use of preparations containing 100 mcg or more of an estrogen. The recommendation of the British Committee was adopted by the F.D.A. in the U.S. who recommended the use of oral contraceptives containing "0.075 mg or less of estrogen".

It is of interest to note that patients in blood group O are rare among cases of thromboembolism in women, and especially in women who were taking oral contraceptives. This difference in blood-group distributions and any possible relationship between blood groups and predisposition to thromboembolism requires further substantiation.

A number of laboratories have investigated the coagulation and fibrinolytic enzyme systems of patients taking oral contraceptives. Beller and Porges (1967) have reviewed these conflicting data and have also described the results of their excellently designed and controlled study in which there was no significant difference among the two groups receiving cyclic progestogen–estrogen mixture and a placebo group. However, in a group of women receiving norethynodrel with mestranol in doses of up to 50 mg per day for a period up to 8 months for the management of endometriosis, an increase in factor VII, fibrogen and plasminogen was seen. This does not imply an increased liability with regard to thromboembolic disease. Blood coagulation factors, such as factor VII, factor X and fibrinogen, are also elevated in pregnancy, but this is not associated with an increased incidence of thrombosis or embolism (Beller, 1956). On the other hand, there is an increase in thromboembolic complications in the immediate postpartum period when blood coagulation factors have returned to normal levels.

A review of additional data describing the results of investigation of the coagulation and fibrinolytic system was summarized by Dugdale and Masi in the report of the Advisory Committee to the United States Food and Drug Administration (1969). A summary of the data is presented in Table 16.

It is recognized that pregnant women have little problem with thromboembolic disorders whereas users of oral contraceptives have excessive

TABLE 16. THE EFFECT OF ORAL CONTRACEPTIVES ON BLOOD COAGULATION

	Oral contraceptives	Estrogens	Progestogens	Pregnancy
Platelets	Increased number and possibly enhanced function	Enhanced function	No effect	Little effect
Coagulation	Definitely accelerated	Accelerated by synthetic steroids	No effect	Slightly accelerated
Level of activity of factors	Increased	No data	No effect	Increased
Fibrinolysis	Increased	Uncertain	Increased	Decreased

disease of this type. Dugdale and Masi suggest that "perhaps the explanation lies in the platelets. Platelets are little affected by pregnancy, whereas the steroid contraceptives increase their number and possibly their tendency to adhere and clump. The increased arterial thrombosis with oral contraceptives could be explained on this basis, although the increased incidence of venous thrombosis might not be so explained. The answer may well lie elsewhere, for example, in changes in the endothelium and vessel wall and in slowing of blood flow."

The changes brought about by the oral steroids are not immediately reversible upon discontinuing the drugs and one to several weeks are required for return to the normal pattern (Donayre and Pincus, 1965; Amris and Starup, 1967; Bolton et al., 1968).

5. VASCULAR EFFECTS AND BLOOD CONSTITUENTS

In a study of twenty cases of fatal thromboembolism in women taking oral contraceptives, Irey et al. (1970) found widely distributed thrombi in arteries and veins, associated with distinctive vascular lesions (endothelial proliferation and internal thickening). In many instances vascular occlusion resulted from locally formed thrombi. These changes were not found in the control patients. Arterial wall changes were also described by Ten Berge (1969) who found a thickening of the intima, together with degenerative changes in the media in the small vessels in the ovaries of pill users (which disappear after cessation of use), and in the uterus. Blaustein et al. (1968) described similar changes in the arteries of the endometrium and also in the skin.

Information regarding the effect of contraceptive steroids on the venous system in humans is limited to clinical observation of increases in the diameter of venous vessels and in venous volume. Animals studied are limited. Goodrich and Wood (1964) noted increase in the distensibility of veins in the calf following administration of contraceptive steroids. An increase in the amount of muscle, a decrease in the amount of collagen, marked fragmentation of the reticulum, apparent loss of elastic tissue and a marked loss of acid mucopolysaccharides in large vessels of rabbits were noted (Danforth et al., 1964). Estrogens seem to be implicated. It was shown in rats that long-term administration of estrogen predisposes to vascular lesions resembling polyarteritis nodosa. Several clinical reports appeared describing neurological complications in oral-contraceptive users as vascular occlusive syndrome of the central nervous system and retina, migraine and other disorders. This is more fully discussed below. In a careful study Connell and Kelman (1968) failed to find any abnormalities (eye vessels) in patients taking combined or sequential preparations.

(a) Blood pressure

Hypertension, in both systolic and diastolic pressure, can occur in users of oral contraceptives. Laragh *et al.* (1967) observed an elevation to hypertensive levels in six normotensive women and an augmentation of hypertension in five additional women receiving oral contraceptives of the combined type. Three of these women showed complete reversal and three more showed considerable reduction in blood pressure upon drug withdrawal. Two of these patients had a re-exacerbation when retaking these oral contraceptives.

Tyson (1968) reported that of forty-five patients receiving ethynoldiol diacetate 1.0 mg plus mestranol 0.1 mg for varying times up to 8 months, seven developed significant elevations in blood pressure. Newton *et al.* (1968) in an extension of the Laragh study found a marked and persistent increase in the concentration of plasma angiotensinogen in women taking oral contraceptives. Less consistently plasma renin and aldosterone were also increased either transiently or persistently. Estrogens were found to increase plasma angiotensinogen (Helmer and Griffith, 1952); both estrogens and progestogens were found to increase the secretion of aldosterone (Layne *et al.*, 1962) and both are also known to enhance the reactivity to endogenous renin (Laragh *et al.*, 1967). Thus it is possible that in susceptible women oral contraceptives may alter the ability of the renin–angiotensin–aldosterone mechanism to respond to normal physiological stimuli.

The most consistent change that may be observed in women taking oral contraceptives is the rise of angiotensinogen in plasma; the values may rise up to 8 times those of normal. The rise is observed within 4 days, reaching a maximum within 2 weeks. After discontinuation of medication the level may remain elevated for more than a month. These changes are reversible even after prolonged use. Changes in the concentration of renin are less consistent. The normal response to an elevation of angiotensinogen is a decrease in renin concentration. Because the quantity of angiotensin that can be generated is limited, a large increase in the concentration of angiotensinogen is accompanied by only a twofold increase in angiotensin.

The clinical implications of these changes in the concentrations of angiotensinogen, renin, angiotensin, and aldosterone remain to be elucidated, since the changes are observed in most patients without a concomitant rise in blood pressure.

(b) *Blood constituents*

Administration of oral contraceptives may lead to decreases in haptoglobin, albumin, and total serum proteins, increases in thyroxine-binding globulin, transcortin (the cortisol binding protein), plasminogen, ceruloplasmin, estrogen-binding proteins, C-reactive protein, renin, factors VII and IX, fibrinogen, β-glucuronidase and isocitrate dehydrogenase. Estrogens were implicated in decreases in lipoprotein lipase, cholinesterase, lactic acid dehydrogenase, and alkaline phosphatase (Aurell *et al.*, 1966; Carruthers *et al.*, 1966; Arturson *et al.*, 1967; Musa *et al.*, 1967; Pulkkinen and Willman, 1967; Spellacy *et al.*, 1967a; Laurell *et al.*, 1968; Song *et al.*, 1970; Horne *et al.*, 1970). Most of these changes seem to be without clinical significance so far.

They must, however, be taken into account in the interpretation of clinical laboratory findings, which may otherwise be misleading. Wilbert *et al.* (1969) have listed more than sixty "normal values" which may undergo changes in women on oral contraception.

Minerals. Increases in serum copper and zinc levels (Carruthers *et al.*, 1966; O'Leary and Spellacy, 1969) and of serum iron and total iron-binding capacity have been noted (Burton, 1967; Mardell *et al.*, 1969). The significance of these observations is not known. Increases of serum copper and ceruloplasmin levels have been linked to estrogens. Oral contraceptives may cause a decrease in serum magnesium levels, suggesting a poorly understood alteration in magnesium metabolism. Concern has been expressed that this could cause an increase of cardiovascular disease but at the present it is only a speculation.

Salt and water metabolism. The effects of oral contraceptives on water and electrolyte metabolism are incompletely understood. Some progestogens cause an increased excretion of sodium followed by retention even while the hormone is administered (see Chapter 31, Subsection 10.3, p. 293). The diuretic effect appears to predominate at higher dose levels, but it is not certain whether long-term progestin administration causes diuresis or retention of sodium. Elimination of sodium by progestogens is opposed by estradiol which at high doses causes sodium retention. In oral contraceptives the estrogen effect appears to predominate and the overall effect appears to be a decrease of sodium excretion (Preedy, 1968). In part, the changes in sodium metabolism (retention) may be reflected in water metabolism, weight gain and figure changes.

6. SKIN AND SKIN APPENDAGES

(a) *Melasma* (*chloasma*)

Melasma, a condition of hyperpigmentation of the skin, particularly over the forehead, the molar eminences and the lower parts of the cheeks, was originally described as a side effect of oral contraceptives in women in Mexico (Rice-Wray *et al.*, 1962) and Puerto Rico (Satterthwaite, 1964). Subsequently, it has also been seen in other countries, in Australia (Carruthers, 1966), in the United States (Resnik, 1967; Hammer, 1968) and in Egypt (Kamal *et al.*, 1968). It is unclear whether this is related to the estrogen or progestogen component of the contraceptives. There is no specific treatment other than withdrawal of the contraceptive agent and protection against sun exposure. The condition does not recede rapidly and becomes a cosmetic problem. Increased skin sensitivity to sunlight has been reported (Erickson, 1968).

(b) *Sebaceous glands and acne*

Strauss and Pochi (1964) have shown that amounts of norethindrone and norethynodrel used currently in the combined oral contraceptives do not influence sebum production. However, lower doses of progestogens in combination with estrogen or estrogen alone, in amounts used in sequential therapy, cause a reduction in sebum production and may have a beneficial effect in the management of acne. Acne has also been reported as a side effect of contraceptive therapy, but these observations lack suitable controls.

(c) *Hair*

There have been reports of alopecia areata or patchy baldness resembling alopecia areata in women taking oral contraceptives (Vollings, 1965; Peterkin, 1965), but others have said that this is no more than coincidence as this is a common condition in women of child-bearing age (Orentreich and Berger, 1966).

7. WEIGHT AND FIGURE CHANGE

Weight gain and weight loss of 6 pounds or more have been reported with the use of all oral-contraceptive agents. In general, with the progestogen–estrogen combinations, those women who gain more than 6 pounds outnumber those who lose more than 6 pounds. In addition to weight changes, there have also been reports that some oral-contraceptive users experience an increase in waist and abdominal circumferential measurements. Bakker and Dightman (1966), in a study over a 4-year period in which women were weighed at every visit, failed to find a significant trend in weight gain or loss. However, in a smaller group of women in whom the pills were discontinued, about 30% showed a distinct and rapid decrease in weight suggestive of fluid loss.

8. CENTRAL NERVOUS SYSTEM AND PSYCHOLOGICAL EFFECTS

In animals estrogens and progesterone are essential for normal sexual behavior. Some investigators suggest that in women the days preceding ovulation coincide with an increase in sexual desire and activity, while the second half of the menstrual cycle is supposedly characterized by a decrease or lack of sexual interest. Such speculations remain unconfirmed at the present and the question whether synthetic steroids may influence libido by antagonistic or synergistic actions remains unanswered (see Subsection (d)). Influences of progesterone and of synthetic progestational compounds on the central nervous system, including thermoregulation, are fully discussed in other chapters (14, 17, 28, 31).

In our studies (Rudel and Kincl, 1966; Rudel, unpublished data) we have found that norethindrone produced a thermogenic effect in a majority of male and female patients treated with a dose of 0.5, 1.2 and 4 mg per day. Chlormadinone acetate was judged to be thermogenic at a dose of 4 mg a day.

Oral contraceptives have been stated to produce a variety of disorders, including headache, depression, loss of libido and a number of neurological symptoms. In most studies samples have been drawn from selected populations, often with characteristics that make such side effects difficult to evaluate. The study of Pincus and co-workers (1959) comparing the incidence of side effects in a selected population is indicative. In this trial one group of patients received placebo tablets and a warning, the second group had oral contraceptives and a warning and the third group had oral contraceptives and no warning. In this study the warnings produced about the same incidence of reactions regardless of whether they had placebo tablets or oral contraceptives. Goldzieher (1968) compared the incidence of "side effects" in a sample of 1064 users of intra-uterine devices and in a series of 165,741 cycles with oral contraceptives. He found the incidence of decreased libido, diarrhea, malaise, headache and dizziness to be about the same in both groups. Nervousness and depression was more frequent in oral-contraceptive users.

The literature on mood and behavioral changes associated with the use of the oral contraceptives was reviewed by Glick (1967). Mental symptoms and sexual adaptation were studied by a group of psychiatrists and gynecologists in Sweden (Nilsson et al., 1967). Psychiatrists are increasingly paying attention to the profound influence of the attitude of the patient with regard to contraception in general on the development of mental reactions, as is shown by an interesting study by Petersen in Switzerland (1969).

(a) *Nausea and vomiting*

Nausea and vomiting, generally agreed to be related to the estrogen component, occur frequently during the initial two or three treatment cycles. In later cycles it tends to diminish. Table 17 lists the incidence of nausea and vomiting with various preparations; for several compounds only the incidence of nausea excluding the incidence of vomiting has been given by the investigators. This may tend to decrease the overall percentage observed.

(b) *Headache*

Mears and Grant (1962) reported that the timing of headaches appeared changed in oral-contraceptive users from the premenstrual period to the interval phase between medication cycles. Similar observations were made by Whitty et al. (1966) regarding the timing of migraine attacks.

Later, Grant (1965) found that 11% of women in their study section developed troublesome headaches for the first time when given progestogen–estrogen contraceptives. The endometrium of these women had a distinct vascular pattern with prominent groups of arterioles, suggesting an etiological correlation. West and West (1966) reported that EEG abnormalities are not caused by oral contraceptives but that they pre-exist, probably indicating a state of latent migraine which can be activated by oral contraceptives. On the other hand, Matsumoto et al. (1966) found EEG changes similar to those in patients with anovulatory cycles believed to be produced by alterations of hypothalamic functions.

(c) *Depression*

There have been reports that women experience an irritability or depression while on contraceptive agents (Kaye, 1963; Tyler, 1964), depression being more frequently associated with women of higher educational background or in young housewives with many small children (Kroger and Peacock, 1968). In general, women who suffer from depression

TABLE 17. INCIDENCE OF NAUSEA AND VOMITING FOR VARIOUS PREPARATIONS

Preparation	Percentage of patients per cycle			Overall incidence	Reference
	Cycle 1	Cycle 2	Cycle 5		
Chlormadinone acetate (2 mg, sequential)	13.7	5.8			(c)
Dimethisterone (25 mg, sequential)[a,b]	6.9	2.2			(c)
Ethynodiol diacetate (1 mg)	15.1	5.8			(c)
Lynestrenol (5 mg)				11.3	Dukes et al. (1963)
(5 mg)				7.5	Turpeinen (1964)
(5 mg)	13.7			1.5	Kopera et al. (1964)
(2.5 mg)				1.8	Strade (1966)
Medroxyprogesterone acetate (10 mg)[a]	30.5	10.6			(c)
Norethindrone (1 mg)	9.6	4.6	2.7		(c)
(2 mg)	13.9	3.3	1.0		(c)
(2 mg, sequential)	11.9	4.9	2.8		(c)
(1 + 80)	4.9	3.2	2.4		(c)
Norethindrone acetate (2.5 mg)	13.3	3.7		0.7	(c)
Norgestrel (0.5 mg)	11.6			3.1	Laurie and Lewis (1968)
Norethynodrel (2.5 mg)[a]	8.1	2.3	2.7		(c)

[a] Nausea only.
[b] Vomiting occurred in 2.3% of patients, sometimes during the course of treatment.
[c] Data obtained from information supplied by the manufacturer to the United States Food and Drug Administration.

before and during the menstrual period seem more susceptible to depression while on contraceptive steroids. Depression and loss of libido are more likely to occur with compounds containing larger quantities of progestins, the lowest incidence of these side effects being observed with the sequential preparations (Grant and Pryse-Davies, 1968). More recent findings are in conflict with previous reports. Bakker and Dightman (1966), using Minnesota Multiphasic Personality Inventory (MMPI) and interviewing techniques, failed to find any causal relationship between oral-contraceptive therapy and episodes of depression. Glick (1967) in a review of the literature found nineteen studies, mostly by obstetricians or gynecologists, in which emotional distress had been noted in women using oral-contraceptive agents. The highest incidence of depression reported was 5%. Subsequently Murawski *et al.* (1968) in a longitudinal study using a variety of psychological and psychiatric interviews and tests failed to observe marked behavioral changes in a group of seventy-two women taking a norethynodrel–mestranol preparation over a 15-month period. Some patients did experience depressive episodes but these were believed to be unrelated to the drug. Kane (1968) reported completely different results from interviewing a group of 139 young, highly educated women of low parity using oral contraceptives. Thirty-four per cent (34%) of them reported depression, 29% irritability, and 24% lethargy. Importantly, about 25% of the subjects felt badly enough to wish to stop taking the drugs. Kane in this report refers to a personal communication from Coppen who conducted a prospective study comparing reactions of oral-contraceptive users to women employing other forms of contraception. He found a 10% incidence of depression serious enough to cause the oral contraceptives from being used further.

Enough concern has now evolved to necessitate a precaution from the Food and Drug Administration of the United States against their use by women with psychic depression.

(*d*) *Libido*

Both an increase and a decrease of libido have been reported by women using oral contraceptives. However, not only is it difficult to give a quantitative value to this appetite, but its very nature almost precludes a correlation of its intensity with any contraceptive practice (Ringrose, 1965; Lidz, 1969). Superficially it is easy to attribute an increase in sexual interest and enjoyment reported with oral contraceptives to the ease of the method and freedom from pregnancy anxiety, while a decrease could be due to guilt and the certainty that pregnancy fulfilment cannot be achieved during their use. A number of studies have been reviewed by Drill (1966). In the study of Nilsson et al. (1967), sexual adaptation was improved in 45.3% of 258 women, impaired in 26%, the majority of these stating a decrease of libido.

(e) *Neurological abnormalities*

In experimental animals, progesterone is known to increase, and estrogens to decrease, the threshold for seizures, induced by electric current. The combination of agents used as contraceptives tends to lower the threshold, and the effect appears to be dependent on the ratio of progestogens to estrogen. It is known that the frequency of epileptic seizures increases in the immediate premenstrual period. This suggests that the observations made in lower species may be applicable to man.

A number of neurological symptoms and syndromes have been randomly reported. In most cases, the etiological significance remains obscure but a number have been linked to underlying vascular problems. The first report of an unexplained cerebrovascular accident was by Lorentz in 1962. Additional reports have appeared since (cf. Illis et al., 1965; Bickerstaff and Holmes, 1967; Gardner et al., 1967; Jennett and Cross, 1967; Salmon et al., 1968). Connell and Kelman (1968) failed to find any eye abnormalities of the cornea, sclera, macula and vessels in 184 patients taking either combined or sequential preparation.

The second report of the Advisory Committee to the U.S. Food and Drug Administration (Masi and Dugdale, 1969) concluded:

1. A review of the major clinical reports of cerebrovascular occlusion in women using the oral contraceptives reveals a notable increase in the number of instances of cerebrovascular disease in healthy women of child-bearing age that have appeared since the introduction of the oral contraceptives.
2. Young women suffering from stroke while using the oral contraceptives almost always have some warning, usually significant headache, prior to the onset of the paretic event. In about one-fourth there is ischemia or infarction in the vertebral and basilar arterial system, a location which was previously considered rare in young healthy women.
3. Cerebral arteries rather than veins are primarily involved. Limited angiographic and autopsy studies suggest intrinsic vascular alterations in addition to possible derangement of the hemostatic mechanisms.
4. Controlled retrospective studies of young women with cerebral thrombosis without a predisposing cause indicate a statistically significant etiologic relation with the oral contraceptives. There is a sixfold estimated increase in the risk of both morbidity and mortality.
5. Notwithstanding available statistical evidence concerning the overall mortality from cerebrovascular disorders in the general population of women of child-bearing age since the time of introduction of the oral contraceptives until 1966 indicates no significant change. There is neither a decrease which one might anticipate due to the

decreased number of pregnancies and deliveries in the general population, nor an increase which might have been evident if the risk from the oral contraceptives *per se* were greater than opposing forces of such mortality operating over this interval.

Another conclusion (Greene, 1969) is that "the lack of a rise in female deaths at reproductive ages from cerebral embolism and thrombosis fails to support an association between the use of oral contraceptives and these conditions barring the possible concealment of an effect by a lowering of pregnancy rates . . .".

9. OTHER EFFECTS

Carcinogenesis

Of the two components of hormonal contraceptives, estrogens have been most widely indicated as potential carcinogens. Prolonged exposure of laboratory animals to estrogens at relatively high dosage may result in the development of certain neo-plastic lesions (Crossen and Suntzeff, 1950; Gardner *et al.*, 1959; Griffiths *et al.*, 1963; Lipschütz *et al.*, 1967; Hertz, 1968). Yet, although all physical and chemical agents believed to be carcinogenic in man produce malignant tumors in experimental animals, the reverse is not always true. Evidence of carcinogenicity in laboratory animals may not be pertinent to man and the question whether estrogens cause cancer in man still remains unresolved. The prime sites of cancer in women are the cervix and the breast. These two organs have been given the greatest attention.

Cervix

Oral contraceptives may produce a variety of epithelial changes in the human cervix of uncertain prognostic significance. One study has revealed a higher prevalence of epithelial abnormalities that the investigators considered to be carcinoma *in situ* among women using oral contraceptives than in those who use the diaphragm (Melamed *et al.*, 1969). The Advisory Committee to the U.S. Food and Drug Administration (1969) which evaluated the study and the inherent epidemiological problems associated with this type of safety studies concluded:

> The prevalence of epithelial abnormalities diagnosed as carcinoma *in situ* was higher among the 6,331 women who had used oral contraceptives for one year or more (9.8 per 1,000) than among the 21,177 women who were using other methods at the time of their first clinic attendance (5.6 per 1,000). There appears to be no further increment with duration of use of the pill. This finding is at variance with what would be expected in the case of a causal relation . . . this study does not prove or disprove an etiologic relation between the oral contraceptives and these cervical changes.

The Committee strongly recommended that additional studies be undertaken and these are currently in progress.

Stern *et al.* (1970) found a higher rate of dysplasia of the cervix in women choosing oral contraceptives in preference to other methods.

In Germany Soost and Baier (1967) evaluated the cytological examinations of 3912 women who used oral contraceptives and arrived at the conclusion that there was no increased incidence of carcinoma of the cervix nor of its potential precursor states.

Breast

Estrogen causes glandular changes in the human breast; its carcinogenic effect on that organ has never been proved. Even in women with frank mammary carcinoma, estrogen produces variable changes in the clinical course of the disease: ovariectomy leads to regression of metastic breast carcinoma in approximately half of premenopausal women; exogenous estrogens cause either regression or stimulation of similar tumors in menstruating women but induce regression in about half of postmenopausal women. The reasons for these paradoxical effects of estrogen on breast cancer are not clear.

There is no method of early detection of mammary carcinoma comparable in efficacy to that of the cervical Papanicolaou smear; also there are no indications of a possible carcinogenic effect of oral contraceptives on the breast. The Advisory Committee to U.S. Food and Drug Administration has concluded in its report in 1969 (p. 7):

> Lacking conclusive information about the applicability of existing animal data to women and sufficient observations of human disease the Committee concludes that potential carcinogenicity of the oral contraceptives can be neither affirmed nor excluded at this time. Clinical surveillance of all women taking oral contraceptives must be continued. A major effort to resolve the questions about steroid-induced neoplasis in human beings should be undertaken.

Some progestogens (not available commercially) and combinations of progestogens and estrogens have induced non-malignant tumors in beagle dogs. Two commercial preparations, medroxyprogesterone combined with ethynyl estradiol (Provest) and mestranol–chlormadione acetate sequential (C-Quens), have produced at a dose 10 and 25 times the human dose these experimental mammary tumors at a more rapid rate than they would occur naturally. Similar studies in mice, rats and monkeys revealed no changes. Despite the lack of direct applicability of the observations in a highly susceptible canine strain to humans the companies concerned withdrew voluntarily these preparations in November 1970 and recommended that women using the two progestogens be transferred to other means of fertility control (Anonymous, 1970). (See also Chapter 28, Subsection 24.2.)

Excretory system

Ureteral dilatation has been seen in oral-contraceptive users (Marshall *et al.*, 1966). Such dilatation disappears after medication ceases and it has been postulated to be due to progestins rather than estrogens. Asymptomatic pyelonephritis is known to occur in some patients. This may be secondary to ureteral dilatation. Acute colonic lesions were observed in a few women on oral contraceptives. It is postulated that these lesions may result from thromboembolic phenomena (Kilpatrick *et al.*, 1968; Ward and Stevensen, 1968).

Lung

Oral contraceptives exert a variety of effects on the respiratory system (Lyons, 1968; Stein *et al.*, 1968). Estrogens appear to inhibit gas transfer to a small degree. Progestogens cause an increase of bronchial resistance, mediated probably by an increase in histamine, a potent bronchial constrictor.

Skeletal maturation

Estrogens have been used to prevent excessive height in otherwise normal girls through the induction of premature epiphyseal closure (cf. Wilkins, 1954). Such observations may lead to concern over the possible effects of oral contraceptives on bone growth in young women. Such fears are unfounded. To be effective at all the estrogen treatment must be started prepuberally, and in much higher dosages than those used for contraceptive purposes.

Effects on the fetus

Several studies in experimental animals implicate synthetic progestogens in masculinization of external genitalia of female fetuses. Masculinization of the external genitals of female fetuses due to oral steroid therapy during the first 16 to 18 weeks of pregnancy were reported (see Chapters 28, Subsection 15.4 and 32, Section B, p. 322). Most of the reported cases appear to occur during the time when oral progestogens in high dosages were used to prevent abortion. With the realization that most of these agents are virtually worthless for this purpose there appears to be little concern of direct effects on the fetus.

Effects on chromosomes

Carr reported in 1967 (see comprehensive article, Carr, 1969) that polyploidy is greatly increased in abortions from women who become pregnant within 6 months of discontinuing oral contraceptives, adding that "fortunately these anomalies are not compatible with live birth". These studies will undoubtedly be a challenge to geneticists and should be followed up by further statistical evaluation.

C. CONCLUSIONS

Ovulation suppression has been considered to be synonymous with hormonal fertility control. The oral contraceptives which are available today and the majority of the new materials now under investigation incorporate estrogens in amounts which are capable of suppressing ovulation. These are usually combined with progestogens in amounts which are also able to inhibit ovulation. Estrogens and progestogens are also used sequentially. In this case, ovulation suppression by the estrogen is the sole antifertility mechanism.

Both preparations may also produce effects other than ovulation inhibition. These include effects on the organs of reproduction and other endocrine and non-endocrine functions. Although highly effective, these methods impose an exogenous hormonal control upon the menstrual cycle, necessitating a greater dependency upon regular drug ingestion to prevent irregular endometrial shedding and breakthrough bleeding. Their administration must also be interrupted at regular intervals to insure withdrawal bleeding. This precludes their use for long-acting parenteral materials. They must be considered more suitable for the sophisticated Western nations where motivation is of a high order.

In the intricate process of female reproduction, there may be no reason to inhibit the hypothalamic–pituitary–gonadal axis to block conception. Temporally imbalancing the cyclic estrogen–progestogen relationships might suffice. Producing a change in the normal estrogen–progestogen ratio at a given time in the menstrual cycle may well interfere with ovum transport, spermatozoal penetration and migration into the uterus and Fallopian tubes, capacitation of sperm, and implantation of fertilized ova.

Antifertility effects may also be accomplished with amounts of continuous progestogen therapy in amounts which do not inhibit ovulation and permit regular menstrual cycle. A further modification and increased effectiveness could be achieved by a pellet implant releasing continuously small quantities of the effective agent to produce prolonged periods of fertility control.

To make significant strides in the solution of the problem of population control, the concept of ovulation suppression as the only hormonal approach must be replaced by the broader concept of creating an estrogen–progestogen imbalance. We believe, with the technical and professional care available in the developing nations, newer contraceptive methods should exert little or no influence on the hypothalamic–pituitary–ovarian axis and on endometrial development and maturation so that they will produce no irregularity of menstrual cycling even though medication may be omitted. Freedom from menstrual and other side effects is more important than absolute effectiveness. Indeed, effectiveness comparable to mechanical or barrier methods of conception control should be eminently acceptable.

REFERENCES

ADVISORY COMMITTEE ON OBSTETRICS and GYNECOLOGY (1969) *Second Report on the Oral Contraceptives*. Food and Drug Administration, Washington D.C.

ALBERT, A. and SMITH, R. A. (1961) Effect of progesterone on HPG. *Human Pituitary Gonadotrophins*, p. 239. Albert, A. (Ed.), Charles C. Thomas, Springfield, Illinois.

ALLAN, J. S. and TYLER, E. T. (1967) Biochemical findings in long-term oral contraceptive usage. 1. Liver function studies. *Fertil. Steril.* **18**: 112–123.

AMRIS, C. J. and STARUP, J. (1967) The coagulation mechanism in oral contraception. *Acta Obstet. Gynec. Scand.* **46**: 78–91.

ANDELMAN, M. B., ZACKLER, J., SLUTSKY, H. L. and JACOBSON, M. M. (1968) Family planning and public health. *Int. J. Fertil.* **13**: 405–414.

ANDREWS, M. C., ANDREWS, W. C. and LeHEW, W. L. (1966) A comparative study of sequential and simultaneous estrogen–progestogen cyclic medication. *Amer. J. Obstet. Gynec.* **96**: 48–56.

ANDREWS, W. C. and ANDREWS, M. C. (1964) Reduction of side effects from ovulation suppression by the use of newer progestin combinations. *Fertil. Steril.* **15**: 75–83.

ANONYMOUS (1970) Two brands of birth control pills are going off the market. *Chem. and Eng. News*, Nov. 2nd, p. 17.

ARNOLD, M., BURCKHARDT-TAMM, E., CLOEREN, S., MALL-HAEFELI, M., MORF, E., RICHTER, R. H. H., ROTH, F., STAMM, H., WEIS, P. and WYSS, H. (1967) Preliminary results of two comparative trials with oral contraceptives (Part I and Part II). In: *Fertility and Sterility*, pp. 1100–1110. Internat. Congress Series No. 133. Westin, B. and Wiqvist, N. (Eds.). Excerpta Medica, Amsterdam, New York.

ARRONET, G. H., ARRATA, W. S. M., LATOUR, J. P. A. and BRODA, S. (1969) A study on ovulation inhibition by quinestrol. One dose a month. *Int. J. Fertil.* **14**: 295–299.

ARTURSON, G., BECHMAN, L. and PERSSON, B. H. (1967) Alterations in serum naphthylamidase isozymes during treatment with oral contraceptives. *Nature* **214**: 1252–1254.

AURELL, M., CRAMER, K. and RYBO, G. (1966) Serum lipids and lipoproteins during long-term administration of an oral contraceptive (Anovlar). *Lancet* **1**: 291–293.

AVENDAÑO, S., TATUM, H. J., RUDEL, H. W. and AVENDAÑO, O. (1970) A clinical study with continuous low doses of megestrol acetate®+ for fertility control. *Amer. J. Obst. Gynec.* **106**: 122–127.

AYDAR, C. K. and GREENBLATT, R. B. (1961) Clinical and experimental studies with a new progestogen—Dimethisterone. *J. Med. Assoc. of the State of Alabama*, **31**: 1–7.
BAČIĆ, M., DE CASPARIS, A. W. and DICZFALUSY, E. (1970) Failure of large doses of ethynyl estradiol to interfere with early embryonic development in the human species. *Amer. J. Obstet. Gynec.* **107**: 531–534.
BAKKER, C. B. and DIGHTMAN, C. R. (1966) Side effects of oral contraceptives. *Obstet. Gynec.* **28**: 373–379.
BALIN, H., WAN, L. S. and RAJAN, R. (1969) Sequential approach to oral contraceptive therapy. *Int. J. Fertil.* **14**: 300–308.
BANKS, A. W., RUTHERFORD, R. N. and COBURN, W. A. (1965) Pregnancy and progeny after use of progestin-like substances for contraception. *Obstet. Gynec.* **26**: 760–762.
BAUNACH, A. and BAUNACH, M. (1964) Erfahrungen mit Ovulen, einem neuen Ovulationshemmer. *Med. Welt.* **41**: 2207–2211.
BEATON, J. H. (1964) Menstrual regulation by sequential hormone therapy. *West. J. Surg. Obstet. Gynec.* **72**: 160–163.
BECK, P. (1969) Effects of gonadal hormones and contraceptive steroids on glucose and insulin metabolism. In: *Metabolic Effects of Gonadal Hormones and Contraceptive Steroids*, pp. 97–125. Salhanick, H. A., Kipnis, J. M. and Van de Wiele, R. L. (Eds.). Plenum Press, New York.
BEHRMAN, S. J. (1964) Norethindrone, 2 mg.: an evaluation. *Obstet. Gynec.* **24**: 101–105.
BELL, E. T. and LORAINE, J. A. (1967) Urinary steroid and gonadotrophin excretion in women following long-term use of oral contraceptives. *Lancet* **2**: 442–444.
BELLER, F. K. (1956) *Die Blutgerinnungsverhaeltnisse bei der Schwangeren und beim Neugeborenen.* Barth, Leipzig.
BELLER, F. K. and PORGES, R. F. (1967) Blood coagulation and fibrinolytic enzyme studies during cyclic and continuous application of progestational agents. *Amer. J. Obstet. Gynec.* **97**: 448–459.
BENJAMIN, F. and COOPER, D. J. (1967) Comparative validity of oral and intravenous glucose tolerance tests in pregnancy. *Amer. J. Obstet. Gynec.* **97**: 488–492.
BICKERSTAFF, E. R. and HOLMES, J. M. (1967) Cerebral arterial insufficiency and oral contraceptives. *Brit. Med. J.* **1**: 726–729.
BLAUSTEIN, A., SCHENKER, L. and POST, R. C. (1968) The effects of oral contraceptives on the endometrium. I: blood vessels. *Int. J. Fert.* **13**: 466–475.
BOCKNER, V. (1963) The contraceptive pill: a clinical evaluation of its long-term use. *Med. J. Aust.* **6**: 809.
BOLTON, C. H., HAMPTON, J. R. and MITCHELL, J. R. (1968) Effect of oral contraceptive agents on platelets and plasma phospholipids. *Lancet* **1**: 1336–1441.
BORGLIN, N. E. (1965) Oral contraceptives and liver damage. *Brit. Med. J.* **1**: 1289–1290.
BOWMAN, J. A. (1968) The effect of norethindrone-mestranol on cervical mucus. *Amer. J. Obstet. Gynec.* **102**: 1039–1040.
BRODY, S., KERSTELL, J., NILSSON, L. and SVANBORG, A. (1968) The effects of some ovulation inhibitors on the different plasma lipid fractions. *Acta Med. Scand.* **183**: 1–7.
BROWN, J. B., FOTHERBY, K. and LORAINE, J. (1962) The effect of norethisterone and its acetate on ovarian and pituitary function during the menstrual cycle. *J. Endocr.* **25**: 331–341.
BROWN, P. S. and BILLEWICZ, W. Z. (1962) The response of immature mice to mixtures of gonadotrophins. *J. Endocr.* **24**: 65–75.
BROWN, P. S., WELLS, M. and CUNNINGHAM, F. J. (1964) A method for studying and mode of action of oral contraceptives. *Lancet* **2**: 446–447.
BROWN, P. S., WELLS, M. and WARNOCK, D. G. (1966) The effect of an oral contraceptive on urinary gonadotrophin in women at mid-cycle. *J. Reprod. Fertil.* **11**: 481–483.

BUCHHOLZ, R., NOCKE, L. and NOCKE, W. (1962) Studies on the mechanism of action of ethinylnortestosterone in the suppression of ovulation. *Geburtsh. Frauenheilk.* **22:** 923–928.

BUCHHOLZ, R., NOCKE, L. and NOCKE, W. (1964) The influence of gestagens on the urinary excretion of pituitary gonadotrophins, estrogens and pregnanediol in women in the post-menopause and during the menstrual cycle. *Int. J. Fertil.* **9:** 231–251.

BUCHLER, D. and WARREN, J. C. (1966) Effects of estrogens on glucose tolerance. *Amer. J. Obstet. Gynec.* **95:** 479–483.

BURTON, J. L. (1967) Effect of oral contraceptives on haemoglobin, packed-cell volume, serum-iron, and total iron-binding capacity in healthy women. *Lancet* **1:** 978–980.

BURTON, J. L., LOUDON, N. B. and WILSON, A. T. (1967) Urinary coproporphyrin excretion and hepatic function in women taking oral contraceptives. *Lancet* **2:** 1326–1327.

CAHAL, D. A. (1965) Safety of oral contraceptives. Committee on Safety of Drugs. *Brit. Med. J.* **2:** 1180.

CARR, D. H. (1969) Chromosomal error and development. *Amer. J. Obstet. Gynec.* **104:** 327–347.

CARRUTHERS, M. E., HOBBS, C. B. and WARREN, R. K. (1966) Raised serum copper and caeruloplasmin levels in subjects taking oral contraceptives. *J. Clin. Path.* **19:** 498–500.

CARRUTHERS, R. (1966) Chloasma and oral contraceptives. *Med. J. Aust.* **2:** 17–20.

COMMITTEE ON SAFETY OF DRUGS (1970) Combined oral contraceptives. A statement. *Brit. Med. J.* **2:** 231–232.

CONNELL, E. B. and KELMAN, C. D. (1968) Ophthalmologic findings with oral contraceptives. *Obstet. Gynec.* **31:** 456–460.

CONNELL, E. B., SEDLIS, A. and STONE, M. L. (1967) Endometrial enzyme histochemistry in oral contraceptive therapy. *Fertil. Steril.* **18:** 35–45.

CORFMAN, P. A. (1969) *Second Report on the Oral Contraceptives.* Advisory Committee on Obstetrics and Gynecology. Food and Drug Administration.

COTTERAL, R. D. (1966) Candida and oral contraceptives. *Lancet* **2:** 830.

COUTINHO, E. M. and DE SOUZA, J. C. (1968) The every-other-day pill. *J. Reprod. Fertil.* **16:** 137–139.

CROCKER, K. M. and STITT, W. D. (1964) Ovulation inhibitors. *Canad. Med. Ass. J.* **90:** 713–716.

CROSSEN, R. J. and SUNTZEFF, V. (1950) Endometrial polyps and hyperplasia produced in an aged monkey with estrogen plus progesterone. *Arch. Path.* **50:** 721–726.

DAHLBERG, B. (1966) Aspects of a new oral contraceptive, Ovulen. *Acta Obstet. Gynec. Scand.* **45:** 43–46.

DANFORTH, D. N., MANALO-ESTRELLA, P. and BUCKINGHAM, J. C. (1964) The effect of pregnancy and of Enovid on the rabbit vasculature. *Amer. J. Obstet. Gynec.* **88:** 952–962.

DEHEJIA, N., PARDANANI, N. S., VAIDYA, R. and PURANDARE, B. N. (1967) Clinical trial with megestrol acetate as an oral contraceptive (Volidan). *J. Obstet. Gynaec. India* **17:** 135–138.

DEVENISH-MEARES, M. (1965) Oral contraceptives. *Med. J. Aust.* **52:** 283.

DICZFALUSY, E. (1965) Probable mode of action of oral contraceptives. *Brit. Med. J.* **2:** 1394–1399.

DICZFALUSY, E., GOEBELSMANN, U., JOHANNISSON, E., TILLINGER, K.-G. and WIDE, L., (1969) Pituitary and ovarian function in women on continuous low dose progestogens; effect of chlormadinone acetate and norethisterone. *Acta Endocrinologica* **62:** 679–693.

DIDDLE, A. W., WATTS, G. F., GARDNER, W. H. and WILLIAMSON, P. J. (1966) Oral contraceptive medication: a prolonged experience. *Amer. J. Obstet. Gynec.* **95**: 489–495.
DINGLE, J. T. (1963) Preliminary report on provest study. *Int. J. Fert.* **8**: 711–719.
DI PAOLA, G., PUCHULU, F., ROBIN, M., NICHOLSON, R. and MARTI, M. (1968) Oral contraceptives and carbohydrate metabolism. *Amer. J. Obstet. Gynec.* **101**: 206–216.
DI SAIA, P. J., DAVIS, C. D. and TABER, B. Z. (1968) Continuous tablet therapy for oral contraception. *Obstetrics and Gynecology* **31**: 119–124.
DOAR, J. W. H., WYNN, V. and CRAMP, D. G. (1969) Studies on venous blood pyruvate and lactate levels during oral and intravenous glucose tolerance tests in women receiving oral contraceptives. In: *Metabolic Effects of Gonadal Hormones and Contraceptive Steroids*, pp. 178–192. Salhanick, H. A., Kipnis, D. M. and Van de Wiele, R. L. (Eds.). Plenum Press, New York.
DODEK, O. I. and KOTZ, H. L. (1967) Syndrome of anovulation following the oral contraceptives. *Amer. J. Obstet. Gynec.* **98**: 1065–1070.
DODEK, O. I., JR., SEGRE, E. J. and KLAIBER, E. L. (1965) Effects of Enovid on cortisol metabolism. *Amer. J. Obstet. Gynec.* **93**: 173–178.
DOLL, R., INMAN, W. H. W. and VESSEY, M. P. (1969) Concerning the British data (letter to the editor). *J. Am. Med. Ass.* **207**: 1150–1151.
DONAYRE, J. and PINCUS, G. (1965) Effects of Enovid on blood clotting factors. *Metabolism* **14** Suppl.: 418–421.
DORFMAN, R. I. and KINCL, F. A. (1963) Steroid anti-estrogens. *Steroids* **1**: 185–209.
DRILL, V. A. (1966) *Oral Contraceptives*. McGraw-Hill Book Co., New York.
DUGDALE, M. and MASI, A. T. (1969) Effects of the oral contraceptives on blood clotting. In: *Second Report on the Oral Contraceptives*, pp. 43–51. Food and Drug Administration, Washington D.C.
DUKES, M. N. G., KOPERA, H. and IJZERMAN, G. L. (1963) Clinical experience with .cyclical administration of lynestrenol in combination with an estrogen for fertility control. *Excerpta Med.* **72**: 336–358.
DUNN, H. P. (1967) Sterility following oral contraceptives. *New Zeal. Med. J.* **66**: 261.
DURANDEAU, A. (1968) Experimentação clinica do produto Ovanon. *Revista Brasiliera de Medicina* **25**: no. 4 (April), Rio de Janeiro.
EDITORIAL (1966) Vaginitis and the pill. *J. Amer. Med. Ass.* **196**: 731–732.
EICHNER, E. (1964) Control of fertility. *J. Kentucky State Med. Ass.* **62**: 195–199.
EISALO, A., JARVINEN, P. A. and LUUKKAINEN, T. (1965) Liver-function tests during intake of contraceptive tablets in pre-menopausal women. *Brit. Med. J.* **1**: 1416–1417.
ERICKSON, L. R. (1968) Sunlight sensitivity from oral contraceptives. *J.A.M.A.* **203**: 178–179.
EVERSE, J. W. R. and ESSELINK, J. (1970) Evaluation of normophasic oral contraceptive (Ovanon). *Clinical Trials Journal* **7**: 249–253.
FELDMAN, E. B. and CARTER, A. C. (1960) Endocrinologic and metabolic effects of 17α-methyl-19-nortestosterone in women. *J. Clin. Endocr. Met.* **20**: 842–857.
FISHER, D. A., ODDIE, T. H. and EPPERSON, D. (1966) Norethynodrel-mestranol and thyroid function. *J. Clin. Endocr. Met.* **26**: 878–884.
FLORSHEIM, W. H. and FAIRCLOTH, M. A. (1964) Effects of oral ovulation inhibitors on serum protein-bound iodine and thyroxine binding proteins. *Proc. Soc. Exp. Biol. Med.* **117**: 56–58.
FLOWERS, C. E., VORYS, N., STEVENS, V., MILLER, A. T. and JENSEN, L. (1966) The effects of suppression of menstruation with ethynodiol diacetate upon the pituitary, ovary, and endometrium. *Amer. J. Obstet. Gynec.* **96**: 784–803.

Foss, G. L. (1968) Oral contraception with continuous microdose of norgestrel. *J. Reprod. Fert.*, Suppl. 5: 145–154.
Francis, W. G. (1964) 2 mg norethindrone-mestranol in contraception and therapy. *Applied Therap.* **6**: 419–423.
Frieden, E. and Osaki, S. (1969) Serum copper and oral estragen. *Science* **163**: 959.
Gall, S. A., Bourgeois, C. H. and Maguire, R. (1969). The morphologic effects of oral contraceptive agents on the cervix. *J. Am. Med. Ass.* **207**: 2243–2247.
Garcia, C. R. (Ed.) (1968) *Oral Contraception. Clinical Obstetrics and Gynecology*, Vol. 11, no. 3. Hoeber Medical Division, Harper & Row, New York.
Garcia, C. and Pincus, G. (1964) Hormonal inhibition of ovulation. *Manual of Contraceptive Practice*, p. 209. Calderon, M. S. (Ed.), The Williams & Wilkins Co., Baltimore, Maryland.
Gardner, J. H., van den Noort, S. and Horenstein, S. (1967) Cerebrovascular disease in young women taking oral contraceptives. *Neurology* **17**: 297–298.
Gardner, W. V., Pfeiffer, C. A. and Trentin, J. J. (1959) Hormonal factors in experimental carcinogenesis. In: *Physiopathology of Cancer*, p. 152. F. Homburger and W. H. Fishman (Eds.). Harper & Row Publishers, Inc., New York.
Gershberg, H., Hulse, M. and Javier, Z. (1968) Hypertriglyceridemia during treatment with estrogen and oral contraceptives. An alteration in hepatic function? *Obstet. Gynec.* **31**: 186–189.
Gershberg, H., Javier, Z. and Hulse, M. (1964) Glucose tolerance in women receiving an ovulatory suppressant. *Diabetes* **13**: 378–382.
Glick, I. D. (1967) Mood and behavioral changes associated with the use of the oral contraceptive agents. A review of the literature. *Psychopharmacologia (Berl.)* **10**: 363–374.
Goldzieher, J. W. (1968) The incidence of side effects with oral or intrauterine contraceptives. *Amer. J. Obst. Gynec.* **102**: 91–94.
Goldzieher, J. W. and Maas, J. M. (1965) Clinical evaluation of a sequential oral contraceptive. Excerpta Med. Presented at the Sixth Pan American Congress of Endocrinology, Oct. 10–15, Mexico City.
Goldzieher, J. W., Maas, J. M. and Hines, D. C. (1968) Seven years of clinical experience with a sequential oral contraceptive. *Int. J. Fertil.* **13**: 399–404.
Goldzieher, J. W., Maqueo, M., Ricaud, L., Aguilar, J. A. and Canales, E. (1966) Induction of degenerative changes in uterine myomas by high dosage progestin therapy. *Am. J. Obstet. Gynec.* **96**: 1078–1087.
Goldzieher, J. W., Becerra, C., Gual, C., Livingston, N. B., Maqueo, M., Moses, L. E. and Tietze, C. (1964) New oral contraceptive. *Amer. J. Obstet. Gynec.* **90**: 404–411.
Goldzieher, J. W., Martinez-Manautou, J., Livingston, N. B., Moses, L. E. and Rice-Wray, E. (1963) The use of sequential estrogen and progestin to inhibit fertility, a preliminary report. *West J. Surg. Obstet. Gynec.* **71**: 187–190.
Goldzieher, J. W. and Nakamura, Y. (1962) A clinical method for the determination of urinary pregnanediol and pregnantriol. *Acta Endocr. (Kbh.)* **41**: 371–380.
Goldzieher, J. W. and Rice-Wray, E. (1966) *Oral Contraception: Mechanism and Management*. Charles C. Thomas, Springfield, Illinois.
Goldzieher, J. W., Rice-Wray, E., Schulz-Contreras, M. and Aranda-Rosell, A. (1962) Fertility following termination of contraception with norethindrone. *Amer. J. Obstet. Gynec.* **84**: 1474–1477.
Goodrich, S. M. and Wood, E. J. (1964) Peripheral venous distensibility and velocity of venous blood flow during pregnancy or during oral contraceptive therapy. *Amer. J. Obstet. Gynec.* **90**: 740–744.
Goolden, A. W. G., Gartside, J. M. and Sanderson, C. (1967) Thyroid status in pregnancy and in women taking oral contraceptives. *Lancet* **1**: 12–15.

GRANT, E. C. (1965) Relation of arterioles in the endometrium to headache from oral contraceptives. *Lancet* **1**: 1143–1144.

GRANT, E. C. G. and PRYSE-DAVIES, J. (1968) Effect of oral contraceptives on depressive mood changes and on endometrial monoamine oxidase and phosphatases. *Brit. Med. J.* **3** (5621): 777–780.

GREANEY, M. O., TABER, B. Z. and BESSLER, S. A. (1968) Methodology in oral contraceptive research. *Fertil. Steril.* **19**: 339–343.

GREENBLATT, R. B. (1961) Antiovulatory drugs and indications for their use. *Med. Clin. N. Amer.* **45**: 973–988.

GREENBLATT, R. B. (1967) One-pill-a-month contraceptive. *Fertil. Steril.* **18**: 207–211.

GREENE, G. R. (1969) Trends in mortality from cerebrovascular diseases. Appendix 2c, *Second Report on the Oral Contraceptives*. Food and Drug Administration, Washington D.C.

GREGG, W. I. (1966) Galactorrhea after contraceptive hormones. *New Eng. J. Med.* **274**: 1432.

GREGOIRE, A. T., RANKIN, J., JOHNSON, W. D., RAKOFF, A. E. and ADAMS, A. (1967) Alpha-amylase content in cervical mucus of females receiving sequential, nonsequential or no contraceptive therapy. *Fertil. Steril.* **18**: 836–839.

GREGOIRE, A. T. and USTAY, K. (1969) Effect of chlormadinone on amount of human cervical mucus and its glycogen content. *Fertil. Steril.* **20**: 938–943.

GRIFFITHS, C. T., TOMIC, M., CRAIG, J. M. and KISTNER, R. W. (1963) Effects of progestins and castration on induced endometrial cancer in the rabbit. *Surg. Forum* **14**: 399–401.

HALLER, J. (1968) *Ovulationshemmung durch Hormone*. Georg Thieme Verlag, Stuttgart.

HALLER, J. (1969) *Hormonal Contraception*. Geron-X, Los Altos, Calif.

HALLER, J. (1970) A review of the long-term effects of hormonal contraceptives. *Contraception* **1**: 233–251.

HAMMER, C. J. (1968) Melasma induced by oral contraceptive drugs. *Northwest Medicine* **67**: 251–254.

HARNECKER, J., CRISOSTO, C., ONETTO, E. and MUÑOZ, L. (1970) Depo-Provera as an injectable female contraceptive agent. In: *Proceedings of the Sixth World Congress on Fertility and Sterility*, pp. 223–228. Gordon & Breach, New York.

HASPELS, A. A. (1969) The "morning-after pill"—a preliminary report. *I.P.P.F. Medical Bulletin.* **3**: 6.

HASS, T. (1963) Provest in private practice. *Int. J. Fert.* **8**: 743–745.

HEANEY, R. P. and WHEDON, G. D. (1958) Impairment of hepatic bromosulphalein clearance by two 17-substituted testosterones. *J. Lab. Clin. Med.* **52**: 169–175.

HEBER, K. R. (1968) Oral contraceptives (Correspondence). *Med. J. Aust.* **2**: 1018.

HECHT-LUCARI, G. (1964) Central and peripheral action of fertility-inhibiting progestogens. *Int. J. Fertil.* **9**: 205–216.

HELMER, O. M. and GRIFFITH, R. S. (1952) The effect of the administration of estrogens on the renin-substrate (hypertensinogen) content of rat plasma. *Endocrinology* **51**: 421.

HERTZ, R. (1968) Experimental and clinical aspects of the carcinogenic potential of steroid contraceptives. *Int. J. Fertil.* **13**: 273–286.

HOLLANDER, C. S., GARCIA, A. AM., STURGIS, S. H. and SELENKOW, H. A. (1963) Effect of an ovulatory suppressant on the serum protein-bound iodine and the redcell uptake of radioactive tri-iodothyronine. *New Eng. J. Med.* **269**: 501–504.

HOLMSTROM, E. G. (1965) The use of Ovulen in clinical practice. *Recent Advances in Ovarian and Synthetic Steroids and the Control of Ovarian Function*, p. 70. Shearman, R. P. (Ed.). Globe Commercial Pty. Ltd., Sydney, Australia.

HOLMSTROM, E. G. (1965) The use of Ovulen in clinical practice. In: *Symposium on Recent Advances in Ovarian and Synthetic Steroids and the Control of Ovarian Function, Oct. 17–18, 1964, Sydney, Australia*, pp. 158–163. Shearman, R. P. (Ed.). Globe Commercial Pty. Ltd., Sydney, Australia.

HOLMSTROM, E. G. (1965) Symposium on long-term safety of progestin–estrogen combinations: the long-term use of Ovulen for contraception. *Metabolism* **14**: 444–445.

HOLZBACH, R. T. and SANDERS, J. H. (1965) Recurrent intrahepatic cholestasis of pregnancy—observations on pathogenesis. *J. Amer. Med. Ass.* **193**: 542–546.

HOMESLEY, H. D. and GOSS, D. A. (1970) Menstrual dysfunction following use of oral contraceptives. *Obstet. Gynec.* **35**: 734–739.

HORNE, C. H. W., HOWIE, P. W., WEIR, R. J. and GOUDIE, R. B. (1970) Effect of combined estrogen–progestogen oral contraceptives on serum-levels of α_2-macroglobulin, transferrin, albumin, and IgG. *Lancet* (1)7637: 49–50.

HOROWITZ, B. J., SOLOMKIN, M. and EDELSTEIN, S. W. (1968) The over-suppression syndrome. *Obstet. Gynec.* **31**: 387–389.

HUTCHERSON, W. P., SCHWARTZ, H. A. and SMITH, L. (1963) Norethindrone with estrogen as an oral contraceptive: a preliminary report. *Southern Med. J.* **56**: 1357–1362.

ILLIS, L., KOCEN, R. S., MCDONALD, W. I. and MONDCAR, V. P. (1965) Oral contraceptives and cerebral arterial occlusion. *Brit. Med. J.* **2**: 1164–1166.

INMAN, W. H. W. and VESSEY, M. P. (1968) Investigation of deaths from pulmonary coronary and cerebral thrombosis and embolism in women of child-bearing age. *Brit. Med. J.* **2**: 193–199.

INMAN, W. H. W., VESSEY, M. P., WESTERHOLM, B. and ENGELUND, A. (1970) Thromboembolic disease and the steroidal content of oral contraceptives. A report to the Committee on Safety of Drugs. *Brit. Med. J.* **2**: 203–209.

IREY, N. S., MANION, W. C. and TAYLOR, H. B. (1970) Vascular lesions in women taking oral contraceptives. *Arch. Path.* **89**: 1–8.

IRIZARRY, S., PANIAGUA, M., PINCUS, G., JANER, J. L. and FRIAS, Z. (1966) Effect of cyclic administration of certain progestin–estrogen combinations on the 24-hour radioiodine thyroid uptake. *J. Clin. Endocr.* **26**: 6–10.

JACKSON, J. L., SPAIN, W. T. and PAYNE, H. (1968) The anti-ovulatory dose of ethynyl estradiol. *Fertil. Steril.* **19**: 649–653.

JACKSON, M. C. N. (1963) Oral contraception in practice. *J. Reprod. Fertil.* **6**: 153–173.

JACKSON, N. H. (1961) Observations in the use of certain orally active progestogens for the control of fertility in women. *Proc. Roy. Soc. Med.* **54**: 984–987.

JAVIER, Z., GERSHBERG, H. and HULSE, M. (1968) Ovulating suppressants, estrogens and carbohydrate metabolism. *Metabolism* **17**: 443–456.

JENNETT, W. B. and CROSS, J. N. (1967) Influence of pregnancy and oral contraception on the incidence of strokes in women of child-bearing age. *Lancet* **1**: 1019–1023.

JOHANNISON, E., TILLINGER, K. G. and DICZFALUSY, E. (1965) Effect of oral contraceptives on the ovarian reaction to human gonadotrophins in amenorrheic women. *Fertil. Steril.* **16**: 292–304.

KAERN, T. (1967) Effect of an oral contraceptive immediately post partum on initiation of lactation. *Brit. Med. J.* **3**: 644–645.

KAMAL, I., HEFNAWI, F., KADRI, S., ASKALANI, H., YOUNIS, N., TAGI, A. and ABDALLA, M. (1968) Sequential oral contraception using a serial regimen. *Egyptian Population and Family Planning J.* **1**: 29–42.

KANE, F. J. (1968) Psychiatric reactions to oral contraceptives. *Amer. J. Obstet. Gynec.* **102**: 1053–1063.

KAUFMAN, R. H. and BOATWRIGHT, B. (1967) The pelvic congestive effects of norethindrone with mestranol. Presented at 23rd Annual Meeting, The American Fertility Society, April 14–16, Washington, D.C.

KAYE, B. M. (1963) Oral contraceptives and depression. *J. Amer. Med. Ass.* **186**: 522.

KILPATRICK, Z. M., SILVERMAN, J. F., BETANCOURT, E., FARMAN, J. and LAWSON, J. P. (1968) Vascular occlusion of the colon and oral contraceptives: possible relation. *New Eng. J. Med.* **278**: 438–440.

KIRCHOFF, H. and HALLER, J. (1964) Klinische Erfahrungen mit einer ovulationsunterdrückenden Oestrogen-Gestagen-Kombination (Anovlar). *Med. Klin.* **59**: 681–687.

KLEINER, G. J., KRESCH, L. and ARIAS, I. M. (1965) Studies of hepatic excretory function. *New Engl. J. Med.* **273**: 420–423.

KOPERA, H., DUKES, M. N. G. and IJZERMAN, G. L. (1964) Critical evaluation of clinical data on lyndiol. *Int. J. Fertil.* **9**: 69–74.

KORA, S. J. (1969) Effect of oral contraceptives on lactation. *Fertil. Steril.* **20**: 419–423.

KORN, G. W. (1961) The use of norethynodrel (Enovid) in clinical practice. *Canad. Med. Ass. J.* **81**: 584–587.

KREEK, M. J. (1969) Cholestasis of pregnancy and during ethynyl estradiol administration in the human and rat. In: *Metabolic Effects of Gonadal Hormones and Contraceptive Steroids*, pp. 40–58. Salhanick, H. A., Kipnis, D. M. and Van de Wiele, R. L. (Eds.). Plenum Press, New York.

KROGER, W. S. and PEACOCK, J. F. (1968) Psychophysiological effects with an ovulation inhibitor. *Psychosomatics* **9[2]**: 67–70.

LAMB, E. J. (1966) Amenorrhea after medroxyprogesterone. *J. Amer. Med. Ass.* **196**: 143–144.

LARAGH, J. H., SEALEY, J. E., LEDINGHAM, J. G. G. and NEWTON, M. A. (1967) Oral contraceptives. Renin, aldosterone and high blood pressure. *J. Amer. Med. Ass.* **201**: 918–922.

LARRANAGA, A. and BERMAN, E. (1970) Clinical study of a once-a-month oral contraceptive: quinestrol-quingestanol. *Contraception* **1**: 137–148.

LARSSON-COHN, U. (1965a) Oral contraception and serum protein-bound iodine. *Lancet* **1**: 317.

LARSSON-COHN, U. (1965b) Oral contraception and liver function tests. *Brit. Med. J.* **1**: 1414–1415.

LARSSON-COHN, U. (1967) Jaundice and oral contraceptives. *Lancet* **1**: 679.

LARSSON-COHN, U. and STENRAM, U. (1965) Jaundice during treatment with oral contraceptive agents. *J. Amer. Med. Ass.* **193**: 422–426.

LARSSON-COHN, U., JOHANSSON, E. D. B. and GEMZELL, C. (1970a) Effects of continuous daily administration of 0.3 mg of norethindrone on the plasma levels of progesterone and on the urinary excretion of pregnanediol and total oestrogens. *Acta Endocr.* **64**: 38–46.

LARSSON-COHN, U., JOHANSSON, E. D. B., WIDE, L. and GEMZELL, C. (1970b) Effects of continuous daily administration of 0.5 mg of norethindrone on the plasma levels of progesterone and on the urinary excretion of luteinizing hormone, pregnanediol and total estrogens. *Acta Endocr.* **63**: 216–224.

LARSSON-COHN, U., JOHANSSON, E. D. B., WIDE, L. and GEMZELL, C. (1970c) Effects of continuous daily administration of 0.5 mg of chlormadinone acetate on the plasma levels of progesterone and on the urinary excretion of luteinizing hormone and total oestrogens. *Acta Endocr.* **63**: 705–716.

LAUMAS, K. R., MALKANI, P. K., BHATNAGAR, S. and LAUMAS, V. (1967) Radioactivity in the breast milk of lactating women after oral administration of ^{3}H-norethynodrel. *Amer. J. Obstet. Gynec.* **98**: 411–413.

LAURELL, C. B., KULLANDER, S. and THORELL, J. (1968) Effect of administration of a combined estrogen–progestin contraceptive on the level of individual plasma proteins. *Scand. J. Clin. Lab. Invest.* **21**: 337–343.

LAURIE, R. E. and LEWIS, E. T. (1968) Fertility control with Ovral: a clinical review. *J. Reprod. Fert.*, Suppl. 5: 95–107.

LAUWERYNS, J. and FERIN, J. (1964) Effects on the ovary of prolonged administration of lynestrenol: a histological study. *Int. J. Fertil.* **9**: 35–39.

LAYNE, D. S., MEYER, C. J., VAISHWANAR, P. S. and PINCUS, G. (1962) The secretion and metabolism of cortisol and aldosterone in normal and steroid-treated women. *J. Clin. Endocr.* **22**: 107–118.

LEACH, R. B. and MARGULIS, R. R. (1965) Inhibition of adrenocortical responsiveness during progestin therapy. *Amer. J. Obstet. Gynec.* **92**: 762–765.

LEBHERZ, T. B., LABUDOVICH, M., SCHIFF, M. and WOOD, J. (1967) Private paper.

LEE, H.-C., FAN, K.-Y., CHOW, C.-M. and CHOW, L.-P. (1966) A study on an oral contraceptive. *J. Formosan Medical Association* **65**: 178–182.

LIDZ, R. W. (1969) Emotional factors in the success of contraception. *Fertil. Steril.* **20**: 761–771.

LIGGINS, G. C. (1967) The effect of variation in estrogen dosage on the pregnancy rate during sequential oral contraception. *Fertil. Steril.* **18**: 191–197.

LIN, T. J., DURKIN, J. W. and KIM, Y. J. (1964) The control of reproduction and of the functions of certain endocrine organs as reflected by biochemical and biological assays. *Curr. Therap. Res.* **6**: 225–248.

LINTHORST, C. (1966) A new progestogen–estrogen combination for gynecologic therapy and contraception. *Int. J. Fertil.* **11**: 35–45.

LIPSCHÜTZ, A., IGLESIAS, R., PANOSEVICH, V. and SALINAS, S. (1967) Ovarian tumors and other ovarian changes induced in mice by two 19-nor-contraceptives. *Brit. J. Cancer* **21**: 153–159.

LIVINGSTON, N. B. (1963) Medroxyprogesterone acetate and estrogen to inhibit fertility. *Int. J. Fertil.* **8**: 699–702.

LLOYD, C. W. (1967) Personal communication.

LORAINE, J. A., BELL, E. T., HARKNESS, R. A., MEARS, E. and JACKSON, M. C. N. (1965) Hormone excretion patterns during and after long-term administration of oral contraceptives. *Acta Endocr. (Kbh.)* **59**: 15–24.

LORENTZ, I. T. (1962) Parietal lesion and "Enovid". *Brit. Med. J.* **2**: 1191.

LUNENFELD, B., SULIMOVICI, S. and RABAU, E. (1963) Mechanism of action of anti-ovulatory compounds. *J. Clin. Endocr.* **23**: 391–395.

LYON, R. A. (1943) Relief of essential dysmenorrhea with ethinyl estradiol. *Surg. Gynec. Obstet.* **77**: 657–660.

LYONS, H. A. (1968) Respiratory effects of gonadal hormones. *Conference on Metabolic Effects of Gonadal Hormones and Contraceptive Steroids, December 1–5, 1968.* Salhanick, H. A. (Ed.).

MAKEPEACE, A. W., WEINSTEIN, G. L. and FRIEDMAN, M. H. (1937) The effect of progestin and progesterone on ovulation in the rabbit. *Amer. J. Physiol.* **119**: 512–516.

MAQUEO, M. and GOLDZIEHER, J. W. (1966) Hormone-induced alterations of ovarian morphology. *Fertil. Steril.* **17**: 676–683.

MAQUEO, M., AZUELA, J. C., CALDERON, J. J., GOLDZIEHER, J. W. (1966) Morphology of the cervix in women treated with synthetic progestins. *Amer. J. Obstet. Gynec.* **96**: 994–998.

MAQUEO-TOPETE, M., SOBERON, J., CALDERON, J. J. and BERMAN, E. (1968) Pill a month contraceptive. *6th World Congress on Fertility and Sterility in Tel Aviv, Israel, May 20–27*, p. 95.

MAQUEO-TOPETE, M., PEREZ-VEGA, E., GOLDZIEHER, J. W., MARTINEZ-MANAUTOU, J. and RUDEL, H. W. (1963) Comparison of the endometrial activity of three synthetic progestins used in fertility control. *Amer. J. Obstet. Gynec.* **85**: 427–432.

MARDELL, M., SYMMONS, C. and ZILVA, J. F. (1969) A comparison of the effect of oral contraceptives, pregnancy and sex on iron metabolism. *J. Clin. Endocr.* **29**: 1489–1495.

MARGULIS, R. R. and LEACH, R. (1966) Effect of prolonged cyclic therapy with estrogen–progestin combinations on thyroid function. *Amer. J. Obstet. Gynec.* **99**: 168–172.

MARSHALL, S., LYON, R. P. and MINKLER, D. (1966) Ureteral dilatation following use of oral contraceptives. *J. Amer. Med. Ass.* **198**: 782.

MARTIN, L. and CUNINGHAM, K. (1961) Inhibition of human pituitary gonadotrophin output by 17-ethinyl 19-nortestosterone. *Human Pituitary Gonadotrophins*, p. 226. Albert, A. (Ed.). Charles C. Thomas, Springfield, Illinois.

MARTINEZ-MANAUTOU, J., GINER, VELASQUEZ, J., CORTEZ-GALLEGOS, V., AZNAR, R., ROJAR, B., GUITTEREZ-NAJAR, A. and RUDEL, W. H. (1967) Daily progestogen for contraception. A clinical study. *Brit. Med. J.* **2**: 730–732.

MARTINEZ-MANAUTOU, J. and RUDEL, H. W. (1966) Antiovulatory activity of several synthetic and natural estrogens. *Ovulation*, pp. 243–258. Robert B. Greenblatt (Ed.). J. B. Lippincott, Baltimore, Maryland.

MASI, A. T. and DUGDALE, M. (1969) Cerebrovascular diseases associated with the use of oral contraceptives: A review of the literature. Appendix 2E, *Second Report on the Oral Contraceptives*. Food and Drug Administration, Washington D.C.

MATSUMOTO, S., ITO, T. and INOUE, S. (1960) Studies on the ovulation-inhibiting effect of 19-norsteroids on laparatomized patients. *Geburtsh. Frauenheilk.* **20**: 250–262.

MATSUMOTO, S. M., SATO, I., ITO, T. and MATSUOKA, A. (1966) Electroencephalographic changes during long term treatment with oral contraceptives. *Int. J. Fertil.* **11**: 195–204.

MATTHEWS, J. G. (1964) Ortho-novum 2 mg in conception control. *J. Amer. Osteop. Ass.* **63**: 1030–1034.

MCCORMICK, W. G., CARLBORG, L. and GEMZELL, C. (1968) Urinary FSH and LH excretion following combined treatment with norethisterone acetate and ethinyl oestradiol and norethisterone acetate only. *Acta Endocr. (Kbh).* **57**: 536–548.

MCDANIEL, E. B. and ZELENIK, J. S. (1970) Field trial results of long-acting injectable medroxyprogesterone acetate as an injectable in 1730 patients. In: *Proceedings of the Sixth World Congress on Fertility and Sterility*, pp. 209–216. Gordon & Breach, New York.

MCGREGOR, M. S. (1968) Amenorrhoea after oral contraceptives. *Lancet* **1**: 643–644.

MEARS, E. (1963) Ovulation inhibition—an assessment of the results of large-scale clinical trials. Second European Meeting of the Int. Fertil. Ass. Brussels, May 2, 3.

MEARS, E. (1964) Ovulation inhibitors: large-scale clinical trials. *Int. J. Fertil.* **9**: 1–9.

MEARS, E. (1965) *Handbook on Oral Contraceptives*. Churchill, London.

MEARS, E. (1966) Oral contraception—U.K. experience. *Proceedings of a Symposium held at Maidenhead, Berkshire, England*, pp. 18–27. Excerpta Medica Foundation, Amsterdam.

MEARS, E. and GRANT, E. C. G. (1962) Anovlar as an oral contraceptive. *Brit. Med. J.* **2**: 75.

MEHRA, L., MOHAPATRA, P. S. and SHARMA, B. B. L. (1970) A report on the oral pill pilot project clinics in India. *CFPI Technical Paper No. 9*, pp. 1–24. Central Family Planning Institute, New Delhi.

MELAMED, M. R., KOSS, L. G., FLEHINGER, B. J., KELISKY, R. P. and DUBROW, H. (1969) Prevalence rates of uterine cervical carcinoma *in situ* for women using the diaphragm or contraceptive oral steroids. *Brit. Med. J.* **3**: 195–200.

MENDEL, E. B. and BRANNON, R. (1968) Oral contraceptive failures. *Ob. Gyn. Digest* **10:** 25–27.

MERRITT, R. I. (1964) The biological effects of 2 mg morethindrone with mestranol. *App. Therap.* **6:** 427–429.

MESTMAN, J. H., ANDERSON, G. V. and NELSON, D. H. (1968) Adrenal pituitary responsiveness during therapy with an oral contraceptive *Obstet. Gynec.* **31:** 378–384.

METCALF, M. G. and BEAVEN, D. W. (1963) Plasma-corticosteroid levels in women receiving oral contraceptive tablets. *Lancet* **2:** 1095–1096.

MISHELL, D. R., TALAS, M., PARLOW, A. F., EL-HABASHY, M. and MOYER, D. L. (1970) Physiologic and morphologic alterations effected by the contraceptive use of depomedroxyprogesterone acetate. In: *Proceedings of the Sixth World Congress on Fertility and Sterility*, pp. 203–208. Gordon & Breach, New York.

MOGHISSI, K. S. (1966) Cyclic changes of cervical mucus in normal and progestin-treated women. *Fertil. Steril.* **17:** 663–675.

MOGHISSI, K. S., ROSENTHAL, A. and MOSS, H. (1963) Provera-ethinyl estradiol for control of conception. *Int. J. Fertil.* **8:** 703–709.

MORRIS, J. McL. and VAN WAGENEN, G. (1966) Compounds interfering with ovum implantation and development. *Amer. J. Obst. Gyn.* **96:** 804.

MORRIS, J. McL. and VAN WAGENEN, G. (1967) Post coital contraception. *Proceed. 8th Int. Conf. of I.P.P.F.*, p. 256. Santiago, Chile.

MORRIS, N. (1965) Oral contraception. *Practitioner* **194:** 478–484.

MOSES, L. E., GOLDZIEHER, J. W. and MOSES, I. G. (1969) Evaluation of a new combination oral contraceptive: lynestrenol–mestranol (Lyndiol). *Fertil. Steril.* **20:** 715–728.

MURAWSKI, B. J., SAPIR, P. E., SHULMAN, N., RYAN, G. M. JR. and STURGIS, S. H. (1968) An investigation of mood states in women taking oral contraceptives. *Fertil. Steril.* **19:** 50–57.

MUSA, B. U., DOE, R. P. and SEAL, U. S. (1967) Serum protein alterations produced in women by synthetic estrogens. *J. Clin. Endocr.* **27:** 1463–1469.

NEVINNY-STICKEL, J. (1964) Inhibition of ovulation determined by estimation of pregnanediol excretion. *Int. J. Fert.* **9:** 57–67.

NEWLAND, D. O., MARSHALL, L. L., RODGERS, L. D., WAY, F. and WEBBER, R. L. (1964) Effectiveness of a low dose oral contraceptive tablet. *Obstet. Gynec.* **23:** 920–924.

NEWLAND, D. O., MINTZER, A. J., KENNEDY, R. F. and KENDALL, T. (1966) Effectiveness of a sequential oral contraceptive tablet. *Obstet. Gynec.* **28:** 516–520.

NEWTON, M. A., SEALEY, J. E., LEDINGHAM, J. G. G. and LARAGH, J. H. (1968) High blood pressure and oral contraceptives. Changes in plasma renin and renin substrate and in aldosterone excretion. *Amer. J. Obstet. Gynec.* **101:** 1037–1045.

NILSSON, Å., JACOBSON, L. and INGEMANSON, C. A. (1967) Side-effects of an oral contraceptive with particular attention to mental symptoms and sexual adaptation. *Acta Obstet. Gynec. Scand.* **46:** 537–556.

NILSSON, I. M. and KULLANDER, S. (1967) Coagulation and fibrinolytic studies during pregnancy. *Acta Obstet. Gynec. Scand.* **46:** 273–285.

OCKNER, R. K. and DAVIDSON, C. S. (1967) Hepatic effects of oral contraceptives. *New Eng. J. Med.* **276:** 331–334.

O'LEARY, J. A. and SPELLACY, W. N. (1969) Zinc and copper levels in pregnant women and those taking oral contraceptives. *Amer. J. Obstet. Gynec.* **103:** 131–132.

ORENTREICH, N. A. and BERGER, R. A. (1966) Oral contraceptives and alopecia areata. *Brit. Med. J.* **1:** 483.

ORR, A. H. and ELSTEIN, M. (1969) Luteinizing hormone levels in plasma and urine in women during normal menstrual cycles and in women taking combined contraceptives or chlormadinone acetate. *J. Endocr.* **43:** 617–624.

PARKINSON, R. W., MCQUARRIE, H. G., ELLSWORTH, H. S. and STONE, R. A. (1966) Evaluation of a new sequential contraceptive agent. *Obstet. Gynec.* **28:** 239–246.

PEARL, R. (1932) Contraception and fertility in 2,000 women. *Human Biology* **4**: 363–407.
PEREZ, V., GOROSDISCH, S., DE MARTIRE, J., NICHOLSON, R. and DI PAOLA, G. (1969) Oral contraceptives: long-term use produces fine structural changes in liver mitochondria. *Science* **165**: 805–807.
PETERKIN, G. A. (1965) Oral contraceptives and alopecia areata. *Brit. Med. J.* **2**: 1124.
PETERSEN, P. (1969) *Psychiatrische und Psychologische Aspekte der Familienplanung bei oraler Kontraception.* Georg Thieme Verlag, Stuttgart.
PETERSON, W. F., STEEL, M. W. and COYNE, R. C. (1966) Analysis of the effect of ovulatory suppression on glucose tolerance. *Amer. J. Obstet. Gynec.* **95**: 484–488.
PINCUS, G. (1956) Some effects of progesterone and related compounds upon reproduction and early development in mammals. *Acta Endocr.* suppl. **28**.
PINCUS, G. (1959) Progestational agents and the control of fertility. *Vitam. and Horm.* **17**: 307–324. Academic Press.
PINCUS, G. (1963) Frontiers in method of fertility control. *Human Fertility and Population Control*, p. 177. Greene, R. O. (Ed.). Schronkman Publ. Co., Cambridge, Massachusetts.
PINCUS, G. (1964) Research involving aspects of mammalian egg development. *The Population Crisis and the Use of World Resources*, p. 258. Mudd, S. (Ed.).
PINCUS, G. (1965) *The Control of Fertility*, p. 231. Academic Press, New York.
PINCUS, G., BIALY, G., LAYNE, D. S., PANIAGUA, M. and WILLIAMS, K. J. H. (1966) Radioactivity in the milk of subjects receiving radioactive 19-norsteroids. *Nature (Lond.)* **212**: 924–925.
PINCUS, G. and CHANG, M. D. (1953) The effects of progesterone and related compounds on ovulation and early development in the rabbit. *Acta physiol. Lat. Amer.* **3**: 177–183.
PINCUS, G. and ROCK, J. (1958) Effects of 19-norsteroids upon reproductive processes. *N.Y. Acad. Sci.* **71**: 677–690.
PINCUS, G., CHANG, M. C., ZARROW, M. X., HAFEZ, E. S. E. and MERRILL, A. (1956) Effects of certain 19-norsteroids on reproduction processes in animals. *Science* **124**: 890–891.
PINCUS, G., GARCIA, C. R., ROCK, J., PANIAGUA, M., PENDLETON, A., LARAQUE, F., NICOLAS, R., BORNO, R. and PEAN, V. (1959) Effectiveness of an oral contraceptive. *Science* **130**: 81–83.
PLATE, W. P. (1968) Ovarian changes after long-term oral contraception. In: *Drug-induced Diseases*, vol. 3, pp. 235–238. Meyler, L. and Peck, H. M. (Eds.). Excerpta Medica, Amsterdam, New York.
POLLER, L., TABIOWO, A. and THOMSON, J. M. (1968) Effects of low-dose oral contraceptives on blood coagulation. *Brit. Med. J.* **3**: 218–221.
PORTER, P. S. and LYLE, J. S. (1966) Yeast vulvovaginitis due to oral contraceptives. *Arch. Derm.* **93**: 402–403.
POTTER, R. G. (1966) Application of life table techniques to measurement of contraceptive effectiveness. *Demography* **3**: 297–304.
PREEDY, J. R. K. (1968) The effects of gonadal hormones on water and electrolyte metabolism in the human. *Conference on Metabolic Effects of Gonadal Hormones and Contraceptive Steroids, December 1–5.* Salhanick, H. A. (Ed.).
PUDDY, E. M. (1967) A clinical trial of the progestational steroid ethynodiol diacetate as an oral contraceptive. *Med. J. Aust.* **1**: 961–967.
PULKKINEN, M. O. and WILLMAN, K. (1967) The effect of oral contraceptives on serum enzymes. *Acta Obstet. Gynec. Scand.* **46**: 526–536.
PUPKIN, M., ROSENBERG, D., GUERRERO, R. and ZAÑARTU, J. (1970) Long-acting injectable steroids as contraceptives. A comparative study of 2 agents, Abstract 12. In: *Sixth World Congress of Gynaecology and Obstetrics. Internat. J. Gynaecol. Obstet.*, Vol. 8.

RESNIK, S. (1967) Melasma induced by oral contraceptive drugs. *J. Amer. Med. Ass.* **199**: 601–605.

RICE-WRAY, E. (1963) Fertility following termination of contraception with norethindrone. Endometrial morphology and conception rate. *Excerpta Med. (Amst.)*, Sect. III, **16**: 272.

RICE-WRAY, E., ARANDA-ROSELL, A., MAQUEO, M. and GOLDZIEHER, J. (1963) Comparison of the long-term endometrial effects of synthetic progestin used in fertility control. *Amer. J. Obstet. Gynec.* **87**: 429–433.

RICE-WRAY, E., AVILA, C. and GUTIERREZ, J. (1968) Norgestrel and ethynyl estradiol. A new low-dosage oral agent for fertility control. *Obstet. Gynec.* **31**: 368–374.

RICE-WRAY, E., CERVANTES, A., GUITIERREZ, J., ARANDA-ROSELL, A. and GOLDZIEHER, J. W. (1965) The acceptability of oral progestins in fertility control. *Metabolism* **14**: 451–456.

RICE-WRAY, E., CORREN, S. and GASTLELUM, H. (1966) Erfahrungen mit dem oralen Kontraceptivum Anovlar. *Med. Klin.* **61**: 959–964.

RICE-WRAY, E., GOLDZIEHER, J. W. and ARANDA-ROSELL, A. (1963) Oral progestins in fertility control: a comparative study. *Fertil. Steril.* **14**: 402–409.

RICE-WRAY, E., PENA, A. and MAQUEO, M. (1968) Ovanon, a new sequential oral contraceptive. *Int. J. Fertility* **13**: 453–459.

RICE-WRAY, E., SHULTZ-CONTREROS, M., GUERRERO, I. and ARANDA-ROSELL, A. (1962) Long-term administration of norethindrone in fertility control. *J. Amer. Med. Ass.* **180**: 355–358.

RINGROSE, C. A. D. (1965) The emotional responses of married women receiving oral contraceptives. *Canad. Med. Ass. J.* **92**: 1207–1209.

RINGROSE, C. and DOUGLAS, E. (1963) Current concepts in conception control. *Canad. Med. Ass. J.* **39**: 246–248.

ROBINSON, R. W. (1967) Effects of estrogen–progestin combinations on clotting factors. *Amer. J. Obstet. Gynec.* **99**: 163–167.

ROCK, J., GARCIA, C. R. and PINCUS, G. (1957) Synthetic progestins in the normal human menstrual cycle. *Recent Progr. Hormone Res.* **13**: 323–346.

ROCK, J., PINCUS, G. and GARCIA, C. R. (1956) Effects of certain 19-norsteroids on the normal human menstrual cycle. *Science* **124**: 891–893.

ROLAND, M., CLYMAN, M. J., DICHER, A. and OBER, W. B. (1964) Classification of endometrial response to synthetic progestogen and estrogen compounds. *Fertil. Steril.* **15**: 143–163.

ROMAN, W. and HECKER, R. (1968) The liver toxicity of oral contraceptives: a critical review of the literature. *Med. J. Aust.* **2**: 682.

ROSEMBERG, E. and ENGEL, I. (1960) The influence of steroids on urinary gonadotrophin excretion in a postmenopausal woman. *J. Clin. Endocr. Metab.* **20**: 1576–1586.

ROTH, F., ANGST-HORRIDGE, A., ARNOLD, M., BURCKHARDT-TAMM, E., CLOEREN, S., MALL-HAEFELI, M., RICHTER, R. H. H. and STREIT-PFENNIGER, M. (1969) Neuere Ergebnisse vergleichender klinischer Versuche mit oralen Kontrazeptiva. *Gynaecologia* **167**: 467–472.

ROVINSKY, J. J. (1964) Clinical effectiveness of a low dose progestogen–estrogen combination. *Obstet. Gynec.* **23**: 840–850.

ROVINSKY, J. J. (1968) Evaluation of ORF-1658, a new formulation for sequential oral contraceptive therapy. *Fertil. Steril.* **19**: 390–404.

ROZIN, S., SALZBERGER, M., DICKSTEIN, S. and SACKS, M. (1966) Inhibition of ovulation with sequence hormone therapy. *J. Reprod. Fert.* **12**: 119–122.

RUBIO, B., BERMAN, E., LARRANAGA, A., GUILOFF, E. and AGUIRRE, J. J. (1970) A new postcoital oral contraceptive. *Contraception* **1**: 303–314.

RUBIO, B. L. and GONZÁLEZ, R. A. (1970) Contraception with medroxyprogesterone acetate. In: *Proceedings of the Sixth World Congress on Fertility and Sterility*, pp. 217–222. Gordon & Breach, New York.
RUDEL, H. W. (1963) Personal observation.
RUDEL, H. W. (1964) Presented at Fifth Annual Meeting of the Mexican Endocrine Society, Ixtapan de la Sal, México.
RUDEL, H. W. and KINCL, F. A. (1966) The biology of anti-fertility steroids. *Acta Endocr. (Kbh.)* **51** Suppl.: 105.
RUDEL, H. W. (1967) *Hormonal Fertility Control—Newer Biological Consideration.* Excerpta Med. Int. Cong. Ser. **133**: 994–998.
RUDEL, H. W. and MARTINEZ-MANAUTOU, J. (1964) Antiovulatory drug evaluation. *Pharmacologic Techniques in Drug Evaluation.* Nodine, J. W. and Siegler, P. E. (Eds.). J. P. Lippincott, Baltimore, Maryland.
RUDEL, H. W. and MARTINEZ-MANAUTOU, J. (1967a) Oral contraceptives. *Topics in Medicinal Chemistry*, p. 11. Rabinowitz, J. L. and Myerson, R. M. (Eds.). Charles C. Thomas, Springfield, Illinois.
RUDEL, H. W. and MARTINEZ-MANAUTOU, J. (1967b) Hormonal fertility control: a working hypothesis for population control. *Fertil. Steril.* **18**: 219–222.
RUDEL, H. W., LEBHERZ, T., MAQUEO-TOPETE, M., MARTINEZ-MANAUTOU, J. and BESSLER, S. (1967) Assay of the antiestrogenic effects of progestogens in women. *J. Reprod. Fert.* **13**: 199–203.
RUDEL, H. W., MARTINEZ-MANAUTOU, J. and MAQUEO-TOPETE, M. (1965) Role of progestogens in the hormonal control of fertility. *Fertil. Steril.* **16**: 158–169.
RUTHERFORD, R. N., BANKS, A. L. and COBURN, W. A. (1964) Deladroxate for the prevention of ovulation. *Fertil. Steril.* **15**: 648–651.
RYAN, G. M., CRAIG, J. and REID, D. E. (1964) Histology of the uterus and ovaries after long-term cyclic norethynodrel therapy. *Amer. J. Obstet. Gynec.* **90**: 715–725.
SALHANICK, H. A., KIPNIS, D. and VAN DE WIELE, R. (Eds.) (1969) *Metabolic Effects of Gonadal Hormones and Contraceptive Steroids.* Plenum Press, New York–London.
SALMON, M. L., WINKELMAN, J. Z. and GAY, A. J. (1968) Neuroophthalmic sequelae in users of oral contraceptives. *Journ. Amer. Med. Assoc.* **206**: 85–91.
SANCHEZ-RIVERA, G., MERLO, J. G., ESCUDERO, M. and BOTELLA-LLUSIA, J. (1968) *Am. J. Obst. Gynec.* **101**: 665–671.
SARTWELL, P. E., MASI, A. T., ARTHES, F. G., GREENE, G. R. and SMITH, H. E. (1969) Thromboembolism and oral contraceptives: an epidemiological case-control study. Appendix 2A to *Second Report on the Oral Contraceptives.* Food and Drug Administration, Washington D.C. Also published in *Amer. J. Epidem.* **90**: 365–380.
SATTERTHWAITE, A. P. (1964) A comparative study of low dosage oral contraceptives. *App. Therap.* **6**: 410–418.
SATTERTHWAITE, A. P. and GAMBLE, C. J. (1962) Conception control with norethynodrel: progress report of a four year field study at Huamoco, Puerto Rico. *J. Amer. Med. Women's Ass.* **17**: 797–802.
SCHERB, J., KIRSCHNER, M. and ARIAS, I. (1963) Studies of hepatic excretory function. The effect of 17α-ethyl-19-nortestosterone on sulfobromophthalein sodium (BSP) metabolism in man. *J. Clin. Invest.* **42**: 404–408.
SCHLEGELMILCH, H. (1964) Erfahrungen mit Anovlar in der Frauenarztpraxis. *Med. Welt* **36**: 1918.
SCHMIDT-ELMENDORFF, H. and KOPERA, H. (1966) The effect of oral contraceptives on gonadotrophin excretion. *Social and Medical Aspects of Oral Contraception. Round Table Conference, Scheveningen, The Netherlands*, pp. 89–94. International Congress Series No. 130.
SEMM, K. and DITTMAR, F. W. (1965) Post partum ovulation: inhibition and milk yield. *Current Therap. Res.* **8**: 48–51.

SENG, P., HASCHE, H. H., REFERSBURG, W. and VOIGT, K. D. (1969) Systematic investigation on the influence of a contraceptive on some biochemical parameters of fat and carbohydrate metabolism. *Acta Endocr. (Kbh.)* **62**: 181–192.

SHAFEY, S. and SCHEINBERG, P. (1966) Neurological syndromes occurring in patients receiving synthetic steroids (oral contraceptives). *Neurology* **16**: 205–211.

SHAH, P. N. (1968) Acceptability and clinical effectivity of the oral progestogens for fertility control in Indian women. *Fertil. Steril.* **19**: 286–293.

SHEARMAN, R. P. (1968a) Amenorrhoea after oral contraceptives. *Lancet* **1**: 817–818.

SHEARMAN, R. P. (1968b) Investigation and treatment of amenorrhoea developing after treatment with oral contraceptives. *Lancet* **1**: 325–330.

SHOKEIR, M. (1968) Oral contraceptives and caeruloplasmin activity. *Lancet* **2**: 1192.

SOBRERO, A. J. (1963) Field trial of Provest as contraceptive. *Int. J. Fertil.* **8**: 721–724.

SONG, C. S., MERKATZ, I. R., RIFKIND, A. B., GILLETTE, P. N. and KAPPAS, A. (1970) The influence of pregnancy and oral contraceptive steroids on the concentration of plasma proteins. *Amer. J. Obstet. Gynec.* **108**: 227–231.

SOOST, H.-J. and BAIER, W. (1967) Influence of ovulation inhibitors on the cervical epithelium. *Dt. Med. Wschr.* **92**: 1799–1804.

SPELLACY, W. N. (1969) The effect of ovarian steroids on glucose, insulin and growth hormone. In: *Metabolic Effects of Gonadal Hormones and Contraceptive Steroids*, pp. 126–143. Salhanick, H. A., Kipnis, D. M. and Van de Wiele, R. L. (Eds.). Plenum Press, New York.

SPELLACY, W. N., BENDEL, R. P., BUHI, W. C. and BIRK, S. A. (1969) Insulin and glucose determinations after two and three years of use of a combination-type oral contraceptive. *Fertil. Steril.* **20**: 892–902.

SPELLACY, W. N., BIRK, S. A., NOER, K. A. and SCHADE, S. L. (1967) Sedimentation rate in the normal menstrual cycle or with oral contraceptives. *Minnesota Med.* **5**: 645–647.

SPELLACY, W. N. and CARLSON, K. L. (1966) Plasma insulin and blood glucose levels in patients taking oral contraceptives. *Amer. J. Obstet. Gynec.* **95**: 474–478.

SPELLACY, W. N., CARLSON, K. L. and BIRK, S. A. (1967a) Carbohydrate metabolic studies after six cycles of combined type oral contraceptive tablets. Measurement of plasma insulin and blood glucose levels. *Diabetes* **16**: 590–594.

SPELLACY, W. N., CARLSON, K. L. and SCHADE, S. L. (1967b) Human growth hormone levels on normal subjects receiving an oral contraceptive. *J. Amer. Med. Ass.* **202**: 451–454.

SPELLACY, W. N., CARLSON, K. L. and SCHADE, S. L. (1968) Effect of a sequential oral contraceptive on plasma insulin and blood glucose levels after six months' treatment. *Amer. J. Obst. Gynec.* **101**: 672–676.

STAEMMLER, H. J. (1964) *Die gestörte Regelung der Ovarialfunktion*, pp. 184–189. Springer, Berlin.

STARUP, J., DATE, J. and DECKERT, T. (1968) Serum insulin and intravenous glucose tolerance in oral contraception. *Acta Endocr.* **58**: 537–544.

STARUP, J. (1966) The mechanism in inhibition of ovulation in oral contraception. I. *Acta. Endocr. (Kbh.)* **51**: 469–480.

STARUP, J. and ØSTERGAARD, E. (1966) The mechanism in inhibition of ovulation in oral contraception. II. *Acta Endocr. (Kbh.)* **52**: 292–304.

STARUP, J., SELE, V. and BUNS, O. (1966) Pituitary–adrenal function in oral contraception. *Acta, Endocr.* **53**: 1–12.

STEIN, M., RARABEIH, A., YASUTAKE, T. and HIROSE, T. (1968) Effects of gonadal hormones and contraceptive steroids on respiration. *Conference on Metabolic Effects of Gonadal Hormones and Contraceptive Steroids.* December 1–5. Salhanick, H. A. (Ed.).

ŠTERBA, R. (1966) Presented at Congress on Anti-fertility Agents, in Prague, Czechoslovakia, November 3.
ŠTERBA, R., DLHOŠOVA, V., DVOŘÁK, K., HAVRÁNEK, F., HECZKO, P., HORÁK, J., HOUDEK, J., HRNEIŘÍK, O., MIŠINGER, I. and PELÁK, Z. (1967) The sequential hormonal contraception by means of Antigest B. *Cs. Gynekologie* **32**: 3–4: 179–181.
ŠTERBA, R., KRÁLOVÁ, A., ULRYCH, J. and VALOVÁ, B. (1965) Die ersten klinischen Erfahrungen mit 17-Methylen-6-dehydro-17-alpha-acetoxyprogesterone (MDAP). *Zentralblatt für Gynäkologie* **87**: 540–548.
STERN, E., CLARK, V. A. and COFFELT, C. F. (1970) Contraceptives and dysplasia: higher rate for pill choosers. *Science* **169**: 497–498.
STEVENS, V. C., GOLDZIEHER, J. W. and VORYS, N. (1968) Effect of mestranol and chlormadinone acetate on urinary excretion of FSH and LH. *Amer. J. Obst. Gynec.* **102**: 95–105.
STEVENS, V. C. and VORYS, N. (1964) The effect of various compounds on urinary FSH and LH excretion. Presented in the *Proceedings of a Symposium held in Sydney*, October 17–18, pp. 49–60.
STOLL, B. A., ANDREWS, J. T. and MOTTERAM, R. (1966) Liver damage from oral contraceptives. *Brit. Med. J.* **1**: 960–961.
STRADE, H. A. (1966) Lyndiol: evaluation of safety and efficacy as an oral contraceptive. *Curr. Therap. Res.* **9**: 265–279.
STRAUSS, J. S. and POCHI, P. E. (1964) Effect of cyclic progestin–estrogen therapy on sebum and acne in women. *J. Amer. Med. Ass.* **190**: 815–819.
STURGIS, S. H. and ALBRIGHT, R. (1940) Mechanism of estrin therapy in the relief of dysmenorrhea. *Endocrinology* **26**: 68–72.
STURTEVANT, F. M. and WAIT, R. B. (1970) High-dose estrogen sequential oral contraception. I. Effectiveness assessed by the Life Table technique. *Contraception* **2**: 187–191.
SURAN, R. R. (1967) Ovulation inhibition with sequential therapy. A continuing clinical study of fertility control. *Fertil. Steril.* **18**: 598–615.
TAUSK, M. (1969) Oral contraceptives and the incidence of thrombosis. In: *Drug-induced Diseases*. Vol. 3: pp. 183–209. Meyler, L. and Peck H. M. (Eds.). Excerpta Medica, Amsterdam and New York.
TAYLOR, H. B., IREY, N. S. and NORRIS, H. J. (1967) Atypical endocervical hyperplasia in women taking oral contraceptives. *J. Am. Med. Ass.* **202**: 637–639.
TAYMOR, M. L. (1964) Effect of synthetic progestins on pituitary gonadotrophin excretion. *J. Clin. Endocr. Metab.* **24**: 803–807.
TAYMOR, J. L. and KLIBANOFF, P. (1962) Laboratory and clinical effects of nortestosterone. *Amer. J. Obstet. Gynec.* **84**: 1470–1473.
TEN BERGE, B. S. (1969) Veränderungen in den Blutgefässen in Ovarien und Uterus nach Anwendung progestativer Stoffe. *Med. Gyn.* **207**: 52–53.
THULIN, K. E. and NERMARK, J. (1966) Seven cases of jaundice in women taking an oral contraceptive, Anovlar, *Brit. Med. J.* **1**: 584–586.
TIETZE, C., GUTTMACHER, A. F. and RUBIN, S. (1950) Time required for conception in 1727 planned pregnancies. *Fertil. Steril.* **1**: 338–346.
TIETZE, C. and LEWIT, S. (1968) Statistical evaluation of contraceptive methods: use-effectiveness and extended use-effectiveness. *Demography* **5**: 931–940.
TOWNSEND, J. F., HALL, D. G., CAVAZOS, F. and LUCAS, F. V. (1965) Uterine peroxidase activity in abnormal human endometrium. *Amer. J. Obstet. Gynec.* **93**: 1013–1017.
TURPEINEN, K. (1964) Ovulation inhibition by lyndiol: a clinical trial. *Int. J. Fertil.* **9**: 137–148.
TYLER, E. T. (1964) Eight years' experience with oral contraceptives and an analysis of use of low dosage norethisterone. *Brit. Med. J.* **2**: 843–847.
TYLER, E. T. (1967) A contraceptive injection study. In: *8th International Conference of I.P.P.F., Chile*. Summaries of papers. Editoria Universitaria, Santiago.

TYLER, E. T. (1970) A contraceptive injection study employing medroxyprogesterone acetate suspension. In: *Proceedings of the Sixth World Congress on Fertility and Sterility*, pp. 197–202. Gordon & Breach, New York.
TYLER, E. T. and OLSON, H. J. (1959) Fertility promoting and inhibiting effects of new steroid hormonal substances. *J. Amer. Med. Ass.* **169**: 1843–1854.
TYLER, E. T., OLSON, H. J., GOTLIB, M., LEVIN, M. and BEHNE, D. (1964) Long term usage of norethindrone with mestranol preparations in the control of human fertility. *Clin. Med.* **71**: 997–1024.
TYLER, E. T., MATSNER, E. M., GOTLIB, M., LEVIN, J., TUCKER, J. S. and PARROTT, F. M. (1966) Oral contraception by sequential approach. *J. Amer. Med. Ass.* **197**: 113–118.
TYSON, J. E. A. (1968) Oral contraception and elevated blood pressure. *Am. J. Obstet. Gynec.* **100**: 875–876.
VAN DER MOLEN, H. J., HART, P. G. and WIJMENGA, H. G. (1969) Studies with 4-^{14}C-lynestrenol in normal and lactating women. *Acta Endocr. (Kbh.)* **61**: 255–274.
VAN LEUSDEN, H. A. (1969) Continuous oral administration of megestrolacetate to women. *J. Reprod. Fertil.* **19**: 537–539.
VESSEY, M. P. and DOLL, R. (1968) Oral contraceptives and thromboembolism. *Brit. Med. J.* **2**: 199–205.
VOLLINGS, R. (1965) Oral contraceptives and alopecia areata. *Brit. Med. J.* **2**: 1005.
VORYS, N., ULLERY, J. C. and STEVENS, V. (1965) The effects of sex steroids on gonadotrophins. *Amer. J. Obstet. Gynec.* **93**: 641–658.
WAIDL, E., FIKENTSCHER, H. and BRUCKNER, W. (1968) Die Interzellulären Strukturen des Endometriums bei der oralen Kontrazeption. *Geburtsh. Frauenheilk.* **28**: 159–166.
WALLACH, E. D., GARCIA, C. R., KISTNER, R. W. and PINCUS, G. (1963) Adrenal function during long-term Enovid administration. *Amer. J. Obstet. Gynec.* **87**: 991–998.
WALSER, H. C., MARGULIS, R. R. and LADD, J. E. (1964) Effects of prolonged administration of progestins on the endometrium and the function of the pituitary, thyroid and adrenal glands. *Int. J. Fertil.* **9**: 189–195.
WAMSTEKER, E. F. (1968) Clinical and laboratory experience with a modified low dosage sequential oral contraceptive. Preliminary Report. *Int. J. Fertil.* **13**: 436–443.
WARD, G. W. and STEVENSEN, J. R. (1968) Colonic disorder and oral contraceptives. *New Eng. J. Med.* **278**: 910.
WEST, J. and WEST, E. C. (1966) The electroencephalogram and personality of women with headaches on oral contraceptives. *Lancet* **1**: 1180.
WESTOFF, C. F., POTTER, R. G., SAGI, P. C., and MISHLER, E. G. (1961) *Family Growth in Metropolitan America*, pp. 83–101. Princeton Univ. Press, Princeton, New Jersey.
WESTOFF, C. F. and RYDER, N. B. (1968) Duration of use of oral contraception in the United States, 1960–65. *Publ. Hlth. Rep. (Wash.)* **83**: 277–287.
WHITELAW, M. J., NOLA, V. F. and KALMAN, C. F. (1966) Irregular menses, amenorrhea and infertility following synthetic progestational agents. *J. Amer. Med. Ass.* **195**: 160–162.
WHITTY, C. W. M., HOCKADAY, J. M. and WHITTY, M. M. (1966) The effect of oral contraceptives on migraine. *Lancet* **1**: 856.
WIDE, L., KAISER, J. and GEMZELL, C. A. (1965) Sequential and combined therapy in oral contraception. Mode of action and efficiency. *Acta Obstet. Gynec. Scand.* **45**: 53–62.
WIED, G. L., DAVIS, M. E., FRANK, R., SEGAL, P. B., MEIER, P. and ROSENTHAL, E. (1966) Statistical evaluation of the effect of hormonal contraceptives on the cytological smear pattern. *Obstet. Gynec.* **27**: 327–334.
WIJMENGA, H. G. and VAN DER MOLEN, H. J. (1969) Studies with 4-^{14}C-mestranol in lactating women. *Acta Endocr. (Kbh.)* **61**: 665–677.

WILBERT, L., HILLMER, T., HUNSTEIN, W., REISERT, P., KABOTH, U. and CREUTZFELDT, W. (1969) Einfluß oraler Ovulationshemmer auf klinisch-chemische Normalwerte. *Dtsh. Med. Wschr.* **94**: 844–849.

WILKINS, L. (1954) Hormonal influences on skeletal growth. *Annals N.Y. Acad. Sci.* **60**: 763.

WILSON, F., LEMMON, F. M. and COUCH, C. (1967) Evaluation of norethindrone 2 mg in the immediate post-partum period. *Memphis and Mid-South Medical J.*, pp. 431–432.

WINIKOFF, D. and TAYLOR, K. (1966) Oral contraceptives and thyroid function tests. *Med. J. Aust.* **53**: 108–112.

WORLD HEALTH ORGANIZATION (1966) Clinical aspects of oral gestogens. *Techn. Report. Ser.* **326**: 1–24.

WYNN, V., DOAR, J. W. H. and MILLS, G. L. (1966) Effect of oral contraceptives on serum lipid and lipoprotein levels. *Lancet* **2**: 720–722.

WYNN, V. and DOAR, J. W. H. (1966a) Some effects of oral contraceptives on carbohydrate metabolism. *Lancet* **2**: 715–719.

WYNN, V. and DOAR, J. W. H. (1966b) Some effects of oral contraceptives on serum-lipid and lipo-protein levels. *Lancet* **2**: 720–723.

WYNN, V. and DOAR, J. W. H. (1969) Fasting serum triglyceride and cholesterol levels during oral contraceptive therapy. In: *Metabolic Effects of Gonadal Hormones and Contraceptive Steroids*, pp. 219–231. Salhanick, H. A., Kipnis, D. M. and Van de Wiele, R. L. (Eds.). Plenum Press, New York.

YAFFEE, H. S. and GROTS, I. (1965) Moniliasis due to norethynodrel with mestranol (Letter to the editor). *New Engl. Med. Mon.* **272**: 647.

YOUNG, C. C. JR., MAMMEN, E. F. and SPAIN, W. T. (1965) The effect of sequential hormone therapy on the reproductive cycle. *Pacific Med. Surg.* **73**: 35–40.

ZAÑARTU, J., RICE-WRAY, E. and GOLDZIEHER, J. W. (1966) Fertility control with long-acting injectable steroids, a preliminary report. *Obstet. Gynec.* **28**: 513.

ZARTMAN, E. R. (1970) Longacting injectable contraception with medroxyprogesterone acetate. In: *Proceedings of the Sixth World Congress on Fertility and Sterility*, pp. 229–236. Gordon & Breach, New York.

ZORRILLA, E., HULSE, M., HERNANDEZ, A. and GERSHBERG, H. (1968) Severe endogenous hypertriglyceridemia during treatment with estrogen and oral contraceptives. *J. Clin. Endocr.* **28**: 1793–1796.

ZUSSMAN, W. V., FORBES, D. A. and CARPENTER, R. J. (1967) Ovarian morphology following cyclic norethindrone-mestranol therapy. *Amer. J. Obstet. Gynec.* **99**: 100–105.

CHAPTER 35

GENERAL SUMMARY

M. Tausk

Utrecht

IN THIS chapter we attempt to summarize the main conclusions as they emerge from the 34 chapters contained in the two volumes of this section of the *International Encyclopedia of Pharmacology*. The time during which those volumes were written and produced spans well over 5 years and although authors have tried to keep their chapters up to date, the reviewer overlooking the whole cannot avoid feeling that here and there the emphasis may have shifted in the light of new facts. It is for this reason that we are not strictly limiting ourselves to a recapitulation of things stated before but are introducing some new matter.

PROGESTERONE (Volume I)

Progesterone as we now know it has all the classical characteristics of a hormone and the knowledge of its actions has enormously deepened our insight into the processes of reproduction, but it has not become a drug of therapeutic value, because of the short duration of its action and its relative inefficacy on oral administration. It has, however, become a model for a great variety of synthetic drugs, more or less mimicking its manifold effects.

MECHANISMS OF ACTION

While great strides have been made in recent years in exploring the mechanisms of action of many hormones—steroids and non-steroids—this cannot be said of progesterone. A number of facts may account for this lack of progress, which this hormone to some extent appears to share with its chemical relatives, the corticosteroids. The greatest advances in the study of the mechanisms of hormone actions have been made in those fields, where hormones—such as estrogens or androgens—cause the growth of certain organs and, in exercising this function, must induce the production of specific enzymes, or where "trophic" hormones activate certain target glands and make *them* produce specific and well-defined substances. Two basic principles of hormone actions, the one involving specific intracellular receptor-proteins and the other the function of cell membranes in the activation of adenylcyclase, have thus been shown to be instrumental in generating biochemically-defined products which mediate biological actions of hormones.

No such chemically-defined effects of progesterone have so far been detected in mammals. Where they have been found is in birds, and the study of the role of progesterone in the production of avidin (see Chapter 9, p. 275 and Chapter 17, p. 384) has indeed been approached by methods of molecular biology, suggesting a mechanism of action at the nuclear level "resulting in new gene transcriptions (RNA) and the eventual *de novo* synthesis of avidin molecules" (O'Malley, 1969).

The difficulties encountered in the study of biochemical progesterone effects in mammals—in the human in particular—have been summarized by Schmidt-Matthiesen in his introduction to Chapter 23. We see morphological and histochemical effects of progesterone in the endometrium, but these are never induced by progesterone *alone* but always in concert with an estrogen. It is for this reason that a whole chapter of Volume I (9) has been devoted to the synergism of progesterone with, and its antagonism to, estrogens. (A finding of interest in this context is that of Falk and Bardin (1970), that estrogen treatment of spayed guinea pigs for 2 days increased the uptake of labeled progesterone seven-fold in the uterus but not in heart or diaphragm.) Besides, the morphological changes produced by progesterone may be very different in different species (see Chapters 2 and 22). While the hormone stimulates epithelial mitoses in the rabbit (hence the adoption of the term "progestational proliferation"), it inhibits them in primates, where proliferation is considered as a characteristic of estrogenic action. But then—as we have just said—what we describe as effects of progesterone in mammalian physiology are always due to its action superimposed on that of estrogens and the result will depend on the quantitative ratio between the two.

The same principle applies not only to morphological changes but also to such phenomena as changes of contractility of the uterus to which—in view of their complexity and their sometimes controversial interpretation—three whole chapters (4, 5 and 24) of Volume I have been devoted. Estrogen dependence and estrogen antagonism are equally involved in the actions of progesterone on the central nervous system, induction and inhibition of ovulation in particular, as reviewed in Chapters 13 and 17, from which it will become clear how important the timing of the administration of progesterone is for the sort of effect that can be produced.

PREOVULATORY PROGESTERONE

The foregoing raises the question of the functional significance of progesterone levels close to the time of ovulation. The possible physiological role of progesterone in inducing ovulation is discussed in Chapter 16 (p. 368). Since the time of its writing new facts have been discovered and this justifies a brief discussion in the present summary.

Throughout the last 10 or 20 years there have been an increasing number of indications, pointing to a preovulatory secretion of progesterone (see Chapter 16, p. 369 and Chapter 21, p. 415). The most recent methods for the determination of very small amounts of progesterone in plasma, in particular those based on competitive protein binding (see Chapter 1, p. 23), have made it possible to reappraise older observations.

Thus it was found in Rhesus monkeys in which the time of ovulation was ascertained by serial laparotomies, that there is "an increase in the plasma progesterone concentration beginning on the third day before ovulation which becomes abrupt and highly significant on the day before ovulation" (Johansson et al., 1968). During this period progesterone concentrations rose from about 0.3 ng/ml to more than 2, whereafter they reached levels close to 4 ng.

When radio-immunological LH determinations had become possible in Rhesus monkeys, Kirton et al. (1970) were able to combine these with laparoscopic inspection of the ovaries and progesterone determinations. Ovulation was found to occur within 30 hours after the LH peak. The increased progesterone concentration (rising to about 1 ng/ml) at the time of the LH surge was thought to be due to secretion by preovulatory granulosa cells as a result of LH stimulation. Thereafter progesterone rose to levels from 4 to 10 ng/ml. Monroe et al. (1970), whose results are essentially in agreement with the foregoing ones, locate ovulation within 24 hours after the LH peak and they conclude that "the initiation of the LH surge in the monkey menstrual cycle cannot be ascribed to an increase in circulating progesterone levels, nor can the functional life span of the corpus luteum be attributed to alterations in LH secretion".

The studies of Stevens et al. (1970) in baboons are in many respects comparable with those in Rhesus monkeys except that they record a rise in "progestins" on the day of the LH peak, which rise they believe to be due to 17α-hydroxyprogesterone, not to progesterone.

This is followed by a fall in "progestins", which has also been observed by Johansson et al. (1968) and by Monroe et al. (1970) in the Rhesus on the day of ovulation.

The same events were observed in normal women by Strott et al. (1969): A preovulatory rise in 17α-hydroxyprogesterone, beginning with that of plasma LH, leading to a peak at about the same time as that of LH, and followed by a decrease. The progesterone rise begins at about the time of the LH peak, becoming steep 1 to 3 days later (17α-hydroxyprogesterone, an intermediate in estradiol synthesis, is presumed to be secreted by the theca interna cells, as discussed in Chapter 1, p. 30, and its fluctuations in the cycle parallel those of the estrogens). Yussman and Taymor (1970), on the other hand, studied LH and progesterone plasma levels at 8-hour intervals and supplemented this by early postovulatory biopsies of the corpora lutea. They report that a demonstrable rise in plasma progesterone (1.5 ng/ml) "occurred 12–24 hours prior to presumed ovulation and from 4–16 hours prior to ovulation at a level of 4.5 ng/ml", which in the opinion of these authors suggests an important preovulatory function for progesterone, perhaps in initiating the ovulatory process itself.

This initiation, as stated before, has been amply documented by the use of *exogenous* progesterone in the rat and it has recently been shown by Gallo and Zarrow (1970) that doses of 0.2–2.0 mg will do this in PMS-treated animals, probably by means of an effect upon the central nervous system controlling the release of LH, i.e. the medial preoptic area.

Endogenous progesterone was determined in ovarian venous blood in the rat during the 4 days cycle by Hashimoto et al. (1968), and the maximum secretion rate (4.4 mcg/hr/ovary) was found in the evening of proestrus, thus clearly preceding ovulation, which occurs during estrus. (The 20-α-hydroxy-derivative of progesterone paralleled progesterone in its secretion rate but at a much higher level.)

A similar behavior of progesterone levels was found in the golden hamster by Lukaszewska and Greenwald (1970). Progesterone production by the corpus luteum (of the 4-day cycle) reached its peak by day 2. Beginning at 4 p.m. of day 4 there was a sharp increase in ovarian progesterone, presumably from extraluteal sources, this being "most likely related to its essentiality for the induction of behavioral estrus". It is unlikely that progesterone elicits the peak secretion of gonadotrophins; on the contrary, "progesterone synthesis is temporally dependent on gonadotrophic stimulation".

This would be in harmony with findings in the rat, described by Hashimoto and Wiest (1969), who induced the formation of a single generation of corpora lutea in immature animals by the injection of PMS-gonadotrophin and found a distinct peak of ovarian vein progesterone before ovulation, which might well be involved in the facilitation of ovulation.

No appreciable concentrations of preovulatory progesterone were found in heifers by Kazama and Hansel (1970) who state that "thus, the cow differs from the guinea-pig, rat, rabbit and possibly also from the red kangaroo, in which appreciable amounts of progesterone are secreted during estrus, and particularly after mating, and from the monkey, in which a preovulatory rise in progesterone has been reported".

In summary, there is a great deal of evidence of a preovulatory secretion of progesterone in a variety of species, the function of which has not been definitely established. It may well be involved in the development of estrous behavior and in facilitating ovulation, but does not appear to bring about the preovulatory LH peak.

POSTOVULATORY FUNCTIONS OF PROGESTERONE

The functions of progesterone, produced postovulatorily by the corpus luteum, have always completely dominated the scene. It has been abundantly shown to be needed for the normal function of the Fallopian tubes (Chapter 7), determining—always in concert with estrogens—the speed of egg transport and the quality and quantity of the fluid surrounding the ovum. Progesterone at the same time transforms the endometrium (Chapters 2, 22 and 23) and brings it into a stage of development that makes it optimally suitable for the reception of a fertilized ovum that has been permitted to develop for exactly the same period, so that nidation can take place (Chapter 6). It could be delayed or prevented by an abnormal ratio between the levels of available estrogen and progesterone. From then on progesterone remains somehow essential for the survival of the fetus. We certainly do not know all the mechanisms involved in this protective action but a large body of evidence makes it reasonable to assume that an influence on myometrial contractility is an important part of it (Chapters 4, 5 and 24).

PREVENTION OF ADDITIONAL OVULATIONS AND OF FERTILIZATION

Another part of the protection given to intrauterine life is undoubtedly represented by the inhibition of ovulation. It has even been stated (Chapter

13, p. 331) that this was the first function hypothetically ascribed to the corpus luteum. It certainly is the one which has led to the most extended use of progestational drugs.

It looks like a double safeguard that apart from the prevention of new ovulations the fertilization of ova would be rendered difficult or even impossible in many species by progesterone-dependent changes in cervical mucus and in sperm capacitation, as discussed in Chapters 8 and 28 (pp. 267 and 143 respectively).

EFFECTS ON THE MAMMARY GLANDS

Not only are the fetuses protected *in utero*. Progesterone is also contributing to the preservation of their early extrauterine life by its effects on the mammary glands, which assure full lobular and alveolar development, as discussed in Chapter 3.

EFFECTS ON THE CENTRAL NERVOUS SYSTEM

Apart from the facilitation and inhibition of ovulation, which are undoubtedly mediated by actions on the hypothalamus and the pituitary, other effects of progesterone on the central nervous system have been demonstrated, manifesting themselves by electrophysiological phenomena, behavioral changes and changes in body temperature, the latter apparently representing a physiological function of progesterone in the human (see Chapters 14 and 17).

Progesterone apparently takes part in the interplay of steroids, which—at least in the rat—in early postnatal life influences the differentiation and maturation of those cerebral functions that determine future sexual behavior and direction of drives (Chapter 11).

OTHER EFFECTS OF PROGESTERONE

In some species progesterone appears to have a physiological effect on appetite, body weight and metabolism (Chapter 15). To these should be added pharmacological actions, which may perhaps be helpful in interpreting certain effects or side-effects of synthetic progestational drugs. In this respect the work of Beck (1969) is discussed in Chapter 28 (p. 172), who found that progesterone enhanced the secretion of insulin in monkeys and slightly reduced its efficacy. Similar observations in humans were reported

General Summary 477

by Kalkhoff *et al.* (1970), who consider the possibility that placental progesterone may contribute to altered plasma insulin responses in pregnancy.

SYNTHETIC SUBSTITUTES FOR PROGESTERONE (Volume II)

While the study of progesterone was of great importance to physiology, that of its synthetic substitutes belongs to the realm of pharmacology. Their field of application can only to a relatively small extent be covered by the concept of substitution, i.e. the administration of drugs with the purpose of making up for a suspected or demonstrated deficiency of a natural hormone.

Progesterone, as its name suggests, was from the beginning considered as a hormone, primarily needed for the preservation of pregnancy and, when it was introduced as a drug, the medical profession expected it to become useful in the treatment of abortion, threatened or habitual. With the same expectations some of its synthetic derivatives or substitutes have been greeted. Whether and to what extent these hopes have been fulfilled is discussed in Chapter 32, to which the reader is referred. It also deals with a number of conditions in which progestational drugs have been used therapeutically, including menstrual disorders, more recently endometrial carcinoma, and those very rare cases of idiopathic sexual precocity in small infants. None of these uses have reached anything like the importance of oral contraceptives. These are appropriately dealt with in Chapter 34, a summary of which is included in the present chapter.

PHARMACOLOGY OF ORALLY ACTIVE PROGESTATIONAL COMPOUNDS

As stated in the concluding remarks of Chapter 28, in which a great number of pharmacological actions of orally active progestational compounds are reviewed, the present summary attempts to present some basic data not according to actions but by compounds. These are grouped by chemical structures, listed in Table 1 of Chapter 28.

N.B. *Tables referred to in this summary are those belonging to Chapter 28 unless otherwise indicated.*

It should be noted that not all the compounds briefly reviewed here are used in oral contraceptives.

PHARMACOLOGICAL PROFILES OF INDIVIDUAL
COMPOUNDS

1. *Derivatives of* 17α-*hydroxyprogesterone*

This group includes anagestone, chlormadinone acetate, medroxyprogesterone acetate, megestrol acetate, melengestrol acetate and superlutin.

1.1. *Anagestone acetate* (AN). Very few pharmacological data have been published on this compound, which was available as a contraceptive drug for several years. It has high progestational potency (Table 2), and a brief statement has been published to the effect that it is able "even in small doses to induce progestational proliferation in the uterus of non-estrogen-primed immature rabbits" (Table 2, note 3). AN inhibits ovulation in the rat (Table 11) and is reported to be "devoid of frank estrogenic or androgenic activity", to be "modestly antiestrogenic" (uterine growth in rats) and not to delay implantation in intact pregnant rats (p. 56). It was found to have the same potency as norethisterone in inducing an increase in carbonic anhydrase concentration in the human endometrium (Nicholls and Board, 1967).

1.2. *Chlormadinone acetate* (CA). A compound with high progestational activity (Table 2). The oral activity in this test is roughly 50 times that of progesterone s.c. It is about 120 times more active than progesterone on topical application in the McGinty test (Table 5). It is active in the deciduoma test in mice and rats (Table 7); it induces nidation of blastocysts in rabbits in doses much lower than those of progesterone (p. 54), but in this respect it is less active in the hamster (Table 9).

CA is very potent in inhibiting reflex ovulation in the rabbit (Table 10), but poorly active in the rat (Table 11). It is a very weak inhibitor of pituitary gonadotrophin secretion in parabiotic rats (Table 16); it has been shown to inhibit the male gonad (Table 17). It is weakly active in facilitating ovulation in the rat (Table 19). CA maintains pregnancy in the rabbit (Table 20) but in rats only in large doses or when combined with estrogen (Table 22).

CA is not estrogenic (Table 25). It inhibits the uterine-growth-stimulating effect of estrogen in mice (Table 26) and in rats (Table 27). It is not androgenic or myotrophic (Table 29) and very weakly active in inducing fetal masculinization in rats (Table 30).

It reduces fertility in mice when implanted in silastic capsules (Table 32)

General Summary

and in rabbits when administered before artificial insemination (Tables 34 and 35). It accelerates egg transport through the Fallopian tube in rabbits (Table 38). CA stimulates mammary gland development in rats (Table 39). It has some adrenal inhibiting activity (Table 40) but no corticoid activity (Table 41). It is active in increasing the plasma insulin response to i.v. glucose (Table 44).

1.3. *Medroxyprogesterone acetate* (MAP). Highly active in Clauberg test, though clearly less than chlormadinone acetate, roughly 10 times more active p.o. than progesterone s.c. (Table 2); 25 times more active than progesterone on topical application in the McGinty test (Table 5); active in the deciduoma test in mice and rats when given s.c. (Table 7). In this test MAP has been found inactive p.o. but very active on percutaneous application. MAP induces nidation of blastocysts in hamsters in lower doses than chlormadinone acetate (Table 9). It is less active than CA in inhibiting ovulation in the rabbit (Table 10) but much more potent in rats (Table 11). It was found not to inhibit ovulation in the hamster. MAP is a potent pituitary inhibitor in parabiotic rats or mice (Table 16) much more than chlormadinone acetate. MAP is very potent in inducing ovulation in PMS-treated rats (Tables 18 and 19) again much more than chlormadinone acetate. It maintains pregnancy in the spayed rabbit (Table 20) and rat (Table 22). It is not estrogenic (Tables 24 and 25) and it antagonizes the effect of estrone on uterine growth in mice (Table 26). It is androgenic and myotrophic (Table 28). MAP has repeatedly been shown to be quite potent in causing fetal masculinization in rats (Table 30), but not so far in the human (Table 31).

MAP reduces fertility and mating behavior in rats and mice on continuous treatment (Tables 32 and 33) and fertilization in rabbits when administered p.o. before artificial insemination (Table 35). It reduces the number of litters when given to pregnant rats (Table 37) and increases the rate of egg transport in the rabbit oviduct (Table 38). It stimulates mammary gland development in rats (Table 39). It is a potent adrenal inhibitor (Table 40) and has relatively high corticoid activity (Table 41). It widens the symphysis pubis in guinea-pigs (p. 98).

1.4. *Megestrol acetate* (MEG). One of the most potent progestational compounds in the Clauberg test, given p.o. it has 50–100 times the activity of progesterone s.c. (Table 2). On intrauterine application (McGinty test) 10 times as active as progesterone (Table 5). Potent inhibitor of (reflex-) ovulation in the rabbit (Table 10) and in rats (Table 11). It inhibits pituitary gonadotrophic activity in parabiotic rats (Table 16). MEG maintains pregnancy in spayed rats, in particular if combined with estrogen (Table 22). It is not estrogenic (Table 25). It antagonizes estrone in mice (vaginal cornification and uterine growth, Table 26), it is neither androgenic nor myotrophic (Table 29) but has been reported to cause fetal masculinization in rats (Table 30) though not in women so far (Table 31). It reduced fertility and mating behavior in rats on continued administration (Tables 32 and 33) and fertilization in rabbits when given before artificial insemination (Tables 34 and 35). It was found not to damage pregnancy in the rat when given from day 15 onwards (Table 37). MEG inhibits the adrenal gland (Table 40) but has no corticoid activity (Table 41).

1.5. *Melengestrol acetate* (MEL). Very potent progestational compound, Clauberg activity (Table 2) of the same order as that of chlormadinone acetate or medroxyprogesterone acetate or even 4 times as potent as the latter according to Duncan *et al.* (1964). It can be inferred that the compound inhibits ovulation in the rat because it inhibits the estrus cycle (0.05 mg p.o. or s.c., daily for 10 days) (Duncan *et al.*, 1964). MEL inhibits pituitary stimulation of the male gonad (Table 17). It maintains pregnancy in spayed rats in low s.c. doses (Table 22). MEL antagonizes estrone in mice (uterine growth, Table 26). It was found to cause slight masculinizing changes in fetal rats (as judged by anogenital distance) without histologically detectable abnormalities (Table 30).

MEL reduces or even prevents fertilization in rabbits when administered before artificial insemination (Table 34). It can interfere with an established pregnancy (Table 37). It has corticoid activity (Table 41).

1.6. *Superlutin*. Highly potent in the Clauberg test (p.o. activity 10 to 25 times that of progesterone s.c., Table 2).

2. *Medrogestone (MED), a derivative of progesterone*

This compound has a distinctly lower progestational potency on oral administration than the 17α-hydroxyprogesterone derivatives. Its p.o. activity in the Clauberg system is roughly equal to that of progesterone s.c. (Table 2). It is also active on intrauterine administration (McGinty test, Table 5) and in inducing deciduomas in rats (Table 7). It inhibits ovulation in the rat (Table 11) and in the hamster (Table 12) and maintains pregnancy in spayed rats (Table 22). It had some androgenic activity when injected daily for 15 days (Table 28) but not, according to another investigator, when given s.c. or p.o. for 7 days (Table 29). It was found distinctly antiandrogenic by Revesz and Chappel (see p. 119). It does not cause fetal masculinization (Table 30). It reduced fertility on continuous administration to female rats (Table 32). It was found not to inhibit the adrenal gland (Table 40), and to increase bodyweight in female rats to the same extent as progesterone (Table 43).

3. *Dydrogesterone* (DY), *a derivative of retroprogesterone*

The pharmacological pattern of this compound differs greatly from that of the progesterone derivatives reviewed so far. Its oral activity is less than that of progesterone s.c. As to its s.c. activity divergent data have been published, but it seems now to be settled at slightly above that of progesterone (Table 3). It is active on intrauterine administration (McGinty test, Table 5), and very weakly deciduomagenic (Table 7). It inhibits ovulation in rabbits in only very high doses (Table 10) but not in rats (nor in the human, Chapter 31). DY facilitates ovulation in rats (Table 19) and maintains pregnancy in rabbits (Table 20) and in rats if combined with estrogen (Table 22). It is not estrogenic (Table 25). It is antiestrogenic in mice (uterine weight, Table 26) and rats (vaginal cornification, Table 27). It is neither androgenic nor myotrophic (Table 29) and does not induce fetal masculinization (Table 30). It does not prevent fertilization when given before artificial insemination in rabbits (Table 35), nor does it interfere with an established pregnancy (Table 37). DY has no corticoid activity. Its influence on bodyweight is equal to that of progesterone (Table 43). It is not thermogenic in the human and has no conspicuous influence on the contractions of the non-pregnant human uterus (Chapter 31).

4. *Derivatives of estrane* (19-*nortestosterone*)

4.1. *Norgestrel* (NG). This compound is included in this series, because it can be described as a substituted homologue of estrane though others prefer to call it a gonane derivative. The term gonane designates a steroid nucleus of seventeen carbon atoms, lacking both angular methyl groups and is in practice used in the nomenclature of some steroids, in which the angular methyl group between the C and the D ring (C-18) has been replaced by a longer alkyl chain. They are usually made by total synthesis, because it is difficult to prepare them from natural steroids. Norgestrel can therefore be described as 13β-ethyl-17α-ethynyl-17β-hydroxy-gon-4-en-3-one or as 18β-methyl-17α-ethynyl-17β-hydroxy-estr-4-en-3-one (and by those who prefer the nortestosterone nomenclature as 18β-methyl-17α-ethynyl-19-nortestosterone).

Norgestrel is one of the progestationally most potent compounds of the estrane series which are, however, all much less active in the Clauberg test than the derivatives of progesterone described as group 1. The total p.o. dose needed for an incomplete transformation of the rabbit endometrium is given as 0.11 mg (see Table 3). It is stated to be 3 times more active p.o. than progesterone given s.c. In the McGinty test (intrauterine administration) in which most members of this series are inactive, NG has been reported to be active, but its potency appears to be very low (see Table 5). It maintains pregnancy in the spayed rat (Table 22), it is not estrogenic (Table 25) but strongly antiestrogenic (mouse vagina and uterine growth, Table 26). NG is also clearly androgenic (Table 28) and has been found to cause fetal masculinization in the rat (Table 30). It prevents pregnancy on prolonged continuous administration in high doses only (Table 32); it does not suppress mating behavior (Table 33). It has, however, an inhibitory effect on the pituitary as shown by the prevention of "compensatory" ovarian hypertrophy following hemicastration in the rat (see p. 78).

NG was found not to interfere with established pregnancy, though the dose tested appears to be very low (Table 37). No adrenal inhibition has been found (Table 42) and no corticoid activity (Table 41).

4.2. *Norethisterone acetate* (NAc). As shown in Table 3, this compound has a relatively high progestational potency, which is equal on s.c. and p.o. administration and is stated to be 25 times the s.c. activity of progesterone. It is inactive in the McGinty test (Table 6). It is a strong inhibitor of ovulation in the rat (Table 11) and of pituitary gonadotrophic stimulation in parabiotic female rats (Table 16) and in ordinary male rats, the latter potency being equal to that of testosterone propionate (Table 17). It is estrogenic though less than the non-esterified parent compound (Table 24) and antiestrogenic (more than the free alcohol, Table 27). NAc is androgenic, though somewhat less than its parent compound norethisterone (Table 28). It causes fetal masculinization (Table 30). It prevents pregnancy when given continuously to rats or mice (Table 32), but not through interference with mating behavior (Table 33). NAc was reported not to interfere with established pregnancy (Table 37). It does not stimulate the mammary glands of spayed rats (Table 39) and it influences bodyweight less than progesterone (Table 43).

4.3. *Norethisterone* (NE). The pattern of activities of this substance is very similar to that of its acetate, but it has been examined in more and broader studies than the latter. The quantitative differences in estrogenic and antiestrogenic behavior between the two have been pointed out in the preceding paragraph 4.2. A number of data referring to NE only are the following. In the subcutaneous Allen–Corner test it was reported to have the same activity as progesterone. It was found inactive in the deciduoma test in mice (Table 8). It induces nidation in the spayed hamster (Table 9), it inhibits ovulation in the rabbit (Table 10) and in the hamster (Table 12) and it facilitates ovulation in the PMS-treated rat (Tables 18 and 19). NE does not maintain pregnancy in the rabbit (Table 21) nor for that matter in the rat (Table 23). It does not inhibit the adrenal (Table 41). It increases the plasma–insulin response to a glucose load, much more than progesterone (Table 44), and was found to be well absorbed through the skin (Table 45).

4.4. *Norvinisterone* (NV). Progestational potency roughly equivalent to that of norethisterone (Table 3). Inactive in McGinty test (Table 6). Interferes with established pregnancy (Table 37).

4.5. *Ethynodiol diacetate* (ETH). One of the most potent compounds in this series, in terms of activity in the Clauberg test, in as much as a dose of 0.1 mg causes a maximum effect, but this decreases as the dose is increased (Table 3, note 10). Inactive on topical application in the uterus (Table 6), inhibits ovulation in the hamster (Table 12). It is estrogenic in the rat, characterized by a shallow curve for uterine growth (Table 24) and at the same time antiestrogenic as assayed by vaginal smears and uterine growth in mice (strongly dose-dependent, Table 26, note 4). ETH is somewhat androgenic (Table 28), it has not been reported to increase significantly the plasma insulin response to glucose (Table 44).

4.6. *Lynestrenol* (LYN). Chemically remarkable for its lack of oxygen on C-3, it holds an intermediate position as regards progestational activity in this series (Table 3). It was found active in the Allen–Corner test (Table 4), inactive in the deciduoma test (Table 8). It inhibits ovulation in rabbits (Table 10) and in rats (Table 11) and hypophyseal stimulation of the ovary in parabiotic rats (Table 16) as well as that of the male gonad in normal rats (Table 17). LYN does not maintain pregnancy in the castrated rat (Table 23). It is estrogenic in the rat (vaginal smears and uterine weight, Table 24), androgenic and myotrophic (Table 28). It prevents fertilization when given to rabbits before artificial insemination (Table 35). LYN was found to interfere with established pregnancy in the rat (Table 37) and with egg transport through the Fallopian tube (Table 38). It does not inhibit the adrenal cortex (Table 42).

4.7. *Allylestrenol* (AL). Chemically related to lynestrenol and of approximately the same progestational activity (Table 3). It was found active in the Allen–Corner test (Table 4) and (weakly) in the McGinty test (Table 5). AL induces the formation of deciduomas in mice (Table 7), it inhibits ovulation in the rabbit (Table 10) and (weakly) in the rat (Table 11). It is a weak inhibitor of pituitary stimulation of the ovaries in parabiotic rats (Table 16) but was reported not to inhibit the male gonad in normal rats (Table 17). AL maintains pregnancy in the spayed rabbit (Table 20) and in the rat (Table 22). It is not estrogenic (Table 25), but has some antiestrogenic activity (uterine growth in mice, Table 26, vaginal smears in rats, Table 27). It was reported to be weakly androgenic (Table 28) and to induce partial persistence of Wolffian ducts in rats (Table 30 and discussion, p. 123). It prevents fertilization in rabbits when administered before artificial insemination (Table 35). AL does not interfere with established pregnancy in rats (Table 37). It does not inhibit the adrenal cortex (Table 42).

4.8. *Normethandrone* (NM). Progestational potency roughly comparable to that of the two preceding compounds, LYN and AL (Table 3), inactive on intrauterine administration (Table 6) and reported to induce deciduomas in rats (Table 7) though not to a significant degree in mice (Table 8). It inhibits ovulation in rabbits (Table 10). NM inhibits overstimulation of the ovary in parabiotic rats (Table 16) and of the male gonad in rats under certain conditions (Table 17). NM was reported to have some protective influence on pregnancy in the spayed rabbit (Table 20) and to maintain pregnancy in rats (Table 22). It is not estrogenic (Table 25) and distinctly antiestrogenic (Table 26), androgenic and myotrophic (Table 28). It has been reported to have caused masculinization of a female baby (Table 31). NM prevents fertilization in rabbits when given prior to artificial insemination (Table 35) and it interferes with established pregnancy in rats (Table 37). It inhibits the adrenal cortex (Table 40). It is absorbed through the rabbit's skin (Table 45).

4.9. *Norgestrienone* (NGT). One of the weaker compounds according to Clauberg assays (Table 3). Maintains pregnancy in the rabbit, when given p.o. (Table 20). Estrogenic (Table 24). Continuous administration to rats (Table 32) prevents pregnancy.

General Summary

4.10. *Quingestanol* (Q). A compound, having a relatively low progestational potency (Table 3). Inhibits ovulation in the rat (Table 11), also overstimulation of the ovary in parabiotic rats (Table 16).

Q does not maintain pregnancy in the spayed rat (Table 23). It is not estrogenic (Table 25). It has androgenic activity (Table 28) and causes fetal masculinization (Table 30). On continuous administration to rats (Table 32) Q prevents pregnancy without suppressing mating behavior (Table 33). It does not inhibit the adrenal cortex (Table 42).

4.11. *Norethynodrel* (NL). The first compound introduced as progestational component of an oral contraceptive. It is amongst the weaker compounds, judged by the Clauberg assay (Table 3). Its behavior in this test is discussed on p. 44. It is more active when given p.o. than s.c. It was found weakly active in the Allen–Corner test (Table 4), inactive in the McGinty test (Table 6). It does not induce deciduoma formation (Table 8). It inhibits ovulation in the rabbit (Table 10), in rats (Table 11) and in hamsters (in high doses, Table 12). It is a strong inhibitor of overstimulation of the ovary in parabiosis (Table 16) and of the normal male gonad (Table 17). It induces ovulation in PMS-treated immature rats (Table 18). NL does not maintain pregnancy in the castrated rabbit (Table 21) nor for that matter in rats (Table 23). It is estrogenic, in fact it has the highest estrogenic potency of all the progestational compounds reviewed (Table 24). It is not antiestrogenic (Table 26). NL is not androgenic or myotrophic (Table 29) but does induce fetal masculinization (Table 30). It was cited as cause of masculinization of a female baby (Table 31). NL prevents pregnancy in rats on continuous administration (Table 32), not suppressing mating behavior in lower doses, only in higher ones (Table 33). It interferes with established pregnancy in rats and mice, causing resorption of fetuses (Table 37). It accelerates egg transport through the oviduct (Table 38). It does not inhibit the adrenal cortex (Table 42) but causes an increase in its weight (see p. 164). NL was found to increase the plasma–insulin response to a glucose load (Table 44).

4.12. *Norgesterone* (NGN). According to the Clauberg assay one of the weakest in the series (Table 3). Inactive on uterine application (Table 6). It inhibits overstimulation of the ovaries in parabiotic rats (Table 16) and of the male gonad in normal rats (Table 17). NGN is practically nonandrogenic (Table 28); it prevents pregnancy in the rat on continuous treatment (Table 32).

5. Derivatives of testosterone

5.1. *Dimethisterone* (DM). A testosterone derivative with relatively low oral potency in the Clauberg assay, as judged by total oral dose, though still reported to have twice the activity of progesterone s.c. (Table 3). DM is inactive in the deciduoma test (Table 8). Combined with an estrogen it is reported to furnish some, though weak, protection to pregnancy in spayed rabbits (Table 20), but not in rats (Table 23). It is not estrogenic (Table 25) and weakly antiestrogenic (uterine growth in mice, Table 26). DM is not androgenic (Table 29) but causes fetal masculinization in rats (Table 30).

5.2. *Ethisterone* (ET). The first synthetic compound ever found to have progestational activity on oral administration though this is lower than that of the newer compounds, except norgesterone (para. 4.12) as shown in Table 3. It was found to be active on intrauterine administration (Table 5); to be inactive in the deciduoma test (Table 8), and not to maintain pregnancy in spayed rats (Table 23). It is not estrogenic (Table 25) but distinctly antiestrogenic in mice (Table 26) though not in rats (Table 27). ET is androgenic and myotrophic (Table 28) and caused fetal masculinization in rats (Table 30) and in the human (Table 31).

PATTERNS OF ACTIVITY

From the profiles of individual compounds certain patterns of activities emerge. Madjerek *et al.* (1960) have suggested a classification of synthetic progestational compounds in gestagens and pregestagens (see Historical Introduction, p. 5) the former, as distinguished from the latter, being able to induce the formation of deciduomas and to maintain pregnancy in spayed rats, apart from the progestational transformation of the rabbits endometrium, which both groups have in common. Overbeek (1968) has used the presence or lack of estrogenicity as a main criterion of classification. The importance of this criterion may be deduced from the synopsis which we present in Table 1.

It will be seen that in the series of derivatives of progesterone, most compounds have high (oral) progestational activity (Clauberg test). As far as has been shown they are not estrogenic. They are active on intrauterine application (McGinty test). Most of the compounds of this group have been found active in maintaining pregnancy in spayed rodents.

In the estrane (i.e. nortestosterone) series, where Clauberg activity is generally lower, some ability to main pregnancy in rabbits or rats has been

TABLE 1. PHARMACOLOGICAL PROFILES OF ORALLY ACTIVE PROGESTATIONAL COMPOUNDS

Compound	Estrogenic	Clauberg Test	McGinty Test	Maint. Pregnancy Rabbit	Maint. Pregnancy Rat	Inhib. Ovulation Rabbit	Inhib. Ovulation Rat	Relax. Symphysis Pubis	Deciduoma	Antiestrogenic	Androgenic	Chemical Classification
Chlormadinone	−	++	++	++	(+)	++	(+)+	+	++	+	−	OHP
Medroxyprogesterone	−	++	++		+(+)	+	+(+)+		+	+	+	OHP
Anagestone	−	++	+		+(+)		++			+	−	OHP
Megstrol	−	++	+				++			+	−	OHP
Melengestrol	−	++	+				(+)			+	−	OHP
Medrogestone	−	+(+)	(+)	+	(+)+			+	(+)	+(+)	(+)	P
Superlutin		+										OHP
Dydrogesterone	−	++	−	−	−		−		−	+	−	Retroprogesterone
Norgestrel	+	++	−		++	(+)	++		+	++	++	E (Gonane)
Norethisterone Acetate	+	++	−	(+)+	++	+	++		+	+	++	E
Norethisterone	−	++	−	+	(+)+	++	++		+	+	++	E
Norvinisterone	++	++	−							+	+	E
Ethynodiol	+	++	(+)				+(+)	(+)			(+)	E
Lynestrenol	−	++	−				++				+	E
Allylestrenol	+	++	−							−	−	E
Normethandrone	++	++	(+)	(+)+						(+)	+	E
Norgestrienone	+	++	−								(+)	E
Quingestanol	−	++	−								−	E
Norethynodrel	+	++	−	(+)							(+)	E
Norgesterone	+	++	+									E
Dimethisterone	−	++	−								−	T
Ethisterone	−	++	+								(+)	T

Symbols: ++ strongly active
+ active
(+) weakly or very weakly active
− inactive

Chemical Classification:
Derivative of:
(P) Progesterone
(OHP) 17α-hydroxy prog.
(E) Estrane (=19 nor test)
(T) Testosterone

demonstrated in four compounds, all of which lack estrogenicity. The same applies to dydrogesterone. Also activity in the McGinty test and in inducing deciduomas was found only in non-estrogenic compounds.

With regard to the importance that has been attached to the estrogen content of oral contraceptives, it should be pointed out that the estrogenic activity of the progestational compounds, as shown in p.o. tests in rats, is in most cases less than 1% of estrone (see Table 24). Only in the case of norethisterone acetate has it been assayed as 3.0% of estradiol (about the same as for norethynodrel s.c.). It is, however, exceedingly difficult to interpret this in terms of human pharmacology. Thus, as shown in Table 24, lynestrenol has been shown to have between 0.1 and 1.0% of the oral estrogenic activity of ethynyl estradiol in the rat and the normal dose of 2.5 mg lynestrenol in a tablet would—in the rat—be comparable with 2.5 to 25 mcg ethynyl estradiol. But the human female is far more sensitive to this estrogen than the rat, both needing about the same absolute dose, to produce an estrogenic effect, while the ratio of their bodyweights may be of the order of 1:500. It is therefore not permissible to express the estrogenic activity of a progestational compound in the human in terms of ethynyl estradiol, quite apart from the fact that the antiestrogenic potency of those weak estrogens may detract from the activity of more powerful estrogens as discussed in Chapter 28, p. 107.

THE PHARMACOLOGICAL CONTROL OF HUMAN FERTILITY ("ORAL CONTRACEPTION")

When the first oral contraceptive came into use it was called "The Pill". The fact that an entirely non-descriptive term has become so very popular illustrates—perhaps more than anything else—the degree of psychological preparedness with which the new method was hailed.

In the 15 years following the first reports by Pincus and his group an enormous literature has appeared dealing with medical and other aspects of oral contraception. Our Chapter 34 summarizes a great deal of clinical data, showing the very high reliability of the method in preventing pregnancy which makes failures exceedingly rare. This is ascribed to the multiple mechanisms involved: inhibition of ovulation and a cervical barrier to the entrance of sperm. To this can be added other effects, each of which may be able to prevent pregnancy but which actually are not called upon to do so in a genital tract into which no ova are shed and no sperm cells can enter.

This high degree of effectiveness and the lack of many of the disadvantages of older methods of birth control have caused such widespread acceptance of oral contraceptives that the question of their medical safety and the significance of their side effects has become a topic of outstanding importance. Discussions are loaded with emotion since many people seem to be unable to view the outcome with cool aloofness. This applies not only to an estimated number of 17 million women using the pill (1970)—not including those who are supplied by government agencies and comparable organizations—but also to their husbands (and often their mothers), to a great part of the medical profession and an increasing number of people concerned with the sociologic problems of growth of the population, not to speak of the small but highly interested group of manufacturers.

As is apparent from Chapter 34, many changes can be observed in women using oral contraceptives, changes undoubtedly caused by the drug but without clinical significance as far as is known today. This group includes biochemical and metabolic parameters of which at least fifty or sixty appear to be affected. A second group may be definitely bothersome and unpleasant but the causal relationship with the pill cannot always be established. In this group are psychological phenomena, changes in sexual adaptation, as well as changes in eating habits and weight.

A third group comprises those conditions which are both serious and recognized as being definitely connected with oral contraception in a cause-and-effect relationship. This group is mainly centered on thromboembolic episodes and their sometimes lethal outcome. It also includes a definite propensity of certain conditions of prediabetes or mild diabetes to become more serious. A fourth group includes changes which are not manifesting themselves in clinical symptoms but which informed observers interpret as potentially dangerous in the long run. Since at the present time the correctness of these interpretations can in general not be proven or disproven by hard facts, it is here that discussions become most heated by fear or hope.

Apart from these emotional factors at least two other major psychological forces are involved. The one originates from religious beliefs and rulings of churches, the other has its roots in a sound and time-honored principle of medical ethics, which condemns any possibly harmful treatment *unless* it is performed in order to avoid a more serious danger.

Medical men have been taught to accept risks of therapy in order to stave off greater risks, due to the illness they treat. But women are often willing to accept risks in order to avoid pregnancy which may under certain conditions be a more serious threat than many an illness.

As an example the present writer may cite the case of a mother of ten who while taking an oral contraceptive developed hemianopsia. When told that this might be due to the pill, she still decided to go on taking it.

At the present time the risk of thromboembolism is certainly the most important one to be considered with regard to the dangers and benefits of oral contraception. The discovery of the cause-and-effect relationship between thromboembolism and the use of the pill represents an illuminating lesson in epidemiology and its methods. For 5 or 6 years reports on an apparent connection between the disease and the drug had been accumulating but they were often dismissed as being probably due to chance. One of the arguments used was that the incidence of thrombosis amongst pill users appeared not to be greater than amongst the female population at large. Authors were comparing the incidence of a very rare event in the treated group with that of a more or less equally rare one amongst a much larger group, in respect to which widely varying figures were utilized.

The decisive turn came when the Royal College of General Practitioners in Great Britain, with the support of the Medical Research Council, set up an investigation, planning to ascertain not the number of thromboses amongst pill users (and other women) but the number of pill users amongst women suffering from thrombosis, and comparing this with the frequency of pill use amongst small groups of carefully matched controls. It was this different approach which eliminated many dubious assumptions and, when followed up by medical statisticians in the United Kingdom and other countries, particularly in the U.S.A., established as a fact what had long been suspected.

One of the leading investigators in this search was Professor Richard Doll, to whose highly interesting Oliver Bird Lecture (Doll, 1970) the reader is referred. It contains the significant statements, that the risk appears not to change with the duration of the use of the method (at least not for the first 3 years) and that risk of death per 100,000 women in Britain (not necessarily in other countries) is 1.5 for users aged 20–34 years as against 0.2 for non-users. The respective figures for the age groups 35–44 are 3.9 against 0.5. In this way the oral contraceptives add about 2% to the annual risk of death from all causes (55.8 per 100,000 for the younger group and 167.6 for the older one).*

As discussed in Chapter 34, it is the estrogenic component of the oral contraceptives that is being indicted for causing this side effect. Estrogens appear to have a double useful function in the combined drugs: they are

---

* Potts and Swyer (1970) have calculated that "the mortality associated with the use of oral contraceptives or the IUD is of the same order of magnitude as the mortality due to unplanned pregnancies when less effective methods are used".

by themselves ovulation inhibitors and by their proliferating—though largely repressed—effect on the endometrium they ensure more normal cyclical bleeding.

Many attempts have been made to design preparations not containing estrogens but a progestational compound only. Their main effect was thought to be on the cervical mucosa, where the estrogens, when given alone, would provide for conditions ideal for fertilization. It is by their estrogen antagonism that progesterone and its synthetic analogues render the cervical mucus impermeable to spermatozoa. The hope was entertained that by giving estrogen-free progestational drugs it would be possible to achieve protection from pregnancy by purely peripheral action and without inhibition of ovulation. So far these preparations have not reached the level of safety provided by the combination drugs, and their side effects, though different from those of the latter, are bothersome. Nevertheless, these attempts have given a new impulse to research on contraception.

The control of human fertility is a sociological necessity—even a prerequisite for the survival of mankind. Experience of the last 15 years has shown that the most desirable methods are those which require no special action close to the time of intercourse and that the pharmacological methods—apart from surgical intervention—provide the highest degree of contraceptive protection. At the same time the development of these methods has greatly stimulated research on human reproduction, a field in which new methods are rapidly being applied. With so much motivation and technology continued joint efforts of academic, industrial and other organizations are bound to produce basic improvements and to find solutions to problems of equal importance to pure physiology and practical birth control.

REFERENCES

BECK, P. (1969) Progestin enhancement of the plasma insulin response to glucose in Rhesus monkeys. *Diabetes* **18**: 146–152.
DOLL, R. (1970) The long term effects of steroid contraceptives. *J. Biosoc. Sci.* **2**: 367–389.
DUNCAN, G. W., LYSTER, S. C., HENDRIX, J. W., CLARK, J. J. and WEBSTER, H. D. (1964) Biologic effects of melengestrol acetate. *Fertil. Steril.* **15**: 419–431.
FALK, R. J. and BARDIN, C. W. (1970) Uptake of tritiated progesterone by the uterus of the ovariectomized guinea pig. *Endocrinology* **86**: 1059–1063.
GALLO, R. V. and ZARROW, M. X. (1970) Effect of progesterone and other steroids on PMS-induced ovulation in the immature rat. *Endocrinology* **86**: 296–304.
HASHIMOTO, I., HENDRICKS, D. M., ANDERSON, L. L. and MELAMPY, R. M. (1968) Progesterone and pregn-4-en-20α-ol-3-one in ovarian venous blood during various reproductive states in the rat. *Endocrinology* **82**: 333–341.

HASHIMOTO, I. and WIEST, W. G. (1969) Correlation of the secretion of ovarian steroids with function of a single generation of corpora lutea in the immature rat. *Endocrinology* **84**: 873–885.

JOHANSSON, E. D. B., NEILL, J. D. and KNOBIL, E. (1968) Periovulatory progesterone concentration in the peripheral plasma of the rhesus monkey with a methodological note on the detection of ovulation. *Endocrinology* **82**: 143–148.

KALKHOFF, R. K., JACOBSON, M. and LEMPER, D. (1970) Progesterone, pregnancy and the augmented plasma insulin response. *J. Clin. Endocr.* **31**: 24–28.

KAZAMA, N. and HANSEL, W. (1970) Preovulatory changes in the progesterone level of bovine peripheral blood plasma. *Endocrinology* **86**: 1252–1256.

KIRTON, K. T., NISWENDER, G. G., MIDGLEY, JR., A. R., JAFFE, R. B. and FORBES, A. D. (1970) Serum luteinizing hormone and progesterone concentration during the menstrual cycle of the rhesus monkey. *J. Clin. Endocr.* **30**: 105–110.

LUKASZEWSKA, J. H. and GREENWALD, G. S. (1970) Progesterone levels in the cyclic and pregnant hamster. *Endocrinology* **86**: 1–9.

MADJEREK, Z., DE VISSER, J., VAN DER VIES, J. and OVERBEEK, G. A. (1960) Allylestrenol, a pregnancy maintaining oral gestagen. *Acta Endocr. (Kbh.)* **35**: 8–19.

MONROE, S. E., ATKINSON, L. E. and KNOBIL, E. (1970) Patterns of circulating luteinizing hormone and their relation to plasma progesterone levels during the menstrual cycle of the rhesus monkey. *Endocrinology* **87**: 453–455.

NICHOLLS, R. A. and BOARD, J. A. (1967) Carbonic anhydrase concentration in endometrium after oral progestins. *Amer. J. Obstet. Gynec.* **99**: 829–832.

O'MALLEY, B. W. (1969) Progesterone: Mechanism of action. In: *Metabolic Effects of Gonadal Hormones and Contraceptive Steroids*, pp. 339–351. Salhanick, H. A., Kipnis, D. M. and van de Wiele, R. L. (Eds.). Plenum Press, New York and London.

OVERBEEK, G. A. (1968) Pharmacology of lynestrenol. In: *Modern Progestational Therapy*, pp. 6–14. Fastner, Z. and Morton, B. (Eds.). Organon Co., Oss, The Netherlands.

POTTS, D. M. and SWYER, G. I. M. (1970) Effectiveness and risks of birth-control methods. *Brit. Med. Bull.* **26**: 26–32.

STEVENS, V. C., SPARKS, S. J. and POWELL, J. E. (1970) Levels of estrogens, progestogens and luteinizing hormone during the menstrual cycle of the baboon. *Endocrinology* **87**: 658–666.

STROTT, C. A., YOSHIMI, T., ROSS, G. T. and LIPSETT, M. B. (1969) Ovarian physiology: relationship between plasma LH and steroidogenesis by the follicle and corpus luteum; effect of HCG. *J. Clin. Endocr.* **29**: 1157–1167.

YUSSMAN, M. A. and TAYMOR, M. L. (1970) Serum levels of follicle stimulating hormone and luteinizing hormone and of plasma progesterone related to ovulation by corpus luteum biopsy. *J. Clin. Endocr.* **30**: 396–399.

AUTHOR INDEX

Page numbers in *italic* type refer to bibliographical lists at the ends of relevant chapters.

Abdalla, M. 297, *297*, *300*, 408, 410, 442, *458*
Abdel Aziz, M. T. 297, *297*
Abdel Hay, A. 297, *297*
Abdel Kader, M. M. 297, *297*
Abrams, C. A. L. 325, 326, *338*
Adam, R. 292, *301*
Adams, A. 423, *457*
Adams, C. E. 145, *194*, 353, *382*
Adlercreutz, E. 318, *327*
Aftergood, L. 170, *194*
Aguilar, J. A. 423, *456*
Ahara, M. 224, 235, *241*
Albert, A. 324, 325, 326, *333*, 395, *452*
Albright, R. 385, *467*
Alexander, J. 237, *239*
Alfin-Slater, R. B. 170, *194*
Allan, J. S. 433, *452*
Allen, G. O. Jr. 134, 135, *194*
Allen, W. M. 46, 54, 93, *194*, *269*, 351, 353, *377*
Allen, W. S. 4, *10*
Altman, K. 290, 291, 295, *299*
Alvarez, R. R. 310, *327*
Amann, W. 316, *327*
Amatsu, M. 227, 228, 233, 237, *241*, 259, *272*
Amris, C. J. 439, *452*
Ånberg, Å. 282, *300*
Andelman, M. B. 407, *452*
Anderson, D. G. 306, *327*
Anderson, G. V. 428, *462*
Anderson, L. L. 474, *491*
Anderson, N. C. Jr. 99, *216*
Andrews, J. T. 434, 435, *467*
Andrews, M. C. 307, *327*, 404, 405, 408, 410, 423, *452*
Andrews, W. C. 307, *327*, 404, 405, 408, 410, 423, *452*
Angee, I. 192, *205*
Angst-Horridge, A. 415, *464*

Anonymous 450, *452*
Antoine, T. 308, *327*
Aoki, Y. 162, 163, 165, *215*
Appelgren, L. E. 177, 182, *194*, *195*
Arai, K. 219, 227, 230, 231, *238*, *240*
Arai, Y. 359, *377*
Aranda-Rosell, A. 249, *272*, 406, 407, 419, 427, 442, *456*, *464*
Arcari, G. 47, 50, 62, 63, 66, 67, 74, 75, 123, 124, 125, 126, 127, 135, 142, *212*, *214*, *215*
Archdeacon, J. W. 80, *201*
Arends, J. 257, 265, *272*
Arias, I. 433, *465*
Arias, I. M. 433, 434, *459*
Arimura, A. 72, 76, *213*, 279, *302*
Arnold, M. 415, *452*, *464*
Aron, M. 324, *338*
Arrata, W. S. M. 416, *452*
Arrighi, L. 312, *327*
Arronet, G. H. 416, *452*
Arthes, F. G. 436, *465*
Arturson, G. 441, *452*
Askalani, H. 408, 410, 442, *458*
Atkinson, L. E. 473, 474, *492*
Auquier, L. 308, *333*
Aurell, M. 441, *452*
Austin, C. R. 372, *377*
Avendaño, O. 413, 415, *452*
Avendaño, S. 413, 415, *452*
Averkin, E. 185, *203*
Aviado, D. M. 192, *195*
Avila, C. 407, *464*
Axelrod, J. 111, *200*, 348, *379*
Ayalon, D. 279, *299*
Aydar, C. 313, *327*
Aydar, C. K. 91, *195*, *269*, 408, *453*
Aznar, R. 393, 411, 413, 419, 423, *461*
Azuela, J. C. 423, *460*

493

Baanders-van Halewijn, E. A. 305, *327*
Baba, Y. 72, *213*, 279, *302*
Babcock, J. C. 29, *33*, 374, 375, *381*
Bačić, M. 392, *453*
Bacigalupo, G. 310, *327*
Backer, M. H. 313, *327*
Baggett, B. 227, 229, 230, *241*
Baginski, S. 306, *337*
Bagnati, E. P. 74, *195*
Baier, W. 449, *466*
Baird, D. 233, *238*
Baker, B. L. 83, 87, 88, 159, 161, 164, 166, 167, 170, 171, 184, 189, *195*, *205*
Baker, K. C. 316, *327*
Bakker, C. B. 443, 446, *453*
Bakker, F. M. 168, *216*
Baldratti, G. 42, 47, 50, 62, 63, 66, 67, 74, 75, 135, 142, *212*, *214*
Balin, H. 409, *453*
Balina, P. A. 308, *327*
Ball, J. 351, *377*
Banik, U. K. 73, *195*, 354, 355, 373, 375, *377*, *383*
Banks, A. L. 415, *465*
Banks, A. W. 427, *453*
Barbosa, J. 292, 293, *297*
Bardin, C. W. 472, *491*
Bardoczy, A. 187, *215*, 323, *343*
Barfield, W. E. 18, 19, *22*, 257, *271*
Barnes, L. E. 7, 8, 10, 29, *33*, 39, 56, 60, *195*, 374, *377*
Barns, D. F. 257, 259, 265, *273*
Barry, R. D. 217, 218, 219, 222, 223, 226, 232, *238*
Bastide, P. 176, *198*
Batres, E. 29, *34*
Battista, J. V. Jr. 161, 162, 166, 167, *214*
Baunach, A. 403, *453*
Baunach, M. 403, *453*
Bayliess, H. 145, *196*
Beach, V. L. 161, 162, 166, 167, *214*, 360, *381*
Beaton, J. H. 428, *453*
Beaven, D. W. 427, *462*
Becerra, C. 395, 408, 409, *456*
Bechman, L. 441, *452*
Beck, P. 172, 173, 174, *195*, 294, *297*, 429, *453*, 476, *491*
Becker, J. 309, *337*
Behne, D. 404, *468*
Behrens, H. 306, *328*
Behrman, S. J. 407, *453*
Beier, H. M. 180, *195*

Bell, E. T. 278, *300*, 392, 395, 396, 426, *453*, *460*
Beller, F. K. 437, *453*
Bellerby, C. W. 357, *382*
Bellman, O. 219, 227, 228, 229, 234, *239*
Belterman, 147, *214*
Benagiano, G. 191, *195*, 296, *297*
Bendel, R. P. 432, *466*
Bengtsson, L. Ph. 318, *328*
Benjamin, F. 429, *453*
Bennett, J. P. 59, 62, 66, 142, 143, 144, 148, 153, 155, *195*, *196*, *216*, 355, *380*
Berger, R. A. 442, *462*
Bergsjö, P. 306, *328*
Berliner, V. R. 39, 40, 56, 63, 106, 116, *196*
Berman, E. 416, *460*
Bern, H. A. 359, *384*
Bernhard, J. 322, *342*
Bernstein, S. 4, *10*
Besch, P. K. 217, 218, 219, 222, 223, 226, 232, *238*
Besemer, D. 83, 87, 167, *195*
Besold, F. 315, *328*
Bessler, S. 267, *273*, 394, *465*
Bessler, S. A. 404, 407, *457*
Betancourt, E. 450, *459*
Beyl, G. 312, *328*
Beyler, A. L. 353, *377*
Bhatnagar, S. 219, 230, *240*, 426, *459*
Bialy, G. 219, 230, *241*, 358, *377*, *383*, 426, *463*
Bianchi, A. 6, 7, *11*
Bickenbach, W. 311, *329*
Bickerstaff, E. R. 447, *453*
Biddulph, C. 350, 370, *377*
Bigger, J. T. 246, *271*
Bigger, J. T. Jr. 282, *299*
Billewicz, W. Z. 393, 395, *453*
Bindon, B. M. 57, *196*
Binks, R. 315, *329*
Birch, A. J. 25, *33*, 370, *381*
Birk, S. A. 430, 432, *466*
Bishop, P. M. F. 278, 282, *297*, 313, *329*
Black, L. J. 112, *206*
Blair, H. A. F. 22, *22*, 227, 228, *239*, 259, *270*
Blanzat-Reboud, S. 186, *196*
Blaquier, J. A. 166, 167, 170, *196*
Blaustein, A. 439, *453*
Bloch, S. 357, *377*
Blye, R. P. 39, 40, 56, 63, 106, 108, 116, *196*

Boake, W. C.   295, *297*
Board, J. A.   478, *492*
Boars, N. F.   362, *377*
Boatwright, B.   424, *459*
Bockner, V.   315, *329*, 406, *453*
Bogdanove, E. M.   349, *377*
Böhnisch, G.   136, *212*
Bolck, F.   309, *329*
Bolton, C. H.   *269*, 295, *297*, 439, *453*
Bonanno, S.   4, *11*
Bongiovanni, A. M.   121, 128, 129, 131, 181, *196*, *202*, 322, *329*
Bonsignori, A.   92, *215*
Bonta, I. L.   92, *196*
Borell, U.   278, 282, *297*, 349, *377*, *378*
Borglin, N. E.   19, *22*, 324, *329*, 433, *453*
Boris, A.   78, 105, 108, 116, 120, *196*
Bork, K. H.   29, 31, *34*
Borman, A.   4, 5, 6, 7, 9, 10, *10*, *11*, 125, 126, *207*, 376, *382*
Borno, R.   426, 443, *463*
Boschann, H.-W.   13, 14, 16, 17, 18, *22*, 246, 259, 267, 268, *269*, *270*, 312, *329*
Botella-Llusia, J.   418, *465*
Bourgeois, C. H.   423, *456*
Boursnell, J. C.   355, *380*
Bowers, C. Y.   71, 76, *213*, 279, *302*
Bowman, B. J.   79, 161, 162, 165, 182, 183, *202*, 324, *333*
Bowman, J. A.   423, 426, *453*
Boxille, G. C.   178, *207*
Boyarski, L. H.   145, *196*
Braaksma, J. T.   285, *298*
Bradbury, J. T.   69, 70, *214*
Bradley, E. M.   291, *300*
Brancaccio, A.   294, *298*
Brannon, R.   403, *462*
Braselton, J. P.   38, 39, 42, 108, 109, *208*
Brennan, D. M.   4, 5, 6, 9, 10, *10*, *11*, 38, 39, 47, 90, 92, 93, 96, 105, 108, 109, 124, 125, 126, 152, 162, 163, 164, 165, *196*, *206*, *207*
Breuer, H.   21, *22*, 221, 227, 228, 233, *238*, *259*, *270*
Briggs, M.   292, *298*
Briggs, M. H.   292, *298*
Brillantes, F. P.   184, *204*
Brittingham, L. C.   294, 296, *302*
Broda, S.   416, *452*
Brodie, H. J.   228, *242*
Brosens, I.   278, 289, *298*, *302*
Brown, J. B.   22, *22*, 227, 228, 237, *239*, *259*, *270*, 395, *453*

Brown, P. S.   393, 395, *453*
Brown, W.   185, *203*
Bruce, H. M.   372, *377*
Bruckner, K.   29, 31, *34*
Bruckner, W.   249, *273*, 419, *468*
Bruinsma, A. H.   305, *330*
Bruni, G.   10, *10*, 46, 74, 75, *201*
Buchholz, R.   391, 395, *454*
Buchler, D.   431, *454*
Buckingham, J. C.   188, *207*, 439, *454*
Buckingham, J. D.   188, *198*
Buhi, W. C.   432, *466*
Bulbrook, R. D.   233, *242*
Bullough, N. S.   350, *378*
Buns, O.   428, *466*
Bur, G. E.   156, 157, *209*
Bur, G. F.   74, *195*
Burckhardt-Tamm, E.   415, *452*, *464*
Burdick, H. O.   353, 354, *378*, *384*
Burns, R. K.   361, *378*
Burrill, M. W.   117, 123, 127, *202*
Burrows, H.   353, *378*
Burt, A.   361, *382*
Burton, J. L.   435, 441, *454*
Buschbeck, H.   310, *330*
Byrnes, W. W.   350, 351, 370, *378*

Cahal, D. A.   435, *454*
Caie, E.   218, *239*
Calderon, J. J.   416, 423, *460*
Calhoun, D. W.   38, 47, 57, 162, 163, 166, *200*
Callantine, M. R.   99, 176, 177, *196*, *216*
Cambourn, P.   315, *329*
Cammanni, F.   288, *298*
Canales, E.   423, *456*
Cargille, C. M.   325, 326, *341*
Carlburg, L.   277, *301*, 393, *461*
Carlburg, L. G.   286, *298*, *301*
Carlson, K. L.   430, 431, 441, *466*
Carpenter, R. J.   418, *469*
Carpentier, P. J.   131, *196*
Carr, D. H.   451, *454*
Carraro, A.   38, 114, 115, 162, 163, 164, *196*
Carriere, B. T.   237, *242*
Carruthers, M. E.   434, 441, *454*
Carruthers, R.   442, *454*
Carter, A. C.   289, *299*, 395, *455*
Carter, D. L.   48, 65, 68, 78, 114, *200*
Carter, W. F.   245, *270*
Carter, W. M.   76, *213*

Casaglia, C.   98, *196*
Casey, A. E.   184, *216*
Casida, L. E.   145, *196*, 221, *241*
Castegnaro, E.   21, *22*, 223, *239*, 290, *298*
Castrén, O.   309, *343*
Cavanagh, D.   154, *215*
Cavazos, F.   420, *467*
Caveng, B.   275, *302*
Čekan, Z.   37, 38, 39, *196*
Cervantes, A.   427, *464*
Cession, G.   279, *299*
Chalkiadakis, J.   80, *197*
Chalmers, J. A.   308, *330*
Chambon, Y.   50, 54, 59, 60, 79, 95, 106, 110, 116, 163, 164, *196*, *197*
Chamorro, A.   348, *380*
Chandra, H.   69, *205*
Chang, C. C.   57, 137, 191, 192, *195*, *197*, *205*
Chang, M. C.   40, 42, 50, 52, 58, 61, 103, 104, 147, 150, 153, 155, *197*, *211*, 355, 356, 365, 366, 372, *378*, 386, *463*
Chang, M. D.   386, *463*
Chapman, J. R.   232, *241*
Chappel, C. I.   38, 39, 45, 47, 48, 50, 63, 66, 75, 95, 114, 116, 119, 125, 134, *197*, *211*
Charles, D.   220, *240*, 265, *271*
Chartier, M.   308, *330*
Chiris, M.   49, *198*
Chow, C. M.   406, *460*
Chow, L. P.   406, *460*
Cittadini, E.   296, *300*
Claassen, V.   41, 61, 85, 86, 105, 108, 116, 165, *197*
Clapp, H. W.   83, 161, *195*
Clapp, M. L.   362, *379*
Clark, J. J.   39, 79, 94, 95, 125, 157, 165, *199*, 376, *379*, 480, *491*
Clark, S. L.   310, *330*
Clark, V. A.   449, *467*
Clinch, J.   295, *298*
Cloeren, S.   415, *452*, *464*
Clyman, M. J.   249, *272*, 419, *464*
Coburn, W. A.   415, 427, *453*, *465*
Cochrane, R. L.   8, *10*
Coffelt, C. F.   449, *467*
Cohen, A. M.   308, *330*
Cohen, M. R.   18, 19, 20, *22*, *23*
Colillas, O. J.   74, *195*
Collins, W. P.   280, *298*
Colton, F. B.   25, 26, 27, *33*, 34, 49, 162, *200*

Cominos, A. C.   80, *197*
Comoy, C.   308, *333*
Connell, E. B.   420, 440, 447, *454*
Connor, F. J.   136, *214*
Consoli, G.   353, *379*
Contamin, R.   319, *330*
Cooke, B. A.   223, 224, *239*
Coombs, M. M.   233, *242*
Cooper, D. J.   429, *453*
Cooper, J. M.   219, 224, 225, *239*
Coppola, J. A.   67, *197*
Cordier, P.   308, *330*
Cordoso, T.   84, *202*
Corette, L.   295, *301*
Corfman, P. A.   426, *454*
Corner, G. W.   353, *377*, *378*
Cornu, C.   308, *330*
Corren, S.   406, *464*
Cortes-Gallegos, V.   393, 411, 413, 419, 423, *461*
Cotteral, R. D.   424, *454*
Cottinet, D.   53, *198*
Couch, C.   407, *469*
Couri, D.   219, 222, 223, *238*
Courrier, M. R.   357, *383*
Courrier, R.   318, *331*
Coutinho, E. M.   296, *298*, 416, *454*
Cowan, M. L.   357, *378*
Cox, M. J. E.   266, *272*
Cox, R. I.   103, 108, *201*, 375, *379*
Coyne, R. C.   430, *463*
Craig, J.   395, 418, 424, *465*
Craig, J. M.   448, *457*
Crain, D. J.   318, *337*
Cramer, K.   441, *452*
Cramp, D. G.   431, *455*
Crane, M. G.   171, *207*, 290, *298*
Creutzfeldt, W.   441, *469*
Crisosto, C.   416, *457*
Crocker, K. M.   407, *454*
Cromer, J. K.   308, *330*
Crone, A.   285, *299*
Cross, J. N.   447, *458*
Crossen, R. J.   448, *453*
Crowley, C. G.   309, *331*
Croxatto, H. B.   65, 71, 89, *203*
Csapo, A. I.   97, *197*
Cunningham, F. J.   393, 395, *453*
Cunningham, K.   310, *331*, 395, *461*
Cupceancu, B.   117, 118, 125, 126, 160, *197*, *198*, *214*
Curchod, A.   306, *331*
Curwen, S.   309, *331*

Cutler, A.   247, 248, *270*, 282, 283, *299*
Czyba, J. C.   49, 53, *198*, *199*

Dahlberg, B.   408, *454*
D'Alessandro, B.   294, *298*
Daly, J. R.   290, *298*
D'Amour, F. E.   353, *384*
Danforth, D. N.   188, *198*, *207*, 439, *454*
Daniel, J. C.   357, *378*
Danon, A.   45, *215*
Dapunt, O.   276, *298*, 318, *331*
Dardenne, U.   227, 228, *238*, 259, *270*
Dargan, A. M.   15, *24*
Darras, P.   295, *301*
Dasgupta, P. R.   134, 137, 180, *212*
Dastugue, G.   176, *198*
Date, J.   430, *466*
Dauria, P.   310, *331*
David, A.   29, *34*, 38, 39, 42, 60, 94, 95, 106, 109, 116, 125, 126, 157, 161, 165, 171, *198*
Davidson, C. S.   434, *462*
Davidson, J. M.   349, *378*
Davis, B. K.   53, 141, 156, *198*
Davis, C. D.   408, *455*
Davis, E.   245, 246, 247, 250, 258, *270*, *273*
Davis, M. E.   4, *10*, 13, 14, 15, 17, 20, 21, *23*, *24*
Deanesly, R.   349, 354, 355, 376, *378*
Debeljuk, L.   72, *213*
De Casparis, A. W.   392, *453*
Decker, A.   249, *272*
Deckers, G. H.   49, *198*
Deckert, T.   430, *466*
de Fremery,   45, *198*
de Groot, C. A.   316, *331*
Dehejia, N.   408, *454*
de Jongh, D. C.   234, *239*
Del Sol, J. R.   15, *24*, 268, *270*
de Martire, J.   433, *463*
De Moor, P.   289, *298*
Dennis, K. J.   219, 227, 233, 234, *239*, *240*
De Phillipo, M.   5, 6, 7, 10, *11*, 125, 126, *207*
De Prospo, N. D.   189, *216*
Der, B. K.   167, 187, 188, *214*
Desaulles, P. A.   39, 40, 41, 46, 47, 48, 62, 63, 74, 75, 90, 91, 94, 95, 114, 115, *198*, 351, 352, 364, 365, 369, *378*, *381*
De Schaepdrijver, A. F.   101, *216*

De Souza, J. C.   416, *454*
Devenish-Meares, M.   406, *454*
de Visser, J.   40, 41, 42, 46, 50, 52, 62, 66, 74, 79, 92, 94, 95, 96, 104, 106, 110, 114, 115, 123, 124, 126, 145, 151, 154. 155, 156, 171, *198*, *207*, *210*, 486, *492*
De Waard, F.   305, 306, *327*, *330*, *344*
De Wachter, A. M.   10, *11*, 123, 124, 125, 126, *213*
Dewar, H. A.   296, *301*
de Wied, D.   168, *216*
de Winter, M. S.   28, *34*
Dhom, G.   84, *198*
Dick, R. G.   186, *208*
Dicker, A.   419, *464*
Dickson, A. D.   57, *198*
Dickstein, S.   410, *464*
Diczfalusy, E.   220, 221, *239*, 246, *273*, 278, 282, *297*, *298*, 392, 393, 395, 396, 415, 417, *453*, *454*, *458*
Diddle, A. W.   418, *455*
Di George, A. M.   121, 128, 129, 131, *196*, 322, *329*
Dightman, C. R.   443, 446, *453*
D'Incerti Bonini, L.   248, *270*, 283, *299*, 306, *331*
Dingle, J. T.   408, *455*
di Paola, G.   431, 433, *455*, *463*
Di Pasquale, G.   161, 162, 166, 167, *214*
Di Saia, P. J.   408, *455*
Dittmar, F. W.   294, *299*, 322, *331*, 425, *465*
Djerassi, C.   25, 27, 29, *34*, 40, 42, 79, 114, 115, *208*, 353, *382*
Doar, J. W. H.   430, 431, 432, *455*, *469*
Döcke, F.   63, 73, *198*, *199*, 349, *379*
Dodds, E. C.   357, *382*
Dodek, O. I.   289, *299*, 426, *455*
Dodek, O. I. Jr.   427, *455*
Doe, J. P.   441, *462*
Doe, R.   292, 293, *297*
Dohrn, M.   349, *383*
Doll, R.   435, *455*, 490, *491*
Domenico, A.   62, 74, 75, 79, 103, 104, 106, 110, *210*
Domm, L. V.   362, *379*
Donayre, J. J.   439, *455*
Donini, S.   296, *297*
Doolittle, D. P.   134, 135, *199*
Dorfman, A. S.   350, *379*
Dorfman, R. I.   9, *10*, 38, 44, 59, 60, 61, 74, 75, 79, 89, 104, 108, 109, 112, 120, 124, 125, 126, 135, 136, 141, 191, *199*,

Dorfman, R. I.—*contd.*
201, *205*, *206*, 217, *239*, 350, 360, 361, 365, 366, 367, 368, 370, *379*, *381*, 394, *455*
Döring, G. K.   311, 313, *329*, 331
Dörner, G.   63, 73, *198*, *199*, 349, *379*
Douglas, E.   407, *464*
Douglas, M. G.   247, *270*
Dreisbach, R. H.   357, *379*
Dresner, M. H.   19, *22*
Drews, R.   16, 17, *22*, 246, 259, 269, *270*
Drill, V. A.   39, 40, 41, 42, 44, 46, 47, 48, 69, 70, 79, 90, 91, 93, 104, 106, 114, 115, 116, 126, 129, *199*, *213*, 315, *332*, 349, *383*, 406, 407, 417, 421, 422, 447, *455*
Dubois, P.   53, *199*
Dubrow, H.   448, *461*
Ducharme, J. R.   128, 130, 131, *202*, 322, *333*
Duckett, G. E.   359, *394*
Dudeck, J.   283, 289, 296, *299*
Dugdale, M.   437, 447, *455*, *461*
Dujovich, A.   308, *332*
Dukes, M. N. G.   404, 407, 421, 445, *455*, *459*
Dulin, W. E.   7, *10*, 29, *33*
Dulin, W. F.   39, 60, *195*
Duluc, A. J.   8, *11*
Dumont, L.   53, *199*
Duncan, G. W.   39, 79, 94, 95, 125, 157, 165, *199*, 374, 375, 376, *379*, *381*, 480, *491*
Dunn, H. P.   426, *455*
Durandeau, A.   410, *455*
Durham, W. C.   20, *23*
Durham, W. D.   308, *332*
Durkin, J. W.   395, *460*
Durruti, M.   316, *335*
Duthie, J. J. R.   318, *332*
Dutt, R. H.   80, *201*
Dutta, N. S.   100, *199*
Dziuk, P. J.   135, 137, *199*

Eben-Moussi, E.   41, 63, 74, 106, 115, *199*
Ectors, F.   83, *199*, *211*
Edelstein, S. W.   426, *458*
Edgren, R. A.   4, 9, *10*, 38, 39, 40, 42, 45, 46, 47, 48, 57, 58, 65, 68, 78, 94, 96, 99, 102, 103, 104, 106, 107, 108, 109, 111, 113, 114, 115, 116, 126, 134, 135, 137, 142, 152, 157, 162, 163, 165, 166, *199*, *200*, *204*, *211*, *213*, 357, 363, 365, 366, *379*, 383
Edwards, K.   38, 39, 42, 60, 94, 95, 106, 109, 116, 125, 126, 157, 171, *198*
Eechaute, W.   176, *207*
Ehrlich, E.   309, *337*
Ehrmann, R. L.   267, *270*
Eichner, E.   408, *455*
Eisalo, A.   433, *455*
Eisenfeld, A. J.   111, *200*, 348, *379*
Ejarque, P. M.   20, 21, *23*
Elce, J. S.   219, 224, 225, *239*
Elger, W.   118, 119, 122, 127, *209*, *210*
El-Habashy, M.   416, *462*
Eliasson, G.   324, *329*
Ellis, B.   29, *34*
Ellis, F.   233, *242*
Ellis, L. T.   315, *333*
Ellsworth, H. S.   409, *462*
El-Safouri, S.   297, *297*
Elstein, M.   290, *298*, 393, 395, 415, *462*
Elton, R. L.   38, 41, 44, 45, 46, 47, 48, 49, 57, 104, 107, 109, 162, 163, *200*, *213*
Emerson, B.   354, *378*
Emmens, C. W.   103, 107, 108, *200*, *201*, 357, 364, 365, 366, 373, 375, 376, *379*, *384*
Engel, I.   391, 395, *464*
Engel, L.   237, *239*
Engelbregt, A.   81, *210*
Engelfried, O.   27, *34*
Engelund, A.   436, *458*
Epperson, D.   428, *455*
Epstein, J. A.   19, *24*, 247, 248, *270*, 282, 283, *299*, 324, *337*
Erb, H.   154, *201*
Ercoli, A.   10, *10*, 27, *34*, 46, 133, 134, 135, 137, *201*, 366, *379*
Erickson, L. R.   442, *455*
Ericsson, R. I.   80, *201*
Erlenmeyer, F.   233, *240*
Ermini, M.   191, *195*, 296, *297*
Escudero, M.   418, *465*
Eskes, T. K. A. B.   285, *299*
Esselink, J.   410, *455*
Esser, R. J. E.   220, 221, *239*
Evans, H. M.   349, *379*
Evans, L. T.   362, *379*
Everse, J. W. R.   410, *455*
Eviator, E.   45, *215*
Exley, D.   73, 76, *201*

Faircloth, M. A. 428, *455*
Fairweather, F. A. 158, 172, *201*, 280, *302*
Falconi, G. 10, *10*, 46, 74, 75, 133, 134, 135, 137, *201*, 366, *379*
Falk, R. J. 472, *491*
Fan, K. Y. 406, *460*
Farman, J. 450, *459*
Faucher, G. L. 245, *270*
Fedden, G. A. 88, 105, *216*
Feenstra, H. 97, *216*
Feierabend, J. F. 227, 230, *241*
Fekete, G. 161, 162, *201*
Feldman, E. B. 289, *299*, 395, *455*
Fellower, K. P. 38, 39, 42, 60, 94, 95, 106, 109, 116, 125, 126, 157, 171, *198*
Ferin, J. 14, *23*. 246, 247, 248, 249, 250, 251, 252, 260, 266, 267, *270*, *271*, *273*, 289, *302*, 308, *332*, 395, 418, *460*
Ferrara, B. 353, *379*
Ferreira, D. A. M. 296, *298*
Ferrero, A. 292, *302*
Feuer, G. 182, *201*
Fikentscher, H. 249, *273*, 419, *468*
Finke, L. 308, *332*
Finn, C. A. 364, 365, *379*
First, N. L. 221, *241*
Fisher, D. A. 428, *455*
Flehinger, B. J. 448, *461*
Flerkó, B. 349, *379*
Florsheim, W. H. 428, *455*
Flowers, C. E. 420, 426, *455*
Fobes, D. C. 308, *338*
Foell, T. J. 234, *239*
Folch-Pi, A. 41, 135, 191, *201*, *206*, 359, 361, *381*
Földi, M. 187, *215*
Fontaine, J. 308, *333*
Foote, C. L. 361, *379*
Foote, L. H. 128, 161, 168, *201*
Foote, W. C. 128, 161, 168, *201*
Foote, W. D. 128, 161, 168, *201*
Forbes, A. D. 473, *492*
Forbes, D. A. 418, *469*
Forbes, T. R. 362, *380*
Forest, A. A. 223, *242*, 251, *273*
Fortner, J. G. 167, 187, 188, *214*
Foss, G. L. 413, *456*
Fotherby, K. 219, 222, 227, 228, 229, 232, 233, 234, 235, *239*, *240*, *241*, 280, *302*, 395, *453*
France E. S. 66, 70, *201*
Franchimont, P. 279, *299*

Francis, W. G. 407, *456*
Frank, R. 19, 22, 424, *468*
Frias, Z. 428, *458*
Frick, H. C. 306, *332*
Fried, 174
Fried, J. 4, *10*, *11*
Friedl, W. 318, *333*
Friedman, M. H. 386, *460*
Fries, K. 312, *332*
Frith, D. A. 72, *201*, *202*
Froewis, J. 312, *332*
Fuchs, F. 99, *202*
Furuhata, T. 41, 94, 106, *206*
Fussgänger, R. 189, *202*

Gaarenstroom, J. H. 362, *380*
Gabbard, R. B. 237, *242*
Gaffney, T. J. 292, *301*
Gagne, W. E. 185, *203*
Gall, S. A. 423, *456*
Gallagher, T. F. Jr. 175, *211*
Gallegos, A. J. 287, *299*
Gallo, R. V. 86, 87, *202*, *216*, 474, *491*
Gamble, C. J. 427, *465*
Gandry, R. 10, *11*
Garcia, A. Am. 428, *457*
Garcia, C. R. 249, *272*, 395, 404, 417, 426, 427, 443, *456*, *463*, *464*, *468*
Garcia, R. 318, *341*
Gardi, P. 27, *34*
Gardi, R. 10, *10*, 46, *201*
Gardner, J. H. 447, *456*
Gardner, W. H. 418, *455*
Gardner, W. V. 448, *456*
Garrett, W. J. 320, *342*
Gartside, J. M. 429, *456*
Gaspard, U. 279, *299*
Gastlelum, H. 406, *464*
Gaudry, R. 48, 125, *197*, *211*
Gawlak, D. 41, 63, 74, 96, 113, 115, *209*
Gay, A. J. 447, *465*
Gazzaniga, P. P. 101, *202*
Gecse, A. 158, *204*
Geipel, K. 312, *332*
Geller, J. 309, *332*
Gellert, R. J. 73, 76, *201*
Gemzell, C. 277, 279, 280, 282, 283, 286, *298*, 300, *301*
Gemzell, C. A. 392, 393, 395, 415, *459*, *461*, *468*
Gerard, G. 84, *202*
Gerard, J. 275, *302*

Gerhards, E.   219, 227, 228, 229, 234, *239*
Gershberg, H.   429, 430, 432, *456, 458, 469*
Geuens, I.   278, *302*
Ghoneim, M.   297, *297, 300*
Giannina, T.   41, 63, 74, 96, 113, 115, 126, 142, 166, 167, *202, 209*
Gibian, H.   284, *299*
Gibson, J.   42, 63, 141, *216*, 365, 366, *384*
Gilbert, R. A.   246, *271, 272*
Gilfrich, H. J.   283, 289, 296, *299*
Gillen, A. L.   107, 109, 111, *200*
Gillette, P. N.   441, *466*
Gillman, J.   351, *380*
Gilmore, D. P.   72, *208*
Giner   393, 411, 413, 419, 423, *461*
Gitsch, E.   310, *333*
Glenn, E. M.   79, 161, 162, 165, 182, 183, *202*, 324, *333*
Glick, I. D.   444, 446, *456*
Goebelsman, U.   278, *298, 300*, 393, 415, *454*
Goisis, M.   83, *202*
Golab, T.   219, 227, 230, 231, *238, 240*
Gold, J. J.   18, 19, 20, *22, 23*
Golding, G. T.   352, *380*
Goldman, A. S.   129, 181, *202*
Goldzieher, J. W.   246, 249, *271*, 315, 321, *333*, 389, 391, 393, 395, 404, 405, 406, 407, 408, 409, 418, 419, 423, 427, 443, *456, 460, 462, 464, 467*
González, R. A.   416, 417, *464*
González-Diddi, M.   287, *299*
Good, R. G.   249, *271*
Goodman, A. L.   309, *333*
Goodrich, S. M.   439, *456*
Goolden, A. W. G.   429, *456*
Gordon, G. G.   290, 291, 295, *299*
Görgey, E.   318, *337*
Gorlitzer, V.   318, *333*
Gorosdisch, S.   433, *463*
Gorski, R.   117, *202*
Gorski, R. A.   359, *380*
Goss, D. A.   426, *458*
Gotlib, M.   404, 410, *468*
Goudie, R. B.   441, *458*
Gould, J.   315, *333*
Gourvès, M.   79, 116, *197*
Grabowich, P.   4, *10, 11*
Grand, L. C.   184, *204*
Granda, V.   182, *201*
Grant, A.   308, *333*

Grant, E. C. G.   315, *338*, 444, 446, *457, 461*
Grant, V.   266, *272*
Gray, C. H.   237, *241*
Gray, L. A.   308, *333*
Greany, M. O.   404, 407, *457*
Greenblatt, R.   313, *327*
Greenblatt, R. B.   18, 19, *22*, 91, *195*, 245, 246, 257, *269, 271*, 282, 283, *299*, 310, 315, *330, 333*, 348, 375, *383*, 396, 408, 416, *453, 457*
Greene, G. R.   436, 448, *457, 465*
Greene, R. R.   117, 123, 127, *202*
Greenwald, G. S.   59, 64, *202*, 351, 353, 354, 355, 369, *380, 474, 492*
Greep, R. O.   351, 352, *380*
Greer, M. V.   246, *271*, 282, *299*
Gregg, W. I.   426, *457*
Gregoire, A. T.   286, *299*, 411, 423, *457*
Gregoire, L.   308, *333*
Greslin, J. G.   374, *380*
Griesbach, W. E.   83, *211*
Griffith, D. R.   158, 159, *202*
Griffith, R. S.   440, *457*
Griffiths, C. T.   448, *457*
Griswold, D. P.   184, *202*
Griswold, D. P. Jr.   184, *216*
Grots, I.   424, *469*
Grumbach, M. M.   121, 128, 129, 130, 131, *196, 202*, 322, *329, 333*
Gual, C.   395, 408, 409, *456*
Gualandi, L.   98, *196*
Guerrero, I.   442, *464*
Guerrero, R.   416, *463*
Guiot, G.   308, *333*
Guiterrez, J.   427, *464*
Guitterez-Najar, A.   393, 411, 413, 419, 423, *461*
Gumbreck, L. G.   350, 370, *377*
Gupta, D.   325, *345*
Gurucharri, C. A.   74, *195*
Gustavson, R. G.   353, *384*
Guterman, H. S.   320, *333*
Gutierrez, J.   407, *464*
Gutsell, E. S.   29, *33*

Hafez, E. S. E.   40, 42, 50, 52, 58, 61, 103, 104, *211*, 355, *380*, 386, *463*
Hahn, H. B.   324, 325, 326, *333*
Hahn, J. D.   118, 122, *209, 210*
Hall, D. G.   420, *467*
Haller, J.   78, 80, 100, 177, *203, 206*, 277,

299, 312, 313, 315, *333*, 404, 415, 416, 417, *457, 459*
Halmi, N. S. 83, *203*
Halterman, D. R. 231, *240*
Haltrecht, I. 73, *195*
Hamada, H. 118, 119, *203*, 312, *333*
Hambourger, W. E. 162, 163, 166, *200*
Hamburger, Chr. 257, 265, *272*
Hamilton, T. 233, *242*
Hammer, C. J. 442, *457*
Hammerstein, F. 316, *335*
Hammond, P. O. 309, *339*
Hampton, J. R. 269, 295, 296, *297, 299,* 439, *453*
Hansel, W. 475, *492*
Hara, K. 50, 51, 52, 53, *209*, 357, *382*
Harkness, R. A. 220, *240*, 265, *271*, 278, *300*, 392, 395, 396, *460*
Harnecker, J. 416, *457*
Harpel, P. C. 180, *203*
Harper, M. J. K. 67, 70, 85, 86, *203*, 355, 356, 365, 366, *378, 380*
Harris, G. W. 73, 76, *201, 203*, 361, *380*
Harris, J. J. 290, *298*
Hart, P. G. 219, 233, *242*, 426, *468*
Harting, J. 120, *206*
Hartley, F. 29, *34*
Hartman, C. G. 351, *377*
Hasche, H. H. 431, 432, *466*
Hashimoto, I. 474, 475, *491, 492*
Haskins, A. L. 310
Haspels, A. A. 391, *457*
Hass, T. 408, *457*
Haterius, H. O. 349, *380*
Hauser, G. A. 312, *334*
Hayashi, H. 220, *241*
Hayles, A. B. 128, 131, *203*, 324, 325, 326, *333, 343*
Hayward, J. N. 65, 71, 89, *203*
Headings, M. 167, *195*
Heany, R. P. 433, *457*
Heap, R. B. 358, *380*
Heber, K. R. 408, *457*
Hecht-Lucari, G. 38, 101, 106, 108, 109, 120, 141, *202, 203*, 245, *271*, 290, *301*, 396, *457*
Heckel, G. P. 351, *377*
Hecker, R. 433, *464*
Hecker, W. 219, 227, 228, 229, 234, *239*
Heckmann, B. 306, *334*
Hefnawi, F. 297, *297, 300*, 408, 410, 442, *458*
Heikel, T. A. J 175, *203*

Hein, P. R. 285, *299*
Helmer, O. M. 440, *457*
Helmreich, M. L. 21, 22, *23*, 223, *240*
Helpap, B. 308, *334*
Hempel, R. 99, 101, *210*
Hendricks, D. M. 474, *491*
Hendrikx, A. 289, *298*
Hendrix, J. W. 39, 79, 94, 95, 125, 157, 165, *199*, 480, *491*
Henzl, M. 312, *334*
Henzl, M. R. 180, *214*, 361, *383*
Herlant, M. 83, *199*
Hernandez, A. 432, *469*
Herr, F. 73, *195*
Herr, M. E. 29, *33*
Herrera Lasso, L. 135, 191, *201*, 359, 360, 361, *381*
Herrmann, U. 18, *23*
Hertig, A. T. 267, *270*
Hertz, R. 40, 42, 178, *203, 215*, 247, *271*, 350, *382*, 448, *457*
Hervey, E. 168, 169, *203*
Hervey, G. R. 168, 169, *203*
Higashi, Y. 224, *241*
Higashiyama, S. 162, 163, 165, *215*, 232, *242*
Hill, R. 185, *203*
Hilliard, J. 65, 71, 89, *203*
Hillmer, T. 441, *469*
Hines, D. C. 405, *456*
Hisaw, F. L. 348, *381, 382*
Hitze, H. 219, 227, 228, 229, 234, *239*
Hobbs, C. B. 434, 441, *454*
Hockaday, J. M. 444, *468*
Hofhansl, W. 313, 318, *334, 335*
Hofmann, D. 308, *334*
Hoge, A. F. 309, *339*
Hogg, J. A. 29, *33*
Hohlweg, W. 281, *301*, 318, *334*, 348, 349, *380, 383*
Hollander, C. S. 428, *457*
Holman, G. H. 128, 129, 130, 131, *216*, 322, *344*
Holmes, J. M. 447, *453*
Holmes, R. L. 63, 82, 135, 140, 167, 170 *204*
Holmstrom, E. G. 404, 408, *457, 458*
Holthaus, F. J. Jr. 372, *382*
Holtkamp, D. E. 374, *380*
Holub, D. A. 83, 161, *204*
Holzbach, R. T. 434, *458*
Holzmann, H. 316, *335, 337*
Homburger, F. 180, *203*

Homesley, H. D.   426, *458*
Homm, R. E.   39, 40, 56, 63, 106, 108, 116, *196*
Hooper, K. C.   72, *201, 202*
Hooton Frayn, A.   186, *205*
Horenstein, S.   447, *456*
Horne, C. H. W.   441, *458*
Horowitz, B. J.   426, *458*
Horský, J.   312, *334*, 361, *383*
Horton, R.   233, *238*
Hosaka, H.   318, *335*
Houki, N.   219, 220, 221, 223, *240, 241*
Houtman, A. C.   220, 221, *239*
Howie, P. W.   441, *458*
Hribar, J. D.   234, *239*
Huggins, C.   182, 184, *204*, 309, *335, 337*
Hughes, G. A.   108, 113, *200*
Hulka, J. F.   187, *204*
Hulse, M.   429, 430, 432, *456, 458,* 469
Humphrey, K. W.   153, *204*
Humphrey, R. R.   176, 177, *196*
Hunstein, W.   441, *469*
Huseby, R. A.   21, 22, *23,* 223, *240*
Husslein, H.   313, *335*
Hutcherson, W. P.   407, *458*
Hvidt, W.   308, *335*

Igarashi, M.   310, 318, *335*
Iglesias, R.   185, *207*, 309, *338*, 448, *460*
Illis, L.   447, *458*
Ingemanson, C. A.   444, 447, *462*
Inman, W. H. W.   435, 436, *455, 458*
Inoue, S.   395, *461*
Irani, N. G.   325, *335*
Irey, N. S.   423, 439, *458, 467*
Iriarte, J.   27, *34*
Irizarry, S.   428, *458*
Ishihara, M.   220, 227, 228, 235, *241*
Ishihara, S.   227, 233, 237, *240, 241,* 259, *272*
Israel, S. L.   282, *299*
Ito, T.   395, 444, *461*
Ivy, A. C.   117, 123, 127, *202*
Iwangoff, P.   316, *335*
Iwasaki, S.   221, 232, *241, 242*

Jackson, J. L.   389, *458*
Jackson, M. C. N.   392, 395, 396, *458, 460*
Jackson, N. H.   396, *458*

Jacobi, J. M.   292, *301*
Jacobsohn, D.   348, *384*
Jacobson, H. I.   348, *381*
Jacobson, L.   444, 447, *462*
Jacobson, M.   477, *492*
Jacobson, M. M.   407, *452*
Jacono, G.   294, *298*
Jacques, J.   373, 375, *383*
Jadrijević, D.   183, *204*
Jaffe, R. B.   278, *300*, 473, *492*
Jailer, J. W.   83, 161, *204*
Jakobovits, A.   158, *204*
Janer, J. L.   428, *458*
Jann, R.   312, *335*
Janssens, J.   285, *299*
Jarvinen, P. A.   433, *455*
Javier, Z.   429, 430, 432, *456, 458*
Jeffery, J. D. A.   168, 169, *203*
Jelinek   78
Jelle, B.   309, *335*
Jellema, M. M.   171, *213*
Jenkins, J. S.   293, *300*
Jennett, W. B.   447, *458*
Jensen, E. V.   348, *381*
Jensen, L.   420, 426, *455*
Jirasek, J.   312, *334*, 361, *383*
Johannisson, E.   278, *298*, 393, 396, 415, 417, *454, 458*
Johansson, E. D. B.   279, 280, 281, 282, 283, *300*, 392, 393, 415, *459*, 473, 474, *492*
John, P. N.   179, *212*
Johnson, S. G.   257, 265, *272*
Johnson, W. D.   423, *457*
Jones, R. C.   4, 9, *10*, 38, 39, 40, 42, 45, 47, 58, 78, 94, 96, 104, 106, 107, 108, 109, 111, 113, 114, 115, 116, 126, 134, 142, 165, 166, *200, 204, 211*
Jones, C. I.   351, 352, *380*
Jones, H. E. H.   224, *239*
Jones, H. W.   322, *344*
Jones, H. W. Jr.   128, 129, 130, 131, *216*
Jongh, S. E. de   81, 102, *204, 210*
Joosse, L. A.   308, *335*
Jost, A.   91, 122, 123, 124, 127, 156, *204*
Julian, P. L.   3, *10*
Jungck, E. C.   246, 257, *271*, 282, *299*
Junkmann, K.   4, 5, 6, 7, 8, *10, 11,* 38, 39, 40, 41, 42, 47, 48, 61, 62, 103, 104, 106, 114, 115, 118, 119, 122, 124, 125, 126, *203, 204, 210, 215,* 303, *335,* 348, *380*
Jürgensen, O.   276, *302*

Kaboth, U.   441, *469*
Kadri, S.   408, 410, 442, *458*
Kaern, T.   425, *458*
Kahn, R. H.   83, 87, 88, 159, 167, 171, 184, 189, *195*, *204*, *205*
Kaiser, J.   395, *468*
Kaiser, R.   21, *23*, 186, *205*, 227, 228, 237, *240*, 247, *271*
Kakushi, H.   50, 51, 52, 53, *209*, 357, *382*
Kalkhoff, R. K.   477, *492*
Kamal, I.   297, *297*, *300*, 408, 410, 442, *458*
Kamboj, V. P.   191, *205*
Kamyab, S.   219, 227, 228, 229, 232, 233, 234, *239*, *240*
Kane, F. J.   446, *458*
Kanematsu, S.   71, *205*, 349, *381*
Kaplan, S. A.   325, *335*
Kappas, A.   175, *211*, 441, *466*
Kar, A. B.   69, 134, 137, 180, 191, *205*, *212*
Karady, M.   158, *204*
Karady, S.   186, *205*
Karpel, W. J.   3, *10*
Kars-Villanueva, E. B.   285, *299*
Käser, O.   308, 310, 318, 319, *335*, *336*
Kaspare, E.   27, *34*
Kastin, A. J.   72, *213*, 279, *302*
Katz, F. H.   83, 161, *204*
Kaufman, C.   303, 311, *336*
Kaufman, R. H.   424, *459*
Kaump, D. H.   171, *213*
Kawakami, M.   88, *205*
Kawasaki, D. M.   309, *341*
Kawashima, S.   361, *381*
Kaye, B. M.   444, *459*
Kazama, N.   475, *492*
Keenan, C. A.   235, *239*
Kelisky, R. P.   448, *461*
Keller, M.   275, *302*
Kellie, A. E.   219, 224, 225, *239*
Kelman, C. D.   440, 447, *454*
Kendall, T.   410, *462*
Kendle, K. E.   143, 153, *205*
Kennedy, R. F.   410, *462*
Kersley, G. D.   318, *336*
Kessler, W. B   4, 9, *10*
Ketchel, M. M.   357, *381*
Kieser, H.   38, 141, *203*
Kilpatrick, Z. M.   450, *459*
Kim, Y. J.   395, *460*
Kincl, F. A.   9, *10*, 38, 39, 40, 41, 42, 44, 57, 59, 60, 61, 62, 65, 67, 68, 70, 74, 75, 79, 85, 86, 87, 89, 104, 108, 109, 117, 124, 125, 126, 135, 136, 137, 138, 141, 191, 192, *195*, *197*, *199*, *201*, *205*, *206*, *208*, *212*, 351, 352, 354, 355, 359, 360, 361, 362, 363, 365, 367, 368, 370, 371, *381*,*382*,*383*, 392,393, *394*, 443,*455*, *465*
King, T. O.   108, 134,135, 171, *194*, *196*, *206*, *207*
Kinnard, J.   92, *214*
Kipnis, D.   417, *465*
Kirchoff, H.   404, *459*
Kirk, D. N.   29, 31, *34*
Kirsch, R. E.   353, *383*
Kirschner, M.   433, *465*
Kirsteins, L.   284, 294, *300*
Kirton, K. T.   473, *492*
Kistner, R. W.   306, 307, *336*, *337*, 427, 448, *457*, *468*
Klaiber, E. L.   289, *299*, 427, *455*
Kleibel, F.   309, *337*
Klein, I.   17, 21, *23*, 304, 311, *340*
Kleiner, G. J.   433, 434, *459*
Klibanoff, P.   392, *467*
Klibansky, Y.   27, *34*
Klimstra, P. D.   25, *34*, 49, *200*
Klinger, R.   38, 114, 115, 162, 163, 164, *196*
Klopper, A.   218, 219, 227, 228, 229, 232, 233, *239*, *240*, 245, *271*
Knobil, E.   473, 474, *492*
Knuppen, R.   221, *238*
Knutsson, F.   282, *300*
Kobayashi, F.   69, 70, *209*
Kobayashi, H.   232, *242*
Kobayashi, T.   41, 61, 94, 105, 106, 116, *206*, 282, *300*
Kocen, R. S.   447, *458*
Koch, F.   99, *202*
Kofler, E.   18, *24*, 312, *341*
Kolstad, P.   309, *337*
König, A.   100, *206*
Kooij, R.   316, *331*
Kopera, H.   278, *302*, 391, 392, 404, 407, 421, 445, *455*, *459*, *465*
Kora, S. J.   425, *459*
Korn, G. W.   406, *459*
Korompay, A.   156, 157, *209*
Korte, W.   308, *337*
Korting, G. W.   316, *335*, *337*
Kosierowski, J.   141, *216*
Koss, L. G.   448, *461*
Kottmeier, H. L.   306, *337*
Kotz, H. L.   426, *455*

Koullapis, E. N.   280, *298*
Kovács, L.   62, 65, 80, 142, *212*, *215*, 323, *343*
Kraay, R. J.   38, 39, 47, 90, 92, 93, 96, 105, 108, 109, 124, 125, 152, 162, 163, 164, 165, *196*, *206*
Kraehahn, G.   69, 70, 81, *206*
Kraft, H. G.   38, 120, 141, *203*, *206*
Krähenbühl, C.   39, 40, 41, 46, 47, 48, 62, 63, 74, 75, 90, 91, 94, 95, 114, 115, *198*, 351, 352, 364, 365, 369, *378*, *381*
Kraicer, J.   83, 171, *207*
Králová, A.   278, *302*, 406, *467*
Kramer, M.   7, *11*, 40, 42, 114, 115, 118, 122, 125, 126, *210*
Krater, J. E.   309, *337*
Kraus, E. J.   348, *381*
Krause, R.   48, 50, *206*
Kreek, M. J.   434, *459*
Krehbiel, R. H.   357, *381*
Kresch, L.   433, 434, *459*
Kridelka, J. C.   246, *273*
Kroc, R. L.   360, *381*
Kroger, W. S.   444, *459*
Krull, P.   84, *198*
Kühn, K.   316, *335*, *337*
Kulin, H. E.   325, 326, *341*
Kullander, S.   293, *300*, 441, *460*
Kuo, M. C.   231, *240*
Kupperman, H. S.   19, *24*, 247, 248, *270*, 282, 283, *299*, 324, *337*
Kur, S.   14, 18, *22*
Kyle, L. H.   318, *337*

Labhsetwar, A. P.   7, *10*, 81, 82, 87, *206*
Lacny, J.   310, *337*
Lacroix, E.   176, *207*
Ladd, J. E.   428, *468*
Lamb, E. J.   420, 426, *459*
Lambert, A.   247, *272*, 283, *301*
Landau, R. L.   309, *337*
Lane, C. E.   348, *381*
Lang, W.   310, *331*
Langecker, H.   20, *23*, 217, 227, 228, *240*, *259*, *271*
Laragh, J. H.   440, *459*, *462*
Laraque, F.   426, 443, *463*
Laron, Z.   324, *337*
Larranaga, A.   416, *459*
Larsson-Cohn, U.   279, 280, 282, 283, *300*, 392, 393, 415, 428, 433, 434, *459*
Lass, F.   306, *343*

Laster, W. R.   184, *202*
László, B.   318, *337*
Lathe, G. H.   175, *203*
Latour, J. P. A.   416, *452*
Laumas, K. R.   219, 230, *240*, 426, *459*
Laumas, V.   219, 230, *240*, 426, *459*
Laurell, C. B.   293, *300*, 441, *460*
Laurie, R. E.   404, 407, 408, 421, 422, 445, *460*
Lauritzen, C.   14, 18, *23*, *24*, 227, *240*
Lauweryns, J.   395, 418, *460*
Lawrence, A. M.   284, 294, *300*
Lawson, J. P.   450, *459*
Lax, H.   308, *338*
Layne, D. S.   219, 227, 229, 230, 231, 232, *238*, *240*, *241*, *242*, 288, *300*, 426, 427, 428, 440, *460*, *463*
Leach, R. B.   427, 428, 429, *460*, *461*
Leathem, J. H.   352, 359, *381*, *384*
Le Bars, S.   60, 163, 164, *196*, *197*
Lebherz, T.   267, *272*, 394, *465*
Lebherz, Th. B.   308, *338*
Lecocq, F. R.   291, *300*
Ledingham, J. G. G.   440, *459*, *462*
Lednicer, D.   374, 375, 376, *379*, *381*
Lee, A. E.   109, *207*
Lee, H. C.   406, *460*
Lee, S. L.   176, 177, *196*
Leeb, H.   312, *332*
Legatt, T.   230, *242*
Legros, J. J.   279, *299*
LeHew, W. L.   404, 405, 410, 423, *452*
Lehmann, W. D.   227, *240*
Leizinger, E.   312, *338*
Lemberger, L.   290, *299*
Lemli, L.   324, *338*
Lemming, G. E.   358, *380*
Lemmon, F. M.   407, *469*
Lemper, D.   477, *492*
Lennon, H. D.   175, *207*
Leonard, S. L.   348, *382*
Leonora, J.   171, *207*
Lerner, L. J.   4, 5, 6, 7, 9, 10, *11*, 112, 125, 126, *207*, 372, 374, 376, *380*, *382*
Leusden, H. A. I. M. van   221, *240*
Leusen, I.   176, *206*
Le Vève, Y.   59, 79, 95, 116, *197*
Levin, J.   410, *468*
Levin, M.   404, *468*
Levine, S.   361, *380*
Levy, J.   308, *333*
Lewin, M.   309, *332*

Lewis, E. T.   404, 407, 408, 421, 422, 445, 460
Lewit, S.   403, *467*
Lidz, R. W.   446, *460*
Lieberman, M. W.   187, *204*
Liggins, G. C.   408, 409, 410, *460*
Lin, H. S.   82, *207*
Lin, T. J.   395, *460*
Lindsay, D. R.   139, *207*
Ling, S. M.   325, *335*
Linthorst, C.   418, *460*
Lipschütz, A.   183, 185, *204*, *207*, 309, *338*, 448, *460*
Lipsett, M. B.   474, *492*
Lisboa, B. P.   21, 22
Lisk, R. D.   349, *382*
Little, B.   233, *240*
Little, K.   188, *207*
Little, V.   259, 265, 269, *273*
Littleton, P.   219, 222, 227, 233, 234, *239*, *240*
Liu, F. T. Y.   82, *207*
Livingston, N. B.   395, 408, 409, *456*, *460*
Lloyd, C. W.   426, *460*
Logothetopoulos, J.   83, 171, *207*
Löhr, G. M. v.   312, *332*
Longcope, C.   233, *238*
Loraine, J. A.   278, *300*, 392, 395, 396, 426, *453*, *460*
Lorentz, I. T.   447, *460*
Loskant, G.   246, *271*
Loudon, N. B.   435, *454*
Lubansky, J.   171, *206*, *207*
Lucas, F. V.   231, *240*, 420, *467*
Luchs, A.   45, *198*
Lucker, W. E.   220, *241*
Ludwig, A. E.   362, *377*
Ludwig, D. J.   352, *382*
Lukaszewska, J. H.   474, *492*
Lumbroso, P.   247, *272*
Lunenfeld, B.   281, *300*, 396, *460*
Lupo, C.   41, 48, 75, 79, 101, 105, 133, 134, 135, *207*, *208*, *212*
Lupu, C. I.   20, 21, *23*
Luraschi, C.   100, *207*
Luukkainen, T.   433, *455*
Lyle, J. S.   424, *463*
Lynch, K. M. Jr.   353, *382*
Lyon, R. A.   385, *460*
Lyon, R. P.   450, *461*
Lyons, H. A.   450, *460*
Lyster, S. C.   39, 79, 94, 95, 125, 157, 165, *199*, 374, 375, 376, *379*, *381*, 480, *491*

Maas, J. M.   405, 409, *456*
MacDonald, J.   309, *331*
Mach, S.   308, *338*
Madjerek, Z.   40, 41, 42, 46, 50, 52, 62, 78, 79, 92, 94, 95, 96, 98, 104, 106, 110, 115, 123, 124, 126, 151, 154, 155, 156, 171, *207*, *210*, 486, *492*
Maekawa, K.   107, *207*
Maguire, R.   423, *456*
Mahesh, V. B.   348, 375, *383*
Mainzer, K.   183, 184, *204*
Makepeace, A. W.   386, *460*
Malkani, P. K.   219, 230, *240*, 426, *459*
Mall-Haefeli, M.   415, *452*, *464*
Manalo-Estrella, P.   188, *198*, *207*, 439, *454*
Mandl, A. M.   63, 82, 135, 140, 167, 170, *204*
Maneschi, M.   296, *300*
Manion, W. C.   439, *458*
Mannhardt, H. J.   29, 31, *34*
Manning, J. P.   178, *207*
Maqueo, M.   79, 124, 135, 191, 201, *206*, *208*, 246, 249, *271*, 360, 361, *381*, 382, 395, 407, 408, 409, 418, 419, 423, *456*, *460*, *464*
Maqueo-Topete, M.   267, *272*, 387, 392, 394, 396, 411, 416, 432, *460*, *465*
Mardell, M.   441, *461*
Mardones, E.   183, *204*
Mares, S. E.   148, 149, *210*
Marescaux, J.   353, *382*
Margulis, R. R.   427, 428, 429, *460*, *461*, *468*
Markle, J.   312, *338*
Marlatt, P. E.   374, 375, *381*
Marois, G.   124, 125, 126, *208*
Marois, M.   46, 47, 94, 98, 106, 110, 116, 156, *208*
Marshall, L. L.   407, *462*
Marshall, S.   450, *461*
Marti, M.   431, *455*
Martin, A. P.   231, *240*
Martin, L.   103, 107, 108, *201*, 357, 364, 375, 376, *379*, *382*, 395, *461*
Martin, S. J.   348, *382*
Martinez-Manautou, J.   246, 249, 267, *271*, *272*, 287, *299*, 386, 387, 388, 389, 392, 393, 394, 396, 408, 411, 413, 419, 423, 432, *461*, 465
Masi, A. T.   436, 437, 447, *455*, *461*, *465*
Mason, B. A.   266, *272*
Mason, D. W.   266, *272*

Mason, M. M. 67, *211*, 368, *383*
Massara, F. 288, *298*
Mastboom, J. L. 305, *327*
Mathews, J. H. 325, 326, *338*
Matscher, R. 41, 48, 75, 79, 101, 105, 115, 133, 134, 135, 168, *208*, *212*
Matsner, E. M. 410, *468*
Matsumoto, S. 310, 314, 318, *335*, *338*, 395, 444, *461*
Matsuo, H. 72, *213*
Matsuoka, A. 444, *461*
Matsuyoshi, K. 221, 229, 237, *240*, *241*
Matthews, J. G. 407, *461*
Mattos, C. E. R. 296, *298*
Mäusle, E. 84, *198*
Mauvais-Jarvis, P. 290, *301*
Mayer, D. L. 249, *271*
Mayer, M. G. 8, *11*
Mazaheri, A. 232, *241*
Mazza, A. 290, *301*
McCarthy, J. D. 184, *208*
McCormack, C. E. 84, 85, 86, *208*
McCormick, W. 286, *298*
McCormick, W. G. 277, 286, *301*, 393, *461*
McDaniel, E. B. 416, *461*
McDonald, P. G. 72, *208*
McDonald, W. I. 447, *458*
McDougall, E. A. 41, 115, 126, 142, 166, 167, *202*
McGinty, D. A. 40, 42, 46, 79, 96, 114, 115, *208*, 353, *382*
McGregor, M. S. 426, *461*
McKelvey, H. A. 267, *270*
McKinney, G. R. 38, 39, 42, 108, 109, 160, 186, 192, *195*, *208*
McQuarrie, H. G. 409, *462*
Mears, E. 315, *338*, 392, 395, 396, 404, 406, 408, 421, 427, 444, *460*, *461*
Mehra, L. 405, *461*
Mehring, M. 118, *214*
Meier, P. 424, *468*
Meinsma, L. 305, *327*
Melamed, M. R. 448, *461*
Melampy, R. M. 474, *491*
Meli, A. 41, 63, 74, 96, 113, 115, 126, 142, 166, 167, *202*, *209*, 220, *241*
Mendel, E. B. 403, *462*
Menon, S. 296, *301*
Merkatz, I. R. 441, *466*
Merklin, R. J. 359, *382*
Merlo, J. G. 418, *465*

Merrill, A. 40, 42, 50, 52, 58, 61, 103, 104, *211*, 386, *463*
Merritt, R. I. 407, *462*
Messinger, A. 309, *341*
Mestman, J. H. 428, *462*
Metcalf, M. G. 427, *462*
Metz, H. 29, 31, *34*
Mey, R. 122, 123, 124, 126, *208*
Meyer, C. J. 288, *300*, 427, 428, 440, *460*
Meyer, E. W. 3, *10*
Meyer, R. K. 8, *10*, 56, 62, 74, 75, 77, 84, 85, 86, 117, 145, *195*, *196*, *208*, *210*, *212*, *214*, 348, 350, 357, 370, 374, *377*, *378*, *382*, *383*
Meyerson, B. J. 138, *208*
Michael, R. P. 138, 139, *209*, 348, *382*
Midgley, A. R. Jr. 278, *300*, 473, *492*
Migliavacca, A. 318, *339*
Mikulásková, J. 37, 38, 39, *146*
Miller, A. T. 420, 426, *455*
Millman, N. 134, 135, *194*
Mills, W. G. 308, *339*
Millson, D. R. 29, *34*, 106, 116, *198*
Mingeot, 247, 250, 260
Minkler, D. 450, *461*
Mintzer, A. J. 410, *462*
Miramontes, L. 25, *34*
Mischler, T. 41, 63, 74, 96, 113, 115, *209*
Mishell, D. R. 416, *462*
Mishler, E. G. 403, *468*
Mitchell, J. R. 439, *453*
Mitchell, J. R. A. *269*, 295, *297*
Mixon, T. 309, *339*
Miyake, T. 8, *11*, 39, 40, 41, 42, 50, 51, 52, 53, 69, 70, 74, 75, 116, *209*, 357, *382*
Mizoguchi, S. 232, *242*
Moggian, G. 41, *209*
Moghissi, K. S. 408, 423, *462*
Mohapatra, P. S. 405, *461*
Mohr, K. 187, *204*
Mohr, U. 186, *205*
Molinatti, G. M. 288, *298*
Moloshok, R. E. 128, 130, 131, *202*
Moloshok, R. E. C. 322, *333*
Mondcar, V. P. 447, *458*
Monroe, S. E. 373, 473, *492*
Montuori, E. 156, 157, *209*
Monzo, O. Z. 310, *339*
Moore, C. R. 348, 351, *382*
Morches, B. 316, *335*
Moreau, M. G. 123, 124, *204*
Moreau-Stinnakre, M. G. 124, 127, 156, *204*

Author Index

Morf, E. 415, *452*
Morishima, A. 325, 326, *338*
Morris, J. McL. 249, 250, *272*, 367, *382*, 391, *462*
Morris, N. 427, *462*
Moses, I. G. 404, 407, *462*
Moses, L. E. 315, *333*, 395, 404, 407, 408, 409, *456*, *462*
Moss, H. 408, *462*
Motta, M. 38, 114, 115, 162, 163, 164, *196*
Motteram, R. 434, 435, *467*
Moyer, D. L. 416, *462*
Mueller, M. N. 175, *211*
Mundy, V. 318, *333*
Muñoz, L. 416, *457*
Munshi, S. R. 135, *209*
Münstermann, A. M. 319, *345*
Murakami, A. 232, *242*
Murata, S. 219, 227, 229, 232, 233, *241*
Murawski, B. J. 446, *462*
Murphy, E. D. 186, *209*
Murray, E. G. 308, *339*
Murray, J. 290, *298*
Musa, B. U. 441, *462*

Nadler, R. D. 73, 76, *201*
Nagra, C. L. 108, 113, 142, 165, *200*
Nair, R. M. G. 72, *213*
Nakamura, Y. 389, 395, *456*
Nalbandov, A. V. 360, *384*
Napp, J. H. 130, 186, *213*, *215*, 312, *339*
Neill, J. D. 473, 474, *492*
Nelson, D. H. 428, *462*
Nelson, W. O. 349, 353, 372, 374, *380*, *382*, *383*
Neri, R. 121, *209*
Nermark, J. 434, *467*
Netter, A. 247, *272*, 283, *301*
Neumann, F. 7, *11*, 40, 42, 44, 49, 62, 74, 75, 79, 99, 101, 103, 104, 106, 110, 111, 114, 115, 117, 118, 119, 122, 123, 125, 126, 127, 136, 160, *197*, *198*, *203*, *204*, *209*, *210*, *212*, *214*, *215*
Nevinny-Stickel, J. 14, 17, *23*, *56*, 210, 246, 248, 251, *272*, 277, 282, *301*, 309, *339*, 391, 392, *462*
Newland, D. O. 407, 410, *462*
Newton, M. A. 440, *459*, *462*
Nicholls, R. A. 478, *492*
Nicholson, R. 431, 433, *455*, *463*
Nicolas, A. 308, *333*

Nicolas, R. 426, 443, *463*
Nieschlag, E. 283, 289, 296, *299*
Nieuweboer, B. 219, 227, 228, 229, 234, *239*
Nilsson, Å. 444, 447, *462*
Nishimura, T. 224, *241*
Nishino, Y. 111, *210*
Niswender, G. G. 473, *492*
Noble, R. L. 348, 349, 357, *382*
Nocke, L. 391, 395, *454*
Nocke, W. 227, 228, *238*, 259, 270, 391 395, *454*
Nolan, R. B. 128, 131, *203*
Norris, H. J. 423, *467*
Novak, E. R. 309, *339*
Noyes, R. W. 353, *382*
Nutting, E. F. 8, *11*, 41, 45, 48, 56, 57, 104, 107, 109, 148, 159, *200*, *210*, 357, *382*

Ober, K. G. 16, 17, 18, 21, *23*, 304, 310, 311, 312, 317, *339*, *340*, *345*
Ober, W. B. 249, *272*, 419, *464*
Ockner, R. K. 434, *462*
Oddie, T. H. 428, *455*
Odell, W. D. 276, *301*
Oettlé, A. G. 306, *344*
Ogawa, Y. 358, *382*
Ogilvie, M. L. 221, *241*
Okada, H. 220, 221, 224, 227, 228, 232, 233, 235, 237, *241*, 259, *272*
O'Leary, J. A. 441, *462*
Oliver, J. T. 162, *211*
Oliveto, E. P. 230, *242*
Olivieri, V. 296, *297*
Olivo, J. 290, 291, 295, *299*
Olson, H. J. 404, 406, *468*
O'Malley, B. W. 472, *492*
Onetto, E. 416, *457*
Orentreich, N. A. 442, *462*
Orino, K. 229, 232, *241*, *242*
Oriol, A. 135, 191, *201*, 360, 361, *381*
Oroján, I. 79, *212*
Orojan, J. 324, *342*
Orr, A. H. 393, 395, 415, *462*
Örstrom, Å. 349, *378*
Østergaard, E. 246, 257, 265, *272*, 280, *301*, 393, 395, *466*
Ota, S. 232, *241*
Overbeek, G. A. 40, 41, 46, 50, 52, 62, 66, 74, 79, 92, 94, 95, 96, 104, 106, 110, 114, 115, 122, 123, 124, 126, 151, 154, 155, 156, 171, *207*, *210*, 486, *492*

Overzier, C. 283, 289, 296, *299*

Paesi, F. J. A. 81, *210*, *211*
Pagani, C. 248, *270*, 283, *299*
Page, D. 294, 296, *302*
Palmer, K. H. 227, 229, 230, *241*
Palmer, R. 309, *340*
Palmer, R. H. 175, *211*
Panasevich, V. I. 185, *207*
Pande, J. K. 134, 137, 180, *212*
Paniagua, M. 219, 230, *241*, 426, 428, 443, *458*, *463*
Panosevich, V. 448, *460*
Papanicolaou, G. N. 267, *273*
Papatheodorou, B. 80, *197*
Papworth, R. A. 315, *329*
Pardanani, N. S. 408, *454*
Parker, A. S. Jr. 315, *340*
Parkes, A. S. 357, *382*
Parkinson, R. W. 409, *462*
Parlow, A. F. 8, *11*, 416, *462*
Parrott, F. M. 410, *468*
Paschen, H. W. 18, *23*
Pasteels, J. L. 83, *199*, *211*
Patanelli, D. J. 353, *383*
Paulsen, C. A. 227, *241*
Payne, H. 389, *458*
Peacock, J. F. 444, *459*
Pean, V. 426, 443, *463*
Pearl, R. 397, *463*
Pegrassi, L. 92, *215*
Pelissier, C. 247, *272*, 283, *301*
Pencharz, R. I. 350, *383*
Pendleton, A. 426, 443, *463*
Perez, V. 433, *463*
Perez Ruelas, J. 29, *34*
Perez-Vega, E. 249, *271*
Perrine, J. W. 67, *197*
Persson, B. H. 441, *452*
Peterkin, G. A. 442, *463*
Petersen, P. 444, *463*
Peterson, D. L. 4, 9, *10*, 38, 39, 40, 42, 47, 48, 58, 78, 94, 96, 99, 104, 106, 107, 108, 109, 111, 113, 114, 115, 116, 126, 134, 135, 137, 166, 200, *211*, 365, 366, *383*
Peterson, W. F. 246, *271*, 430, *463*
Peterson Clancy, D. 107, 142, 152, 157, 165, *200*, *211*
Petrov, V. 29, 31, *34*, 132, *211*, 223, *241*
Petry, R. 295, *301*

Pfeiffer, C. A. 448, *456*
Picard, F. 106, 110, *197*
Pincus, G. 39, 40, 41, 42, 44, 50, 52, 58, 60, 61, 66, 67, 70, 103, 104, 133, *201*, *209*, *211*, 219, 227, 230, 231, *238*, *240*, *241*, 249, *272*, 288, *300*, 318, *341*, 353, 354, 355, 357, 358, 368, 373, 375, *377*, *378*, *381*, *382*, *383*, 386, 395, 404, 408, 417, 425, 426, 427, 428, 439, 440, 443, *455*, *456*, *458*, *460*, *462*, *463*, *464*, *468*
Piukovich, I. 158, *204*
Planck, S. 18, *24*
Plate, W. P. 418, *463*
Platt, W. R. 296, *302*
Plotz, E. J. 20, 21, *23*, 321, *331*
Plotz, J. 304, 320, *340*
Plummer, J. M. 38, 39, 42, 60, 94, 95, 106, 109, 116, 125, 126, 157, 171, *198*
Pochi, P. E. 442, *467*
Poel, W. E. 187, *211*
Poggi, G. 101, *207*
Polenz, B. 309, *340*
Poller, L. 296, *301*
Popper, A. 27, *34*
Porges, R. F. 437, *453*
Porter, P. S. 424, *463*
Possanza, G. 228, *242*
Possanza, G. J. 162, *211*
Post, R. C. 439, *453*
Pots, G. O. 353, *377*
Pots, P. 18, 19, *23*, 247, *272*, 303, 311, *340*, *345*
Potter, R. G. 403, *463*, *468*
Potts, D. M. 490, *492*
Powell, J. E. 473, *492*
Powell, L. W. 292, *301*
Prates, H. 296, *298*
Preedy, J. R. K. 441, *463*
Présl, J. 312, *334*, 361, *383*
Preucel, R. W. 316, *342*
Price, D. 351, 348, *382*
Priedkalns, J. 177, *211*
Priest, C. M. 296, *301*
Prill, H. J. 312, *340*
Pryse-Davies, J. 446, *457*
Pschyrembel, W. 309, 318, *340*
Psychoyos, A. 357, *383*
Puchulu, F. 431, *455*
Puck, A. 309, *340*
Puddy, E. M. 408, *463*
Pujohl, J. M. 310, *341*
Pulkkinen, M. O. 434, 441, *463*

Pullen, D.   315, *341*
Pulliam, A. L.   223, *242*, 251, *273*
Pupkin, M.   416, *463*
Purandare, B. N.   408, *454*
Purshottam, N.   67, *211*, 368, *383*
Purves, H. D.   82, 83, *211*

Quartararo, P.   296, *300*
Quincy, R. V.   237, *241*

Rabau, E.   281, *300*, 396, *460*
Raffelt, E.   40, 42, *203*
Rajan, R.   409, *453*
Rakoff, A. E.   423, *457*
Ramella, J. E.   309, *339*
Ramirez, F. T.   352, *380*
Ramirez, V. D.   111, *211*
Rand, J.   290, *299*
Rankin, J.   423, *457*
Rannie, G. H.   296, *301*
Rapcsák, V.   79, *212*, 324, *342*
Raspé, G.   7, *11*
Rassaert, C. L.   41, 115, 126, 142, 166, 167, *202*
Rauscher, H.   18, 19, *24*, 96, 110, 114, 115, *213*, 284, *301*, 312, 313, 317, 319, *341*
Rausch-Stroomann, J. G.   295, *301*
Rayford, P. C.   325, 326, *341*
Redding, T. W.   72, *213*
Reerink, E. H.   33, *34*
Rees, R. W. A.   234, *239*
Reeves, J. J.   279, *302*
Refersburg, W.   431, 432, *466*
Reid, D. E.   395, 418, 424, *465*
Reifenstein, E. C.   321, *341*
Reiffenstuhl, G.   281, *301*, 318, *334*
Reisert, P.   441, *469*
Renard, M. P.   176, *198*
Resch, B.   65, 142, *212*
Resnik, S.   442, *464*
Revesz, C.   4, 5, 9, 10, *11*, 38, 39, 45, 47, 48, 50, 63, 66, 75, 95, 114, 116, 119, 125, 134, *197*, *211*
Rhodes, L. S.   227, 229, *241*
Ricaud, L.   423, *456*
Rice-Wray, E.   249, *271*, *272*, 404, 406, 407, 408, 409, 419, 427, 442, *456*, *464*
Richards, M. P. M.   88, *212*
Richardson, S. L.   79, 161, 165, 182, 183, *202*, 324, *333*

Richter, K.   309, 341
Richter, R. H. H.   156, *212*, 415, *452*, *464*
Riddle, O.   363, *383*
Riegel, B.   41, 47, 48, *199*
Rifkind, A. B.   325, 326, *341*, 441, *466*
Riisfeldt, O.   310, *341*
Ringler, I.   191, *212*
Ringold, H. J.   26, 27, 29, *34*, 108, 109, *199*
Ringrose, C.   407, *464*
Ringrose, C. A. D.   446, *464*
Riva, H. L.   309, *341*
Robey, M.   312, *341*
Robin, M.   431, *455*
Rock, J.   249, *272*, 318, *341*, 386, 395, 426, 443, *463*, *464*
Rodgers, L. D.   407, *462*
Rodriguez, R.   84, *202*
Rogers, A. W.   179, *212*
Rohrbach, C.   268, *270*
Rojar, B.   393, 411, 413, 419, 423, *461*
Roland, M.   249, 266, *272*, 286, *301*, 321, *341*, 419, *464*
Roman, W.   433, *464*
Romberg, G.   312, *341*
Rongone, E. L.   237, *242*
Root, C. A.   374, *380*
Rorig, K.   373, 375, *383*
Rosati, P.   353, *379*
Rose, F. D.   315, *333*
Rosemberg, E.   391, 395, *464*
Rosenberg, D.   416, *463*
Rosenkranz, G.   25, 26, *34*
Rosenthal, A.   408, *462*
Rosenthal, E.   424, *468*
Ross, F. T.   227, 229, *241*
Ross, G. T.   325, 326, *341*, 474, *492*
Roth, F.   415, *452*, *464*
Rothermich, N. O.   267, *272*
Roussel,   41, 91, 105, 135, *212*
Routier, G.   295, *301*
Rovinsky, J. J.   407, 408, 410, *464*
Rowson, L. E.   355, *380*
Roy, S.   348, 375, *383*
Rozin, S.   410, *464*
Rubio, B. L.   416, 417, *464*
Rudel, H.   249, *271*
Rudel, H. W.   40, 41, 42, 62, 63, 65, 67, 68, 70, 192, *205*, *206*, *212*, 267, *272*, 351, 352, 354, 355, 359, 360, 368, 370, 371, *383*, 386, 387, 388, 389, 392, 393, 394, 396, 408, 411, 413, 415, 425, 432, 443, *452*, *461*, *465*

Rudel, W. H.   393, 411, 413, 419, 423, *461*
Ruggieri, P. de   41, 48, 75, 79, 105, 115, 133, 134, 135, *212*
Ruiz Gijon, J.   41, *212*
Rummel, H. R.   308, *343*
Rumney, G.   324, *343*
Russel, T. J.   178, *207*
Russfield, A. B.   186, *196*
Rust, W.   310, *341*
Rutherford, R. N.   415, 427, *453*, *465*
Ryan, G. M.   395, 418, 424, *465*
Ryan, G. M. Jr.   446, *462*
Rybo, G.   282, *300*, 441, *454*
Ryder, N. B.   415, *468*

Saad el Din, J.   297, *297*
Sabe, F.   4, *10*
Sacks, M.   410, *464*
Sager, D. B.   77, *212*
Sagi, P. C.   403, *468*
Saha, N. N.   229, 230, 232, *242*
Saito, M.   76, *213*
Sakinen, F. M.   136, *214*
Sala, G.   21, *22*, 47, 50, 135, 142, *212*, 223, *239*, 290, *298*
Salhanick, H. A.   46, *212*, 417, *465*
Salinas, S.   185, *207*, 448, *460*
Salloch, R. R.   136, *212*
Salmon, M. L.   447, *465*
Salzberger, M.   410, *464*
Sanchez-Rivera, G.   418, *465*
Sandberg, A. A.   22, *24*, 219, 222, *242*
Sanders, J. H.   434, *458*
Sanderson, C.   429, *456*
Santano, A. R.   296, *298*
Santi, F.   292, *302*
Sanwal, P. C.   134, 137, 180, *212*
Sanyal, R. K.   100, *199*
Sapir, P. E.   446, *462*
Sartwell, P. E.   436, *465*
Sas, M.   65, 79, 142, *212*, 323, 324, *342*, *343*
Sato, I.   444, *461*
Satterthwaite, A. P.   406, 408, 427, 428, 442, *465*
Saunders, F. J.   42, 44, 46, 47, 48, 69, 70, 79, 81, 90, 91, 93, 104, 133, 135, 137, 140, 141, 151, 156, 160, *199*, *212*, *213*, 349, 363, 364, 365, 373, 375, *383*
Sawyer, C. H.   65, 71, 88, 89, 111, 185, *203*, *205*, *211*, *213*, 349, *378*, *381*

Sawyer, M. J.   162, *211*
Scaramuzzi, R. J.   139, *207*
Scarpellini, L.   245, *271*
Schabel, F. M. Jr.   184, *202*
Schack, S. L.   430, 431, 441, *466*
Schally, A. V.   71, 72, 76, *213*, 279, *302*
Schardein, J. L.   171, *213*
Schenk, M.   27, *34*
Schenker, L.   439, *453*
Scherb, J.   433, *465*
Schermund, H. J.   186, *213*
Schild, W.   18, *23*
Schlegelmilch, H.   406, *465*
Schlikker, E.   247, 248, 249, 250, 260, *271*
Schlösser, W.   312, *342*
Schlough, J. S.   374, *383*
Schmidt, F. L.   7, *10*, 39, 60, *195*
Schmidt Elmendorff, H.   278, *302*, 391, 392, *465*
Schmidt Matthiesen, H.   306, 312, *342*
Schneider, W.   96, 110, 114, 115, *213*, 284, *301*
Schneller, O.   282, *299*
Schoeller, W.   349, *383*
Schoen, E. J.   325, 326, *342*
Schofield, B. M.   99, *213*, 363, *383*
Schöler, H. F. L.   10, *11*, 41, 94, 97, 123, 124, 125, 126, *213*
Schreibman, P. H.   294, *302*
Schuetz, A. W.   77, *212*
Schulz-Contreras, M.   419, 427, 442, *456*, *464*
Schwartz, E.   178, *207*
Schwartz, H. A.   311, *342*, 407, *458*
Schwarz, F.   306, *344*
Sciaky, R.   223, *242*
Scott, R. B.   152, 156, *216*, 309, *342*
Scrascia, E.   62, 63, 66, 67, 74, 75, *214*
Seahle,   310, *327*
Seal, U. S.   292, 293, *297*, 441, *462*
Sealy, J. E.   440, *459*, *462*
Sebok, L.   257, 259, 265, *273*
Seda, M.   37, 38, 39, *196*
Sedlis, A.   420, *454*
Sefgar, G.   311, *342*
Segal, P. B.   424, *468*
Segal, S. J.   372, 374, *383*
Segaloff, A.   114, *213*, 237, *242*
Segre, E. J.   289, *299*, 427, *455*
Seidl, J. E.   19, *24*
Sele, V.   428, *466*
Selenkow, H. A.   428, *457*
Self, L. W.   171, *214*

Selye, H. 350, 351, *383*
Semm, K. 319, 322, 323, *331*, *342*, *344*, 425, *465*
Seng, P. 431, 432, *466*
Senge, Th. 295, *301*
Setty, B. S. 134, 137, 180, 191, *205*, *212*,
Shah, P. N. 410, *466*
Shapiro, E. L. 230, *242*
Sharma, B. B. 83, 171, *207*
Sharma, B. B. L. 405, *461*
Shearman, R. P. 320, *342*, 426, *466*
Shelley, W. B. 316, *342*
Sherrat, R. M. 76, *203*
Shipley, E. G. 7, 8, *11*, 49, 50, 54, 55, 60, 61, 62, 74, 75, 117, 189, 190, *214*, 351, *384*
Shipley, G. C. 357, 363, *379*
Shokeir, M. 434, *466*
Shorr, E. 267, *273*
Shraders, S. 234, *239*
Shulman, N. 446, *462*
Sichuk, G. 167, 187, 188, *214*
Sickles, J. S. 87, *206*, 361, 362, 363, *381*
Siegmann, C. M. 28, *34*
Silverman, J. F. 450, *459*
Simpson, M. E. 349, *379*
Skipper, H. E. 184, *202*
Skov Jensen, T. 306, *343*
Slaunwhite, W. R. 22, *24*, 219, *222*, *242*
Slutsky, H. 407, *452*
Smith, B. D. 69, 70, *214*
Smith, D. L. 223, *242*, 251, *273*
Smith, D. W. 324, *338*
Smith, H. 25, *33*, 48, 78, 108, 113, 114, *200*, 234, *239*
Smith, H. E. 436, *465*
Smith, J. C. 360, *384*
Smith, L. 407, *458*
Smith, M. G. 357, *384*
Smith, R. A. 395, *452*
Smith, R. E. 180, *214*
Snaith, L. 309, *343*
Sneddon, A. 233, *242*
Snijder, F. F. 145, *216*
Soberon, J. 416, *460*
Sobrero, A. J. 408, *466*
Soderwall, A. L. 136, *214*
Soiva, K. 309, *343*
Sollman, P. B. 8, *11*, 57, *210*
Solomkin, M. 426, *458*
Sommerville, I. F. 280, *298*
Sondheimer, F. 25, 26, 27, *34*
Song, C. S. 441, *466*

Sonnino, F. F. 101, *202*
Soost, H. J. 449, *466*
Southren, A. L. 290, 291, 295, *299*
Spain, W. T. 389, *458*
Sparks, S. J. 473, *492*
Spazzoli, G. 41, 48, 75, 79, 105, 133, 134, 135, *212*
Spellacy, W. N. 429, 430, 431, 432, 441, *462*, *466*
Spencer, J. 353, *384*
Spiegel, E. 89, *214*
Spoont, St. S. 316, *342*
Staemmler, H. J. 18, *24*, 310, 313, 318, *343*, 396, *466*
Stamm, H. 415, *452*
Stamm, O. 275, 283, *302*
Staples, R. E. 374, *384*
Starkey, W. F. 352, *384*
Starup, J. 280, *301*, 393, 395, 417, 428, 430, 439, *452*, *466*
Stecher, K. H. 316, *335*
Steel, M. W. 430, *463*
Steeno, O. 289, *298*
Stegner, H. E. 147, *214*
Stein, M. 450, *466*
Steinbeck, H. 177, 118, 119, 122, 127, *198*, *209*, *210*, *214*
Steinberger, E. 359, *384*
Steinetz, B. G. 41, 115, 126, 142, 161, 162, 166, 167, *202*, *214*, 220, *241*, 360, *381*
Stempfel, R. S. 322, *344*
Stempfel, R. S. Jr. 128, 129, 130, 131, *216*
Šterba, R. 278, *302*, 406, 409, 421, *467*
Stern, E. 449, *467*
Stevens, V. C. 217, 218, 226, 232, *238*, 389, 391, 392, 393, 420, 426, *455*, *467*, *468*, 473, *492*
Stevensen, J. R. 450, *468*
Stevenson, R. H. 78, 105, 108, 116, 120. *196*
Stimmel, B. F. 267, *273*
Stitt, S. L. 92, *214*
Stitt, W. D. 407, *454*
Stoll, B. A. 434, 435, *467*
Stoll, P. 308, *343*
Stolte, L. A. M. 278, 285, *299*, *302*
Stone, G. M. 357, *384*
Stone, M. L. 420, *454*
Stone, R. A. 409, *462*
Strade, H. A. 407, 421, 422, 445, *467*
Strauss, A. F. 307, *327*

Strauss, A. J.   113, *215*
Strauss, J. S.   442, *467*
Streit-Pfenniger, M.   415, *464*
Strenram, U.   434, *459*
Strott, C. A.   474, *492*
Strube, R.   84, *198*
Stucki, J.   93, 94, 95, 96, 97, *214*, 375, *379*
Stucki, J. C.   29, *33*
Sturgis, S. H.   385, 428, 446, *457*, *462*, *467*
Sturtevant, F. M.   405, 409, *467*
Suchowsky, G.   6, 10, *11*
Suchowsky, G. K.   42, 62, 63, 66, 67, 74, 75, 92, 94, 95, 122, 123, 124, 125, 126, 127, 184, *214*, *215*
Sulimovici, S.   281, *300*, 396, *460*
Sulman, F. G.   45, *215*
Sumi, M.   220, 235, *241*
Sundaram, K.   191, *195*
Suntzeff, V.   448, *453*
Suran, R. R.   410, *467*
Surti, N. R.   324, *343*
Swanson, J.   46, *212*
Swelheim, T.   348, 351, *384*
Swerdloff, R. S.   276, *301*
Swyer, G. I. M.   257, 259, 265, 269, *273*, 281, *302*, 490, *492*
Syhora, K.   29, *34*, 37, 38, 39, *196*
Symmons, C.   441, *461*
Szeberényi, S.   161, 162, *201*
Szereday, Z.   323, *343*
Szontagh, F. E.   62, 80, 142, 158, 187, *204*, *212*, *215*, 323, *343*
Szóny, I.   186, *215*
Szpilfogel, S. A.   28, *34*

Tabachnik, I. A.   141, *216*
Taber, B. Z.   404, 407, 408, *455*, *457*
Tabiowa, A.   296, *301*
Taft, P.   294, 296, *302*
Tagi, A.   408, 410, 442, *458*
Tagui, A.   297, *297*, *300*
Tait, J. F.   233, *238*, *240*
Tait, S. A. S.   233, *240*
Takasugi, N.   359, 360, *384*
Take, H.   221, *241*
Take, K.   232, *241*
Takewaki, K.   361, *381*
Talaat, M.   297, *297*, *300*
Talas, M.   416, *462*
Tange, M.   362, *383*
Tatum, H.   296, *298*
Tatum, H. J.   413, 415, *452*

Taubert, H. D.   57, *215*, 276, *302*
Tausk, M.   45, 123, *198*, *215*, 435, *467*
Tavolga, M. C.   362, *384*
Taylor, H. B.   423, 439, *458*, *467*
Taylor, K.   294, 296, *302*, 429, *469*
Taylor, R. J.   45, *204*
Taymor, J. L.   392, *467*
Taymor, M. L.   18, *24*, 393, 395, *467*, 474, *492*
Telford, J. M.   143, 153, *205*
Ten Berge, B. S.   439, *467*
Tenhaeff, D.   295, *301*
Terragno, A.   154, *215*
Terragno, N.   154, *215*
Thamdrup, E.   324, *343*
Thijssen, J. H. H.   219, 235, *242*
Thoma, R. W.   4, *11*
Thomas, H. H.   18, *24*, 309, 311, *343*
Thomas, J. A.   113, 174, *215*
Thomas, L. B.   247, *271*
Thompson, C. R.   372, *382*
Thompson, D. L.   350, 351, *383*
Thomsen, K.   130, *215*, 319, *344*
Thomson, J. M.   296, *301*
Thorell, J.   293, *300*, 441, *460*
Thulin, K. E.   434, *467*
Tietze, C.   395, 403, 408, 409, *456*, *467*
Tillinger, K. G.   220, 221, *239*, 246, *273*, 278, 282, *297*, *298*, 393, 396, 415, 417, *454*, *458*
Tochimoto, S.   290, *299*
Tokuda, G.   162, 162, 165, *215*, 227, 228, 232, 233, 237, *241*, *242*, 259, *272*
Tolksdorf, S.   42, 63, 141, *216*, 365, 366, *384*
Tomic, M.   448, *457*
Tonkers, E.   305, *327*
Tornaben, J. A.   178, *207*
Torralra, Y.   183, 184. *204*
Tóth, F.   171, 172, 186, *215*
Townsend, J. F.   420, *467*
Townsley, J. D.   228, *242*
Traub, A.   323, *343*
Treger, A.   180, *203*
Trentin, J. J.   448, *456*
Trmal, Th.   78, 105, 108, 116, 120, *196*
Tronconi, G.   292, 296, *302*
Troop, R. C.   162, *211*
Tsuyuguchi, M.   41, 94, 106, *206*
Tucker, J. S.   410, *468*
Tucker, M. J.   170, 174, 175, *215*
Tullner, W.   40, 42, 178, *203*, *215*
Turkheimer, A. R.   6, 7, *11*, 376, *382*

Turner, C. W. 158, 159, *202*
Turolla, E. 123, 124, 125, 126, 127, 179, *215*
Turpeinen, K. 404, 407, 445, *467*
Tyler, E. T. 317, 320, *344*, 404, 405, 406, 407, 410, 416, 433, 444, *452*, *467*, *468*
Tyson, J. E. A. 440, *468*

Ufer, J. 309, 318, *344*
Uhlarik, S. 62, 80, 166, *215*
Ullery, J. C. 217, 218, 219, 222, 223, 226, 232, *238*, 389, 392, *468*
Ulrych, J. 406, *467*
Ungar, F. 217, *239*
Unger, R. 284, *299*
Upton, R. D. 309, *344*
Ustay, K. 286, *299*, 411, *457*

Vaidya, R. 408, *454*
Vaishwanar, P. S. 288, *300*, 427, 428, 440, *460*
Vallance, D. K. 59, 62, 66, 142, 143, 144, *195*, *196*, 223, 224, *239*
Valová, B. 278, *302*, 406, *467*
Van de Lely, M. A. 316, *331*
Van den Driessche, J. 41, 63, 74, 106, 115, *199*
Van den Noort, S. 447, *456*
Van der Molen, H. J. 219, 232, 233, *242*, 426, *468*
Van der Vies, J. 41, 46, 49, 50, 52, 53, 79, 94, 95, 96, 97, 106, 110, 113, 115, 123, 124, 126, 156, 163, 166, 168, 171, *198*, *207*, *216*, 486, *492*
Van de Wiele, R. 417, *465*
Van Kessel, H. 278, *302*
Van Leusden, H. A. 266, *273*, 415, *468*
Van Rees, G. P. 81, *211*
Van Wagenen, G. 249, 250, *272*, 367, *382*, 391, *462*
Varga, L. 187, *215*
Velardo, J. T. 5, 6, 9, *11*, 88, 105, *216*
Velasquez, J. 393, 411, 419, 423, *461*
Vermeulen, A. 289, *302*
Vessey, M. P. 435, 436, *455*, *458*
Vickery, B. H. 59, 62, 66, 142, 143, 144, 148, 155, *195*, *196*, *216*
Vignolo, W. H. 84, *202*
Vinegra, M. 42, 63, 141, *216*, 365, 366, *384*
Viski, S. 62, 80, *215*

Voigt, K. 284, *301*
Voigt, K. D. 431, 432, *466*
Voigt, K. H. 73, *198*, *199*
Vokaer, R. 246, *273*
Volk, H. 309, *332*
Vollings, R. 442, *468*
Von Berswordt-Wallrabe, R. 69, 70, 81, 118, 119, 122, *206*, *209*, *210*
Vorbeck, M. L. 231, *240*
Vorys, N. 217, 218, 219, 222, 223, 226, 232, *238*, 389, 391, 392, 393, 420, 426, *455*, *467*, *468*

Waidl, E. 249, *273*, 294, *299*, 322, *344*, 419, *468*
Wait, R. B. 405, 409, *467*
Waite, J. H. 247, *271*
Wakeling, A. 135, 136, *216*
Wall, M. E. 227, 229, 230, *241*
Wallace, C. 353, *384*
Wallach, E. D. 427, *468*
Waller, I. R. 3, *10*
Walser, H. C. 428, *468*
Walther, R. A. 296, *302*
Walton, A. 353, *382*
Wamsteker, E. F. 411, *468*
Wan, L. S. 409, *453*
Wang, D. Y. 233, *242*
Ward, C. J. 189, *216*
Ward, G. W. 450, *468*
Warnock, D. G. 393, *453*
Warren, J. C. 431, *454*
Warren, R. K. 434, 441, *454*
Watanabe, H. 229, 230, 232, *242*
Watanabe, M. 310, 314, *338*
Waterhouse, B. 29, *34*
Waters, H. W. 315, *344*
Watnick, A. S. 42, 63, 141, *216*, 365, 366, *384*
Watts, G. F. 418, *455*
Way, F. 407, *462*
Webb, W. K. 186, *208*
Webber, R. L. 407, *462*
Weber, M. 17, 21, *23*, 304, 311, *340*
Webster, H. D. 39, 79, 94, 95, 125, 157, 165, *199*, 480, *491*
Weichert, C. K. 357, *384*
Weifenbach, H. 78, *216*
Weightman, D. 296, *301*
Weikel, J. H. 160, 186, *208*
Weikel, J. H. Jr. 171, *216*
Weinstein, G. L. 386, *460*

Weir, R. J.   441, *458*
Weis, P.   415, *452*
Weisburger, E. K.   184, *216*
Weisburger, J. H.   184, *216*
Weissman, G.   181, *216*
Wellers, H.   306, *342*
Wells, M.   393, 395, *453*
Wenner, R.   154, *201*
Werder, F. V.   29, 31, *34*
Werle, E.   322, *344*
Wesselius-de Casparis, A.   278, *302*
West, E. C.   444, *468*
West, J.   444, *468*
Westerhof, P.   33, *34*
Westerholm, B.   436, *458*
Westman, A.   348, 349, *377*, *378*, *384*
Westoff, C. F.   403, 405, *468*
Wharton, L. R.   152, 156, *216*, 309, *342*
Whedon, G. D.   433, *457*
Wheeler, A. G.   171, *216*
Wheeler, M.   237, *239*
White, W. F.   279, *302*
Whitelaw, M. J.   420, *468*
Whitney, R.   353, 354, *378*, *384*
Whitty, C. W. M.   444, *468*
Whitty, M. M.   444, *468*
Wide, L.   278, 279, 282, 283, *298*, *300*, 392, 393, 395, 415, *454*, *459*, *468*
Wied, G. L.   4, *10*, 13, 14, 15, 17, *23*, *24*, 245, 246, 247, 250, 258, *270*, *273*, 303, *331*, 424, *468*
Wiedhaup, K.   219, 232, 233, *242*
Wiendl, H. J.   322, *342*
Wiest, W. G.   97, *197*, 310, *345*, 475, *492*
Wijmenga, H. G.   219, 232, 233, *242*, 426, *468*
Wilbert, L.   441, *469*
Wilcox, W. S.   184, *202*
Wilkins, L.   128, 129, 130, 131, *216*, 322, 324, *344*, 450, *469*
Willems, J. L.   101, *216*
Williams, B. F. P.   309, *344*
Williams, K. I. H.   219, 230, *241*, 426, *463*
Williams, P. C.   109, *207*
Williams, R.   158, 159, *202*
Williamson, D. M.   29, 31, *34*
Williamson, P. J.   418, *455*
Willman, K.   434, 441, *463*
Wilson, A. T.   435, *454*
Wilson, F.   407, *469*
Wilson, G.   227, 232, 233, 234, *239*, 240

Wilson, H.   309, *341*
Wilson, J. G.   359, *384*
Windbichler, H.   276, *298*
Winikoff, D.   294, 296, *302*, 429, *469*
Winkelman, J. Z.   447, *465*
Winter, G. F.   303, *345*
Wislocki, G. B.   145, *216*
Wolf, R. C.   352, *381*
Wolff, A.   220, *241*
Wood, E. J.   439, *456*
Woosley, E. T.   171, *213*
Wright, J. B.   375, *379*
Wright, St. W.   280, *302*, 309, *345*
Wu, D. H.   46, 54, 91, 93, *194*, *216*, 269
Wycis, H.   89, *214*
Wynn, V.   430, 431, 432, *455*, *469*
Wyss, H.   415, *452*

Yaffee, H. S.   424, *469*
Yamamoto, H.   220, 232, 233, *241*, 242
Yanagimachi, R.   355
Yaneva, H.   247, *272*, 283, *301*
Yiacas, E.   4, 5, 6, 7, 9, 10, *11*, 125, 126, 207
Yoshimi, T.   474, *492*
Younis, N.   297, *297*, *300*, 408, 410, 442, *458*
Yussman, M. A.   474, *492*
Yzerman, G. L.   404, 407, 421, 445, *455*, *459*

Zackler, J.   407, *452*
Zanartu, J.   416, *463*, *469*
Zander, J.   14, *24*, 310, 319, 320, 321, *345*
Zanotti, D. B.   159, 167, 170, 189, *195*, 205
Zapati, A. C.   74, *195*
Zarrow, M. X.   5, *11*, 40, 42, 50, 52, 58, 61, 86, 87, 99, 103, 104, *202*, *211*, *216*, 386, *463*, 474, *491*
Zatrman, E. R.   416, *469*
Zderic, J. A.   25, *34*
Zelenik, J. S.   416, *461*
Zichella, L.   101, *202*
Zilva, J. F.   441, *461*
Zimprich, H.   325, *345*
Zorrilla, E.   432, *469*
Zorn, H.   312, *345*
Zussman, W. V.   418, *469*

SUBJECT INDEX

Abortion, hormonal treatment 319
Absorption, progestogens 189, 190, 251
Acetoxy progesterone, feminization of fetuses 129
3-Acetoxy-6,7,-dichloroestra-1,3,5(10)-triene-17-one, antifertility activity of 366
17α-Acetoxy-21-fluoro-6α-methyl progesterone, delaying nidation 56
3β-Acetoxy-16-methyl pregna-5,16-diene-20-one, steroid synthesis 30, 31
17α-Acetoxy-4,1,19nor-pregnadiene-3,20-dione
  effect on endometrium 253
  progestational effects 253, 261
17α-Acetoxy-19-nor progesterone, effect on ovary 418
17α-Acetoxy-progesterone (17α-Acetoxy pregn-4-ene-3,20-dione)
  antiestrogenic effect 9
  compounds related to 29 ff.
  effect
    on human endometrium 252, 258, 259
    on uterine contractility 101
  feminizing effect 129
  progestational activity 258
  with mestranol in sequential therapy 410
6α-Acetoxy-progesterone acetate, anticonvulsant effect 89
17α-Acetoxy-progesterone-cyclopentyl-enol-ether
  maintenance of pregnancy 46
  postponing menstruation 259
Acetylcholine
  oviduct contraction 154
  uterine contraction 100
Acne
  and oral contraceptives 442
  effect of progesterone on 316

ACTH
  effects of MAP on 83, 160
  effects of oral contraceptives on 428
ACTH response, effects of steroids on 289
Adrenal
  effect of contraceptive drugs on 427
  effect of MAP on 326
  effect of progestational compounds on 160 ff, 288
  effect of oral contraceptives 427
Aldosterone action, effect of progesterone on 293
Aldosterone excretion, effect of MAP on 290
Aldosterone levels, effect of oral contraceptives on 440
Allen–Corner test, progestational compounds in 45, 46
17α-Alkyl-19-norprogestogens, effect on BSP 433
4-Allyl-estradiol, antifertility effect of 366
Allylestrenol (17α-allylestrenol-4en-17β-ol)
  and compensatory ovarian hypertrophy (parabiosis) 78
  and deciduoma formation 50
  and pregnancy maintenance 91, 94, 97
  antiandrogenic activity 115, 120
  antiestrogenic activity 108, 110
  antifertility effect 146
  antiovulatory effect 277
  effect
    on acne 316
    on adrenal 166
    on body temperature 281
    on BSP test 175
    on estrous cycle 118
    on mammary gland 160
    on oxytocin-induced parturition 99
    on oxytocinase (serum) 323
    on uterine contractility 100, 101
  estrogenic activity 106

Allylestrenol—cont.
  estrogenic activity 106
  excretion 219
  in Allen–Corner test 45, 46
  in McGinty test 47
  in pregnancy 154
  masculinization 123, 124
  mating behaviour 118, 138
  metabolism of 219 ff, 235
  ovulation inhibition 59, 61, 63
  profile of 484, 487
  progestational effect 256
  synthesis of 28
  toxicity of 171
17α-Allyl-19-nortestosterone in McGinty test 47
Ambystoma tigrinum, effect of estrogens on 362
Amenorrhea
  and oral contraceptives 420
  and progestational compounds 310
Aminolevulinic acid synthetase (ALA) and oral contraceptives 435
Anabolic activity of steroids 112 ff.
Anagestone (acetate)
  androgenic activity 116
  antiestrogenic activity 106
  estrogenic activity 106
  nidation 56–58
  ovulation inhibition 63
  toxicity 171
  with mestranol, sequential 140
Androgenic activity, of progestational compounds 133 ff.
Androstane derivatives, chemistry of 25 ff.
Angiotensinogen, effect of estrogens on 440
Anolis, effect of estradiol in 362
Anovlar®
  antiovulatory effect 277
  composition of 398
  effect
    on ovary 418
    on oviduct 158
    on premenstrual tension 315
    on vaginal sialic acid 286
  number of pregnancies 106
Anovulatory cycles, effect of progestational compounds on 311
Antiandrogenic effects of progestational compounds 9, 118 ff.
Antiestrogenic effects of progestational compounds 9, 103 ff.
Antifertility
  activity of steroids 6 ff., 363 ff.
  mechanism of 141 ff.
Antigest A®
  composition of 400
  number of pregnancies 409
Antigest B
  composition of 402
  number of pregnancies 406
α-receptors in uterus, effect of various compounds on 101
Arthritis, effect of progesterone on 318
Arylesterase in ovary, effect of lynestrenol on 76
Aschheim–Zondek reaction and lynestrenol 66
AY-11483, ovulation inhibition and MAP 73

"3β-enzyme", inhibition by progestogens 81
Behavior
  aggressive, and steroids 92
  human sexual, and steroids 118
  mating, and steroids 118
Benzyl-benzoate-sesame oil, effect on onset of HP-caproate activity 4
Blood, chemistry of, and oral contraceptives 292, 435
Blood coagulation and oral contraceptives 295, 435 ff.
Blood pressure and oral contraceptives 440
Blood vessels
  oral contraceptives and 439, 447
  progestational compounds and 188
Body mass
  oral contraceptives 442
  progestational compounds 168 ff., 291
Body temperature and progestational compounds 16, 19, 282, 303, 443
Bone marrow, progestational compounds and 188
Boron trifluoride in steroid synthesis 28
β-receptor in uterus, effects on 101
Breast *see* Mammary gland
9α-Bromo-4-androstene-3,11,17-trione
  in metabolism 226
9α-Bromo-3α,21-dihydroxy-5β-pregnane-11,20-dione in metabolism 226

Subject Index

9α-Bromo-11-ketoprogesterone
  effect of endometrium 258
  metabolism of 226, 227
9α-Bromo-4-pregnene-3,11,20-trione,
    metabolism of 226
BSP retention
  and oral contraceptives 443
  and progestational compounds 175, 294

Candidiasis, vulvovaginal, and oral contraceptives 424
Carboanhydrase, uterine, effects of oral contraceptives on 420
Carbohydrate metabolism
  effects of oral contraceptives on 443
  effects of progestational compounds on 88 ff., 293
  effects of progesterone on 476
Carcinogenesis and oral contraceptives 448
Carcinoma
  endometrium, and steroids 305 ff.
  mammary gland 309
Central nervous system
  effect of oral contraceptives on 443
  effect of progesterone 476
  effect of progestogens on 88 ff.
Cervix
  effect of chlormadinone acetate on 412
  effect of estrogen–progestogen combination on 396
  effect of estrogens on 358 ff.
  effect of MAP on 416
  effect of oral contraceptives on 423
  effect of progestational compounds on human 258, 260, 265 ff., 286
  effect of progestational compounds on rabbit 143
Chloasma and oral contraceptives 442
Chloramiphene, antifertility activity of 374
Chlormadinone acetate
  and amenorrhea 421
  and intermenstrual bleeding 422
  and nausea 445
  androgenic activity 116
  antiandrogenic activity 119 ff.
  antiestrogenic effects 108, 110
  antifertility effects 141–143 ff.
    continuously administered 413
  antiovulatory effects 277 ff., 392

concentration in different parts of body 287
diabetic effect of 174
early androgen syndrome 117
effect
  on adrenal 163, 164
  on blood, cholesterol 175
  on blood, coagulation 295
  on body temperature 282, 443
  on body weight 169, 170, 291
  on carbohydrate metabolism 172 ff., 430
  on central nervous system 89
  on cervical mucus 147, 286, 412
  on deciduoma 49, 50
  dysfunctional bleeding 311
  on egg transport 156
  on ejaculation volume 80
  on endometrium 180, 252, 414, 419
  on endometriosis 308
  on estrogen receptors in uterus 101
  on estrous cycle 117
  on fertilization 147
  on fetus 124 ff.
  on 20-hydroxy-progesterone acetate in ovarian vein blood 73, 76
  on hypothalamus 73
  on LH plasma level release 76, 77, 85, 279
  on mammary gland tumors 158, 159, 184 ff.
  on mating behavior 139
  on nidation 54, 55
  on ovulation, induced inhibition 59, 60, 63, 65, 277, 392
  on oxytocin induced parturition 99
  on oxytocinase activity in hypothalamus 72
  on pituitary
    FSH–LH content 82
    inhibition 77
  on progesterone plasma level 279
  on uterus
    contractility 100
    receptors 112
  with mestranol on
    glucose tolerance test 430
    mating behavior 139
in McGinty test 47
intermenstrual bleeding 422
percutaneous activity 189, 190
pregnancy
  maintenance of 90, 94

Chlormadinone acetate—contd.
  pregnancy—contd.
    rates (continuously administered) 134
  profile of 478, 487
  synthesis of 29, 30
6α-Chloro-17α-acetoxy-4-pregnene-3,20-dione in steroid synthesis 29, 30
6α-Chloro-1,2α-methylene-Δ-4,6-pregnadiene-17α-ol-3,20,dione 17 acetate see Cyproterone acetate
6α-Chloro-17α-acetoxy-6-dehydroprogesterone, effect on endometrium 252
16α-Chloroestra-1,3,5(10)-trien-17-one, antifertility effect 365
6-Chloro-9β,10α,4,6-pregnadiene-3,20-dione, effect on endometrium 253
6-Chloro-9β-16α-1,4,6-pregnatriene-3,20-dione
  effect on endometrium 252
  relative progestational potency 260
Cholecystopathy, effect of progesterone on 318
Cholesterol
  and chlormadinone acetate 175
  and Enovid® 174
  and oral contraceptives 429, 432
Chromosomes and oral contraceptives 451
Clauberg test
  potency in
    and ovulation inhibition 59
    and percutaneous administration 190
  progestational compounds in 38 ff.
Clomiphene
  and hypothalamus 281
  in pregnant rats 374
  in return to fertility 426
Composition of steroid contraceptives 398
Concentration of 17β-estradiol in tissues 348
Conovid E®
  composition of 398
  effect
    on number of pregnancies 407
    on premenstrual tension 315
Copper, blood levels
  and oral contraceptives 441
  and progestational compounds 292

Coproporphyrin in urine, and oral contraceptives 425
Corpus luteum
  effect of
    estrogens on 350
    progestational compounds on 7, 8, 87
    progestogen–estrogen combination on 395
  extracts of, effect on endometrium 45
  insufficiency of, and progestational compounds 317
  removal and substitution in pregnancy 317
Corticosterone
  and ovulation induction 87
  and steroids 161
Cortisol
  and progestogen–estrogen combination 427
  level of, effect of different compounds on 288
  steroids, and gluconeogenic effect of 174
Coturnix coturnix japonica
  effect of estrogens on 361
  effect of mestranol on 363
  ovulation induction in 87
C-quens®
  and mammary tumors 449
  composition of 398
  number of pregnancies 405, 409
  toxicity of 406
2α-Cyano-4,4,17α-trimethyl-androst-5-en-17β-ol-3-one inhibiting "3β-enzyme" 181
Cyproterone acetate
  antiandrogenic activity 118
  feminizing fetus 129
  structural formula 119

Decidua, effect of various steroids on 20
Deciduoma
  effects of estrogens on 357
  effects of percutaneous steroid treatment 190
  effects of progestational compounds 48 ff., 50, 52
Dehydroandrosterone and clitoral hyperplasia 132
11-Dehydroprogesterone
  and glycogen deposition 14

effect on endometrium 14
6-Dehydro-retroprogesterone *see* Dydrogesterone
Deladroxate-w with estradiol enanthate, antifertility effect 415
Depression, oral contraceptives and 444
Desoxycorticosterone and deciduoma formation 49
17-Desoxyestrone in neonatal animals 360
3-Desoxy-19-nortestosterone, synthesis 28
$3\beta,17\beta$-Diacetoxy-17α-ethynyl-3,5-estradiene in steroid synthesis 27
1,3-Diacetoxy-16α-hydroxyestra-1,3,5(10)-trien-17-one, effect on uterine carbonic anhydrase 358
1,4-Diacetoxy-1,3,5(10)-trien-17-one, effect on uterine carbonic anhydrase 358
2,4-Diallylestradiol, antifertility effect 366
Diazocine, antifertility activity 375
3,4-Dicoumarine and antifertility effects 375
Diethylstilboestrol
  antiestrogenic effect of 107
  effect
    on carbohydrate metabolism 174
    on endometriosis 307
    on fetus (feminization) 119
    on fetus (masculinization) 121, 125, 322
    on follicular development 369
    on ovarian weight DNA/RNA content 176
    on pituitary gonadotrophin contents 81
  vaginal epithelium 268
  with delalutin, effect on endometriosis 307
3,4-Dihydronaphthalenes, antifertility activity of 377
17α-Dihydroxy-progesterone (DP)
  DP acetofuran
    effects of antiandrogenic 9
    effects of antiestrogenic 9
    effects of teratological 10
    pregnancy maintenance 5
    progestational activity 4
  DP acetonide
    pregnancy maintenance 5
    progestational activity 4
  DP acetophenone
    effects of antiandrogenic 9
    effects of antiestrogenic 9
    effects of teratological 10
    effects on estrous cycle 6
    effects on pregnancy maintenance 5
    metabolism of 220
    progestational activity 4
17α-(2'ξ,3'-Dihydroxypropyl)-17β-acetoxy-4-estrene in metabolism of allylestrenol 236
Dimethisterone
  and amenorrhea 421
  and deciduoma 52
  and intermenstrual bleeding 422
  and maintenance of pregnancy 90, 94, 96
  and nausea 445
  androgenic activity 116
  antiandrogenic activity 120 ff.
  antiestrogenic activity 108
  effects
    adrenal cortex 161
    on body weight 168
    on emphysema 192
    on fetus 124 ff.
    on LH plasma level 76, 77
  menstruation, postponement of 259
  profile of 486, 487
  synthesis of 28, 29
7,12-Dimethyl benzanthracene inducing mammary carcinoma 184
6,16α-Dimethyl-6-dehydro-17α-acetoxyprogesterone, effect on endometrium 253
6,17α-Dimethyl-6-dehydroprogesterone, effect on ovary 418
6α-21-Dimethyl-ethisterone, effect on endometrium 254
Dimethylpolysiloxane membranes and release of crystalline steroids 191
Dimethylstilbestrol *see* DMS
2,3-Diphynyl indene, substitution in molecule and antifertility activity 374
Diuresis
  oral contraceptives and 440
  progestational compounds and 293
DMS (dimethylstilbestrol)
  antiestrogenic effect of 107
  effect on sperm transport 143
DMSO steroids dissolved in, in Clauberg test 45
DNA, content of mammary gland and steroids 159

DP see Dihydroxyprogesterone
Duphastone (see Dydrogesterone)
 composition of 398
 synthesis 33
Dydrogesterone
 and body temperature 282
 and deciduoma 49, 50
 androgenic activity 116
 antiandrogenic activity 120
 antifertility effect 146
 antiovulatory effect 278
 corticoidlike effect 165
 effect
  on body weight 169
  on dilatation of symphysis pubis 98
  on endometrium 19, 250, 253
  on fertilization 165
  on oxytocin-induced parturition 99
  on uterine contractility 285
 estrogenic and metrotrophic effect 103 ff.
 excretion of 219
 in Clauberg test 41
 in Corner–Allen test 45
 in dysmenorrhea 313
 in McGinty test 47
 in pregnancy 154
 masculinizing effect on fetus 125 ff.
 mating behavior 138
 menstruation, postponement of 259
 metabolism of 220 ff., 222
 ovarian hypertrophy in parabiosis 78
 ovulation
  induction 85, 86
  inhibition 59, 61
 profile of 484, 487
 synthesis 33
Dysfunctional bleeding and progestational compounds 311
Dysmenorrhea and progestational compounds 313, 408

Early androgen syndrome and various steroids 117
EEG, effect of various compounds on 88
Egg transport, effects of various steroids on 148, 153 ff.
Embolism
 and oral contraceptives 435
 see also Thromboembolism
Emphysema and steroids 195
Endometriosis, effect of progestational compounds on 306 ff.
Endometrium
 human
  antiestrogenic effects on 267, 394
  carcinoma of, effect of progestational compounds on 304, 419
  effect of oral contraceptives 396, 409, 419
  progestational effects of injectable compounds 13 ff., 304, 416
  progestational effects of orally active compounds 252, 258, 259, 269
 mouse, enzyme changes 180
 rabbit
  activity of progestogens in Clauberg test 37 ff.
  histochemical effects 180
 rat, histological and histochemical effects 179
Enovid
 composition of 398
 effect on
  blood vessels 188
  body mass 170
  cortisol level 288
  dysfunctional bleeding 312
  endometriosis 307
  fetus 151
  lactation 151
  lipid metabolism 174
  milk flow 425
  ovary 418
  oviduct 156
  plasminogen activator 180
  pregnancies, incidence of 406
  pregnancies, prevention 11, 135
  premenstrual tension and 315
Epinephrine, uterine contractility and 101
Estradiol
 accumulation of 348
 and deciduoma 53, 357
 and gonadotrophin secretion 350
 and implantation of ovum 58
 and ovulation 368, 389
 antifertility effects of 141, 363 ff., 366
 effect
  on aggressive behavior 92
  on blastocyst development 356
  on carbonic anhydrase 358
  on central nervous system 92
  on deciduoma 53, 357
  on egg transport 354

on endometrium 180
    with norethynodrel 44
on liver function 175
on mating behavior 138
on neonatal animals 360
on nidation 357, 358
on ovary 349 ff.
on ovulation 87, 352
on pituitary gonadotrophin content 81
on tumors (mamma) 183
on uterus 357 ff.
on vagina 286
effects in nonmammals 362
with progestogens
    effect on mammary gland 158, 159
    effect on symphysis pubis 98
Estradiol cyclopentenyl propionate
antifertility effect 365
effect
    on blastocyst development 356
    on cervix 360
    on follicle development 369
Estradiol dibenzoate and uterine carbonic anhydrase 358
Estradiol dipropionate
effect on ovary 350
in neonatal animals 359
pregnancy maintenance 97
Estradiol enanthate with Deladroxate-w®, antifertility effect 415
Estradiol-3-methyl ether in neonatal animals 360
Estradiol monobenzoate, corpus luteum substitution 317
Estradiol valerate (Delestrogen®)
effect on ovary 351
with delalutin, effect on endometriosis 307
with 17-hydroxy-progesterone effect
    on habitual abortion 320
    on menstrual disorders 310 ff.
with various steroids, effect on uterine contractility 100
Estrane derivatives
chemistry of 25 ff.
intermenstrual bleeding and 421
nidation and 54 ff.
1,3,5(10)-Estratrien-3-ol, anterfertility effect of 367
1,3,5(10)-Estratrien-17-ol, antifertility effect of 365
1,3,5(10)-Estratrien-17-one, antifertility effect of 365, 366
4-Estrene-3,7-dione, metabolite of norethisterone 229
Estrenol, derivates of, effect on endometrium 252
Δ^4-Estrenolone, derivates of, effect on endometrium 252
$\Delta^{5(10)}$-Estrenolone, derivates of
effect on endometrium 83
effect on uterovaginal tract 85
Estriol
antifertility effects 365
antiovulation effect 389 ff.
effect
    on carbohydrate metabolism 172 ff.
    on deciduoma 357
    on gonadotrophin secretion 350
    on neonatal animals 360
    on ovulation 309
    on uterine carbonic anhydrase 358
inhibition of estradiol 112
Estrogens
activity in young animals 347
and carcinogenesis 448
and carcinoma
    endometrii 305
    mammae 449
and glucose level 429
and implantation of ovum 357
and thrombosis 435
antifertility effects 347 ff., 388 ff.
concentration in tissues 348
effect
    on caeruloplasmine oxidase 439
    on egg transport 354 ff.
    on endometrium 249 ff.
    on pituitary gonadotrophins 81
    on plasma angiotensinogen level 440
with progestogens, antiovulatory effect 395
Estrone
and gonadotrophin secretion 350
and implantation 56
and pregnancy interruption 363
antifertility effect 363 ff., 365
effect
    in birds 362
    in neonatal animals 359, 360
    on blastocyst development 356
    on carbonic anhydrase 358
    on follicle development 369
    on ovary in parabiosis 78
    on ovulation 352, 369

Estrone—contd.
  effect—contd.
    on pituitary gonadotrophin content 81
    on uterus 357.
17α-Ethynyl-19-nortestosterone see Norethisterone
17α-Ethynyl-19-nortestosterone acetate see Norethisterone acetate
Ethisterone
  and body temperature 282
  and deciduoma 52, 53
  and pregnancy maintenance 96
  and superovulation in parabiosis 78
  androgenic activity 114
  antiandrogenic effect 120
  effect
    on BSP retention 175
    on endometrium 250, 254, 258, 259
      withdrawal bleeding 178
    on fructose concentration in prostate 113
    on tumors 183 ff.
    on uterine contractility 100, 101
  estrogenic activity 106
  fetus and 125, 130, 322
  profile of 486, 487
  progestational effect in man 258
16α-Ethoxy-9α,10α-4,6-pregnadiene-3,20-dione, effect on endometrium 254
17α-Ethyl-estrenol, effect on uterovaginal tract 264
13-Ethyl-17α-ethynyl-3α,17β-dihydroxy-5β-gonane in norgestrel metabolism 234
1-13β-Ethyl-17α-ethynyl-17-hydroxy-gon-4-ene-3-one, in progestational activity 257
17α-Ethyl-19-nortestosterone, effect on endometrium 259
  see also Norethandrone
16α-Ethyl progesterone, effect on endometrium 14, 18
17α-Ethyl progesterone, effect on body temperature 19
Ethynodiol-acetate see Ethynodiol diacetate
Ethynodiol-diacetate
  and amenorrhea 421
  and deciduoma 49
  and intermenstrual bleeding 422
  and nausea 445
  and nidation 56

  and pregnancy rate 404
  androgenic effects 115
  antiestrogenic activity 103 ff., 266
  effect
    on estrous cycle 118
    on glucose level 172, 173, 430
    on mating behavior 118
    on plasma LH level 76, 77
  estrogenic activity 103 ff.
  excretion 219
  in Clauberg test 41
  in McGinty test 48
  in sequential therapy 410
  intermenstrual bleeding 136
  menstruation 259
  metabolism of 219 ff., 232
  ovulation inhibition 64
  profile of 483, 487
  progestational effect in man 255
  percutaneous absorption 191
  toxicity of 171
  uterine contractility 100
  with EE in sequential therapy 410
  with lynestrenol, effect on ovary 418
  with mestranol
    effect on blood pressure 440
    effect on glucose tolerance 430
    effect on mating behavior 138
    effect on ovary 419
    effect on thyroid 428
  with norethynodrel, percutaneous absorption 191
17α-Ethynyl-5α-androst-2-en-17β-ol, antifertility effect of 141
17α-Ethynyl-3β,17β-diacetoxyestr-4-ene see Ethynodiol diacetate
17α-Ethynyl-3α,17β-dihydroxy-5β-estrane, metabolite of lynestrenol (rabbit) 233
17α-Ethynyl-3β,17β-dihydroxy-5α-estrane, metabolite of lynestrenol and norethisterone 233
17α-Ethynyl-3β,17β-dihydroxy-5β-estrane, metabolite of lynestrenol and norethisterone (rabbit) 229, 233
17α-Ethynyl-3,17β-dihydroxy-5(10)-estrene, metabolite of norethynodrel 230
17α-Ethynyl-10β,17β-dihydroxy-4-estrene-3-one, metabolite of norethynodrel 230
Ethynyl estradiol

Subject Index

antifertility activity 365
antifertility effect 148, 356, 367
antiovulatory effect 389 ff.
effect
  in pregnancy 152
  in sequential therapy 408
  on blood chemistry 292
  on carbohydrate metabolism 172
  on egg transport 153, 355
  on endometrium, with progestogens 107, 250
  on fertilization and sperm transport 143
  on fetus 152
  on FSH/LH ratio in women 356
  on LH level 72, 76, 77
  on liver function 175, 434
  on MAP inhibited ovulation 73
  on milk flow 425
  on neonatal animals 360
  on ovarian enzymes 176
  on ovulation 59, 369
  on oxytocin content of hypothalamus 72
  on pregnancy 15
  on vagina 123
in ovulation inhibition 59, 73, 369
in sequential therapy 410
interaction with norgestrel 107, 111
metabolite of norethisterone 22
"morning after" pill 391
reversing effects of MAP 73
with chlormadinone acetate on adrenal 164
with delalutin, effect on endometriosis 258–259
with dydrogesterone in maintenance of pregnancy 97
with norethindrone acetate 430
with norethisterone acetate, vagina 286
with norgestrel 107, 152, 416
with 17α-progesterone caproate, dysfunctional bleeding 312
with quingestanol, endometrium 178 ff.
with various compounds in sequential therapy 410
17α-Ethynylestradiol 233
17α-Ethynylestradiol-17β, and norethisterone metabolism 228
Ethynylestradiol-3-methyl ether, antiovulatory effect in women 389
see also Mestranol
17α-Ethynylestradiol-3,17-bis-tetrahydropyranylether, antifertility effect 367
17α-Ethynyl-5α-estrane-3α,17β-diol, metabolite of norethisterone 228, 229
17α-Ethynyl-5α-estrane-3β,17β-dione, metabolite of norethisterone 228, 229
17α-Ethynyl-5β-estrane-3α,17β-diol, metabolite of norethisterone 228, 229
17α-Ethynyl-5β-estrane-3β,17β-dione, metabolite of norethisterone 228, 229
17α-Ethynyl-1,3,5(10)-estratrien-17β-ol, antifertility effect 367
17α-Ethynylestr-4-en-17β-ol, synthesis of 28
see also Lynestrenol
17α-Ethynyl-17β-hydroxy-5α-estrane-3-one, metabolite of lynestrenol 233
17α-Ethynyl-17β-hydroxy-5β-estrane-3-one, metabolite of lynestrenol 233
17α-Ethynyl-estrenol-phenyl prionate, effect on endometrium 14, 17, 19
17α-Ethynyl-17β-hydroxy-5β-estrane-3-one, metabolite of norethisterone 229
17α-Ethynyl-17β-hydroxyestr-4-en-3-one, synthesis of 25, 26
see also Norethisterone
17α-Ethynyl-17β-hydroxyestr-5(10)-en-3-one, synthesis of 25, 26
see also Norethynodrel
17α-Ethynyl-19-nortestosterone see Norethisterone
17α-Ethynyl-19-nortestosterone-enanthate see Norethisterone enanthate
effect on endometrium 14, 15, 16, 17, 18, 19, 259
metabolism of 22
17α-Ethynyl-3α,10β,17β-trihydroxy-5α-estrane, metabolite of norethynodrel 230
17α-Ethynyl-3α,10β,17β-trihydroxy-5β-estrane, metabolite of norethynodrel 230
17α-Ethynyl-3β,10β,17β-trihydroxy-5α-estrane
metabolite of ethynodiol diacetate 232
metabolite of norethynodrel 230
17α-Ethynyl-3β,10β,17β-trihydroxy-4-estrene 230

Excretory system, effect of oral contraceptives on 450

Fallopian tubes *see* Oviduct
Fatty acids, nonesterified
  effect of Enovid-E on level of 174
  effect of oral contraceptives on 430, 432
Feces, radioactive progestogens in 219 ff.
Fertility, return to, after use of contraceptives 426, 427
Fetus, oral contraceptives and 121 ff., 450
Fibroids, abdominal, effect of progestogens on 182 ff.
Fibromyoma
  effect of oral contraceptives on 423
  effect of progestational compounds on 309
9α-Fluoro-17α-acetoxy-4-pregnene-3,11,20-trione, effect on endometrium 253
Fructose in prostate, effect of various steroids on 113
FSH
  effect
    of estrogens in women 389 ff.
    of progestogen–estrogen combination in women 395
    of progestogens in women 389 ff.
  pituitary content
    effect of norethisterone acetate 81
    production in Haller's test 80
    secretion of, in parabiosis 78

Galactorrhea and oral contraceptives 420
Gestafortin *see* Chlormadinone acetate
Gestonoron caproate, effect on mammary gland 160
Glucose
  metabolism of, effect of progestogens on 172 ff., 293
  tolerance and oral contraceptives 429
β-Glucuronidase
  effect of oral contraceptives on 420, 433
  effect of progestogens, in ovary 176, 177
Glutamic oxalacetic transaminase, effect of progestogen on 434

Glycogen
  antiestrogen activity 267
  in cervical mucus, and progestogens 286
  in endometrium, effect of different compounds on 14, 477
Gonadotrophin releasing factor, effect of steroids on 72, 349,
Gonanes, synthesis of 32
Growth hormone, level of, and norethynodrel–mestranol combination 432
Gynovlar®
  composition of 398
  effect of, on ovary 418

Hair and oral contraceptives 442
Haller's test 80
HCG-induced ovulation, effect of various steroids on 65, 67, 68
Headache and contraceptive drugs 444
Histochemical effects of steroids, in different organs 175 ff.
Hohlweg effect, suppression of 73
Hormone screening tests 193
HP caproate *see* 17α-Hydroxy-progesterone-caproate
1-Hydroxy-estradiol, effect on uterine carbonic anhydrase 358
1-Hydroxy-estradiol-triacetate, effect on uterine carbonic anhydrase 358
17β-(2′-Hydroxy)-ethoxyestra-1,3,5(10)-triene-3-methoxy, antifertility effect of 367
2α-Hydroxy-melengestrol, metabolite of melengestrol acetate 225
1β-Hydroxy-19-norandrostenedione in norethisterone metabolism 228
20β-Hydroxy-19-nor-pregnene-3-one-20β-phenyl-propionate, effect on endometrium of derivatives of 19
17α-Hydroxy-19-nor-progesterone caproate
  effect in carcinoma endometrii 360
  effect on human endometrium 14, 17
  metabolism and excretion 21
17α-Hydroxy-pregn-4-ene-3,20-dione caproate *see* 17α-Hydroxyprogesterone caproate
20α-Hydroxy-pregn-4-ene-3-one, effect of, in ovarian vein blood 76
3β-Hydroxy-5,16-pregnadien-20-one in progestogen synthesis 3

Subject Index

17α-Hydroxy progesterone
  and induced parturition 99
  effect on endometrium 252
  esters of 2, 3
  in steroid synthesis 29, 30
  LH peak and 474
20α-Hydroxy progesterone and induction of ovulation 87
20β-Hydroxy progesterone and induction of ovulation 87
10α-Hydroxy-progesterone acetate
  in ovarian vein blood 73, 76
  induction of ovulation 87
17α-Hydroxy-progesterone acetate
  and body temperature 282 ff.
  and pregnancy maintenance 97
  effect on endometrium 13, 15, 17
17α-Hydroxy-progesterone-p-butoxy-phenyl-propionate in carcinoma endometrii 306
17α-Hydroxy-progesterone-caproate
  and body temperature 282 ff.
  antiestrogenic activity 9
  antiuterotropic activity 9
  effects
    on abortion 320
    on acne 316
    on corpus luteum 7, 8
    on endometrium 13 ff., 59, 304, 307
    on estrous cycle 6, 7
    on maintenance of pregnancy 5
    on mammary carcinoma 309
    on mastopathia cystica 309
    on menstrual disorders 310
    on menstruation postponement 21
    on premenstrual tension 315
    on sclerodermia 316
    on serumoxytocinase 323
    on sterility 317
  in treatment of endometriosis 307
  metabolism and excretion 21
  substitution for corpus luteum 317
Hydroxy prolin, excretion of, effect of 17α-hydroxyprogesterone-caproate on 316
10β-Hydroxy-16α-n-propyl-19-nortestosterone acetate, effect on utero-vaginal tract 255
Δ5-3β-Hydroxy-steroid dehydrogenase, inhibited by progestational compounds 129, 177, 181
17-Hydroxy steroids, excretion of, and oral contraceptives 428

17β-Hydroxy steroid dehydrogenase, effect of Lyndiol® on 290
Hypertension and oral contraceptives 440
Hypothalamus and estrogens 349 ff.
see also Pituitary

ICSH in pituitary, and steroids 80
Immunological reactions, effects of progestational compounds on 187 ff.
Insulin
  and oral contraceptives 429 ff.
  effect of progestational compounds
    on level of 172, 173
    on secretion of 294
  effect of progesterone on level of 172
Intermenstrual bleeding and oral contraceptives 421
Iodine uptake
  influence of progestational compounds on 179
  influence of norethynodrel and mestranol on 428
Iron, plasma level of, influenced by
  oral contraceptives 441
  progestational steroids 292
Isocitric acid dehydrogenase
  hepatic, effect of oral contraceptives on 433
  placental, and antiestrogenic activity 112
16α-17α-(Isopropylidenedihydroxy)-9β, 10α-4,6-pregnadiene-3,20-dione, effect on human endometrium 254

Jaundice and oral contraceptives 434

17-Keto steroids, excretion of
  effect of MAP on 290
  effect of oral contraceptives on 428
Kidney, effect of progestational compounds on 188

Lactation
  effect of oral contraceptives on 425
  effect on, by lynestrenol 297
Lactic dehydrogenase in liver, effect of oral contraceptives on 433

Leydig cells
  effect of estrogens on   353
  effect of norethisterone   80
LH
  effects
    of chlormadinone on release of   85
    of estrogens on, in woman   388 ff.
    of MAP on production of   8, 81–82
    of megestrol acetate on secretion of   76, 77
    of norethisterone on release of   79
    of ortho novum® on release of   65, 71
    of progestational compounds
      on contents of pituitary   8
      on plasma level of   76, 77
    of progestogen–estrogen combination in women   395
  peak, and progesterone   474
Libido
  effect of MAP in man on   291
  effect of oral contraceptives on   443 ff., 446
Lipase in ovary
  effect of ethynyl estradiol on   176, 177
  effect of lynestrenol on   176, 177
Lipid metabolism, effect of progestational compounds on   174, 429
Lipoproteins and oral contraceptives   432
Liver functions
  effects of oral contraceptives on   432, 433 ff.
  effects of progestational compounds on   175, 189
LRF in ovulation inhibition studies   76, 77
Lumisterol in steroid synthesis   33
Lung, effect of progestational compounds on   195, 450
Lyndiol
  and carbohydrate metabolism   431
  and mating behavior   142
  composition   398
  effect
    on LH–FSH in women   391
    on lipoprotein level   432
    on metabolism of steroids   290
    on milk flow   425
    on nonpregnant uterus, contractility   285
    on ovary   418
    on pregnancies
      incidence of   407
      prevention   142
    on sarcoma   186
Lynestrenol (17α-ethynyl estr-4-en-17β-ol)
  amenorrhea by   421
  and deciduoma formation   52, 53
  and intermenstrual bleeding   422
  and nausea   445
  and pregnancy
    maintenance of   96, 97
    rate   404
  androgenic and myotrophic activity   115
  antifertility effect   146
  antiovulatory effect in women   392
  on damaging fetus   151
  effects
    on adrenal   166
    on BSP   175
    on bone marrow   188
    on cortisol binding capacity of plasma   289
    on dysfunctional bleeding   311
    on egg transport   156
    on endometriosis   308
    on fertilization   146
    on immunological reaction   187
    on lactation   425
    on mating behavior   138
    on metabolism of DHAS   290
    on ovarian enzymes   176
    on ovary   418
    on oviduct   156
    on ovulation
      HCG induced   65
      inhibition   54, 60, 62
    on pituitary–gonadotrophic function   74, 79
    on pituitary–CSH content   80
    on progestational activity   256
    on uterine contractility   100, 285
    on uterovaginal tract   260
  estrogenic activity   103, 104
  excretion of   219
  in milk   426
  in pregnancy   154
  intermenstrual bleeding   421
  metabolism of   219 ff., 232, 234
  profile of   483, 487
  synthesis of   28
  toxicity of   171
Lynestrenol acetate, effect on uterovaginal tract   260
Lysosomal enzymes, effect of steroids on, in endometrium   180

Magnesium, effect of oral contraceptives on level of 441
Mammary gland
 effect
  of oral contraceptives on size of 425
  of progestational steroids on 158 ff.
 mastopathia cystica, effect of progestational drugs on 309
 tumors of, and steroids 183, 184, 309
MAP (medroxy progesterone acetate)
 amenorrhea by 420
 anaesthesia and 138
 androgenic activity 114
 antiestrogenic effect 109
 antifertility effect 142, 146, 148, 150
 antiinflammatory effect of 161
 early androgen syndrome 117, 118
 biological halflife 22
 effect
  in jaundice-prone women 295
  in pregnancy 155
  of antiandrogenic 9
  of antiestrogenic 9
  on ACTH 160
  on adrenal function 160 ff., 288
  on blood chemistry 292
  on body temperature 282
  on body weight 170
  on carcinoma endometrii 305
  on central nervous system 88–92
  on corpora lutea 7, 8, 177
  on deciduoma formation 40, 50, 52
  on dilatation of symphysis pubis 98
  on diuresis 293
  on egg transport 153 ff.
  on endometrium 179 ff., 252
  on endometriosis 307
  on fertilization prevention 142, 146
  on fetus 129, 125, 296
  on fibroadenoma mammae 183
  on glucose tolerance test 294
  on gonadotrophin excretion 326
  on immunological reaction 188
  on intermenstrual bleeding 422
  on LH content of pituitary 81–82
  on LH plasma level 76–77
  on mammary gland 156, 158, 183
  on mating behavior 118, 137, 138
  on nidation 8, 54, 55
  on ovary
   growth 76
   in parabiosis 77
  on ovulation 7, 60, 62, 64, 67, 73, 81, 87
  on oxytocin-induced parturition 99
  on pituitary 8, 81, 83, 326
  on pituitary-gonadotrophic function 75, 79
  on pituitary histology of 82–83
  on precocious puberty 324
  on pregnancy, maintenance of 5, 90, 93, ff. 95
  on testosterone metabolism 291
  on thyroid 296
  on uterus histology 179 ff.
 estrogenic activity 105, 106
 excretion 21, 219
 McGinty test, activity in 47
 metabolism of 21, 219 ff., 221, 223
 pregnancy (prevention, continuously administered) 134
 profile of 479, 487
 progestational activity 4, 15 ff., 39
 relative progestational activity in human endometrium 260
 structure formula 37
 synthesis of 29, 30
 toxicity of 171
Masculinization
 of female fetuses by steroids 121
 oral contraceptives 450
 signs of, in rats 122 ff.
Mating behavior, influence of steroids on 133 ff.
McGinty test
 and maintenance of pregnancy 97
 steroids in 45, 46, 47, 48
Mechanism
 of antifertility drugs in human 388
 of antifertility in rabbit 142
 of ovulation inhibition 65 ff.
 of pituitary inhibition 71
Median eminence extracts see MEE
Medrogestone
 and body weight 169
 and deciduoma formation 50
 and ovulation inhibition 64
 and pregnancy
  maintenance of 95
  prevention of, continuously administered 134
 androgenic effect 115, 116, 120
 effect
  on adrenal cortex 163, 164
  on fibromyomata 425

Medrogestone—cont.
  effect—contd.
    on HCG induction of ovulation 66
    on pituitary-gonadotrophic function 75
  in McGinty test 47
  masculinization effect 125 ff.
  profile of 480, 487
  progestational potency 381
Medroxy progesterone acetate see MAP
MEE (median eminence extracts)
  effect on ovulation 72, 73, 76
  effect on pituitary 71
Megestrol acetate (6-methyl-17α-acetoxy-pregna-4,6-diene-3,20-dione)
  and body temperature 282
  and implantation 57
  androgenic effect 116
  antiestrogenic activity 109
  antifertility activity 143, 144, 146
  anti-HCG effect 67
  antiandrogenic effect 120
  continuously administered, and pregnancy rate 413
  corticoidlike function 165
  diabetogenic effect of 174
  distribution of, in uterus 179
  early postnatal administration 117
  effect
    on adrenal cortex 161, 163
    on body weight 169, 282
    on carbohydrate metabolism 174
    on egg transport 156 ff.
    on emphysema 95
    on endocervical mucosa 266
    on endometrium 253, 414
    on fertilization, prevention 143 ff.
    on LH plasma level 76–77
    on mating behavior 137
    on ovulation 66, 67
    on pituitary gonadotrophic function 75
  estrogenic activity 106
  excretion of 219
  in DPS capsules 57, 191
  in McGinty test 47
  in pregnancy 155
  in sequential therapy 410
  masculinization and 125 ff.
  metabolism of 219 ff., 223, 225
  ovulation, inhibition of 59, 60, 62
  postponement of menstruation 259
  pregnancy
    maintenance of 95
    prevention of, continuously administered 134
  profile of 479, 487
  synthesis of 29, 31
  toxicity of 171
  uterus 179
  with ethynyl estradiol, in sequential therapy 410
  with mestranol
    effect on glucose level 431
    effect on gonadotrophins 395
Melasma 442
Melengestrol acetate (6α-methyl-16-methylene-17α-acetoxy-pregna-4,6-diene-3,20-dione)
  and fertility 143, 144
  antiandrogenic activity 120
  antiestrogenic effect 109
  corticoidlike function 165
  effect
    on adrenal cortex 161, 163
    on body weight 282
    on ovary 177
    on pituitary function 79
  excretion of, in urine 219
  masculinizing effect 125 ff.
  metabolism of 224, 226
  postponement of menstruation 259
  pregnancy
    effect in 155
    maintenance of 94
  profile of 480, 487
  synthesis of 31
Menstruation
  disorders of, and oral contraceptives 310 ff.
  missed, and oral contraceptives 420
  postponement of, by different steroids 21, 259, 265, 269
MER-25 [1-(p-2-diethylaminoethoxyphenyl)-1-phenyl-2-p-methoxyphenyl], antifertility activity of 372
Mestranol (ethynyl estradiol 3-methyl ether)
  antifertility effect 141, 147, 365
  damaging effect on fetus 151
  effect
    in coturnix quail 362
    in neonatal animals 360
    in nonmammals 362
    in sequential therapy 390

on carbohydrate metabolism 172 ff.
on egg cleavage 357
on endometrium 267
on fetus 151
on FSH–LH in women 389
on glucose tolerance 429
on kidney 188
on lipid metabolism 429
on mating behavior, with ethynodiol acetate and chlormadinone acetate 133 ff.
on milk flow 425
on ovary 418
on ovulation 65, 352, 389, 368
on testes 353
in milk 426
LH plasma level 76, 77
sterilizing neonatal animals 360
with 17-acetoxy progesterone in sequential therapy 410
with chlormadinone in sequential therapy 390
with different progestogens, effect on body mass 168 ff., 282
with different steroids, effect on postponement of menstruation 265
with ethynodiol diacetate
  effect on blood pressure 440
  effect on deciduoma formation 49
  effect on endometrium 267
  effect on glucose level 430
  effect on mating behavior 133 ff.
  effect on thyroid 428
  in sequential therapy 408
with lynestrenol, antiovulatory effect 277
with megestrol acetate
  effect on glucose level 431
  effect on gonadotrophins 395
with norethisterone, effect on ovulation 65
with norethynodrel
  effect on adrenal cortex 168
  effect on amenorrhea 420
  effect on blood coagulation 437
  effect on body weight 170
  effect on central nervous system 92
  effect on cervical mucus 396
  effect on galactorrhea 426
  effect on growth hormone level 432
  effect on mamma 159
  effect on ovary 417
  effect on thyroid 428

Metabolism
  carbohydrate and lipid, effect of oral contraceptives on 172 ff., 429 ff.
  general metabolic effects of steroids 291 ff.
  glucose, effect of steroids on 293
  of progestational compounds 217 ff.
  of salt and water, effect of oral contraceptives on 441
17α-($2'$-Methallyl)-9β-10α-4-6-androstadiene-17-ol-3-one, effect on human endometrium 254
17α-($2'$-Methallyl)-$9\beta,10\alpha$-androst-4-en-17-ol-3-one, effect on human endometrium 254
17α-Methallyl-estrenol, progestational effect of 14, 19
17α-($2'$-Methallyl)-17-hydroxy-9β-10α-androsta-4,6-diene-3-one, effect on endometrium 260
Methallyl-19-nortestosterone
  effect on mating behavior 133
  effect on rabbit endometrium 45
Methandrolone, antifertility effect of 146
3-Methoxy-17β-cyanoethoxy-1,3,5(10)-estratrien, antifertility effect of 366, 367
6-Methoxy-1,2-diphenyl-(1-p-ethoxy pyrrolidine)-3,4-dihydro-naphthalene hydrochloride (V-11100A), antifertility activity of 375
3-Methoxy-2,5(10)-estradiene-17β-ol in synthesis of norethisterone 25, 26
3-Methoxy-estradiol
  antifertility effect of 365
  in steroid synthesis 25
3-Methoxy-13β-ethyl-1,3,5(10)-gonatriene-17-one, synthesis 32
3-Methoxy-17α-fluoro-1,3,5(10)-estratriene, antifertility 366
3-Methoxy-17β-methoxyformyl,1,3,5(10)-extratriene, antifertility effect of 366
3-Methoxy-16α-methyl-1,3,5(10)-estratriene-16β-17β-diol, antifertility effect of 365
3-Methoxy-16α-methyl-16β-hydroxy-1,3,5(10)-estratriene-17-one, antifertility effect of 365
6-m-Methoxyphenyl-1-hexen-3-one in steroid synthesis 32
6-Methyl-17α-acetoxy-6-dehydro-progesterone see Megestrol acetate

1-Methyl-3-acetoxy-1,3,5(10)6-estratetra-en-17-one, antifertility 366
6-Methyl-17α-acetoxy-pregna-4,6-diene-3,20-dione
  formula 31
  see also Megestrol acetate
6α-Methyl-17α-acetoxy-pregn-4-ene-3,20-dione see MAP
6α-Methyl-17α-acetoxy-progesterone see MAP
Methyl androstene diol, masculinizing effect of 128
17α-Methyl-3α,17β-dihydroxy-5α-estrane in normethandrone metabolism 237
16-Methylene-17α-acetoxy-pregna-4,6-diene-3,20-dione see Superlutin
2-Methyl-estradiol, antifertility effect of 366
Methylestrenolone see Normethandrone
17α-Methyl-17β-hydroxy-5α-estrane-3-one in normethandrone metabolism 237
6α-Methyl-17α-hydroxy progesterone acetate see MAP
17-Methyl-normethandrone see Normethandrone
17α-Methyl-19-nortestosterone see Normethandrone
17α-Methyl-progesterone and deciduoma formation 49
6α-Methyl-17α-1-propyne-17β-hydroxy-4-androsten-3-one, synthesis of 28, 29
Methyl-testosterone
  effect of endometrium 254
  effect on fructose concentration in prostate 113
Metopirone®, response and contraceptive drugs 428
Metrotrophic activity of progestogens 102 ff.
Metrulen®, effect on human oviduct 156
Milk
  effect of lynestrenol on protein and fat content of 296
  excretion of oral contraceptive in 425
  excretion of radioactive progestational compounds in 219
MLA (musculus levator ani) as indicator of myotrophic and anabolic activity 113 ff.
"Morning after" and progestational compounds 391
Mucopolysaccharides
  in blood vessels, effect of steroids on 188
  in endometrium, effect of steroids on 180
Myotrophic activity of progestational compounds 113

Nausea and oral contraceptives 444, 445
Neurological abnormalities and oral contraceptives 447
Nidation
  effects of estrogens on 357
  effects of hypophysectomy on 57
  effects of MAP on 8
  effects of progestational compounds on 54 ff., 55
  percutaneously administered 190
Nitrogen retention
  and chlormadinone acetate 291
  and norethynodrel 291
19-Nor-androstenedione in steroid synthesis 25
18-Nor-estrone-3-methyl-ether, effect on uterine carbonic anhydrase 358
Norethandrolone see Norethandrone
Norethandrone (17α-ethyl-19-noretesto-sterone)
  and deciduoma formation 49
  and maintenance of pregnancy 96
  progestational activity 255
Norethindrone see Norethisterone
Norethisterone
  and body temperature 282, 443
  and compensatory ovarian hypertrophy in parabiosis 78
  and deciduoma formation 52, 53
  and early androgen syndrome 117
  and jaundice 295
  and maintenance of pregnancy 94
  androgenic and myotrophic activity 113, 114, 115
  antiandrogenic activity 120
  antiestrogenic effect of 107, 110, 111, 267
  antifertility effect 141, 146
  antiovulatory effect in women (dose) 396
  effect
    in pregnancy 154
    on adrenal cortex 161, 166

on aggressive behavior 92
on body temperature 443
on body weight 170
on BSP retention 175, 433
on carbohydrate metabolism 172, 173
on central nervous system 88, 89
on fetus 152, 154
on fibromyomas 423
on fructose concentration in prostate 113
on glucose level 173
on human endometrium 250, 255, 259
on human endometrium during continuous administration 414
on hypothalamus 72
on immunological reactions 188
on LH plasma level 41, 44, 76, 77, 279
on liver functions 175
on mammary gland 158, 159,
on menstruation (postponement) 259
on nidation 54, 55
on ovarian growth 69, 176
on ovarian hypertrophy in biosis 78
on oxytocinase in hypothalamus 72
on pituitary gonadotrophic content 81
on pituitary gonadotrophic function 74, 79
on plasma level of progesterone 280
on precocious puberty 325
on sodium excretion 293
on testis 79, 80
on tumors 183 ff.
on uterus 178 ff., 181
on uterine contractility 100, 101
on withdrawal bleeding 178
estrogenic and metrotropic activity 103, 104
excretion in urine 219
feminizing effect 152–156
implanted in hypothalamus, effect on ovulation 71
in Allen–Corner test 45
in Clauberg test 41–44
in Haller test 80
in McGinty test 48
in pregnancy 152
inhibiting 3-hydroxy-steroid dehydrogenase 181

intermenstrual bleeding 422
masculinizing effect 131, 125 ff.
mating behavior 118, 138
metabolism of 22, 227, 229
metabolite
 of lynestrenol 232
 of norethynodrel 230
nausea 445
ovulation
 induction 72, 85, 87
 inhibition 60 ff., 392
 inhibition, mechanism of 72
percutaneous activity 189, 190
pregnancy, maintenance of 93, 94, 97
pregnancy rate during continuous administration 413
profile of 482, 487
progestational effect of 255
synthesis 25 ff., 26
toxicity of 171
with estradiol benzoate, effect on dilatation of symphysis pubis 98
with menstrual bleeding (amenorrhea) 420
with mestranol
 effect on insulin excretion 294
 effect on lactation 425
 effect on prevention of pregnancy 134, 404
Norethisterone acetate
and nausea 445
and nidation 56
and ovulation 62, 396
androgenic effect 115
early postnatal administration 118
effect
 in pregnancy 155
 on blood chemistry 292
 on body weight 169, 171
 on dysfunctional bleeding 311
 on endometriosis 308
 on human endometrium 255, 259
 on liver functions 175
 on mammary gland 158, 159
 on mating behavior 137, 138
 on ovarian growth 176
 on oxytocin-induced parturition 99
 on pituitary FSH–LH content 81
 on pituitary gonadotrophic function 74, 79
 on pituitary histology 84
 on uterine contractility 100

Norethisterone acetate—*contd.*
  estrogenic and metrotrophic activity 103, 104
  in McGinty test 48
  in sequential therapy 411
  intermenstrual bleeding 422
  masculinizing effect on fetus 125, 131
  postponement of menstruation 259
  pregnancy, prevention of, by continuous administration 134
  pregnancy rate 404
  profile of 482, 487
  progestational effect of 255
  synthesis 27
  with ethynyl estradiol, effect on glucose tolerance 392
  with mestranol, effect on lactation 421
Norethisterone enanthate
  and body temperature 282, 303
  effect
    on adrenal 288
    on blood coagulation 295
    on endometrium 14, 15, 16, 17, 18, 19, 295
    on liver function 295
    on mammary gland 158
  metabolism 22
Norethynodrel (Enovid)
  absorption, percutaneous 191
  and body mass 170
  and body temperature 282
  and deciduoma formation 52, 53
  and nausea 445
  and nidation 56
  and pregnancy maintenance 93
  and pregnancy prevention 135
  and pregnancy rate 404
  androgenic effect of 116
  antiestrogenic activity 109, 111
  antifertility effects 140 ff.
  antiovulatory effect in women 392
  distribution of, in rat 111
  effect
    on adrenal cortex 166
    on aggressive behavior 92
    on blood vessels 188
    on body mass 170
    on bone marrow 188
    on BSP retention 175
    on carbohydrate metabolism 172, 173
    on central nervous system 89, 92
    on corpus luteum 87
    on egg transport 157
    on endometriosis 307
    on fructose concentration in prostate 113
    on glucose level 173
    on immunological reaction 188
    on kidney 188
    on lactation 425
    on LH plasma level 72, 76
    on liver functions 175
    on mammary gland 159
    on mating behavior 133, 137, 138
    on ovarian growth 176
    on ovarian hypertrophy in parabiosis 78
    on pituitary, gonadotrophic function 74, 79
    on pituitary, histology 82 ff.
    on plasminogen activator in uterine fluid 180
    on postponement of menstruation 259
    on thyroid 189
    on tumor (mammary) 183
    on uterine contractility 100
  estrogenic and metrotrophic activity of 10
  excretion of 219
  in Clauberg test 41, 44
  in Corner–Allen test 46
  in endometriosis 308
  in McGinty test 48
  in milk 426
  in pregnancy 154
  intermenstrual bleeding 422
  masculinizing effect on fetus 126 ff.
  metabolism of 229 ff.
  ovulation
    induced by HCG 65 ff.
    inhibition 58 ff.
  percutaneous absorption 191
  profile of 485, 487
  progestational activity of 255
  prolactin content of pituitary 83, 87
  synthesis of 25 ff.
  toxicity of 171
Norethynodrel with mestranol
  and galactorrhea 426
  and pelvic thrombi 424
  effect
    on amenorrhea 420
    on blood coagulation 437
    on cervical mucus 396

on fertility 135
on glucose tolerance 430
on growth hormone, level 432
on lactation 425
on ovary 418
on thyroid 428
Norgesterone
and body temperature 282
and uterine contractility 100
androgenic effect 115
effect on pituitary gonadotrophic function 75
in McGinty test 48
in treatment of carcinoma endometrii 306
pituitary inhibition and 79
postponement of menstruation 259
pregnancy, prevention by continuous administration 134
profile of 485, 487
Norgestrel
amenorrhea caused by 421
and nausea 445
and pregnancy rate 404, 413
androgenic and myotrophic activity 113
antiestrogenic activity of 103, 106, 108
antifertility effect 141
corticoidlike function 165
early postnatal administration 117
effect
on adrenal cortex 166
on blood chemistry 292
on cervix 266, 286
on fetus 152
on LH plasma level 76, 77
on mammary gland 158 ff.
on mating behavior 137
on ovulation 280
on oxytocin-induced parturition 99
on progesterone plasma level 280
on uterovaginal tract 260
implanted in silastic capsules 296
in McGinty test 48
in pregnancy 155
intermenstrual bleeding 422
metabolism of 233
postponement of menstruation 259
pregnancy, prevention of, by continuous administration 134
pregnancy rate 413
profile of 481, 487
synthesis of 32

toxicity of 172
d-Norgestrel
effect on ovulation 280
excretion in urine 219
Norgestrienone
and body temperature 282
and maintenance of pregnancy 92
estrogenic and metrotrophic activity 104
implanted in silastic capsules 296
prevention of pregnancy by continuous administration 135
profile of 484
relative progestational effect on human endometrium 255
Norinyl 2
composition of 398
incidence of pregnancies 407
Norlestin®
composition 398
effect on tumor growth (mammary) 184
number of pregnancies 407
Norlutin®
effect on dysfunctional bleeding 312
effect on endometriosis 307
Normethandrolone see Normethandrone
Normethandrone
and body temperature 282
and compensatory ovarian hypertrophy in parabiosis 78
and deciduoma formation 48, 50, 52
and maintenance of pregnancy 91, 94, 96
androgenic and myotrophic activity 113, 114
antiestrogenic activity of 103, 106, 108
antifertility effect 146
effect
in pregnancy 155
on adrenal cortex 163
on adrenal function 289
on BSP retention 175
oxytocin-induced parturition 99
on pituitary gonadotrophic function 74, 79
on tumor growth 184
uterine contractility 100, 101
in McGinty test 48
inhibition of ovulation 61
masculinization of fetuses 131
mating behavior 138
metabolism of 237
percutaneous activity of 189, 190

Normethandrone—contd.
　profile of 484, 487
　relative progestational effect on human endometrium 260
　toxicity of 172
　with ethynyl estradiol, dilatation of symphysis pubis 98
19-Nor-pregnanediol-20-one, metabolite of 17α-hydroxy-19-nor-progesterone-17-caproate 21
19-Nor-progesterone
　delaying withdrawal bleeding 178
　effect
　　on central nervous system 89
　　on human endometrium 14, 253
　　on tumors 183
19-Nortestosterone (17β-hydroxy-estr-4-en-3-one)
　derivatives of, relative progestational activity 255 ff.
　in steroid synthesis 25
19-Nor-testosterone-17β-methyl ether, effect on human endometrium 14
Norvinisterone
　effect in pregnancy 155
　effect on liver functions (BSP) 175
　in McGinty test 48
　profile of 483

Oracon®
　composition 398
　pregnancy rate 405, 409
Orgametril® see Lynestrenol
Ortho-Novum®
　composition 398
　effect
　　on adrenal weight 168
　　on ovarian weight 168
　　on ovary 418
　　on pituitary weight 168
　　on premenstrual tension 315
　incidence of pregnancies 407
　LH release, suppression 71
　LH rise, suppression 65
　preventing reflex ovulation 65
Ortho-Novum SQ®
　composition 391
　pregnancy rate 405, 409
Ovanon®
　composition 398
　pregnancy rate 405, 409

Ovary
　atrophy by dihydroxyprogesterone-acetophone 6
　compensatory hypertrophy and progestational drugs in parabiosis 78
　effect
　　of contraceptive drugs on 396, 417 ff.
　　of diethyl stilbestrol on weight of 176
　　of estrogens on 349, 350
　　of progestational compounds on human 277 ff.
　enzymes, effect of progestational compounds on 176, 177
　fluid retention in, and norethisterone 69
　venous blood, concentration of progesterone 474
Oviduct, rate of egg transport, effects of different steroids on 153 ff.
Ovral®
　and antifertility 142
　composition of 398
　effects in pregnancy 152
　incidence of pregnancies 407
Ovulation
　after use of oral contraceptives 426
　and progestogens in women 391 ff.
　and sequential therapy 390
　effect
　　of different steroids on reflex, in rabbits 61
　　of estrogens on 352
　　of estrogens on, in human 389
　　of hypothalamic implant of norethisterone 71
　　of percutaneously administered steroids on 190
　　of steroids on induction of 277 ff.
　facilitation of, by steroids 84 ff.
　inhibition of
　　by sequential therapy 390, 408 ff.
　　by steroids 368, 369
　　in different animals 58 ff.
　　mechanism of inhibition 65 ff.
Ovulen®
　composition 398
　effect on human oviduct 156
　incidence of pregnancies 408
Ovum transport, effect of estrogens on 353 ff.
Oxogestone, relative duration of effect on human endometrium 19

Oxytocin
  induced parturition and progestogens 98 ff.
  progestogen effect on uterine contractility 100 ff.
  threshold of, in pregnancy 363
Oxytocinase
  activity, influenced by steroids 72
  in pregnancy 322

Parturition, oxytocin induced, and progestogens 100
PBI and contraceptive drugs 428
Pearl formula 397
Pelvic vasculature, effect of contraceptive drugs on 424
Pentobarbital, effect on ovulation 85
Phloretin (β-(p-hydroxyphenyl)-2,4,6-trihydroxy-propiolone), antifertility effect of 376
Phosphatases
  effect of lynestrenol on, in ovary 76, 77
  effect of oral contraceptives on 433
  effect of progestogens on, in endometrium 178 ff., 180
Pituitary
  and oral contraceptives 429
  gonadotrophic function, influence of different compounds on 71, 74 ff., 348
  histology of, and steroids 82 ff., 349
  ICSH contents and steroids 80
  prolactin contents, effect of norethynodrel on 83, 87
  tumors, effect of progestogens on 187
  weight of
    and norethynodrel 168
    effect of Ortho-Novum® on 168
Planovin®
  composition 398
  effect on ovary 48
Plasma proteins, effect of progestational drugs on 293
Platelets, effect of oral contraceptives on 439
Platypoecilius, effect of estradiol benzoate in 362
PMS (pregnant mare's serum) and induction of ovulation 84, 85
Precocious puberty, effect of progestational compounds on 324
9β,10α-Pregna-4,6-diene-3,20-dione *see* Dydrogesterone
Pregnancy
  and blood coagulation 438
  effect
    of continuous progesterone administration 411
    of steroids in pregnancy 151 ff.
  interruption of, by estrogens 363
  maintenance of
    by different compounds 92 ff.
    percutaneously administered compounds 190
    progesterone and DP derivatives 5
    symphysis pubis relaxation and 98
  prevention of, by continuously administered compounds 133
  rate 319, 397 ff.
    with combined compounds 404
    with progesterone continuously administered 411
    with sequential therapy 405
  serum oxytocinase and 322
  test for, by MAP 297
  therapeutic use of progestational compounds in 319 ff.
Pregnanediol
  in metabolism of progestational compounds 220
  in sequential therapy, excretion of 390
4-Pregnene-3-one-20α-ol cyclopentenyl propionate, relative progestational activity 15
Premarin®
  antiovulatory effect in women 389
  effect on follicle development 369
  masculinizing effect in human fetus 131
Primolute-nor® *see* Northisterone acetate
Progestational potency of different compounds 37 ff.
20α-Progesterol, progestational activity of 14
20β-Progesterol, progestational activity of 14
Progesterone
  and carcinoma endometrii 305 ff.
  and ovarian hypertrophy in parabiosis 78
  and ovulation inhibition 58 ff.
  and pituitary
    gonadotrophic function 75
    gonadotrophin content 81

Progesterone—contd.
  and PMS activity in monkey 69
  androgenic activity 117
    early androgen syndrome and 117 ff.
  antiandrogenic activity 119 ff.
  antifertility effect 141, 145, 149
  deciduoma induction and 20, 53
  delaying withdrawal bleeding 178
  duration of action in endometrium 8
  effect
    in pregnancy 319
    on adrenal cortex 163
    on arthritis 318
    on body weight 168, 291
    on carbohydrate metabolism 172
    on central nervous system 88 ff., 479
    on cervix 258
    on cholecystopathy 318
    on corpus luteum 7, 8, 87, 317
    on egg transport 153
    on ejaculatory volume 16 ff., 80
    on emphysema 195
    on endometrium 178 ff., 252 ff.
    on estrous cycle 6
    on fetus 129 ff.
    on fibromatosis 309
    on fructose concentration in prostate 113
    on glucose blood level 172
    on insulin level 172 ff.
    on iodine uptake 179
    on lungs 192
    on mating behavior 133 ff., 138 ff.
    on nidation 54 ff., 357
    on ovary growth 176
    on ovary weight in parabiosis 78
    on ovulation 58 ff., 84 ff.
    on pregnancy, maintenance of 5, 90 ff., 319 ff.
    on pruritus vulvae 316
    on relaxin 98
    on sialic acid in vagina 286
    on sodium excretion 293
    on sperm transport 149
    on tumors 183 ff.
    on uterine contractility 100 ff.
  feminizing effect 129
  masculinizing effect 130
  mechanisms of action 471
  menstruation, postponement of by 21
  percutaneous activity of 189, 190
  plasma level, effect of different compounds on 279
  postovulatory functions 475
  pregnancy prevention by continuous administration 135
  pregnancy, therapeutic use of, in 317 ff.
  preovulatory secretion 473
  profile of 471
  vaginal smear, effect on 258
  with estrone in parabiosis 78
  with ethynyl estradiol, effect on dilatation of symphysis pubis 98
  with stilbestrol, effect on fetus 131
Progesterone cyclopentenyl-3-enolether
  effect on endometrium 252
  metabolism of 218 ff.
Progestin, effect on egg transport 153
Progestogens
  antiovulatory effect 391 ff.
  with estrogens 395
Prolactin
  excretion
    influenced by norethynodrel 83, 87
    influenced by progesterone 87
  pituitary contents of, and norethynodrel 159
17α-Propargyl-estrenol, relative progestational effect on human uterovaginal tract 260
17α-Propynyl-19-nortestosterone, relative progestational effect on human endometrium 260
Prostate, influence of different compound on 113
Provest®
  and mammary tumors 449
  and toxicity 406
  composition 398
  effect on premenstrual tension 315
  number of pregnancies 408
Pruritus vulvae, effect of progesterone on 316
Pseudopregnancy, induction by steroids 87 ff.
Psychological effects of oral contraceptives 443
Pyruvate, level of, in blood, and oral contraceptives 430

Quinestrol, antifertility effect with progestogens 416

Quingestanol acetate
  and antifertility effect 142
  androgenic activity of 115
  effect
    on adrenal 166
    on maintenance of pregnancy 96
    on mating behavior 137
    on phosphatases in endometrium 178 ff.
    on pituitary gonadotropic function 74
  estrogenic activity 106
  inhibition of ovulation 63
  masculinizing effect 126
  pregnancy, prevention by continuous administration 135
  profile of 485, 487
  synthesis 27
  with quinestrol, antifertility effect of 416

Relaxin and progestogens 98
Renin, plasma level, effect of oral contraceptives on 440
Retroid®, effect on ovulation 276
Retroprogesterone (9β-10α-pregn-4-ene-3,20-dione)
  metabolism of 220, 222
  synthesis of 33
RO-4-8347, effect on ovulation 276

Salt metabolism and oral contraceptives 441
Sceloporus, effect of estrone in 362
SCH 12600, antiandrogenic activity 121
Sclerodermia, effect on progestogens on 316
Screening tests 193
Sebaceous glands, effect of oral contraceptives on 442
Seizures and oral contraceptives 447
Sequential therapy, effects of 390, 408 ff., 428
Sialic acid in vagina, and steroids 286
Side effects of oral contraceptives 417 ff.
Skeletal maturation and oral contraceptives 450
Skin
  diseases, effects of progestational compounds 316
  effect of oral contraceptives on 442
Sperm transport, effect of different compounds on 143, 144, 149
Stein–Leventhal syndrome, lynestrenol, influence on 290
Sterility produced in neonatal animals by various steroids 360
9β-10α-Steroids in steroid synthesis 32, 33
Stilbestrol
  antifertility effect 367
  antiovulatory effect in women 389 ff.
  effect
    on blastocyst development 356
    on liver functions 175
    on ovarian atrophy 350
    on ovulation 372
    on testis regeneration 353
    on uterine carbonic anhydrase 358
  influence of substitution in molecule 373
  masculinizing effect 129, 131
  "morning after" pill 391
  with 17-α-hydroxy-progesterone-caproate, effect on endometriosis 308
  with progesterone, masculinizing effect 131
Streptomyces roseochromogenus, 16α-hydroxylation in progestogen synthesis 4
Superlutin (16-methylene-17α-acetoxy-pregna-4,6-diene-3,20-dione)
  amenorrhea by 421
  and body temperature 282
  and compensatory ovarian hypertrophy in parabiosis 78
  antiovulatory effect in women 278
  profile of 480, 487
  synthesis of 29, 31
Symphysis pubis, relaxation of, and steroids 98

Teratological effects of progestational compounds 10, 121 ff.
Testis
  atrophy of, by gonadotrophic inhibition of steroids 79, 80
  effect of estrogens on 348 ff., 351, 352
Testosterone
  effect
    on central nervous system 89
    on fructose concentration in prostate 113

Testosterone—contd.
  metabolism of
    effect of Lyndiol on 290
    effect of MAP on 290
Testosterone propionate
  and deciduoma formation 49
  and fibroadenoma mammae 183
  and induction of ovulation 87
  and sterilization 361
  effect
    on behavior 92
    on rabbit endometrium 44
Tests, screening, for compounds 193
1,2,3,4-Tetrahydro-1-naphthols, antifertility activity of 377
Therapeutic applications of progestational drugs 303 ff.
1-ξ-Thiomethylestra-1,3,5(10)-trien-17-one, effect on uterine carboanhydrase 358
Thromboembolism and oral contraceptives 423, 424, 435 ff., 439, 447
Thyroid, effect of oral contraceptives on 428
Thyroxin
  effect of, on effects of norethynodrel 189
  effect of oral contraceptives on 428
Thyroxin-binding globulin, effect of steroids on 296
Tolbutamide, effect of progesterone on effect of 172
Toxicity
  of progestational compounds 171 ff., 406
  studies 194
TPN, effect of MAP on oxidation of 182
Transaminases, effect of oral contraceptives on 433
Transcortin, effect of steroids on 288
Trengestone and body temperature 282
Triglycerides in serum, and oral contraceptives 432
6-β-17α-21-Trihydroxy-6α-methyl-pregna-4-ene-3,20-dione acetate in MAP metabolism 21
TSH secretion, effect of oral contraceptives on 428
Tubal transport
  effect of estrogens on 353 ff.

effect of norethynodrel on 136
effect of progestational compounds 153 ff.
Tumors
  and oral contraceptives 448
  effects of steroids on 182 ff.

U-11100A, antifertility activity of 375
Urine, excretion of radioactive progestational compounds in 219 ff.
Uterus
  α- and β-receptors in, and progestogens 101
  contractility of (nonpregnant), and progestogens 100 ff., 285
  cramps of, and estradiol valerate 307
  effects
    of estrogens on 357 ff.
    of progestogens on 178 ff.
  hypoplasia of, and progestogen–estrogen treatment 317
  tumors in, and effects of progestational compounds on 185 ff.

Vagina
  absorption from 60, 192
  effect of oral contraceptives on 424
  sialic acid in, and steroids 286
  vaginal smear, effect of different steroids on 258, 260 ff., 266, 268
Vascular effects of contraceptive agents 439
Vestalin® see Norgesterone
Vinyl estrenolone see Norgesterone
Vitamin E in pregnancy 319
Volidan®
  composition 398
  number of pregnancies 408

Water metabolism and oral contraceptives 441

Zinc level in serum, effect of oral contraceptives on 441

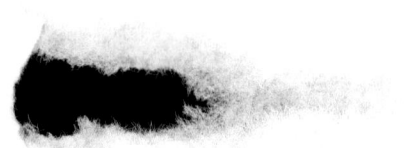